Contents

Resources for Nursing Research

An Annotated Bibliography

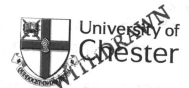
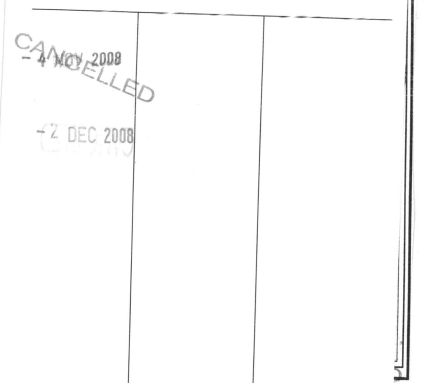

This book is dedicated with sincere gratitude to
Lisbeth Hockey – an outstanding nurse,
researcher and a very special friend

First edition © The Library Association 1991
Second edition © The Library Association 1994
Third edition © Cynthia G.L. Clamp and Stephen Gough 1999

First published 1991
Second edition 1994
Third edition 1999

The rights of Cynthia G.L. Clamp and Stephen Gough to be
identified as authors of this work have been asserted by them in
accordance with the Copyright, Designs and Patents Act 1988.

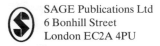

SAGE Publications Ltd
6 Bonhill Street
London EC2A 4PU

SAGE Publications Inc
2455 Teller Road
Thousand Oaks, California 91320

SAGE Publications India Pvt Ltd
32, M-Block Market
Greater Kailash - I
New Delhi 110 048

British Library Cataloguing in Publication data

A catalogue record for this book is available from the British Library

ISBN 0 7619 6065 1
ISBN 0 7619 6066 X (pbk)

Library of Congress catalog card number 99–071274

Typeset by Type Study, Scarborough, North Yorkshire
Printed in Great Britain by The Cromwell Press Ltd, Trowbridge, Wiltshire

Foreword

To have produced yet another edition, the *third*, of this master resource of resources for nursing research is no small feat. Having had the privilege of writing the foreword to the first two editions and realizing the amount of work undertaken, I did not consider a third edition humanly sustainable. I am amazed and delighted that it came about.

Not only has this latest edition been brought up to date, which, in view of the rapid proliferation of literature, is an enormous achievement, it has also been enriched by the inclusion of Internet websites and many currently used databases, including CD-ROM. The international aspect of the sources has been widened further, thus reflecting the extension of research effort world-wide.

I would like to stress that the main purpose of this book is to *direct* the reader to appropriate sources. With the bewildering increase of possibilities, the clear 'signpost' function of this new treasure promises to be extremely valuable – probably indispensable.

Because of my age, I remember the time-consuming and frustrating grappling for sources to help me with my early research. What an enormous difference this book would have made to me and has since to countless nurse researchers and users! Anne Marie Rafferty, who is at present at the very centre of nursing research development, is better able to speculate on the potential of this book for the future.

As we move closer to the 'information society', skills in accessing and utilizing information come to the fore. To have assembled and synthesized the myriad entries within this singular volume reflects an achievement of significant magnitude and commitment. One may wonder whether this accelerated age justifies the publication of a resource in paper form? Such doubts will be dispelled since this 'route map' through the disciplinary highways and by-ways of research still has much to offer the would-be and seasoned researcher. Not surprisingly, the section on electronic sources has been expanded and others up-dated. The volume is unique in the sense of providing an historical record and reference point for analysing 'growth areas', through the development of research resources and categories over time.

The sign-post approach adopted helps to take the 'sting' out of searching for those new to the field, as well as leading the reader on an investigative trail that points the path from 'novice to expert'. The result of a creative collaboration between a librarian and nurse researcher, an attempt is made to address different audiences' needs in the text. The international dimension provides a further index of the topical and methodological interests and investments in nursing research over time. Many useful pointers are provided on policy and funding opportunities, frameworks, career structures and contexts that can make or break research. As a reflection on one such career, Lisbeth Hockey's legacy lives through this text.

Lisbeth Hockey
Anne Marie Rafferty

Acknowledgements

Many relatives, friends and colleagues have assisted in the development of this resource book and we would like to record our sincere thanks to them all. In particular I would like to express gratitude to my co-author Stephen Gough for his patience, kindness and support at times of frustration and crisis!

Lisbeth Hockey and Anne Marie Rafferty, both highly respected nurse researchers, have kindly written the foreword and we appreciate this very much. To have their endorsement of our work is praise indeed.

Staff at libraries in Birmingham, London, New York and Vancouver have been most helpful. Roy Pearce taught me how to use the Internet and Graham Martin, Professor and Head of the University of Birmingham School of Continuing Studies, gave me continuing access. For this privilege I am most grateful. We also thank all the librarians who have now made the Internet a virtual library for everyone to use.

Three people have given many hours of their time to compiling the indexes – David Clamp, Philippa Jordan and Raymond Poland. I cannot thank them enough. Many others have also contributed in various ways: Debra Evans, David Gill, Pam Griffin, Lucy Land, Hazel Lloyd and Roy Sladden.

Stephen Gough sends a particular thank you and much love to Kyle, Calum, Kathryn, Tom and Joshua.

The staff at Sage Publications have answered our every question and given continuing support, particularly Sarah Bury, Rosemary Campbell, Melissa Dunlop, Nerida Harrowing, Susie Home and Susan Worsey, and we thank them all.

Introduction

'Nursing research involves a systematic search for knowledge about issues of importance to the nursing profession.... [Although it] has experienced remarkable growth in the past three decades . . . many health questions remain to be answered . . . and many answers remain to be utilized. . .' (Polit & Hungler, 1995: 3)

This book is an annotated bibliography that provides a guide to sources of literature, research methodology and the background to research in nursing. It is designed to complement existing texts on research methods and its aim is to act as a 'signpost' to literature, mainly from the disciplines of nursing and the social sciences. It is intended for all those with an interest in nursing research, students, teachers, researchers and practitioners of nursing.

Increasingly, nurses are gaining access to the Internet and CD-ROM databases but, however desirable this may be, it is not yet universal. Communication with colleagues has become easier via the Internet, but it may never replace the printed text as the primary source of information.

The book includes over 2760 entries, 64 per cent of which are new and cite material written since 1994. Most of these have been annotated. In addition, websites have been included with their URL (Uniform Resource Locator — the 'address' of a document on the World Wide Web). The rapid growth in electronic sources is reflected in the much-expanded section, 1.8. For all entries the criteria for inclusion are current usage, focus and relevance.

The book is divided into: Part 1: Sources of literature, Part 2: Methods of inquiry, and Part 3: The background to research in nursing, with author and subject indexes at the end of the book. Details of the book's structure, format and numbering system are explained on page xvii in 'How to use this book'.

The entries have been extensively cross-referenced and in addition examples are given in most sections in Part 2 to show where a particular element of the research process has been used. Definitions are also included from published sources (Appendix D).

All books have been checked for the latest editions but not all remain in print. Material on research methods dates only slowly and in many instances has not been superseded. The number of entries varies considerably between sections and this largely reflects the state of the literature. Breadth rather than depth has governed the choice of sources, from which readers can follow their own interests.

Well over 350 journals from around the world have been scanned, giving international coverage, and a list of those containing research material is included in Appendix B. In addition to extensive use of the Internet, the following databases were searched: ASSIA (Applied Social Sciences Index and Abstracts), British Nursing Index, CINAHL (Cumulative Index to Nursing and Allied Health Literature), DHSS-Data, Dissertation Abstracts, Global Books in Print, Health Service Abstracts, HealthSTAR, Medline, Sage Publications/SRM Database of Social Research Methodology and Ulrich's Periodicals Directory. Other sources consulted were reference lists in books and journals, book reviews and publishers' catalogues.

The varying amount of literature included from different countries reflects the length of time in which nurses have been undertaking research and also the ways in which they have been educated. A high proportion of the citations are from Britain and America. Literature from Australia, Canada, China, Europe, India, New Zealand and South Africa is also included. As more nurses are educated to diploma and degree level, or perhaps in 'Cybercourses', and develop research literacy, the number of publications in any given country will gradually increase.

A fairly recent development is that of full-text, on-line journals and specialized resources, enabling those with Internet access to search and retrieve literature from any location. For example, the *Online Journal of Issues in Nursing*, *New England Journal of Medicine* and *Nursing Research* are either available as full text, abstracts and contents pages or most recent issues.

Based on the comments from readers of previous editions, it is clear that the book can be used in a variety of ways, e.g. both as a conventional bibliography or as a dictionary. It may also provide an overview of research processes, and a basis for developing group exercises.

The authors hope that use of this book will save time during the initial searching process for any nurse undertaking or evaluating research, so contributing to our goal of the best patient care based on research findings.

How to use this book

INDEXES

There are two indexes in this book, author and subject, which will be found at the end. At the beginning, an expanded contents list will enable readers to see its structure and quickly find the relevant sections.

STRUCTURE OF THE BOOK

The book is divided into three major parts:

Part 1   Sources of literature
Part 2   Methods of inquiry
Part 3   The background to research in nursing

FORMAT OF SECTIONS

The format of each section follows a similar pattern, although not all sections include each item. Entries are listed in alphabetical order. Where more than one reference by individual authors are cited, these are listed in date order.

Title
Introductory statement
Definition(s)
Example
Original or major text/article [specific to sub-section]
Annotations

NUMBERING SYSTEM

The numbering system used in the book should enable items to be found easily.

Part 1   items are numbered 1.1 to 1.9
Part 2   items are numbered 2.1 to 2.102
Part 3   items are numbered 3.1 to 3.23

Within each section entries have individual numbers, e.g. 1.1.1, 2.1.2 or 3.1.3, and this number is also used in the cross-referencing system.

CROSS-REFERENCING SYSTEM

Many books and articles contain information which comes under several headings in the book. Where this occurs, other item reference number(s) are given at the end of the annotation so that further relevant entries can be found. The number may indicate a whole section, e.g. CR 2.15, or a particular annotation, e.g. CR 2.15.6. In general, cross-referencing has not been done within sections as so many items relate to each other.

NOTES

Every effort has been made to ensure the accuracy of entries, but the authors would like to know of any errors.

British English has been used throughout the text, except in book and journal titles, in order to achieve consistency.

International Standard Book Numbers (ISBNs) have been included for most books. Occasionally it has not been possible to find this number, or the book does not have one.

The authors' policy has been to see most of the books and articles and these have been annotated. In a few instances this has not been possible, but the bibliographical data is included so that readers can still follow up the reference.

Where website addresses (URLs or Uniform Resource Locators) have been included, they were correct at the time of going to press.

PART 1:   SOURCES OF LITERATURE

LITERATURE SEARCHING AND LIBRARIES

1.1   LITERATURE SEARCHING AND LIBRARIES

The purpose of this section is to highlight material which will be helpful in identifying sources of research methodology and other literature, and general guides to using libraries and special collections. It is not an exhaustive list and where there are no guides the sources themselves have been documented.

Annotations

1.1.1   Akinsanya, J. (1984) Learning about nursing research. *Nursing Times*, 29 August 80 (16) 59–61 Occasional Paper   10 References

Describes a small-scale survey of theses and dissertations in the Steinberg Collection at the Royal College of Nursing, London. The study, carried out by Diploma in Nursing students, aimed to show the range and scope of nursing literature in this collection.

1.1.2   Anonymous (1995) How to search for information on trans-cultural nursing and health. *Michigan Nurse*, 68 (9) 27–8

This article gives tips and advice as well as describing several of the main sources, and suggests a strategy for performing an effective search on transcultural subjects and health.

1.1.3   Anonymous   (1996)   Literature searches: part 3. *Practice Nurse*, 11 (1) 35–7 1 Reference

This article describes how to organize a search of the literature.

1.1.4   Burnard, P. (1993) Facilities for searching the literature and storing references. *Nurse Researcher*, 1 (1) 56–63   4 References

Article discusses the use of computers to search for references and store bibliographical information.

1.1.5   Dale, P. (ed.) (1997) *Guide to Libraries and Information Sources in Medicine and Health Care*. London: British Library. ISBN 0712308393

Provides basic information on individual libraries plus the major literature-searching services and sources.

1.1.6   Duffel, P.G.S. (1995a) Focus. Finding information in the medical literature. *Insight*, 20 (2) 21–4   7 References

Gives an overview of the literature and main sources of information available to ophthalmic nurses.

1.1.7   Duffel, P.G.S. (1995b) Searching for articles in the medical literature. *Insight*, 20 (3) 20–7   8 References

Describes literature searching and how to structure a search with the emphasis on ophthalmic nursing.

1.1.8   Gash, S. (1989) *Effective Literature Searching for Students*. Aldershot: Gower. ISBN 0566057492

A general guide to the principles and practice of literature searching. It is not applied to any particular subject area and covers preparation, searching, online searching, keeping records, writing references and citing references in the text.

1.1.9   Grossman, S. & Schedel, M. (1992) Locating information in the nursing literature. *ANNA Journal*, 19 (2) 197

Article covers computerized literature searching, use of nursing indexes and the nursing literature.

1.1.10   Mason, C. (1993) Doing a literature review. *Nurse Researcher*, 1 (1) 43–55 15 References

Provides a step-by-step guide to searching and reviewing the literature.

1.1.11   Morton, L.T. & Wright, D.J. (1990) *How to Use a Medical Library* 7th edition. London: Clive Bingley. ISBN 0851574661

Provides an introduction to medical libraries for practitioners, research workers and specialist librarians. The main sources of bibliographical data are given together with information on the catalogues, classification schemes, periodicals, indexes and abstracting services, manual and computer literature-searching and audio-visual aids.

1.1.12   Shepherd, T. (1996) The RCN Library at your service. *Paediatric Nursing*, 8 (8) 11

An overview guide to the services of the Royal College of Nursing.

1.1.13   Smith, J.P. (1983) Steinberg Collection of Nursing Research. *Journal of Advanced Nursing*, 8 (5) 357 Editorial

Outlines the history and background of this internationally important collection.

1.1.14   Strauch, K.P. (ed.) (1992) *Guide to Library Resources for Nursing*. New York: Oryx. ISBN 0897744918

This book is designed to identify a variety of current materials in nursing, how to locate and evaluate them easily and quickly. Features include: comprehensive listings of general reference sources, annotated lists of nursing literature organized by subject, separate listings of periodicals related to nursing, a list of audio-visual material and names and addresses of publishers.

1.1.15   Summers, A. (1996) *How to Find Source Materials: British Library Collections on the History and Culture of Science, Technology and Medicine*. London: British Library, Science Reference and Information Service

This work is based on the collections of the British Library and is particularly useful for any researcher of the history and philosophy of health care.

1.1.16   Williams, R.M., Baker, L.M. & Marshall, J.G. (1992) *Information Searching in Health Care*. Thorofare, NJ: Slack Inc. ISBN 1556420935   References

Book, designed for health professionals, provides a foundation in information searching skills. It also includes guidance on the critical appraisal of research evidence. Chapters include the process – knowing where to start; the resources – putting them to work; and analysing the information. An appendix gives advice on reading clinical journals (CR 2.95).

1.1.17   Wilson, M.E. (1988) How to do a literature search. *Nursing Standard*, 8 October 2 (3) 39

Briefly covers the use of abstracts and indexes.

1.2   SOURCEBOOKS/GUIDES

Sourcebooks and guides give information about primary (original information) and secondary (indexes, information centres, libraries) sources.

Annotations

1.2.1   Advisory Committee for the Co-ordination of Information Systems (ACCIS) (1992) *ACCIS Guide to United Nations Information Sources on Health*. New York: United Nations. ISBN 9211003636

A guide to sources of information within the United Nations (UN) system on health. Intended for all health workers, planners and researchers. Covers programmes of the World

Health Organization (WHO) together with other UN organizations outside HQ locations. Short organizational descriptions are included, information sources in 11 subject categories, a list of health reference libraries for WHO publications – 700 worldwide. Subjects include disease prevention and control, environmental health, health promotion and care, health systems infrastructure, humanitarian assistance, disaster management, maternal and child health, nutrition and food control, occupational safety and health, population, statistics and epidemiology.

1.2.2 Allan, B. (1988) *Guide to Information Sources in Alternative Therapy.* Aldershot: Gower. ISBN 0566056119

Contents includes introduction to alternative therapy, searching for information, a bibliography of general and specialized sources and people, organizations and activities.

1.2.3 Association for Information Management *Forthcoming International Scientific and Technical Conferences.* London: Aslib

Gives details of forthcoming conferences, both national and international in the fields of science and technology, and nursing is included. Issued quarterly with the main issue in February and supplements in May, August and November (CR 1.7.3).

1.2.4 Auger, C.P. (1998) *Information Sources in Grey Literature* 4th edition. London: Bowker-Saur. ISBN 1857391942

Only British book on grey literature, i.e. literature published by local and national government agencies and other organizations not usually available through booksellers and often difficult to trace.

1.2.5 Davinson, D. (1977) *Theses and Dissertations as Information Sources.* London: Clive Bingley. ISBN 0851572278 (Published in the USA by Linnet Books ISBN 0208015396)

A general guide to theses and dissertations. Contents include: history of theses medium; nature and purposes of theses; bibliographical control; access and research in progress. An additional section lists guides to thesis preparation (CR 3.17).

1.2.6 Health Education Authority (1994) *Health Related Resources for Black and Minority Ethnic Groups.* London: Health Education Authority ISBN 0752100335

This work starts with an index which is divided by subject and then by format. Each entry in the main resources list gives clear information on format, language, target audience, producer, distributor and a detailed description including commentary on content. There is also a list of distributors with addresses.

1.2.7 Li, T.-C. (1990) *Social Science Reference Sources: a Practical Guide* 2nd edition. New York: Greenwood Press. ISBN 0313255393

A guide to basic, important reference sources in the social sciences. Comprises two parts: social science in general and sub-disciplines. Information on online databases, CD-ROM and other sources are included. Part 1 includes the nature of social science, bibliographical needs of social scientists, research resources in the social sciences, access to sources, sources of information, statistical sources periodicals, government publications, archives and unpublished materials. Part 2 includes additional reference sources and subjects of relevance to nursing – cultural anthropology, education, psychology and sociology.

1.2.8 Peretz, A., Steryan, A. & Terry, F. (eds) (1990) *Core Collections in Nursing and the Allied Health Sciences: Books, Journals, Media.* Phoenix, AZ: Oryx Press. ISBN 0897744640

Lists approximately 1,000 books and media programmes in health sciences. Entries are non-critically annotated. Contains periodicals indexes, periodicals, yearbooks, annuals, media sources, collection development and a directory of publishers, distributors and producers.

1.2.9 Shockley, J.S. (ed.) (1988) *Information Sources for Nursing: a Guide.* New York: National League for Nursing. ISBN 0887373860 Publication No. 41–2200

Provides an overview of the current state of information sources, discusses the role and scope of libraries, lists actual resources, gives guidelines for planning a search and strategies for accessing online sources of data. Other chapters cover clinical information systems and how information may be organized. Appendices contain (a) bibliography of selected resources for nursing; (b) regional medical libraries; (c) selected additional printed indexes and abstracts; (d) file management software for organizing information.

1.2.10   Thomson, I. (1989) *The Documentation of the European Communities: a Guide.* London: Mansell. ISBN 0720120225

Describes the range of printed information which is publicly available. This includes primary and secondary legislation through working documents and research reports, together with explanatory and background sources. References to health care are included.

1.2.11   Walford's Guide to Reference Material: Volume 1. Science and Technology (1996) 7th edition. Edited by Mullay, M. & Schlicke, P. London: Library Association. ISBN 1856041654

An introductory resource to the principal texts including medicine and nursing.

1.2.12   Wortzel, M. & Brody, L.D. (1995) Information sources on Child Welfare Archives: how to identify, locate, and use them for research. *Child Welfare*, 74 (1) 305–19   31 References

A detailed description of information sources for child welfare.

1.3   DIRECTORIES

Directories are useful and often essential for identifying sources of information, people and possible assistance. However, not all are truly comprehensive as questionnaire returns are often the method used for compilation. The entries here are not intended to be comprehensive. ISBN numbers and editions have been excluded for titles where the frequency of publication is regular.

Annotations

1.3.1   American   Libraries   Directory

1992–1993. (1992) 45th edition. New Providence, NJ: R.R. Bowker ISBN Volume 1 0835231585; Volume 2 0835231593

Gives the history of public, academic, government and specialized libraries in the USA and Canada. Names and addresses of all libraries are listed and these include health and information science.

1.3.2   Associations Unlimited. Detroit: Gale Research

Available both on CD-ROM and the Internet via GaleNet, this suite of databases is based on the Gale series the Encyclopedia of Associations. The three main elements are National, International, and Regional, State and Local. There are over 400,000 organizations listed. Updates are three times a year on GaleNet and annually for the CD-ROM (CR 1.3.20, 1.3.30).

1.3.3   Centres, Bureaux & Research Institutes. (1996) 13th edition. Beckenham: CBD Research. ISBN 0900246723

Lists over 2,000 establishments indexed by subject.

1.3.4   City and State Directories in Print. Edited by Towell, J.E. & Montney, C.B. Detroit: Gale Research

1.3.5   Councils, Committees and Boards: a Handbook of Advisory, Executive and Similar Bodies in British Public Life. (1995) 5th edition. Beckenham: CBD Research. ISBN 0900246790

Arranged alphabetically, each entry gives details of structure and purpose.

1.3.6   Current Asian and Australasian Directories. Beckenham: CBD Research

1.3.7   Current British Directories. (1993) 12th edition. Beckenham: CBD Research. ISBN 0900246561

A guide to major directories covering Great Britain. Sections include: local directories, specialized directories, publishers and subject indexes.

1.3.8   Current British Journals: a Bibliographic Guide. (1992) 6th edition. Edited by Toase, M. Boston Spa: British Library Document Supply Centre. ISBN 0712320881

Arranged in ten sections including social sciences, humanities and science, which includes nursing.

1.3.9 Current European Directories: a Guide to International, National, City and Specialized Directories. (1994) 3rd edition. Beckenham: CBD Research. ISBN 0900246618

3,000 directories are listed with subject indexes in English, French and German and of publishers with full addresses and publications.

1.3.10 Current Research in Britain, Social Sciences. London: Longman

A national register of current research being carried out in universities, colleges and other institutions in the UK. The series is divided into four areas: physical sciences (annual – 2 parts); biological sciences (annual – 2 parts); social sciences (annual); humanities (biennial). Contains a department index, lists research in progress and has name, study area and keyword indexes. Social sciences covers nursing and medicine.

1.3.11 Directory of British Associations and Associations in Ireland. (1998) 14th edition. Beckenham: CBD Research

Arranged alphabetically, each entry includes a statement of purpose, publications, whether there is a library and gives website and e-mail addresses. A subject index is also included (CR 1.3.7).

1.3.12 Directory of British Official Publications: a Guide to Sources. (1984) 2nd edition. Compiled by Richard, S. London: Mansell. ISBN 0720117062

Directory identifies the full range of publications by official organizations and sources of supply. The book's introduction describes the pattern of official publications, bibliographical sources, HMSO and its services, cataloguing and information services, forthcoming publications and bookselling services. It also outlines the types of material published. The publications of the Department of Health and other bodies concerned with health and nursing are included.

1.3.13 Directory of European Medical Organizations. (1993) Beckenham: CBD Research. ISBN 0900246626

Lists government and other official health bodies, international and pan-European organizations. The subject index is in English, French and German.

1.3.14 Directory of European Professional and Learned Societies. (1995) 5th edition. Beckenham: CBD Research. ISBN 0900246707

Directory is a complementary volume to the Directory of British Associations. Arrangement is by subject with an index in French, English and German (CR 1.3.5).

1.3.15 Directory of Health Services Libraries. Pacific North West Region and Selected Canadian Provinces. Seattle, WA: National Network of Libraries of Medicine

A geographical arrangement of academic, hospital and specific libraries with significant biomedical collections. Information includes name, address, telephone, fax, Internet, ariel addresses, NUC codes and an NUC code index.

1.3.16 Directory of Libraries in Canada. Toronto: Micromedia. ISSN 1191-1603

Includes over 7,000 listings of libraries and branches, information and resource centres, archive and learning centres. Health science libraries are included at numbers 436–40.

1.3.17 Directory of Medical and Health Care Libraries in the United Kingdom and Republic of Ireland 1997–8. (1997) 10th edition. London: Library Association. ISBN 1856042197

Each entry includes the name, address and telephone number, type of library, opening hours, stock policy, holdings, classification system, publications and network membership.

1.3.18 Directory of Members' Research Interests and Projects, The Canadian Nursing Research Group. Vancouver, BC, Canada: Board of Directors [Contact Ann Hilton, School of Nursing, University of British Columbia, Vancouver, BC, Canada V6T 2B5]

Directory lists members of research group 1993/94, together with details of current projects and methods used.

1.3.19 Directory of Social Research Organizations in the United Kingdom. (1993) Edited by Sykes, W. London: Mansell. ISBN 0720121655

Main body of the book contains details of 1,050 social research organizations which returned a questionnaire. Organizations include central and local government, health authorities/trusts, higher education and independent institutions, management consultancies, charities, trades unions, quangos and public limited companies. Also listed are individuals offering freelance services, foundations supporting research in the UK and a range of courses. Entries provide name, address, director, number of researchers, fields and methods of research, details of recent projects, training opportunities and contact information. Short articles on each of the main sectors are included. Section 8, Health research, outlines the problem of definition, scope and purpose of health care research, recent developments and principal themes in the health research agenda.

1.3.20 Encyclopedia of Associations: Regional, State and Local Organizations. (1998) 8th edition. Gale Research. ISBN 078761386X

Volume 1: Great Lakes States ISBN 0787613908
Volume 2: Northeastern States ISBN 0787613878
Volume 3: Southern and Middle Atlantic States ISBN 0787613886
Volume 4: South Central and Great Plains States ISBN 0787613916
Volume 5: Western States ISBN 0787613894

Includes professional and social welfare non-profit membership organizations giving detailed information for each entry (CR 1.3.2, 1.3.30).

1.3.21 General Clinical Research Centers – a Research Resources Directory. (1988) National Institute of Health NIH Pub No. 88–1433

1.3.22 Government Research Centers Directory 1996–97: a Descriptive Guide to more than 4,200 U.S. and Canadian Government Research and Development Centers, Institutes, Laboratories, Bureaus, Test Facilities, Experiment Stations, Data Collection and Analysis Centers, and Grants Manage- ment and Research Coordinationg Offices in Agriculture, Commerce, Education, Energy, Engineering, Environment, the Humanities, Medicine, Military Science, and Basic and Applied Sciences. (1996) 9th edition. Edited by Barrett, J.K. & Hubbard, M.M. New York: Gale Research. ISBN 0810349418 (CR 1.3.30)

1.3.23 International Directories in Print. Edited by Towell, J.E. & Montney, C.B. Detroit: Gale Research

1.3.24 International Directory of Bioethics Organizations. Edited by Nolen, A.L. & Coutts, M.C. Washington, DC: National Reference Center for Bioethics Literature, Kennedy Institute of Ethics. ISBN 188391311X

Lists organizations engaged in the study, teaching, research or practice of bioethics or health care ethics. Information given is names, addresses, telephone, fax, director, purpose, e-mail, educational programmes and publications.

1.3.25 International Research Centres Directory. Edited by Piccirelli, A. Detroit: Gale Research (CR 1.3.30)

1.3.26 Libraries in the UK and Republic of Ireland. Edited by Harrold, A. London: Library Association

Gives names and addresses of all public, university, selected government, national and specialized libraries. It also includes departments of librarianship and information science. Published annually.

1.3.27 Medical and Health Information Directory, 1998: a Guide to Organizations, Agencies, Institutions, Programs, Publications, Services, and other Resources concerned with Clinical Medicine, Basic Biomedical Sciences, and the Technological and Socioeconomic Aspects of Health Care. (1998) 9th edition. Edited by Travers, B. Detroit: Gale Research. ISBN 0787615560

1.3.28 Medical Research Centres: a World Directory of Organisations and Programmes. (1988) 8th edition. London: Longman. ISBN Volume 1 A–N Y6622895 0582017777; Volume 2 O–Z + Index Y6622903

A comprehensive reference source giving

profiles of industrial centres, official laboratories and major university or technical college laboratories which carry out or fund research into medical specialities and medically orientated elements of other disciplines. Information includes address/telephone/status/staff/director, activities and publications.

1.3.29 Pan-European Associations. (1996) 3rd edition. Beckenham: CBD Research. ISBN 0900246731

More than 2,300 entries indexed by subject.

1.3.30 Ready Reference Shelf. Detroit: Gale Research

The *Ready reference shelf* is available on CD-ROM and the Internet via GaleNet. Entries are drawn from the Encyclopedia of Associations, Publishers Directory, Directories in Print, Gale Directory of Databases, Directory of Special Libraries and Information Centers, Research Centers Directory, International Research Centers Directory and Government Research Centers Directory (CR 1.3.2, 1.3.20, 1.3.22, 1.3.25, 1.8.6).

1.3.31 Research Services Directory. (1995) 6th edition. Detroit: Gale Research. ISBN 0810379058

Gives details of the services, facilities and expertise of over 4,500 for-profit research and development companies in the USA, and includes geographical and subject indexes.

1.3.32 UK Publishers Directory. Edited by Rocco, E. Detroit: Gale Research

1.3.33 Ulrich's International Periodicals Directory 5 volumes. New York: Bowker

Arranged by subject, each entry includes title, publisher, year first published, frequency, special features, where indexed, online availability, title changes and a brief description of typical contents.

1.4 STATISTICS

This section gives details of guides to statistics.

Annotations

1.4.1 Central Statistical Office. *Guide to Official Statistics.* London: HMSO

Enables one to trace sources of official statistical data. There are periodic updates.

1.4.2 Eurostat: Your Partner for European Statistics: a Guide to the Statistical Office of the European Communities. (1994) Luxembourg: Office for Official Publications of the European Communities. ISBN 9282673073

A detailed guide to the type and range of European Communities statistics as well as the sources.

1.4.3 Eurostat Index: a Detailed Subject Index to the Series Published by the Statistics Office of the European Communities. (1989) 4th edition. Compiled by Ramsay, A. Stamford, Lincs: Capital Planning Information

A detailed keyword subject index to assist the layperson in finding European Community statistics. Online access is publicly available via the Euronet DIANE network. It also contains a bibliography enabling Eurostat titles to be traced, lists other published titles, European documentation centres and depository libraries.

1.4.4 Flemming, T. & Kent, D. (1990) *Sourcebook of Canadian Statistics.* Toronto: Canadian Health Libraries Association. ISBN 0969217129

Documents publications offering information of a statistical nature about health and health care in Canada. Covers hospital morbidity, chronic conditions and life-style concerns, health care expenditure and utilization, supply of personnel and education. It also includes journal literature, aquisitions aids, general bibliography and a strategy for locating statistical information.

1.4.5 Minister of Industry, Science and Technology (1993) Statistics Canada Catalogue Cat. No. 11–204E. ISSN 0823-4223

A guide to the wide range of print and electronic products and services from Statistics Canada.

1.4.6 Mort, D. (1997) *Sources of Unofficial UK Statistics* 3rd edition. Aldershot: Gower. ISBN 0566076721

Comprises 1,059 entries of bodies publishing statistics. Included are name, address, telephone & telex numbers, title, frequency, date of first issue, general description, number of tables, availability of source, cost, ISSN/ISBN numbers and who to contact for further information.

1.4.7   Population Statistics: a Review of UK Sources. (1989) Edited by Benjamin, B. Aldershot: Gower. ISBN 056605731X

1.4.8   Radical Statistics Health Group. (1980) *Unofficial Guide to Official Health Statistics.* London: Radical Statistics Health Group. ISBN 0906081033

Outlines the types of official health statistics collected and where they may be found. Reliability of these data are questioned as they are collected and used for political purposes.

1.4.9   State and Local Statistic Sources. (1990) Edited by Balachandran, M. Detroit: Gale Research

1.4.10   Statistic Sources. (1991) 14th edition. Edited by O'Brien, J.W. & Wasserman, S.R. Detroit: Gale Research. ISBN set 0810373750; Volume 1 0810373769; Volume 2 0810373777

Includes a selected bibliography of key statistical sources and a dictionary of statistics sources. The bibliography includes statistical databases online, almanacs and international sources as well as US statistical sources. Topics covered include financial, business, social, educational and health.

1.4.11   Statistics Europe. (1996) 6th edition. Beckenham: CBD Research. ISBN 0900246731

1,250 statistical sources are listed covering social, economic and market research in all European countries. Arranged by country and indexed by subject.

1.4.12   US Bureau of the Census Statistical Abstract of the US. Washington, DC: US Bureau of the Census. ISBN 0160420474

Standard summary of statistics on social, political and economic organizations of the USA. Published annually.

1.4.13   Vital and Health Statistics Series: an Annotated Checklist and Index to Publications of the 'Rainbow Series'. (1991)

Compiled by Walsh, J. & Bothmer, A.J. New York: Greenwood Press. ISBN 0313272603

Lists, annotates and indexes all reports (853) from 1958 to 1991 of the four series of National Center for Health statistics. Subject and title indexes are included.

1.4.14   World Health Statistics Quarterly. Geneva: World Health Organization

Published quarterly, it provides health guidance based on what can be learned from statistical data. Each issue focuses on a selected theme or topic of current public health interest which will be a prime source for health planners.

1.5   BIBLIOGRAPHIES

Bibliographies are listings of books and other materials which can be grouped by a common factor, hence the British National Bibliography is based primarily on items received by the Copyright Receipt Office of the British Library.

Annotations

1.5.1   AIDS bibliography.
Publisher: National Library of Medicine.
Frequency: Monthly (from January 1989) In June & December a final section lists all new serial titles added in the previous six months Format similar to Index Medicus.

Contains citations added to MEDLINE, CANCERLIT, CATLINE and AVLINE.

1.5.2   Bibliography of Nursing Literature 1859–1960: with an Historical Introduction. (1968) Edited by Thompson, A.M.C. London: Library Association. ISBN 0853654700
and

1.5.3   Bibliography of Nursing Literature 1961–1970. (1974) Edited by Thompson, A.M.C. London: Library Association. ISBN 085365316X
and

1.5.4   Bibliography of Nursing Literature 1971–1975. (1985) Edited by Walsh, F.

London: Library Association. ISBN 0853656231
and

1.5.5 Bibliography of Nursing Literature 1976–1980. (1986) Edited by Walsh, F. London: Library Association. ISBN 0853657467

These bibliographies are of value to anyone researching the history of nursing. The entries include journal articles as well as books. The listings are, however, not comprehensive.

1.5.6 Books in Print.
Publisher: Bowker-Saur.
Frequency: Monthly. Available on microfiche and CD-ROM.

Contains author, title and publisher indexes. Covers books published in North America only.

1.5.7 British National Bibliography.
Publisher: British Library.
Frequency: Weekly, with four monthly and annual cumulations.

BNB is a subject catalogue of all the titles published in Britain, received by the Copyright Receipt Office of the British Library. Published since 1950, it forms a reasonably comprehensive listing of nursing titles, but caution is needed as not all titles listed actually reach the booksellers' shelves.

1.5.8 International Books in Print.
Publisher: Saur, Munich

Contains author and title indexes. Lists English-language titles published in Canada, Continental Europe, Latin America, Oceania, Africa, Asia and the Republic of Ireland.

1.5.9 Library of Congress Catalogue (National Union Catalogue).
Publisher: Library of Congress, Washington, DC.
Frequency: Monthly.

Available on microfiche since 1983 and covers books and audio-visual materials. Includes the following indexes: name, title, subject and series (i.e. monographs, symposia, reports, periodicals, papers, occasional papers, intermittent publications and conference proceedings).

1.5.10 Medical & Health Science Data

Book. (1993) Edited by Forbes, C.D. Mansion Publishing. ISBN 1874545049

This service provides bibliographical data on over 20,000 titles. Arranged by subject and author, it includes contents, new title descriptions, publishers and distributors.

1.5.11 Whitaker's Books in Print (formerly *British Books in Print*).
Publisher: Whitaker.
Frequency: Monthly.

Available on microfiche and has author, title and subject indexes. Also contains forthcoming books.

1.6 CURRENT AWARENESS SERVICES

Current awareness services are produced to provide up-to-date listings, sometimes annotated, of items usually of interest to a specific group.

Annotations

1.6.1 Ethnic Minorities Health: a Current Awareness Bulletin.
Publisher: Bradford Health Authority.
Frequency: Quarterly, with annual subject index.

Arranged by broad subject categories, each entry includes a brief annotation where the item's title does not make the content clear.

1.6.2 Health Visitors' Association Current Awareness Bulletin.
Publisher: Health Visitors' Association.
Frequency: Quarterly.

Lists articles of interest to health visitors and their managers. Each entry includes a brief annotation. Journals indexed in the bulletin are listed.

1.6.3 Midwives' Information and Resource Service (MIDIRS).
Publisher: MIDIRS.
Frequency: 3 times a year.

An unusual service in that it includes original source material. Would be useful to teachers of midwifery, midwives, health visitors and students (CR 1.9.4).

1.6.4   Nursing Bibliography.
Publisher: Royal College of Nursing.
Frequency: Monthly.

A useful source of information but the lack of an annual cumulation makes searching slow. Available as part of the British Nursing Index on CD-ROM and via the Internet (CR 1.7. 4).

1.6.5   Royal College of Midwives Current Awareness Service.
Publisher: Royal College of Midwives.
Frequency: Quarterly.

Gives lists of journals and available bibliographies. Also included are book reviews of items in the current awareness service, information on books, reports, press releases, useful addresses and journal holdings of the library.

1.7   INDEXING SERVICES

Indexing services give brief details of items, most often periodicals, published during a specified period and are usually arranged by subject. Many of these services are now available on CD-ROM and via the Internet.

Annotations

1.7.1   British Education Index.
Publisher: Leeds University Press.
Frequency: Quarterly, with annual cumulation.

Issues are divided into two sections: author list and subject list. Entries in the author list include subject descriptor terms and the type of document. Subject list entries are more brief. Lists all periodicals indexed.

1.7.2   British Humanities Index.
Publisher: Bowker-Saur.
Frequency: Quarterly, with annual cumulations.

Covers a wide range of social science subjects and is particularly useful for community subjects.

1.7.3   British Library Monthly Index of Conference Proceedings.
Publisher: British Library.

Frequency: Monthly, with annual cumulations.

Covers all types of conference proceedings including those published in serial and book form. Nursing conferences are also included (CR 1.2.3).

1.7.4   British Nursing Index.
Publisher: BNI Publications.
Frequency: Monthly.

Generated from UK-based journal collections. Terminology for the subject headings follows British practice.

1.7.5   Cumulative Index of Nursing and Allied Health Literature.
Publisher: CINAHL.
Frequency: Bimonthly, with annual cumulations.

Subject headings follow a very similar pattern to Medical Subject Headings (MeSH). Entries are similar to the International Nursing Index but are expanded to include qualifiers for the title and subject descriptors.

1.7.6   Current Technology Index (replaces British Technology Index).
Publisher: Library Association.
Frequency: Monthly, with annual cumulation.

Covers all branches of engineering and chemical technology. Some subjects related to medicine are included, e.g. health foods, health hazards, hearing, heart, medical equipment and medical photography.

1.7.7   Index Medicus.
Publisher: National Library of Medicine (USA).
Frequency: Monthly, with annual cumulations.

The major service in the field of health sciences.

1.7.8   Index to Social Sciences and Humanities Proceedings.
Publisher: Institute for Scientific Information Inc. Philadelphia.
Frequency: 3 quarterly issues with an annual cumulation.

Index publishes the most significant proceedings worldwide in a range of disciplines in the social sciences and humanities. Nursing is included.

1.7.9 Index to Theses: with Abstracts accepted for Higher Degrees by the Universities of Britain.
Publisher: Aslib.
Frequency: Each volume covers a calendar year.

Contains abstracts of all theses accepted for higher degrees in the UK.

1.7.10 International *Nursing Index*.
Publisher: American Journal of Nursing Company.
Frequency: Quarterly, with annual cumulation.

International Nursing Index (INI) uses Medical Subject Headings (MeSH), the authoritative list of terms produced by the United States National Library of Medicine. Entries are limited to title, author, journal title, date, volume/issue and page numbers. Where the original is not in English the language is noted.

1.7.11 Popular Medical Index.
Publisher: Mede Publishing.
Frequency: 3 issues per year plus cumulation.

An index to articles on medical subjects written specifically for the layperson, appearing in popular magazines. Arranged alphabetically by subject headings.

1.7.12 Royal College of Midwives (1987) *Midwifery Index: a Source of Journal References on Midwifery and Related Topics 1980–1986.* (With selective coverage of 1976–79) Edited and compiled by Ayres, J. London: Royal College of Midwives. ISBN 1870822005

A cumulation of the main sections of the Royal College of Midwives Library's Current Awareness Service. A list of subject headings is given together with an author index. Journals only are covered and these are not listed.

1.7.13 Social Sciences Citation Index.
Publisher: ISI.
Frequency: 3 times per year with an annual cumulation.

Social Sciences Citation Index comprises a citation index, source index, permuterm subject index and a corporate index. Citation services rely on the citations given by authors and are of particular use in establishing a body of literature on a subject and identifying key authors or seminal works. Nursing journals are covered by this service.

Guide

1.7.14 Strickland-Hodge, B. (1986) *How to Use Index Medicus and Excerpta Medica.* Aldershot: Gower. ISBN 0566035321

This manual aims to improve the search techniques of students and others needing to use medical literature. It discusses all aids to searching *Index Medicus* and *Excerpta Medica*, and gives guidance on the use of Medical Subject Headings (MeSH), both public and annotated, permuted MeSH and supplementary Chemical Records.

Article

1.7.15 Gooch, P.M. (1996) Databases: Hom-Inform bibliographical database and information service for homeopathic literature. *Complementary Therapies in Medicine,* 4 (1) 63–6 4 References

This article describes the Hom-Inform Library Information Service (Glasgow Homeopathic Hospital) database of homeopathic literature.

1.8   ELECTRONIC SERVICES

Electronic services are those based on the use of a computer. The greatest growth area is in CD-ROM (Compact Disc-Read Only Memory) and the use of the Internet. It is now possible, and will become increasingly so, to perform a literature search and gather the source material from one integrated service.

Many of the CD-ROM publishers are making their services available on the Internet either through commercial, fee-based providers, or free. For example, Medline via the National Institutes of Health and the National Library of Medicine is now available free on the Internet. This section does not provide a list of databases and services as it would be out of date before publication. Instead, it identifies some of the key directories and articles on particular services together with those which discuss strategies for searching. Directories are defined, in the context of this section, as any service, whether on paper, CD-ROM or Internet/website, which lists systematically services of interest to those searching the literature.

URLs given are correct at time of publication.

Directories

1.8.1 American Nurses' Association Nursing World
Source: American Nurses' Association
URL: http://www.nursingworld.org/index.htm

Largely centred on the activities of the American Nurses' Association, this website includes links to the *Online Journal of Issues in Nursing*, nursing-related resources and State Nursing Associations.

1.8.2 Gale Research (1998) *CD-ROM's in Print 1998*. Detroit: Gale Research. ISBN 0787614459

Includes subject and distributor indexes.

1.8.3 Gale Research (1998) *Cyberhound's Guide to Internet Databases* Volume 4. 4th edition. Detroit: Gale Research. ISBN 0787611891

Includes information on over 5,000 databases and indexes arranged by subject and host/provider as well as a glossary of Internet terms.

1.8.4 Gale Research (1996) *Cyberhound's Guide to Internet Discussion Groups* Volume 1. Detroit: Gale Research. ISBN 0787610194

Discussion groups can provide a very useful source of information and help for the researcher. This guide features a subject index.

1.8.5 Gale Research (1996) *Cyberhound's Guide to Internet Libraries* Volume 1. Detroit: Gale Research. ISBN 0787610240

An evaluative guide to libraries on the Internet. Includes information on special collections, catalogue addresses, a bibliography and a glossary of Internet terms.

1.8.6 Gale Research Directory of Databases. Detroit: Gale Research (CD-ROM).

Over 13,000 databases available online, on CD-ROM, diskette or magnetic tape are

listed. Possible to search by subject. It is updated twice yearly (CR 1.3.30).

1.8.7 Gale Research (1998) *Gale Guide to Internet Databases*. Detroit: Gale Research

A new serial guide from Gale.

1.8.8 Hardin Meta Directory of Health Internet Sites
Source: University of Iowa, Hardin Library for the Health Sciences
URL: http://www.lib.uiowa.edu/hardin/md/index.html

This website is structured as an index and is designed to provide easy access to leading websites that act as 'directories' in the health sciences. It has general and subject-specific listings.

1.8.9 HealthWeb – Nursing
Source: University of Michigan, Taubman Medical Library
URL: http://www.lib.umich.edu/hw/nursing.html

Organized in seven categories: career information; clinical nursing; communication; education; organizations; research and resources, this website aims to provide a comprehensive index to online information for nurses.

1.8.10 Mental Health Network
Source: CMHC Systems
URL: http://www.opd.state.md.us/mhnet.htm

Self-help mental health resources and links to related websites are provided. There is clear subject distinction in the structure of the site but with overlapping links between categories.

1.8.11 NursingNet
Source: NursingNet
URL: http://www.nursingnet.org/allied.htm

A subject directory to nursing on the World Wide Web. Includes subject categorization of links.

1.8.12 OMNI – Organizing Medical Networked Information
Source: OMNI Consortium (National Institute for Medical Research Library, Nottingham University, Cambridge University, Royal Free Hospital School of Medicine, King Edward's Hospital Fund, Wellcome Centre for Medical Sciences)
URL: http://omni.ac.uk

Emphasis on the UK but with international coverage, its aim is a comprehensive catalogue of networked biomedical and health-related resources. The database is fully browsable, using alphabetical listings, National Library of Medicine Classification and Medical Subject Headings (MeSH). Includes an invaluable section on evaluating Internet resources.

1.8.13   Resources for Nurses and Families
Source: Dr Diane Wink, School of Nursing, College of Health and Public Affairs, University of Central Florida
URL: http://pegasus.cc.ucf.edu/~wink/home.html

Aimed at family health services' nurses and families, this website provides links to sites based around the needs of these two groups.

1.8.14   Royal College of Nursing, Research & Development Co-ordinating Centre: Dissemination & Utilisation Databases
Source: Royal College of Nursing
URL: http://www.man.ac.uk/rcn/d&udata base.html

Lists databases used to disseminate information about research and development within the field of nursing, midwifery and health visiting. Bias is towards British-based services.

1.8.15   UK Directory: the Definitive Guide to UK Internet Sites Winchester: UK Directory. ISSN 1368-8510

1.8.16   University of Central England: Library Home Page
Source: University of Central England
URL: http: //www.uce.ac.uk/library/public

This website is included as an example of a typical academic institution's set of pages which provide links to resources on the Internet. The structured links give access to general search engines, health care and nursing-specific sites, government departments and agencies, databases, library catalogues and source material. Most institutions now have home pages with this type of structure which can serve as a good starting point for any search of the Internet.

Articles/books

1.8.17   Aker, P.D., McDermaid, C., Opitz,

B.G. & White, M.W. (1996) Searching chiropractic literature: a comparison of three computerized databases. *Jmpt (Journal of Manipulative & Physiological Therapeutics)*, 19 (8) 518–24

A comparison of CHIROLARS, Index to Chiropractic Literature (ICL) and MEDLINE.

1.8.18   Andrews, M. (1995) A guide to searching on-line for information on transcultural nursing and health. *Journal of Transcultural Nursing*, 7 (1) 36–9

1.8.19   Anonymous (1998) Patient education materials off the Net. *Patient Education Management*, 5 (1) 10–12

Teaching materials available via the Internet.

1.8.20   Anonymous (1998) Resources. Websites of interest to RNs. *Chart*, 95 (1) 4

A brief but very useful article which lists and describes a number of websites.

1.8.21   Anthony, D. (1996) *Health on the Internet*. Oxford: Blackwell Science. ISBN 0632040726

Includes information on what the Internet is, connecting, health-related resources, libraries, electronic publishing, e-mail, World Wide Web and searching for information.

1.8.22   Barnsteiner, J.H. (1994) The Online Journal of Knowledge Synthesis for Nursing. *Reflections*, 20 (2) 10–11

A description of the journal, one of the first in nursing to be exclusively available on the Internet.

1.8.23   Behm, K. & Baier, M. (1998) News, notes & tips. Evaluating online literature searches. *Nurse Educator*, 23 (2) 9 –10

Looks at the techniques researchers can use to ensure that their literature search, using electronic resources such as CINAHL and Medline, has been comprehensive.

1.8.24   Benner, J. (1997) Nursing the Net. Researching health care topics on the Internet. *Nursing*, 27 (9) 28–9

1.8.25   Booth, A. (1991) The place of CINAHL within the British context. *Health Libraries Review*, 8 (4) 220–3

Highlights the differences in terminology and organizational practice which affect search strategies in Britain when executed on a database from North America. Many of the points made are applicable internationally.

1.8.26   Brown, C.M. (1998) The benefits of searching EMBASE versus MEDLINE for pharmaceutical information. *Online & Cdrom Review*, 22 (1) 3–8

This article demonstrates the difference in search results from using the same strategy on two apparently similar databases.

1.8.27   Burg, B. & Kautzmann, A.M. (1998) Web versus CD-ROM: format follows function. *Searcher: The Magazine for Database Professionals*, 6 (1) 59–63   11 References

The choice between CD-ROM and Internet-based services is becoming less easy to make. This article highlights the differences based on their functions.

1.8.28   Cox, J. (1991) *Online and CD-ROM Database Searching*. London: Mansell. ISBN 0720120934

Covers a rapidly developing area of information science and includes a survey of online and CD-ROM information sources, an annotated bibliography and directory of organizations.

1.8.29   Curl, D.D. & Shapiro, C.S. (1998) Health information and other useful facts on the World Wide Web. *Jmpt (Journal of Manipulative and Physiological Therapeutics)*, 21 (2) 126–7

1.8.30   Delozier, E.P. & Lingle, V.A. (1992) MEDLINE and MeSH: challenges for end users. *Medical Reference Services Quarterly*, 11 (3) 29–46

Discusses the problems encountered by end users with MeSH strategies using search software. Includes a review of the literature.

1.8.31   Devitt, M. (1998) Getting started on the Internet. Digital headlines: news sites on the Web. *Dynamic Chiropractic*, 16 (4) 42–3

Often overlooked by researchers, news sources can provide much information of value. This article outlines some of the main news websites.

1.8.32   DeZelar-Tiedman, C. (1997) Known item searching on the World Wide Web. *Internet Reference Services Quarterly*, 2 (1) 5–14

A comparison of search engine effectiveness using a known item as the test.

1.8.33   Ferguson, T. (1996) *Health Online: How to Find Health Information, Support Groups, and Self-help Communities in Cyberspace*. Reading, MA: Addison-Wesley. ISBN 0201409895

1.8.34   Fikar, C.R. (1997) Childhood asthma resources on the Internet. *Health Care on the Internet*, 1 (1) 23–33

1.8.35   Fryer, R.K., Baratz, N. & Helenius, M. (1991) Important full-text databases for the health sciences. *Cd-Rom Professional*, 4 (6) 92–6

Introduces full-text databases useful to anyone researching in the health sciences.

1.8.36   Gibbs, S., Sullivan-Fowler, M. & Rowe, N.W. (eds) (1996) *Mosby's Medical Surfari: a Guide to Exploring the Internet and Discovering the Top Health Care Resources*. St Louis: Mosby. ISBN 0815148178

Includes chapters on getting started, choosing a service, searching, security, medical networks, general health care resources and other health care resources.

1.8.37   Grainger, F. & Lyon, E. (1991) A comparison of the currency of secondary information sources in the biomedical literature: weekly current awareness services part 1. *Health Libraries Review*, 8 (3) 150–6

A comparative study of three services distributed on floppy disc.

1.8.38   Grainger, F. & Lyon, E. (1992) A comparison of the currency of secondary information sources in the biomedical literature: MEDLINE online and on CD-ROM part 2. *Health Libraries Review*, 9 (4) 138–43

The speed at which journal articles appear in the indexing services can make a considerable difference to the currency of a literature search. This study highlights the time taken for each of the index services.

1.8.39   Graves, J.R. (1993) Data versus information versus knowledge. *Reflections*, 19 (1) 4–5

The   Virginia   Henderson   International

Nursing Library is an electronic library. This article outlines its conceptual basis.

1.8.40 Graves, J.R. (1997) The Virginia Henderson Library: resource for nurse administrators. *Nursing Administration Quarterly*, 21 (3) 76–83   8 References

Provides a description of the Registry of Nursing, including a comparson of an example retrieval from a typical bibliographical database and the Registry.

1.8.41 Hancock, L. (1996) *Physicians' Guide to the Internet.* Philadelphia: Lippincott. ISBN 0397516347

1.8.42 Hock, R.E. (1998) Precision searching with Web search engines. *Cyberskeptic's Guide to Internet Research*, 3 (1) 4

This article looks at getting the best from using search engines to find information on the World Wide Web.

1.8.43 Hsu, P.P. (1993) ClinPSYC, PsycLIT, and MEDLINE for health professionals. *Medical Reference Services Quarterly*, 12 (4) 7–22   12 References

A comparison of the three databases.

1.8.44 Hutchinson, D. (1997) A nurse's guide to the Internet. *RN*, 60 (1) 46–52 6 References

A general guide to the Internet.

1.8.45 Hutchinson, D. (1997) The Internet for healthcare professionals. *ORL–Head and Neck Nursing*, 15 (3) 9–14   28 References

Provides a summary of different types of Internet resource and suggests a basic strategy for its use. The emphasis is on Otolaryngology and several sites are listed and described.

1.8.46 Keeping, D. (1998) The Internet: uses for the laboratory technologist. *Canadian Journal of Medical Laboratory Science*, 60 (11) 11–15

1.8.47 Kilby, S. (1991) Database searching made easy. *Nurse Educators' Microworld*, 5 (3) 18

A useful introduction to database searching.

1.8.48 Kleyman, P. (1998) Media currents.

Using the Net for good health . . . assessing Web sites. *Aging Today*, 19 (1) 18–19

Based around consumer health information, this article gives advice on the assessment of the efficacy of websites.

1.8.49 Korn, K. (1998) Diabetes mellitus information on the Internet. *Journal of the American Academy of Nurse Practitioners*, 10 (2) 61–3   4 References

Links to World Wide Web sites are listed in the references.

1.8.50 Korn, K. (1998) Pharmacology resources on the Internet. *Journal of the American Academy of Nurse Practitioners*, 10 (1) 29–30

1.8.51 LaBruzza, A.L. (1997) *The Essential Internet: a Guide for Psychotherapists and other Mental Health Professionals.* Northvale, NJ: Jason Aronson. ISBN 0765701057

A very useful guide for those working in the field of mental health.

1.8.52 Lingle, V.A. (1997) Journal searching in non-MEDLINE resources on Internet Web sites. *Medical Reference Services Quarterly*, 16 (3) 27–43   10 References

Provides a review of a selection of non-MEDLINE-based searches and sources on the Internet.

1.8.53 Makulowich, J.S. & Bates, M.E. (1995) 10 tips on managing your Internet searching. *Online*, 19 (4) 32–4, 36–7   2 References

1.8.54 McGuire, T.J. (1997) Medlineing: why and how to conduct a literature search. *Jems: Journal of Emergency Medical Services*, 22 (4) 56–7, 59–60   7 References

1.8.55 McKenzie, B.C. (1996) *Medicine and the Internet: Introducing Online Resources and Terminology.* Oxford: Oxford University Press. ISBN 0192627058

1.8.56 Mendelsohn, S. (1996) First person: CDROM, online or the Internet? *Information World Review*, 114 30–1

A useful comparison of three electronic services.

1.8.57 Munoz, M.B., Sanchez, A.G. & Sanchez, M.M. (1997) How to make a bibliographical search in rehabilitation [Spanish]. *Rehabilitation*, 31 (2) 108–17   32 References

Provides a thorough comparison of many of the main databases and sources with particular emphasis on Spanish sources such as Indice Médico Español.

1.8.58 Nahl-Jakobovits, D. & Tenopir, C. (1992) Databases online and CD-ROM: how do they differ, let us count the ways. *Database*, 15 (1) 42–50

A comparison of online and CD-ROM searching, with particular regard to cost and time factors.

1.8.59 Nicholson, L. (ed.) (1997) *The Internet and Healthcare.* Chicago, IL: Health Administration Press. ISBN 1567930603

Concentrates on health care administration sources.

1.8.60 Nicoll, L.H. (1992) Grateful Med: an easy to use information tool. *Reflections*, 18 (3) 40–1

Describes the Grateful Med software package.

1.8.61 Notess, G.R. (1996) On the nets. Searching the Web with Alta Vista. *Database*, 19 (3) 86–8   2 References

1.8.62 Notess, G.R. (1997) On the net. Internet search techniques and strategies. *Online*, 21 (4) 63–6

1.8.63 O'Brien, K. (1998) Web-site review: occupational health and safety. *Collegian: Journal of the Royal College of Nursing, Australia*, 5 (1) 43

1.8.64 Okuma, E. (1994) Selecting CD-ROM databases for nursing students: a comparison of MEDLINE and the Cumulative Index to Nursing and Allied Health Literature (CINAHL). *Bulletin of the Medical Library Association*, 82 (1) 25–9

A research study to produce a systematic method of comparing databases. This is important when choosing the most appropriate database on which to execute a search.

1.8.65 Osenga, A. (1997) The Cochrane Library, a reference work on CD-ROM. *Journal of Chiropractic Education*, 11 (1) 33–4

The Cochrane Library is an essential index of clinical trials.

1.8.66 Partin, R.L. (1998) *Prentice-Hall Directory of On-line Social Studies Resources: 1,000 of the Most Valuable Social Studies Web Sites, Electronic Mailing Lists and Newsgroups.* Paramus, NJ: Prentice-Hall. ISBN 013679887X

1.8.67 Peters, R. & Sikorski, R. (1998) The X(ray) files: radiology resources on the Internet. *Jama: Journal of the American Medical Association*, 279 (7) 561–2

1.8.68 Potter, L.A. (1995) A systematic approach to finding answers over the Internet. *Bulletin of the Medical Library Association*, 83 (3) 280–5   6 References

1.8.69 Poynder, R. (1998) Patent information on the Internet. *Online and Cdrom Review*, 22 (1) 9–17

Suggests strategies for searching for patent information on the Internet as well as some of the services available.

1.8.70 Reed, K.L. & Cunningham, S. (1997) *Internet Guide for Rehabilitation Professionals.* Philadelphia: Lippincott. ISBN 039755463X

1.8.71 Ryer, J.C. (1997) *HealthNet: Your Essential Resource for the Most Up-to-date Medical Information Online.* New York: John Wiley. ISBN 0471137693

Covers all aspects of health.

1.8.72 Schneider, D. (1993) Internet: linking nurses, scholars libraries. *Reflections*, 19 (1) 9

Describes the use of the Internet computer network with particular reference to the Virginia Henderson International Nursing Library.

1.8.73 Smith, R.P. & Edwards, M.J.A. (1997) *The Internet for Physicians.* New York: Springer. ISBN 0387949364

1.8.74 Walker, C.J., McKibbon, K.A., Haynes, R.B. & Ramsden, M.F. (1991) Problems encountered by clinical end users of

MEDLINE and GRATEFUL MED. *Bulletin of the Medical Library Association*, 79 (1) 67–9

Looks at end-user behaviour, analysing why search strategies were unproductive.

1.8.75 Yensen, J. (1998) Connecting points: electronic nursing resources. Systematic, fast, comprehensive search strategies in nursing. *Computers in Nursing*, 16 (1) 23–9   23 References

A very useful article describing in detail some of the possible strategies to adopt to get the best from searching the Internet.

1.9   ABSTRACTING SERVICES

Abstracting services provide a source for identifying relevant material in a literature search. They tend to be less comprehensive as an index but the abstracts (summaries) give details of item content which can save time in checking original sources.

Annotations

1.9.1 ASSIA – Applied Social Sciences Index and Abstracts
Publisher: Library Association.
Frequency: Bi-monthly with an annual cumulation.

Arrangement is by subject and author with the abstracts appearing in the subject listings. Includes nursing and newspapers, and is of particular interest to the researcher who requires current or past coverage of issues.

1.9.2 Dissertation Abstracts International
Publisher: University Microfilms Inc.
Frequency: Monthly.

Contains abstracts of doctoral dissertations submitted by institutions. It is divided into three major sections:
A   Humanities and Social Sciences
B   Science and Engineering
C   Worldwide

Each entry contains title, author, degree, date, name of institution, number of pages, location adviser and order number. Author's abstract is included. Theses related to all aspects of health sciences are included in section B.

1.9.3 Health Service Abstracts
Publisher: Department of Health Library.
Frequency: Monthly.

Covers a broad range of subjects of interest in the health service.

1.9.4 Midwifery Research Database (MIRAID)
Publisher: National Perinatal Epidemiology Unit, Oxford.
Frequency: Annual.

A new national register, in the form of a computerized database, of all completed and ongoing research in midwifery in the UK. Information will be published 3 times a year from mid-1990 and includes an abstract, keywords, details of the researchers, funding and publications (CR 1.7.12).

1.9.5 Nursing Abstracts
Publisher: Nursing Abstracts Company.
Frequency: Bi-monthly with annual author, subject and publication indexes.

Individual issues are arranged by subject. Entries include bibliographical data and a concise abstract. Exclusively uses North American journal sources.

1.9.6 Nursing Research Abstracts
Publisher: Department of Health Index of Nursing Research.
Frequency: Quarterly with an annual index.

Enables the tracing of completed and ongoing research in the UK, but relies on the authors or interested organizations for its information on unpublished and published projects. The abstracts are precise, making judgements on the source materials of the users' work more accurately than is the case with indexing services. This service has now ceased publication.

1.9.7 Psychological Abstracts
Publisher: American Psychological Association.
Frequency: Monthly with an expanded annual cumulation of the indexes.

The monthly issues are divided into subject index, author index and abstracts. The abstracts are divided into 16 major categories with sub-categories where appropriate. As well as the standard bibliographical material, the entries include the affiliation of the first-named author, the number of references and the abstract source. This is the major abstracting service in the field of psychology.

1.9.8 Research into Higher Education Abstracts
Publisher: Carfax Publishing.
Frequency: 3 times per year – February, June October.

Of particular use to researchers in education.

1.9.9   Social Science Abstracts
Publisher: Department of Social Security Library.
Frequency: Monthly.

Uses the same system of abstracts and indexes as Nursing Research Abstracts, and includes a broad range of subjects of particular interest to community nurses and service managers.

1.9.10   Sociological Abstracts
Publisher: Sociological Abstracts.
Frequency: 6 issues per year, published in April, June, August, October and 2 in December.

Divided into four sections: subject, author and source indexes and a main section of abstract entries. Sociological Abstracts is the major abstracting service in the social sciences.

1.9.11   Sociology of Education Abstracts
Publisher: Carfax Publishing.
Frequency: Quarterly with annual subject and author indexes.

The quarterly issues are divided into five sections: journal abstracts, book abstracts, journals covered, author index and subject index. This service will be of particular interest to educational researchers but it should be noted that no nursing journals are covered.

Article

1.9.12   Stodulski, A.H. & Stafford, S.M. (1982) Disseminating nursing research information in the UK: Nursing Research Abstracts from the Index of Nursing Research. *International Journal of Nursing Studies*, 19 (4) 231–6   4 References

Describes the development of the Index of Nursing Research and the resultant Nursing Research Abstracts.

PART 2: METHODS OF INQUIRY

AN INTRODUCTION TO RESEARCH

2.1 RESEARCH TEXTS

Two major categories of research methodology texts are included in this section, those written for nurses, and general texts suitable for use by any discipline. Some texts include both quantitative and qualitative methods, but those exclusively on the latter may be found in section 2.36.

Annotations

2.1.1 Abbott, P. & Sapsford, R. (1998) *Research Methods for Nurses and the Caring Professions.* Buckingham: Open University Press. ISBN 0335096204 References

An introductory text which will assist those undertaking or evaluating research for the first time. Small-scale social research papers are discussed and exercises are given.

2.1.2 Babbie, E. (1997) *The Practice of Social Research* 8th edition. Pacific Grove, CA: Brooks Cole Publishing Co. ISBN 053450468X References

This revised and updated edition provides a comprehensive text on research methods for social science and other students (CR 2.2).

2.1.3 Baker, T.L. (1994) *Doing Social Research* 2nd edition. New York: McGraw-Hill. ISBN 0070034923 References

Book aims to give students insight into the techniques of social research and the motivation behind various studies. Many chapters have been revised, new topics included and a wide range of methods is discussed (CR 2.2).

2.1.4 Bernard, H.R. (1994) *Research Methods in Anthropology: Qualitative and Quantitative Approaches* 2nd edition. Thousand Oaks, CA: Sage. ISBN 0803952457 References

Book covers the major methods of designing research, collecting and analysing data in a systematic way. Traditional methods of doing anthropological research are covered and current concerns of applied work, quantification, sampling and validity are all discussed. Information on the positivist/interpretativist debate, ethics, sampling, and the use of methods for theory development is given. The use of computers for doing library searches, managing field notes and analysing data are also discussed (CR 2.7, 2.17, 2.22, 2.25, 2.29, 2.36, 2.84, 2.86, 2.87).

2.1.5 Blaxter, L., Hughes, C. & Tight, M. (1996) *How to Research.* Buckingham: Open University Press. ISBN 0335194524 References

Written for the less experienced researcher, this book is about the practical aspects of doing research. The style is jargon-free and it contains exercises, examples and practical hints for all stages of a project. Also included are extensive annotated bibliographies (CR 2.16).

2.1.6 Bouma, G.D. & Atkinson, G.B.J. (1995) *A Handbook of Social Science Research* 2nd edition. New Zealand: Oxford University Press. ISBN 0198280017 References

Book is intended for tertiary-level students undertaking an introductory research methods course. Activities are given to encourage learning and the approach is non-statistical and non-mathematical. A new chapter on qualitative research is included (CR 2.36).

2.1.7   Bowling, A. (1997) *Research Methods in Health: Investigating Health and Health Services.* Buckingham: Open University Press. ISBN 0335198856   References

Text is written for students and researchers of health and health services, together with policy-makers who have responsibility for applying research findings in practice. Its major sections are: investigating health services and health; the philosophy, theory and practice of research; quantitative research and the tools which may be used; qualitative and combined research methods and their analysis. Chapters include questions for discussion, an overview, key terms and further reading (CR 2.2, 2.29, 2.36).

2.1.8   Breakwell, G.M., Hammond, S. & Fife-Schaw, C. (eds) (1995) *Research Methods in Psychology.* London: Sage. ISBN 0803977654   References

Book presents a non-technical introduction to the key research methods employed in psychology and the social sciences. The relationship between psychological theory and research methodology is discussed, together with all stages of the research process. Examples are given from current research. Step-by-step advice, exercises, projects and lists for further reading are also included (CR 2.34, 2.35, 2.67, 2.92).

2.1.9   Brink, P.J. & Wood, M.J. (1998) *Basic Steps in Planning Nursing Research: from Question to Proposal* 5th edition. Sudbury, MA: Jones & Bartlett Inc. ISBN 0867206772 References

Book is intended for students undertaking a first course in research methods and deals solely with the beginning phase, the research plan. It begins with identifying a research topic and ends with the written proposal. There is recommended reading at the end of each chapter with four sample research proposals as appendices (CR 2.96).

2.1.10   Brockoff, D.Y. & Hastings-Tolma, M.T. (1989) *Fundamentals of Nursing Research.* Glenview, IL: Scott Foreman & Co. ISBN 0673398404   References

Book is intended for nursing students and practising clinicians. Units cover the nurse as

scientist, asking and answering the question. Both qualitative and quantitative research designs are included, together with many examples. Each chapter includes exercises, working definitions and critical appraisal (CR 2.2, 2.29, 2.36).

2.1.11   Burnard, P. & Morrison, P. (1994) *Nursing Research in Action: Developing Basic Skills* 2nd edition. Basingstoke: Macmillan Press. ISBN 0333608763   References

Book aimed at beginners wishing to develop basic research skills. Each chapter is in the format of a 'Do it yourself' manual and comprises suggested reading, aims, information boxes, exercises and learning checks.

2.1.12   Burns, N. & Grove, S.K. (1997) *The Practice of Nursing Research: Conduct, Critique and Utilization* 3rd edition. Philadelphia: W.B. Saunders. ISBN 0721630545 References

Instructor's manual ISBN 072163057X. Study guide ISBN 0721625878.

This revised and updated text, reflecting advances in nursing research, is intended for undergraduates, graduates and those practising in the field. It is organized into four units: an introduction to nursing research which includes discussion on quantitative and qualitative research; the research process; the pragmatics of research; and the implications of research for nursing. A chapter on outcomes research, a new paradigm in nursing, is included. Examples are given throughout the text (CR 2.2, 2.29, 2.36, 2.43).

2.1.13   Burns, N. & Grove, S.K. (1999) *Understanding Nursing Research* 2nd edition. Philadelphia: W.B. Saunders. ISBN 0721681009   References

Written for a course in undergraduate nursing research, this textbook teaches students the steps of the research process. The importance of critique and utilization of findings in clinical practice is emphasized using examples from published studies (CR 2.95, 2.102).

2.1.14   Chisnall, P.M. (1996) *Marketing Research: Analysis and Measurement* 5th edition. London: McGraw-Hill. ISBN 0077091752   References

Provides a comprehensive and authoritative text on marketing research. Parts cover the methodologies used in this type of research, basic techniques, specific applications and the handling and interpretation of data.

2.1.15 Christensen, L.B. (1996) *Experimental Methodology* 7th edition. Boston, MA: Allyn & Bacon. ISBN 0205263658 References

Book focuses on experimental methodologies. Two topic areas, quasi-experimental and single-subject designs, have undergone change and development so separate chapters are included in this edition. Evaluation research is also explored in depth. Although intended mainly for students of psychology, nurses will readily identify with the examples given (CR 2.29, 2.34, 2.35, 2.43).

2.1.16 Clifford, C. (1997) *Nursing and Health Care Research: a Skills Based Introduction* 2nd edition. London: Prentice-Hall. ISBN 0132297418 References

This book, which has been updated and expanded, is intended for students undertaking health care studies. It traces the research process from the initial idea to dissemination and the implementation of findings. There is increased coverage of qualitative research and the focus is on practical skills needed for small-scale projects (CR 2.36).

2.1.17 Cohen, L. & Manion, L. (1994) *Research Methods in Education* 4th revised edition. London: Routledge. ISBN 0415102359 References

Book will serve both researchers and consumers of research evidence. A wide range of traditional and more recent approaches are included, together with many examples of British research reported since 1980. Additional material has been added to this edition and references have been updated.

2.1.18 Cormack, D.F.S. (ed.) (1996) *The Research Process in Nursing* 3rd edition. Oxford: Blackwell Science Inc. ISBN 063204019X References

Text includes writings by a group of research specialists to guide nurses step by step through the research process.

2.1.19 Couchman, W. & Dawson, J. (1995) *Nursing and Health Care Research: a Practical Guide* 2nd edition. Harlow, Middlesex: Scutari. ISBN 1873853289 References

A self-instruction workbook, designed to introduce research to nurses who are in the initial stages of learning, and it would also be useful for updating and professional development. An extended fictitious nursing research project is used to illustrate each step in the process and chapters contain exercises and references.

2.1.20 Crombie, I.K. & Davies, H.T.O. (1996) *Research in Health Care*. New York: John Wiley. ISBN 0471962597 References

Provides health care professionals with a comprehensive guide to the design, conduct and interpretation of health care research. The range of problems which may be encountered are discussed.

2.1.21 Dempsey, P.A. & Dempsey, A.D. (1996) *Nursing Research* 4th edition. New York: Little, Brown. ISBN 0316181889 References

Text, written for undergraduates and graduates, covers basic nursing research principles and techniques. Quantitative and qualitative approaches are included, together with applied activities. Appendices contain examples of historical, descriptive, ethnographic, experimental and quasi-experimental research proposals; abstracts of two studies; guidelines for writing a proposal; evaluating reports and a statistical primer (CR 2.2, 2.29, 2.36, 2.96).

2.1.22 DePoy, E. & Gitlin, L.N. (1994) *Introduction to Research: Multiple Strategies for Health and Human Services*. St Louis: Mosby. ISBN 0801662842 References

Provides the reader with an understanding of how researchers use both naturalistic and experimental research methods. Philosophical foundations are discussed together with the thinking and action processes of research (CR 2.2, 2.5).

2.1.23 Fitzpatrick, J.J. (ed.) (1998) *Encyclopedia of Nursing Research*. New York: Springer. ISBN 082611170X

Encyclopedia contains over 300 articles by the world's leading authorities in nursing research and will be of value to all who have an interest in improving patient care through research. Key terms and concepts are comprehensively explained and an extensive cross-referenced index is included. Entries include applied and clinical nursing research, concept analysis, data management, ethics of research, the Internet, journals in nursing research, measurement and scales, qualitative and qualitative research, statistical techniques and research utilization (CR 1.8, 2.2, 2.5, 2.17, 2.29, 2.36, 2.79, 2.80, 2.85, 2.102, Appendix B).

2.1.24   Frankfort-Nachmias, C. & Nachmias, D. (1996) *Research Methods: the Social Sciences* 5th edition. London: St Martin's Press. ISBN 0312137745   References

Gives a non-technical introduction to research methods. Examples are given from classic social science studies and current social issues. Book concentrates mainly on quantitative approaches (CR 2.2, 2.29, 2.88, 2.91).

2.1.25   Gilbert, N. (ed.) (1993) *Researching Social Life*. London: Sage. ISBN 0803986823 References

A comprehensive guide to methods of social research. It is intended as a first course for students in many disciplines including nursing and health studies. Each chapter includes exercises and suggested further readings.

2.1.26   Hek, G., Judd, M. & Moule, P. (1996) *Making Sense of Research: an Introduction for Nurses*. London: Cassell. ISBN 0304333387   References

Book, which is intended for students and qualified nurses just starting out on research, aims to demystify research by explaining its role, giving an overview of the process and presenting a range of approaches. The emphasis is on developing critical skills, ethical issues, disseminating and implementing findings (CR 2.17, 2.95, 2.98, 2.102).

2.1.27   Hoskins, C.N. (1998) *Developing Research in Nursing and Health*. New York: Springer. ISBN 0826111858   References

Book contains the basic elements of conducting and understanding nursing research for students at BSN and Masters level, and by practising nurses (CR 2.29, 2.36).

2.1.28   Isaac, S. & Michael, W.B. (1995)

Handbook in Research and Evaluation 3rd edition. San Diego, CA: Edits. ISBN 0912736321   References

A collection of principles, methods and strategies useful in the planning, design and evaluation of studies in education and the behavioural sciences.

2.1.29   Jackson, W. (1995) *Methods: Doing Social Research*. Hemel Hempstead: Prentice-Hall. ISBN 013064031X   References

Book covers aspects of both qualitative and quantitative research methods. Exercises and a bibliography are included together with appendices on ethical guidelines and commands for SPSSX and SPSSPC+ (CR 2.2, 2.17, Appendix A).

2.1.30   Leedy, P.D. (1996) *Practical Research* 6th edition. Hemel Hempstead: Prentice-Hall. ISBN 0132414074   References

A practical text which encourages learning by doing, with assignments linked to each chapter. Book is suitable for all courses in basic research methodology and references are given from different disciplines, including nursing. Examples of research are given in each chapter, and there is a series of discussions on the computer as a tool of research. Appendix contains an annotated research proposal (CR 2.96).

2.1.31   Leong, F.T.L. & Austin, J.T. (eds) (1996) *The Psychology Research Handbook: a Guide for Graduate Students and Research Assistants*. Thousand Oaks, CA: Sage. ISBN 0803970498   References

Book follows all aspects of the research process and also includes a special topic section covering co-ordinating a research team, applying for research grants and using theory in research (CR 2.7, 3.13, 3.16).

2.1.32   LoBiondo-Wood, G. (1997) *Nursing Research: Methods, Critical Appraisal and Utilization* 4th edition. St Louis: Mosby Year Book Inc. ISBN 0815123906   References

Text prepares nursing students and practitioners to become knowledgeable research consumers. It addresses the role of the research consumer, teaches the fundamentals of the research process as well as critical appraisal. Each chapter relating to the research process includes lists of critiquing criteria and examples to illustrate each stage (CR 2.2, 2.95, 2.102, 3.16).

2.1.33 Mark, R. (1996) *Research Made Simple: a Handbook for Social Workers.* Thousand Oaks, CA: Sage. ISBN 0803974272 References

This 'how to' guide discusses the scientific method, fundamental terms and the research process from initial idea to completion. Both quantitative and qualitative approaches are considered.

2.1.34 May, T. (1997) *Social Research: Issues, Methods and Process.* Buckingham: Open University Press. ISBN 0335200052 References

Book is designed as a complete course of study for sociology and social policy students and aims to bridge the gap between theory and methods.

2.1.35 Mertens, D.M. (1997) *Research Methods in Education and Psychology: Integrating Diversity with Quantitative and Qualitative Approaches.* Thousand Oaks, CA: Sage. ISBN 0803958285 References

Book explains both quantitative and qualitative methods and incorporates the view of various research paradigms into the descriptions of these methods – the post-positivist and interpretative/constructivist paradigms and a relative newcomer, the emancipatory paradigm which includes the perspectives of feminists, ethnic/racial minorities and people with disabilities. In each chapter, a step of the research process is explained from the literature through to analysis and reporting (CR 2.9, 2.10, 2.29, 2.36).

2.1.36 Mouton, J. & Marais, H.C. (1992) *Basic Concepts in the Methodology of the Social Sciences.* Pretoria: Human Sciences Research Council. ISBN 0796906483 References

Book discusses the fundamental methodological concepts which underlie decision-making in the research process, rather than the methods and techniques themselves (CR 2.7, 2.9, 2.14, 2.16, 2.64, 2.96, 2.97).

2.1.37 Notter, L.E. & Hott, J.R. (1994) *Essentials of Nursing Research* 5th edition.

New York: Springer. ISBN 0826115985 References

A concise introductory guide for nurses embarking on a research project or attempting to evaluate published research. The text makes reference to many American clinical nursing studies to illustrate each step of the research process (CR 2.2).

2.1.38 Oliver, P. (1997) *Research for Business, Marketing and Education.* London: Hodder & Stoughton. ISBN 034069081X

Book takes the reader through the research process from beginning to end. Examples are given from business, industry, education and everyday life. It stresses the practical uses of research and will meet the needs of college and university students learning research methods (CR 2.2).

2.1.39 Parahoo, K. (1997) *Nursing Research: Principles, Process and Issues.* Basingstoke: Macmillan Press. ISBN 0333699181 References

Written for students with little or no previous knowledge of research, this book aims to equip readers with a comprehensive understanding of the concepts and principles of research so that it may be read critically, and utilized where appropriate (CR 2.2, 2.95).

2.1.40 Polgar, S. & Thomas, S.A. (1995) *Introduction to Research in the Health Sciences* 3rd edition. Melbourne: Churchill Livingstone. ISBN 0443050392 References

Text is intended for all health science students. It covers quantitative research methods and readers are led through the research process. No prior knowledge of statistics is assumed. New features in this edition are section introductions which will facilitate an overview of the research process together with discussion questions inviting examination of more complex issues (CR 2.2, 2.29).

2.1.41 Polit, D.F. & Hungler, B.P. (1995) *Study Guide for Nursing Research: Principles and Methods* 5th edition. Philadelphia, PA: Lippincott. ISBN 0397551398

Book complements the 5th edition of *Nursing Research: Principles and Methods.* It comprises matching, complementary and application exercises and study questions related to each chapter. Special projects are also included.

2.1.42   Polit, D.F. & Hungler, B.P. (1998) *Accompany Nursing Research: Principles and Methods* 6th edition. Philadelphia, PA: Lippincott-Raven. ISBN 0781715636

2.1.43   Polit, D.F. & Hungler, B.P. (1999) *Nursing Research: Principles and Methods* 6th edition. Philadelphia: Lippincott. ISBN 0781715628   References

This book retains all the features of previous editions and also includes a balanced presentation of both qualitative and quantitative methods. A new chapter on qualitative research design and approaches is included together with expanded discussion of multimethod research. A study guide and instructor's manual and testbank are available to complement the text (CR 2.2, 2.36, 2.84).

2.1.44   Reid, N.G. & Boore, J.R.P. (1987) *Research Methods and Statistics in Health Care.* London: Edward Arnold. ISBN 0713145226   References

Text written for nurses discusses research in the practice context and illustrates the practical aspects of conducting such studies. Statistical tests are used, clearly explained and again applied to practice.

2.1.45   Robertson, J. (ed.) (1994) *Handbook of Clinical Nursing Research.* Melbourne: Churchill Livingstone. ISBN 0443048665 References

Book, intended for students and new researchers, has been designed to facilitate the conduct of research in the clinical setting. It concentrates on the practical aspects of research, and is intended to complement existing texts. Additional printed and software resources are included.

2.1.46   Sarantakos, S. (1998) *Social Research* 2nd edition. Basingstoke: Macmillan Press. ISBN 0333738683   References

This text, designed for undergraduates, introduces the methods and techniques of social research and their theoretical frameworks. This new edition includes quantitative and qualitative methods and guidance is given on computer-aided analysis (CR 2.29, 2.36, 2.84).

2.1.47   Schutt, R.K. (1995) *Investigating the Social World: the Process and Practice of Research.* Thousand Oaks, CA: Pine Forge Press. ISBN 0803990103   References

A textbook on research strategy for undergraduate students which covers both qualitative and quantitative methods. A disk and exercises are included (CR 2.29, 2.36).

2.1.48   Seale, C. (ed.) (1998) *Researching Society and Culture.* London: Sage. ISBN 0761952772   References

Book aims to provide a comprehensive overview, and introduction to, the research methods used in the social sciences and cultural studies. Intended for undergraduates and graduates, the book gives tools with working examples of actual research, together with examining methodological and theoretical issues.

2.1.49   Wilson, H.S. & Hutchinson, S.A. (1996) *Consumer's Guide to Nursing Research: Exercises, Learning Activities, Tools and Resources.* Albany, NY: Delmar Publishing. ISBN 0827362641   References

Book is designed to complement existing texts and will facilitate the acquisition of skills and knowledge required by the novice researcher, practitioners and graduate students. It provides an action-orientated approach and deals with quantitative and qualitative studies in an unbiased fashion. Each aspect of the research process is covered, relevant exercises are given and sources for further reading are included (CR 2.2, 2.29, 2.36).

2.2   THE LANGUAGE OF RESEARCH AND STATISTICS

Research, as with any other discipline, has its own terminology, and this section makes reference to dictionaries, chapters and articles where words or phrases are defined. Because no one source contains all words to be found in this bibliography, definitions, taken from the literature, are given in each section where appropriate. Their original sources may be found in Appendix D.

Annotations

2.2.1 Berger, R.M. & Patchner, M.A. (1988) Research vocabulary, in Authors, *Planning for Research: a Guide for Helping Professions*. Beverly Hills, CA: Sage. ISBN 080393033X Chapter 2, 29–47

Chapter defines some research terms using a narrative format.

2.2.2 Brand, K.P. (1991) A crossword puzzle can teach research terms. *Western Journal of Nursing Research*, 13 (2) 278–83 12 References

Suggests a different way of assisting nurses to learn research terminology.

2.2.3 Cambridge Dictionary of Statistics in the Medical Sciences. (1995) Edited by Everitt, B.S. Cambridge: Cambridge University Press. ISBN 0521479282

Provides simple definitions and explanations of statistical concepts, especially those used in biomedicine.

2.2.4 Collins Dictionary of Sociology. (1995) Edited by Jary, D. & Jary, J. New York: HarperCollins. ISBN 0004708040

Covers terms and concepts used in sociology and related language in psychology, economics, political science and anthropology.

2.2.5 Davitz, J.R. & Davitz, L.L. (1997) The language of research: definitions and applications, in Authors, *Evaluating Research Proposals in the Behavioural Sciences: a Guide* 2nd edition. Englewood Cliffs, NJ: Prentice-Hall. ISBN 0133485668 References

Research and some statistical terms and concepts used in the behavioural sciences are defined and an example of use is given for each one (CR 2.96).

2.2.6 Dictionary of Nursing Theory and Research. (1995) 2nd edition. Edited by Powers, B.A. & Knapp, T.R. Thousand Oaks, CA: Sage. ISBN 0803956266

A compilation of definitions and discussion of both research and statistical terms likely to be encountered in the nursing scientific literature. Examples of where terms are used are included and citations are provided to books and articles where they are more fully explained.

2.2.7 Dictionary of Social and Market Research. (1996) Edited by Koschnick, W.J. London: Gower Technical Press. ISBN 056607611X

2.2.8 Dictionary of Social Science Methods. (1990) Edited by Miller, P.McC. & Wilson, M.J. Chichester: John Wiley. ISBN 0471900362

Collects in one source accounts of current methods of inquiry which the empirical social sciences share in common. Definitions and explanations are also given and a cross-referencing system leads to other relevant items. Many statistical terms are also included.

2.2.9 Dictionary of Statistics. (1998) Edited by Porkes, R. London: Collins. ISBN 0004343549

Book is intended for the student and informed layperson and is encyclopaedic in nature, with 426 entries. The text contains definitions, graphs, diagrams and worked examples of more advanced topics. Appendices include lists of symbols, formulae and statistical tables.

2.2.10 Dictionary of Statistics and Methodology. (1999) 2nd edition. Edited by Vogt, W.P. Thousand Oaks, CA: Sage. ISBN 0761912746

This dictionary has been thoroughly revised and includes 600 additional new terms and definitions.

2.2.11 Gubrium, J.F. & Holstein, J.A. (1997) *The New Language of Qualitative Method*. New York: Oxford University Press. ISBN 019709994X

2.2.12 Presly, A. (1996) Common terms and concepts in nursing research, in Cormack, D.F.S. (ed.), *The Research Process in Nursing* 3rd edition. Oxford: Blackwell Science Inc. ISBN 063204019X Chapter 2, 14–21

Chapter explains some of the terms commonly used in research (CR 2.1.18).

2.2.13 Schwandt, T.A. (1997) *Qualitative Inquiry: a Dictionary of Terms*. Thousand Oaks, CA: Sage. ISBN 0761902546

Book considers the key concepts and issues that help to shape the field of qualitative research. The definitions acknowledge the multiple and often contested points of view which characterize these research approaches. It focuses primarily on philosophical and methodological concepts rather than on the technical aspects of methods and procedures (CR 2.36).

2.2.14   Sweeney, M.A. & Olivieri, P. (1981) *An Introduction to Nursing Research: Research, Measurement and Computing in Nursing.* Philadelphia, PA: Lippincott. ISBN 0397542631 Chapter 2, 32–42   References

Chapter explains the use of research terms by describing the process in a general way.

2.3   THE NATURE AND PURPOSE OF RESEARCH IN NURSING

'As nurses we want to be able to give the very best care to our patients and clients. In order to do this we need to know what is the best and how to give it. Research findings and evidence can give us some of the knowledge to help us decide what is best and therefore to deliver the highest standards of care possible.' (Hek, Judd & Moule, 1996: 9)

Definitions

Applied research – research without emphasis on theory, explanation or prediction but rather on application and development of research-based knowledge
Basic research – . . . primarily concerned with developing the knowledge base and extending the theory in academic and/or practice disciplines . . . findings cannot always be applied directly to practice
Clinical research – . . . investigating questions emerging from clinical experience, paying attention to and revealing any underlying values and assumptions . . . and directing the results towards clinical participants
Community health nursing research – research which attempts to prevent potential patients from becoming actual patients and to promote the health and well-being of both groups outside an institutional setting
Empirical research – . . . data-based investigations in which researchers systematically study some aspect of human behaviour

Nursing research – research into those aspects of health care which are the appropriate and predominant responsibility of nurses
Research – an attempt to extend the available knowledge by means of a systematically and scientifically defensible process of inquiry
Research methodology – . . . the methods for collecting, processing and analysing research data
Research-mindedness – . . . implies a critical, questioning approach to one's work, the desire and ability to find out about the latest research in that area, and the ability to assess its value to the situation and apply it as appropriate. It also implies a recognition of the importance of research to the profession and to patient care, and a willingness to support nurse-researchers in their work

Annotations

2.3.1   Chapman, J. (1991) Research: what it is and what it is not, in Perry, A. & Jolley, M. (eds), *Nursing: a Knowledge Base for Practice.* London: Edward Arnold. ISBN 0340514922 Chapter 2, 28–51   25 References

Provides an overview of research in nursing and outlines ways in which researchers explore problems to generate knowledge (CR 2.6, 2.14, 2.95, 3.7).

2.3.2   Gage, N.L. (1993) 'The obviousness of social and educational research results', in Hammersley, M. (ed.), *Social Research: Philosophy, Politics and Practice.* London: Sage. ISBN 0803988052 Chapter 17, 226–37 11 References

Chapter discusses the obviousness of research and whether therefore it should be undertaken. Critiques, positions and studies by several researchers are cited to illustrate the points made (CR 2.36.25).

2.3.3   Hockey, L. (1981) Knowledge is a precious possession. *Nursing Mirror*, 23 September, 152 (13) 46–9   1 Reference

Examines what nursing research is and what it is not. The scepticism and enthusiasm of some nurses for research is contrasted, together with the value of and necessity for research as a basis for practice.

2.3.4   Hockey, L. (1996) The nature and

purpose of research, in Cormack, D.F.S. (ed.), *The Research Process in Nursing* 3rd edition. Oxford: Blackwell Science. ISBN 063204019X 20 References

Chapter explores the nature, purpose and urgency of nursing research. Nurses' research involvement is discussed and the author speculates about the future (CR 2.1.18).

2.3.5 Holden, J.E. (1996) Physiological research is nursing research. *Nursing Research*, 45 (5) 312–13 1 Reference

Author believes that what should drive nursing research is the question asked, not the bodily category in which it falls. Some of the confusion may have come from the struggle of nursing to gain autonomy as a separate profession from medicine. Nurses should take a holistic view so physical, psychosocial, spiritual and environmental factors are all important.

2.3.6 Hutchins, S.A. & Eckes, R. (1996) Clinical research: considerations for prospective participants. *Nursing Clinics of North America*, 31 (1) 125–35 17 References

Article describes the purpose and process of clinical research, the patient's perspective, ethical considerations and the role of the nurse in biomedical research (CR 2.17, 2.22, 3.16).

2.3.7 Martin, P.A. (1995) Is it research? *Applied Nursing Research*, 8 (4) 199–201 11 References

Discusses some of the differences between research and organization improvement processes which can sometimes cause confusion. The pitfalls are highlighted when there is no clarity about which process is being used and the terminology is different. The implications of these problems are discussed.

2.3.8 Nolan, M. & Behi, R. (1995) What is research? Some definitions and dilemmas. *British Journal of Nursing*, 4 (2) 111–15 24 References

Issues are addressed concerning the meaning and purpose of research and some of the principal differences between the major approaches are described (CR 2.2).

2.3.9 O'Brien, M. (1993) Social research and sociology, in Gilbert, N. (ed.), *Research-*

ing Social Life. London: Sage. ISBN 0803986823 Chapter 1, 1–17 References

Chapter outlines some of the key features of sociology as an approach to understanding social life. The role of theory in social research is discussed and two examples of research are given as illustrations (CR 2.1.25, 2.7).

2.4 RESEARCH PROCESSES

Although the phrase research process is frequently used, the practice of research often involves a series of processes. Science does not occur in stages, or follow a linear path, but instead consists of overlapping processes in all parts of the investigation. Literature in this section provides brief overviews of these processes.

Definitions

Research approaches – ,,, a set of methods and techniques for designing a study and collecting and analysing data: quantitative data for quantitative research, and qualitative data in qualitative research

Research processes – the use of quantitative and qualitative methods to collect and analyse data for the purpose of prediction and explanation [adapted]

Annotations

2.4.1 Arber, S. (1993) The research process, in Gilbert, N. (ed.), *Researching Social Life*. London: Sage. ISBN 0803986823 Chapter 3, 32–50 References

Gives a personal account of a survey as an example of planning the research process. It also discusses the realities of research which are not always in accord with the ideas set out in manuals on methods (CR 2.1.25, 2.14, 2.16).

2.4.2 Barzun, J. (1998) *The Modern Researcher* 6th edition. San Diego, CA: Harcourt Brace College Publishers. ISBN 0155055291 References

Contains detailed information for researchers

with particular reference to historical research. Advice is given on all aspects of writing reports (CR 2.46, 2.97).

2.4.3 Bush, C.T. (1997) Understanding nursing research, in Chitty, K.K. (ed.), *Professional Nursing: Concepts and Challenges* 2nd edition. Philadelphia: W.B. Saunders. ISBN 0721668836   18 References

Chapter outlines the research process, how it may contribute to practice and its relationship to nursing theory and practice. Sources of support are identified and the roles of nurses in research discussed (CR 3.16).

2.4.4 Fitch, M.I. (1995) Introduction to the process of research: a focus on oncology nursing research. *Canadian Oncology Nursing Journal*, 5 (4) 130–5   41 References

Article offers a user-friendly approach for oncology nurses to instil confidence about some of the terminology and concepts used in research (CR 2.2).

2.4.5 Kirk, K. (1996) Embarking on the research process: a guide. *Health Visitor*, 69 (9) 370–2   11 References

Readers are taken through the research process from inspiration to dissemination. Useful sources to support each stage are described.

2.4.6 Rees, C. (1994) A step-by-step guide to the research process. *British Journal of Midwifery*, 2 (10) 479–84   4 References

Outlines the stages involved in the research process.

CONCEPTUALIZING NURSING RESEARCH

2.5 PHILOSOPHICAL BASES FOR RESEARCH

'... a plurality of philosophies may be necessary to reflect the many facets of nursing science, that is, no one view may be sufficient to embrace or drive nursing knowledge in its totality.' (Omery, Kasper & Page, 1995: x)

Definitions

Concept – an abstraction based on observations of certain behaviours or characteristics (e.g. stress, pain)
Conceptual framework – lays out the key factors, constructs and variables and the presumed relationship between them
Constructivism – ... a philosophical perspective interested in the ways in which human beings individually and collectively interpret or construct the social and psychological world in specific linguistic, social and historical contexts
Hermeneutics – the science or art of interpretation
Ontology – the branch of philosophy that deals with the nature of being and first principles
Operationalization – the process of figuring out how to measure concepts using empirical evidence
Paradigm – the basic belief or world-view that guides the investigator, not only in choices of method but in ontologically and epistemologically fundamental ways
Philosophy – love and pursuit of wisdom by intellectual means

Annotations

2.5.1 Allen, D.G. (1995) Hermeneutics: philosophical traditions and nursing practice research. *Nursing Science Quarterly*, 8 (4) 174–82 50 References

Article traces some of the main themes in philosophical hermeneutics and their potential for developing nursing practice research. The relationship between hermeneutic philosophy and research methods used in interpretative traditions and the role of experimental design in addressing such questions is discussed (CR 2.29).

2.5.2 Annells, M. (1996) Hermeneutic phenomenology: philosophical perspectives and current uses in nursing research. *Journal of Advanced Nursing*, 23 (4) 705–13 52 References

Discusses the contemporary use of hermeneutic phenomenology within the discipline of nursing. Author believes it has considerable potential for improving nursing practice.

2.5.3 Appleton, J.V. & King, L. (1997) Constructivism: a naturalistic methodology for nursing inquiry. *Advances in Nursing Science*, 20 (2) 13–22 28 References

Article explores the philosophical underpinnings of the constructivist research paradigm. Fundamental issues surrounding this methodology are debated and differences between method and methodology are highlighted.

2.5.4 Draper, P. (1996) Nursing research and the philosophy of hermeneutics. *Nursing Inquiry*, 3 (1) 45–52 50 References

Paper explores some of the implications of hermeneutic philosophy for nursing research. Using material from a study into the quality of life of older people in nursing homes, the paper shows that hermeneutics can provide a perspective to examining the literature which guides data collection and interpretation.

2.5.5 Edwards, S. (1997) Philosophy in nursing. *Nursing Times*, 17–23 December 93 (51) 48–9   14 References

Article identifies three ways in which the term philosophy is commonly used in the context of nursing. The four main areas of philosophical inquiry are described, together with the kind of questions which are relevant to nursing.

2.5.6 Flew, A.G. (1995) *Thinking about Social Thinking* 2nd edition. London: Prometheus Books. ISBN 0879759542 References

Book challenges the methodology of social science and its applications in the form of contemporary social policies. Illustrative material is provided from recent and classical literature.

2.5.7 Gift, A.G. (ed.) (1997) *Clarifying Concepts in Nursing Research*. New York: Springer. ISBN 0826199801   References

Book presents a critique of concept development in nursing and makes suggestions for improving traditional methods. It is a guide to the evolving and dynamic nature of concept development and stresses the importance of a sustained programme of nursing research.

2.5.8 Hindess, B. (1977) *Philosophy and Methodology in the Social Sciences*. Hassocks, Sussex: Harvester Press. ISBN 0855273445 References

Book provides a systematic critique of epistemological and philosophical interventions in the social sciences and of prescriptive methodology in general. The works of Weber, Schutz, Husserl, Mills and Popper are analysed and discussed (CR 2.6).

2.5.9 Holmes, C.A. (1990) Alternatives to natural science foundations for nursing. *International Journal of Nursing Studies*, 27 (3) 187–98   68 References

Paper discusses some of the philosophical assumptions associated with humanistic and holistic approaches to nursing and outlines their impact on nursing theory, education and practice. Author believes nursing should concentrate on phenomenological and humanistic methodologies.

2.5.10 Hughes, J. (1997) *The Philosophy of Social Research* 3rd edition. London: Longman. ISBN 0582311055   References

An introductory text which examines some philosophical views arising from social research practices. Ways of evaluating both current and historical research in the social sciences are discussed (CR 2.46).

2.5.11 Hupcey, J.E., Morse, J.M., Lenz, E.R. & Tason, M.C. (1996) Wilsonian methods of concept analysis: a critique. *Scholarly Inquiry for Nursing Practice*, 10 (3) 185–210   50 References

The evolution and modifications of Wilsonian methods of concept analysis are discussed and compared using examples. Authors believe that these methods have been eroded because of modifications made to them. Priority needs to be given to the significance of concept development for the nursing profession and the evaluation of conceptual inquiry.

2.5.12 Kikuchi, J.F. & Simmons, H. (1994) *Developing a Philosophy of Nursing*. Thousand Oaks, CA: Sage. ISBN 0803954239 References

Book explores several important questions: What is a philosophy of nursing? What is required for its development? How is it related to contemporary conceptualizations of nursing? It will help nurses to understand what is necessary to establish a sound philosophical basis for the development of nursing practice, education, research and administration.

2.5.13 Koch, T. (1996) Implementation of a hermeneutic inquiry in nursing: philosophy, rigour and representation. *Journal of Advanced Nursing*, 24(1) 174–84   39 References

Discusses the process of a hermeneutic inquiry as a research methodology in seeking to understand the experiences of older people admitted to an acute hospital.

2.5.14 Morse, J.M. (1995) Exploring the theoretical basis of nursing using advanced techniques of concept analysis. *Advances in Nursing Science*, 17 (3) 31–46 45 References

Article critiques the traditional methods of concept development and presents alternative ways which use qualitative methods of inquiry. Variations of concept development techniques, appropriate to the maturity of the concept being explored, are described, including methods of concept delineation, comparison, clarification, correction and identification. An illustration is given of the application of concept development to theory through a research programme to delineate the construct of comfort.

2.5.15 Morse, J.M., Hupcey, J.E., Mitcham, C. & Lenz, E.R. (1996) Concept analysis in nursing research: a critical appraisal. *Scholarly Inquiry for Nursing Practice*, 10 (3) 253–77 104 References

Article compares the four methodological approaches to concept analysis: Wilson-derived methods, qualitative methods, critical analysis of the literature and quantitative methods. The particular value of each is described and authors present criteria for the selection of an appropriate research approach for concept analysis and its evaluation (CR 2.29, 2.36).

2.5.16 Morse, J.M., Mitcham, C., Hupcey, J.E. & Tason, M.C. (1996) Criteria for concept evaluation. *Journal of Advanced Nursing*, 24 (2) 385–90 25 References

Paper presents the anatomy of a concept. Methods of concept analysis are critiqued and criteria for the level of maturity of a concept are suggested. Factors necessary for the evaluation of criteria are discussed and authors argue that this process should precede concept development research.

2.5.17 Nolan, M. & Behi, R. (1995) Research in nursing: developing a conceptual approach. *British Journal of Nursing*, 4 (1) 47–50 17 References

Authors argue that research, like nursing, is best understood by the practical application of ideas, but that action should not be taken until a basic research appreciation or literacy is attained.

2.5.18 Packard, S.A. & Polifroni, E.C. (1992) The nature of scientific truth. *Nursing Science Quarterly*, 5 (4) 158–63 30 References

Article discusses authors' views on the need for a philosophical foundation in nursing scholarship. Nursing epistemology will not develop as good science until all theorists, thinkers and philosophers identify their positions prior to the discovery of theory through research and other scientific endeavours (CR 2.6, 2.8).

2.5.19 Phillips, D.C. (1987) *Philosophy, Science and Social Inquiry: Contemporary Methodological Controversies in Social Science and Related Applied Fields of Research.* Oxford: Pergamon. ISBN 0080334113 References

Discusses the contemporary debates concerning the scientific status of research in the social and human sciences. It provides a clear exposition of the relevant developments in philosophy against which research needs to be seen. Also discussed are the works of Kuhn, Winch, Lakatos, Feyerhand and especially Popper, the demise of positivism, the rise in interest in hermeneutical approaches, relativism and holism. A detailed case study illustrates the main ideas (CR 2.2).

2.5.20 Popper, K.R. (1991) *The Poverty of Historicism* 2nd edition. London: Routledge. ISBN 0415065690 References

Historicism as an approach to the social sciences assumes that historical prediction is the principal aim. The book exposes this idea in order to account for the unsatisfactory state of the theoretical social sciences. It is contrasted with scientific empiricism and suggestions are made as to what the character and methods of social science should be.

2.5.21 Reed, J. & Ground, I. (1997) *Philosophy for Nursing*. London: Arnold. ISBN 034061028X References

Book provides an overview of nursing and philosophy – philosophies of knowledge, mind, science, language, moral and political. Authors draw on everyday experiences to enlighten the philosophies explored.

2.5.22 Riegel, B., Omery, A., Calvillo, E., Elsayed, G., Lee, P., Shuler, P. & Siegal, B.E.

(1992) Moving beyond: a generative philosophy of science. *Image: Journal of Nursing Scholarship*, 24 (2) 115–20   28 References

Describes an alternative philosophy of science, influenced by several major existing philosophies, in particular that advocated by Thomas Kuhn, called the generative philosophy. Authors believe this has a special significance for nursing. Major concepts, relationships among concepts and implications for nursing research are discussed (CR 2.8).

2.5.23 Swartz, O. (1997) *Conducting Socially Responsible Research.* Thousand Oaks, CA: Sage. ISBN 0761904999   References

Volume describes where philosophy ends and application begins. Based in the field of communication studies, the book describes an understanding of theory, criticism and pedagogy with the vocabulary of neo-pragmatism and argues that rhetorical scholars can assume a cultural importance in life.

2.5.24 Thorne, S.E. (1997) Pearls, pith and provocation. Phenomenological positivism and other problematic trends in health science research. *Qualitative Health Research*, 7 (2) 287–93   13 References

Author challenges readers to consider the philosophical positions from which qualitative methods are derived and, in so doing, to reconsider the necessity for methodological integrity towards the overall purpose of knowledge development (CR 2.6, 2.36).

2.5.25 Walsh, K. (1996) Philosophical hermeneutics and the project of Hans Georg Gadamer: implications for nursing research. *Nursing Inquiry*, 3 (4) 231–7   22 References

Gives an overview of the historical roots of philosophical hermeneutics grounded in the work of Husserl and Heidegger. The work of Gadamer is then discussed under the four concepts of prejudice, the fusion of horizons, the hermeneutic circle and play, and their implications for nursing research. Illustrations are given from the author's own work.

2.5.26 Williams, M. & May, T. (1996) *Introduction to the Philosophy of Social Research.* London: UCL Press. ISBN 1857283120   References

Examines the relationship between social research and philosophy, addressing the questions of theory and method. Two central approaches are explored: naturalism and interpretativism. Objectivity and values are analysed to show how they have shaped research.

2.5.27 Wolper, L. (1992) *The Unnatural Nature of Science.* London: Faber & Faber. ISBN 0571169724

An introduction to what science is and what it is not – a philosophy of science not written by a philosopher.

2.6   EPISTEMOLOGY

'Knowledge progresses not by absolute establishment of conclusions, but by the exposing of conjectures or hypotheses to criticism and to the possibility of refutation. However not even this process yields certainty, for a position that is soundly criticizable today might undergo resuscitation tomorrow. Progress follows a tentative and meandering course.' (Phillips, D.C., 1987: 116)

Definitions

Epistemology – a concept in philosophy that relates to the theories of knowledge or how people come to have knowledge of the world
Human becoming theory – a school of thought within the discipline of nursing
Praxis – practical application or exercise of a branch of learning
Realism – . . . the doctrine that there are real objects that exist independently of our knowledge of their existence

Example

O'Brien, B. & Pearson, A. (1993) Unwritten knowledge in nursing: consider the spoken as well as the written word. *Scholarly Inquiry for Nursing Practice*, 7 (2) 111–24   39 References

Reports a study which examined the therapeutic potential of nursing in an embryonic unit through nurses' unwritten and orally transmitted knowledge. Quality assurance measures showed an acceptable standard of care delivery was being maintained despite absence of written documentation. The research intent and methodology are discussed in the context of distinctions between written and unwritten knowledge (CR 2.37).

Annotations

2.6.1 Allen, M.N. & Jenson, L.A. (1996) Knowledge development in nursing, in Kerr, J.C. & MacPhail, J. (eds), *Canadian Nursing: Issues and Perspectives* 3rd edition. St Louis: Mosby. ISBN 0815152256 Chapter 8, 85–103 81 References

Examines a world-view of nursing knowledge, its substantive structure, sources, levels, classification and modes of inquiry in nursing. Criteria for credibility of nursing knowledge and future directions for development are discussed.

2.6.2 Antrobus, S. (1997) Developing the nurse as a knowledge worker in health: learning the artistry of practice. *Journal of Advanced Nursing*, 25 (4) 829–35   27 References

Paper argues that health has been inadequately conceptualized and the knowledge base required by nurses is poorly defined. An epistemology for nursing is proposed that considers knowledge to be a construction of empirical, clinical and personal ways of knowing. The difficulties in defining and developing this epistemology are discussed and the author makes suggestions for advancing the situation.

2.6.3 Baumann, S.L. (1996) Parse's research methodology and the nurse researcher – child process. *Nursing Science Quarterly*, 9 (1) 27–32   35 References

Discusses use of the Parse research method when exploring various aspects of childhood, regarding them as partners in the study.

2.6.4 Behi, R. & Nolan, M. (1995a) Sources of knowledge in nursing. *British Journal of Nursing*, 4 (3) 141–2, 159   12 References

Article provides a brief overview of the various sources and types of nursing knowledge, highlighting the similarities and differences. The underlying principles and strengths and weaknesses of such knowledge are explored.

2.6.5 Behi, R. & Nolan, M. (1995b) The nature of scientific knowledge: fact or theory? *British Journal of Nursing*, 4 (4) 221–4 24 References

The complex and confusing literature on nursing theories and theory-building are discussed and the distinctions between facts and theories explained (CR 2.7).

2.6.6 Booth, K., Kenrick, M. & Woods, S. (1997) Nursing knowledge, theory and method revisited. *Journal of Advanced Nursing*, 26 (4) 804–11   54 References

Paper considers the contemporary status of nursing knowledge, theory and method and describes a framework which is able to accommodate the great diversity of ideas and practices within nursing, and which is accessible to the entire spectrum of nursing experience.

2.6.7 Bowers, R. & Moore, K.N. (1997) Bakhtin, nursing narratives and dialogical consciousness. *Advances in Nursing Science*, 19 (3) 70–7   28 References

Reports the dialogical narrative approach put forward by Mikhail Bakhtin, a key philosopher in the 20th century which is directly related to nursing concepts of narrative, interaction and personhood, and suggestive of a postmodern clinical epistemology. Authors relate this approach to nursing practice (CR 2.89).

2.6.8 Bradley, S.F. (1996) Processes in the creation and diffusion of nursing knowledge: an examination of the developing concept of family-centred care. *Journal of Advanced Nursing*, 23 (4) 722–7   33 References

Paper outlines processes of creation and diffusion and discusses the influence of factors inside and outside the nursing profession on the epistemology of its knowledge base.

2.6.9 Carboni, J.T. (1995) The Rogerian process of inquiry. *Nursing Science Quarterly*, 8 (1) 22–37   33 References

Article presents a Rogerian process of inquiry which aims to understand the nature of human evolution and its multiple, unpredictable potentialities (CR 2.36).

2.6.10 Copnell, B. (1998) Synthesis in nursing knowledge: an analysis of two approaches. *Journal of Advanced Nursing*, 27 (4) 870–4   43 References

Paper examines two approaches to the synthesis of nursing knowledge development: the use of multiple paradigms and the possible emergence of a new paradigm based on chaos theory. Both approaches have flaws but they may be able to make significant contributions to nursing knowledge.

2.6.11   Cushing, A. (1994) Historical and epistemological perspectives on research and nursing. *Journal of Advanced Nursing*, 20 (3) 406–11   26 References

Examines problematic issues concerning nursing, nursing scholarship and the social sciences. The search for a knowledge base in nursing is explored and an historical context provides key developments between qualitative and quantitative approaches in nursing. Difficulties in applying qualitative methodologies are also discussed (CR 2.29, 2.36).

2.6.12   Dancy, J. & Sosa, E. (eds) (1993) *A Companion to Epistemology*. Oxford: Blackwell. ISBN 0631192581   References

This volume, in the Blackwell 'Companion to Philosophy' series, is organized as a standard reference book with 250 alphabetically arranged entries. It contains contributions from leading epistemologists and includes summaries of technical terms and extended essays on major topics (CR 2.2).

2.6.13   Dean, H. (1995) Science and practice: the nature of knowledge, in Omery, A., Kasper, C.E. & Page, G.G. (eds), *In Search of Nursing Science*. Thousand Oaks, CA: Sage. ISBN 0803950942   Chapter 20, 275–90 31 References

Chapter explores the relationship among beliefs about science and the nature of scientific inquiry and practice, especially as this relationship exists in professional disciplines such as nursing (CR 2.8.11).

2.6.14   Fitzpatrick, J.J. (1998) *Building Nursing Knowledge: Selected Writings of Joyce Fitzpatrick*. New York: Springer. ISBN 0826112277   References

Book draws together some of Dr Fitzpatrick's most significant writings on nursing research, theory, education and international health care.

2.6.15   Gadow, S. (1995a) Clinical epistemology: a dialectic of nursing assessment. *Canadian Journal of Nursing Research*, 27 (2) 25–34   12 References

Clinical assessment in nursing combines general knowledge from theory and research with particular knowledge about a client. A philosophical account of this synthesis is given to elucidate the paradox of knowledge that is both general and particular. A dialectical model is suggested which may help to solve these inconsistencies.

2.6.16   Gadow, S. (1995b) Narrative and exploration: towards a poetics of knowledge in nursing. *Nursing Inquiry*, 2 (4) 211–14 12 References

Author believes that the dualism of subject and object which has been the traditional model for nursing knowledge is inappropriate. It is suggested that narrative inquiry offers nursing an epistemology that is both ethically and aesthetically congruent with its practice of engagement (CR 2.89).

2.6.17   Geanellos, R. (1995) Storytelling: what can it reveal about the knowledge of mental health nursing? *Australian New Zealand Journal of Mental Health Nursing*, 4 (2) 87–94   34 References

Paper examines nurses' stories from the literature using a hermeneutic approach. This raises epistemological issues surrounding questions of both practical and theoretical nursing knowledge. Author believes that examining the stories, holistically and selectively, can support the knowledge claims of mental health nursing and provide opportunities for theory development or testing (CR 2.7).

2.6.18   Geanellos, R. (1997) Nursing knowledge development: where to from here? *Collegian: Journal of the Royal College of Nursing, Australia*, 4 (1) 13–21   64 References

Discusses issues related to nursing epistemology including logical positivism, empiricism and interpretative–emancipatory paradigms and how they may influence the construction of knowledge and its methods of derivation and verification. Changes in the conceptualization of science and how scientific realism may help the discipline of nursing to develop are discussed. The development of nursing knowledge, and the use of borrowed theories is considered. Author believes that nursing science should develop a dialectic between research and practice to assist the move towards meaningful nursing theories and philosophies (CR 2.8).

2.6.19 Gibbons, M., Limoges, C., Nowothny, H., Schwartman, S., Scott, P. & Trow, M. (1994) *The Production of New Knowledge: the Dynamics of Science and Research in Contemporary Societies.* London: Sage. ISBN 0803977948 References

2.6.20 Horsfall, J.M. (1995) Madness in our methods: nursing research, scientific epistemology. *Nursing Inquiry,* 2 (1) 2–9 30 References

Paper critiques some of the research methods seen in current nursing literature. Four difficulties are discussed which the author believes can be traced back to the use of scientific methodology by many researchers. These are: the absence of overt conceptual frameworks; an avoidance of complex social contexts within which research subjects live; an apparent lack of empathy and an apolitical articulation of research problems and data analyses. The problems these create for nursing are examined.

2.6.21 Ketefian, S. & Redman, R.W. (1997) Nursing science in the global community. *Image: Journal of Nursing Scholarship,* 29 (1) 11–15 27 References

Examines the development of knowledge in nursing in a global context and addresses the degree to which Western values and the social environment in the USA shape nursing theory development. Three perspectives illustrate the influence of American values and contextual factors. Questions are raised about the relevance of knowledge to other cultural or national contexts. Recommendations are made for nursing inquiry which will make knowledge more applicable to the global community.

2.6.22 Kikuchi, J.F., Simmons, H. & Romyn, D. (eds) (1996) *Truth in Nursing Inquiry.* Thousand Oaks, CA: Sage. ISBN 0761900993 References

Book depicts the epistemological problems with which nursing as a discipline is struggling, particularly the notion of truth in

nursing inquiry. The three parts cover speculative and prescriptive truth; measures of truth such as the individual, the community or tradition; and expressions of truth such as story-telling and poetics. Questions are included to assist readers in identifying and clarifying the issues and concepts being discussed.

2.6.23 Kuhn, T.S. (1970) *The Structure of Scientific Revolutions* 2nd edition. Chicago: University of Chicago Press. ISBN 0226458040 References

Author argues that science is not a gradual accumulation of knowledge, but a series of developments interrupted by 'intellectually violent revolutions'. He believes science is often influenced in apparently non-rational ways and new theories develop which may appear more complex but are not any nearer to the truth.

2.6.24 Landesman, C. (1997) *An Introduction to Epistemology.* Cambridge, MA: Blackwell Publishers Inc. ISBN 0631202137 References

Provides an introduction to the fundamental problems and issues of epistemology. No prior knowledge is assumed and the text is suitable for students. Sections cover sense awareness, appearance and reality, steps to self-knowledge, beyond basic belief, a priori knowledge and epistemology.

2.6.25 Lauzon, S. (1995) Gortner's contribution to nursing knowledge development. *Image: Journal of Nursing Scholarship,* 27 (2) 100–3 28 References

Paper is a synthesis of Gortner's views on science, nursing science and its creation. It is based on her publications and emphasizes her contributions (CR 2.8).

2.6.26 Lutz, K.F., Jones, K.D. & Kendall, J. (1997) Expanding the praxis debate: contributions to clinical inquiry. *Advances in Nursing Science,* 20 (2) 23–31 29 References

Article examines the differences in interpretative and critical approaches to clinical inquiry relative to praxis, expanding on how praxis can be used to inform nursing practice. Differences in the nature of knowledge, goals of inquiry and claims to praxis are discussed.

2.6.27 Macmillan Open Learning (1995)
London: Macmillan Magazines Ltd. References
Understanding your Nursing Knowledge
R1   Part 1   Types of knowledge
R1   Part 2   Nursing   knowledge.   ISBN
0333651995
Exploring Nursing Knowledge
R2   Part 1   Sources of knowledge
R2   Part 2   Rubbing   shoulders   with
research. ISBN 0333652002

Forms part of the Professional Practice Study
Unit series which is an open learning system
for students and practitioners. Learning
materials include work planners, information,
activities and a specific focus for further work
This unit examines the types, sources and
nature of knowledge.

2.6.28   Mullen, E.J. (1995) Pursuing knowledge through qualitative research. *Social Work Research*, 19 (1) 29–32   18 References

Discusses the differing views of qualitative
research as a coalition of interests and a
movement towards diversity of inquiry. This
movement rejects the view that practice
knowledge is derived from scientific research
and believes that it is achievable in many
ways, including some that are subjective,
interpretative and case-specific. The soundness of a profession's knowledge base is critical to its effectiveness and researchers are
urged to carefully consider the consequences
of movement towards subjectivity and pluralism in a society which increasingly applies
scientific criteria to knowledge claims (CR
2.36).

2.6.29   Parse, R.R. (1996) Building knowledge through qualitative research: the road less travelled. *Nursing Science Quarterly*, 9 (1) 10–16   65 References

Author specifies the ontological, epistemological   and   methodological   differences
among selected qualitative methods and
three extant nursing research methods. A
further distinction is made between general
and nursing knowledge. Building knowledge
requires both existing nursing theories and
frameworks (CR 2.36).

2.6.30   Parse, R.R. (1997) Transforming
research and practice with the Human
Becoming Theory. *Nursing Science Quarterly*,
10 (4) 171–4   19 References

Article focuses on the Human Becoming
Theory as a guide to the transformation of
research and practice. The research method,
knowledge from the theory, transferring practice and research related to practice are all
discussed.

2.6.31   Rafferty, A.M. (1996) *The Politics of
Nursing Knowledge*. London: Routledge.
ISBN 0415114926   References

This book, based on a doctoral thesis, identifies the pressures that have shaped nursing
education and policy-making in England and
Wales between 1860 and 1948. It also considers the role that ideas about the educability of nurses and the status of nursing have
played in the genesis of nursing knowledge.

2.6.32   Reed,   P.G. (1996) Transforming
practice knowledge into nursing knowledge –
a revisionist analysis of Peplau. *Image:
Journal of Nursing Scholarship*, 28 (1) 29–33
52 References

Author focuses on a specific strategy and
philosophical perspective, as derived from
Peplau, for integrating nursing practice more
fully into today's knowledge development.
Emphasis is on the need for nursing practice-based theory as well as nursing theory-based
practice.

2.6.33   Retsas, A. (1994) Knowledge and
practice development: towards an ontology of
nursing. *Australian Journal of Advanced
Nursing*, 12 (2) 20–5   31 References

Author believes there is a crisis in the
development of nursing knowledge and practice. The patterns and dependencies in the
way modern nursing has been constructed
have contributed to a lack of clarity about the
significance of its ontological dimensions.
Ways forward are suggested.

2.6.34   Rolfe, G. (1994) Towards a new
model   of   nursing   research. *Journal of
Advanced Nursing*, 19 (5) 969–75   18 References

Paper argues that whereas nursing research is
generally located in social science research
which seeks to develop knowledge, the aim of
research in nursing is to improve practice. An
alternative model is offered which categorizes
research according to the extent to which it is
likely to bring about change.

2.6.35 Rolfe, G. (1995) Playing at research: methodological pluralism and the creative researcher. *Journal of Psychiatric and Mental Health Nursing*, 2 (2) 105–9 16 References

Drawing on ideas from several authors writing about the philosophy of social science, the author argues that a rigid approach to methodology stifles creativity. A new and anarchistic epistemology is suggested which would enable formerly untried methods to be used and later validated.

2.6.36 Rolfe, G. (1998) *Expanding Nursing Knowledge: Understanding and Researching Your Own Practice.* Oxford: Butterworth-Heinemann. ISBN 0750630132 References

Book explores ways in which nurses and other health care practitioners can carry out personal research studies into their own practice. A new paradigm of nursing is advocated, the type of knowledge and theory needed are discussed, and suggestions made as to how this can be acquired (CR 2.13, 2.34, 2.37, 2.39).

2.6.37 Rose, P. & Parker, D. (1994) Nursing: an integration of art and science within the experience of the practitioner. *Journal of Advanced Nursing*, 20 (6) 1004–10 33 References

Paper argues that nursing is a unique discipline as its knowledge is underpinned by the philosophies of art and science. These are explored in relation to nursing (CR 2.8).

2.6.38 Sarvimäki, A. (1994) Science and tradition in the nursing discipline. *Scandinavian Journal of Caring Sciences*, 8 (3) 137–42 39 References

Article clarifies the role of practical and theoretical knowledge in nursing and develops a concept of the roles of tradition and science in the discipline of nursing (CR 2.8).

2.6.39 Schon, D.A. (1992) The crisis of professional knowledge and the pursuit of an epistemology of practice. *Journal of Interprofessional Care*, 6 (1) 49–63 16 References

A seminal paper which, although not focusing on social and health care professionals, introduces the concept of the reflective practitioner. Paper analyses the contemporary loss of confidence in professional knowledge

and argues that professional education is based on positivistic philosophy which privileges the technical, testable and the objective, separates ends from means, yet fails to train for the real problems of practice. Author suggests a model of an epistemology of practice based on reflection in and on practice.

2.6.40 Sherman, D.W. (1997) Rogerian science: opening new frontiers of nursing knowledge through its application in quantitative research. *Nursing Science Quarterly*, 10 (3) 131–5 33 References

Discusses the theoretical and methodological considerations in selecting Roger's science of unitary human beings as a framework for quantitative research. It shows how Rogerian science guided the research process in selected studies (CR 2.29).

2.6.41 Steier, F. (ed.) (1991) *Research and Reflexivity.* London: Sage. ISBN 0803982399 References

Explores the implications of reflexivity and self-reference in social science research including issues of responsibility raised for researchers. A range of theoretical issues and perspectives about the nature of knowledge and reflexive learning are discussed. Key themes are the role of language in constructing scientific and everyday knowledge and the significance of the 'multiple conversations' of reflexive research (CR 2.7).

2.6.42 Thorne, S., Kirkham, S.R. & Mac-Donald-Emes, J. (1997) Interpretive description: a non-categorical qualitative alternative for developing nursing knowledge. *Research in Nursing and Health*, 20 (2) 169–77 51 References

Authors believe that a non-categorical description, drawing on principles grounded in nursing's epistemological mandate, may be an appropriate methodological alternative for credible research towards the development of nursing knowledge. They propose a set of strategies for conceptual orientation, sampling, data construction, analysis and reporting (CR 2.22, 2.36, 2.64, 2.79, 2.97).

2.6.43 Thorne, S.E. & Hayes, V.E. (eds) (1997) *Nursing Praxis: Knowledge and Action.* London: Sage. ISBN 076190011X References

As nursing theory and knowledge evolve,

relationships between ideas and actions become blurred. Contributors to this book present some of the ways in which nursing scholars are confronting this problem by reflecting on the nature of nursing knowledge and the application of theory in practice.

2.6.44   Wainwright, S.P. (1997) A new paradigm for nursing: the potential of realism. *Journal of Advanced Nursing*, 26 (6) 1262–71 120 References

Paper argues that both positivism and constructivism are seriously flawed as philosophies of social and natural science. Author proposes the use of realism which is a philosophy of both to unify biopsychosocial nursing.

2.6.45   White, J. (1995) Patterns of knowing: review, critique, and update. *Advances in Nursing Science*, 17 (4) 73–86   40 References

Article explores the degree to which Carper's patterns of knowing represent nursing knowledge in the 1990s. The addition of socio-political knowing is suggested. Modifications are suggested to ideas put forward by Jacobs-Kramer and Chinn for exploring processes of inquiry into nursing knowledge and practice.

2.7   DEVELOPMENT OF THEORY

The nature of nursing as a science and an art requires a strong theoretical basis which needs translating into practice. Nurse researchers are now developing this base which will inform all subsequent studies.

Definitions

Facet theory – a meta-theoretical approach to scientific research
Taxonomy – the science, laws or principles of classification
Theoretical frameworks – a set of integrated hypotheses designed to explain particular classes of events
Theoretical substruction – a powerful tool for conceptualizing and assessing congruence between the theoretical and operational components of research

Theory – a set of statements that tentatively describes, explains or predicts relationships between concepts that have been systematically selected and organized as an abstract representation of some phenomena

Annotations

2.7.1   Algase, D.L. & Whall, A.F. (1993) Rosemary Ellis's view on the substantive structure of nursing. *Image: Journal of Nursing Scholarship*, 25 (10) 69–72 26 References

Drawing largely from work of the late Rosemary Ellis, this paper summarizes her views on the substantive structural nature of nursing which raises implications for the development of nursing theory.

2.7.2   Blegen, M.A. & Tripp-Reimer, T. (1997) Implications of nursing taxonomies for middle-range theory development. *Advances in Nursing Science*, 19 (3) 37–49   34 References

Article suggests using concepts in the newly developing taxonomies of nursing knowledge as building blocks. These are nursing diagnoses, interventions and outcomes (CR 2.6).

2.7.3   Chinn, P.L. & Kramer, M.K. (1995) *Theory and Nursing: a Systematic Approach* 4th edition. St Louis: Mosby. ISBN 0801679478   References

Book examines the relationships between theory and nursing and discusses ways in which nursing research studies can be theoretically sound.

2.7.4   Clarke, H.F. (1996) Theory testing and theory building: research in nursing, in Kerr, J.C. & MacPhail, J. (eds), *Canadian Nursing: Issues and Perspectives* 3rd edition. St Louis: Mosby. ISBN 0815152256 Chapter 9, 105–17 26 References

Explores research issues involved in theory development including its generation and testing.

2.7.5   Denzin, N.K. (1989) *The Research Act: a Theoretical Introduction to Sociological Methods* 3rd edition. Englewood Cliffs, NJ: Prentice-Hall.   ISBN   0137743815   References

Book offers an interpretative, symbolic interactionist view of sociological theory and research methodology. With roots in hermeneutics, critical theory, feminist theory, pragmatism and symbolic interactionism, the self-reflective political nature of everyday and scientific conduct is stressed. This new edition aims to shed light on old issues and assists in bringing theory and method in research activities together again (CR 2.17, 2.26, 2.29, 2.52, 2.68, 2.71, 2.72).

2.7.6 Donald, I. (1995) Facet theory: defining research domains, in Breakwell, G.M., Hammond, S. & Fife-Schaw, C. (eds), *Research Methods in Psychology*. London: Sage. ISBN 0803977654 Part II, Chapter 9, 116–37

Chapter discusses the components of domain definition and mapping sentences (CR 2.1.8).

2.7.7 Dudley-Brown, S.L. (1997) The evaluation of nursing theory: a method for our madness. *International Journal of Nursing Studies*, 34 (1) 76–83   21 References

Paper attempts to define theory, including nursing theory, and then analyses criteria for its evaluation. A more comprehensive set of criteria is proposed which may stimulate more informed decision-making regarding the choice of nursing theory for use in practice, education and research, and from which new ones may emerge.

2.7.8 Estabrooks, C.A., Field, P.A. & Morse, J.M. (1994) Aggregating qualitative findings: an approach to theory development. *Qualitative Health Research*, 4 (4) 503–11   18 References

Authors suggest that the findings of independent, similar research articles may be aggregated into a cohesive study. This increases the generalizability of the original studies and produces a relatively solid mid-range theory. The criteria for selecting studies, possible problems and potential areas for application are discussed (CR 2.28, 2.36).

2.7.9 Fawcett, J. & Downs, F.S. (1992) *The Relationship of Theory and Research* 2nd edition. Philadelphia: FA Davis. ISBN 0803634153   References

Book fills a major gap in the literature and presents a detailed discussion of the relationship between theory and research. Emphasis

is placed on information needed by novices and scholars for analysing and evaluating research reports and proposals for new studies. This edition has been extensively revised and new examples included. Appendices contain analyses and evaluation of descriptive, correlational and experimental studies. Chapter 15 contains a comprehensive bibliography related to nursing theory and theorizing in nursing (CR 2.29, 2.36, 2.40, 2.95, 2.96, 2.99).

2.7.10 Gigliotti, E. (1997) Use of Neuman's Lines of Defence and Resistance in nursing research: conceptual and empirical considerations. *Nursing Science Quarterly*, 10 (3) 136–43   26 References

Operationalization of the Neuman system model concepts, the flexible lines of defence and resistance are explored. Conceptual and empirical concerns imposed on the researcher when employing the model are discussed.

2.7.11 Gilbert, N. (ed.) (1993) Research, theory and method, in Author, *Researching Social Life*. London: Sage. ISBN 0803986823 Chapter 2, 18   31 References

Chapter looks at what counts as good social research and how the various methods described in this book fit into the research process (CR 2.1.25, 2.14).

2.7.12 Heslop, L. (1997) The (im)possibilities of post-structuralist and critical social nursing inquiry. *Nursing Inquiry*, 4 (1) 48–56   59 References

Paper discusses the differences between and within poststructural and critical social theory and their relevance to nursing research. A reflexive approach to discourse analysis provides insight into some of the methodological challenges arising in each methodology.

2.7.13 Jaarsma, T. & Dassen, T. (1993) The relationship of nursing theory and research: the state of the art. *Journal of Advanced Nursing*, 18 (5) 783–7   20 References

Study analysed the role of theory in nursing practice research by examining papers published in six journals between 1986 and 1990. The use of nursing theories showed a slight increase when compared with earlier analyses but testing of theories is minimal (CR 3.6).

2.7.14 Levine, M.E. (1995) The rhetoric of nursing theory. *Image: Journal of Nursing Scholarship*, 27 (1) 11–14   22 References

Author believes that theory is the intellectual life of nursing and in order to further research and gain insights into the discipline, theorizing must be encouraged. The language of theorizing, antecedents of nursing theory and scholarship related to it are all discussed (CR 2.2).

2.7.15 Lindeman, C.A. & McAthie, M. (eds) (1990) *Nursing Trends and Issues.* Springhouse, PA: Springhouse Corporation. ISBN 0874342325 Unit 2 Discipline issues, nursing research: theory and practice. 146–200   References

Chapters explore the relationship between theory, research and practice, evaluating research and the role of the clinician in the development and use of knowledge. Study questions and assignments are included (CR 2.95, 2.101, 2.102).

2.7.16 McQuiston, C.M. & Campbell, J.C. (1997) Theoretical substruction: a guide for theory testing research. *Nursing Science Quarterly*, 10 (3) 117–23   19 References

Article guides readers through the process of substruction for theory testing nursing research, beginning at the proposal stage and continuing through analysis and results. An example is given for illustration.

2.7.17 Meleis, A.I. (1997) *Theoretical Nursing: Development and Progress* 3rd edition. Philadelphia: Lippincott. ISBN 0397552599   References

A comprehensive text which explores, discusses, analyses, critiques, compares and contrasts different epistemologies, theories of truth and nursing theories. Although the focus is on nursing theories, it is emphasized that nursing is based on philosophy, theory, practice and research. The theory-research/theory-strategy is explained, abstracts of theoretical writing in nursing are given and there is an extensive bibliography on theory and meta-theory (CR 2.5, 2.6).

2.7.18 Moody, L.E. (1990) *Advancing Nursing Science through Research.* Newbury Park, CA: Sage. ISBN Volume 1 080393811X; Volume 2 0803938128

Two volumes intended for graduates and doctoral students which cover major advances in theory and research. Many examples are given together with questions for further study. Volume 2 discusses statistical approaches to theory-building and applications are described. Clinical trials, meta-analyses, causal modelling and time-series approaches are discussed. Non-statistical approaches include case studies, foundational, hermeneutical and sociolinguistic inquiry (CR 2.20, 2.29, 2.39, 2.92).

2.7.19 Morse, J..M. (1995) Exploring the theoretical basis of nursing using advanced techniques of concept analysis. *Advances in Nursing Science*, 17 (3) 31–46   45 References

Author critiques the traditional methods of concept analysis and presents alternative methods which use qualitative methods of inquiry. Concept delineation, comparison, clarification, correction and identification are explored and described. To illustrate the application of concept development methods to nursing theory, a research programme to delineate the construct of comfort is described.

2.7.20 Morse, J.M. (1996) Nursing scholarship: sense and sensibility. *Nursing Inquiry*, 3 (2) 74–82   47 References

Paper explores the relationship between nursing theory, research and practice. The difficulties in operationalizing, testing and implementing nursing theories perhaps shows their lack of suitability for clinical practice. Author urges that research which supports the exploration and identification of nursing concepts and the development of theory will guide both research and practice.

2.7.21 Mouzelis, N. (1995) *Sociological Theory: What Went Wrong?* London: Routledge. ISBN 0415076943   References

Book analyses the central problems of sociological theory today and suggests ways in which they may be resolved.

2.7.22 Murphy, E. & Freston, M.S. (1991) An analysis of theory–research linkages in published gerontologic nursing studies. *Advances in Nursing Science*, 13 (4) 1–13 26 References

Authors examined 142 gerontological studies

using the Theory–Research Linkage Inventory to assess the extent to which theory and research were interrelated. Forty-six per cent were related in varying degrees to a specific theory or model. Strengths and limitations were identified for various stages of the studies. Factors influencing the linkages were examined and recommendations made for the development of nursing science in gerontology.

2.7.23 Newman, M.A. (1994) Theory for nursing practice. *Nursing Science Quarterly*, 7 (4) 153–7   26 References

Describes the development of nursing theory and research over the past 30 years. After many early difficulties, the author believes that the focus and paradigm of the discipline are now clear with the core purpose and societal commitment of nursing as a practice discipline being captured in the phrase, 'caring in the human health experience'. Appropriate research methods make it possible to develop theory that structures practice.

2.7.24 Nolan, M. & Behi, R. (1995) Induction: moving from the specific to the general. *British Journal of Nursing*, 4 (5) 279–82. 15 References

Article discusses theory-building, together with the processes of induction and deduction. Use of the Meleis model is explored (CR 2.36).

2.7.25 Norris, A. (complier) (1996) *Nursing Research Theory*. Winchester, MA: Book Tech Inc. ISBN 1577900138

2.7.26 Poggenpoel, M. (1996) Psychiatric nursing research based on nursing for the whole person theory. *Curationis: South African Journal of Nursing*, 19 (3) 60–2 6 References

Author believes that the whole person theory has a set of meta-theoretical, theoretical and methodological assumptions which can provide direction to psychiatric nurses undertaking research. The application of this theory is demonstrated by using a completed study as an example.

2.7.27 Sandelowski, M. (1993) Theory unmasked: the uses and guises of theory in qualitative research. *Research in Nursing and Health*, 16 (3) 213–18   26 References

The uses and manifestations of theory at the substantive and paradigmatic levels of research, and as they pertain to different qualitative approaches, are described. Consideration is given to the various sources, centrality, temporal placement and functions of theory in qualitative research (CR 2.36).

2.7.28 Walker, L.O. & Avant, K.C. (1995) *Strategies for Theory Construction in Nursing* 3rd edition. Stamford, CT: Appleton & Lange. ISBN 0838586880   References

Aims to provide a developmental approach to theory. A general overview of the state of the art is given, followed by concept, statement and theory development using three approaches: analysis, synthesis and derivation. The nature of theory in nursing is discussed together with its relevance to practice (CR 3.6).

2.7.29 Ward, R. (1993) The search for meanings in nursing: could Facet Theory be a way forward? *Journal of Advanced Nursing*, 18 (4) 549–57   27 References

Paper explains the use of Facet Theory as a systematic method for the examination of embodied knowledge which will enable research to develop insights into practice (CR 2.5, 2.64).

2.8 SCIENCE AND THE SCIENTIFIC METHOD

The major components of the scientific method are asking questions, defining problems, obtaining and interpreting data and drawing conclusions. These allow researchers to complete work according to a set of rules so that a series of workable ideas is generated. Over time, better ideas and theories emerge, which is the ultimate goal of science.

Definitions

Applied science – that which is orientated towards the solution of practical problems
Basic science – study of phenomena from a purely epistemological viewpoint, regardless of any practical applications the findings might happen to have

Deductive reasoning – the process of developing specific predictions from general principles

Inductive reasoning – the process of reasoning from specific observations to more general rules

Objectivity – . . . the extent to which two independent researchers would arrive at similar judgements or conclusions (i.e. judgements not biased by personal values or beliefs)

Science – an activity that combines research (the advancement of knowledge) and theory (explanation for knowledge)

Scientific method – a way of pursuing knowledge that presumes a logical, observational and cautious approach

---

Annotations

2.8.1   Behi, R. & Nolan, M. (1995) Deduction: moving from the general to the specific. *British Journal of Nursing*, 4 (6) 341–4 12 References

Article considers the issue of theory-testing, using the hypothetico-deductive model. The nature and purpose of hypotheses are explored and the varying types described (CR 2.20).

2.8.2   Chalmers, A.F. (1995) *What is this Thing called Science: an Assessment of the Nature and Status of Science and its Methods* 3rd edition. Indianapolis, IN: Hackett Publishing Co. Inc. ISBN 0872201996   References

Provides an introduction to the new philosophy of science. The shortcomings of the empiricist accounts of science are explored and modern writings which replace these are discussed.

2.8.3   Chitty, K.K. (ed.) (1997) The scientific method, in Author, *Professional Nursing: Concepts and Challenges*. Philadelphia: W.B. Saunders. ISBN 0721668836   References

Chapter differentiates between pure and applied science, describes development of the scientific method, gives examples of inductive and deductive reasoning, explains its steps and highlights its limitations.

2.8.4   Closs, J. (1994) What's so awful about science? *Nurse Researcher*, 2 (2) 69–83 11 References

Author believes that the art-versus-science debate should be buried and discusses the concept of 'complexity', which she believes holds great promise for future nursing research.

2.8.5   Couvalis, G. (1997) *The Philosophy of Science: Science and Objectivity*. London: Sage. ISBN 0761951016   References

Textbook provides a clear, non-technical guide to the philosophy of science. The works of key thinkers and debates which define the field are all discussed (CR 2.5).

2.8.6   Fitzpatrick, J. & Martinson, I. (eds) (1996) *Selected Writings of Rosemary Ellis: In Search of Meaning of Nursing Science*. New York: Springer. ISBN 0826194001   References

Book is a collection of many previously unpublished writings, as well as several classic publications of Rosemary Ellis. She tries to get to the very essence of nursing science, and to lay the philosophical groundwork for the development of theory and research to improve nursing practice (CR 2.5, 2.7, 3.17).

2.8.7   Frederickson, K. (1992) Research methodology and nursing science. *Nursing Science Quarterly*, 5 (4) 150–1   8 References

Author states that most nursing research which purports to add to the science of nursing utilizes theories or conceptual models from other disciplines. Nursing scholars are challenged to develop new methodologies consistent with extant theories and frameworks.

2.8.8   Hinshaw, A.S. (1990) National Centre for Nursing Research: a commitment to excellence in nursing, in McCloskey, J.C. & Garce, H.K. (eds), *Current Issues in Nursing* 3rd edition. St Louis: Mosby. ISBN 0801655250 Chapter 49, 357–62   17 References

Chapter discusses the characteristics of 'good' science and strategies for promoting excellence. A brief history is given of the National Centre for Nursing Research (CR 3.5, 3.10, 3.14).

2.8.9   Lerheim, K. (1991) Nursing science – does it make a difference? *International Nursing Review*, 38 (3) 73–8   18 References

Describes a study which focused on the relationship between nursing science and nursing service in a service perspective, and the impact each had upon the other.

2.8.10 Nolan, M. & Behi, R. (1995) Induction: moving from the specific to the general. *British Journal of Nursing,* 4 (5) 279–82 15 References

The scientific method comprises two main processes: deduction (theory-testing) and induction (theory-building). The main emphasis in this article is on theory-building, using the Meleis model to illustrate some of the steps and stages involved.

2.8.11 Omery, A., Kasper, C.E. & Page, G.G. (eds) (1995) *In Search of Nursing Science.* Thousand Oaks, CA: Sage. ISBN 0803950942 References

Book analyses the major schools of thought in contemporary Western science in order to arrive at a philosophy (or philosophies) of science consistent with the discipline of nursing. The traditional views of science are examined and the contributors then focus on schools which challenge them, for example feminism, phenomenology, critical theory and poststructuralism. Each discussion is followed by an exploration of how particular tenets of the school have influenced the development of nursing knowledge and nursing science (CR 2.5, 2.6, 2.10, 2.49).

2.8.12 Packard, S.A. & Polifroni, E.C. (1991) The dilemma of nursing science: current quandaries and lack of direction. *Nursing Science Quarterly,* 4 (1) 7–13 22 References

Paper examines factors which influence the conception of nursing as emerging, the notion of applied science, the debate over methodologies and the social policy statement.

2.9 QUANTITATIVE AND QUALITATIVE RESEARCH METHODS

'The roots of the qualitative and quantitative quandary can be traced to two opposed Greek philosophical visions of human science

that emphasize number (Pythagoras) and meaning (Socrates) as the essence of mind, and we may yet have something to learn about improving qualitative validity from the idiographic question-and-answer method of studying meaning systems by Socrates.' (Wakefield, 1995: 9)

Definitions

Qualitative research – this is usually inductively derived and seeks to name and describe categories into which observations belong, e.g. grounded theory or ethnomethodology
Quantitative research – this mode of research is often deductively derived and seeks to confirm the construct validity and internal structure of a research instrument designed to measure a particular concept

---

Annotations

2.9.1 Allen-Meares, P. (1995) Applications of qualitative research: let the work begin. *Social Work Research,* 19 (1) 5–7   13 References

Article reviews the methodological debate between qualitative and quantitative research and concludes that they should be integrated to further the exploration and application of social work issues (CR 2.29, 2.36).

2.9.2 Avis, M. & Robinson, J. (1996) Continuing dilemma in health care research. *NT Research,* 1 (1) 9–11 9 References Editorial

Authors discuss the conflicting arguments relating to quantitative and qualitative research. They suggest that health care professionals could develop an approach that considers the credibility of particular research evidence and its application to specific problems.

2.9.3 Baum, F. (1995) Researching public health: behind the qualitative–quantitative methodological debate. *Social Science and Medicine,* 40 (4) 459–68   67 References

Paper argues that issues underlying the use of both quantitative and qualitative methods are crucial to current debates about public health research, but they are simply tools to further knowledge and have no inherent status in themselves. Because public health issues are complex, a range of methods needs to be chosen (CR 2.14, 2.29, 2.36).

2.9.4 Bryman, A. (1992) *Quantity and Quality in Social Research*. London: Routledge. ISBN 0415078989   References

This book, which is intended for graduates and undergraduates, focuses on the debate about quantitative and qualitative research together with the nature and relative virtues of each perspective. Underlying philosophical positions are also discussed and research from a wide range of social issues is used for illustrative purposes (CR 2.13, 2.27, 2.28).

2.9.5 Carr, L.T. (1994) The strengths and weaknesses of quantitative and qualitative research: what method for nursing? *Journal of Advanced Nursing*, 20 (4) 716–21 38 References

Paper explores the controversy over the methods by which truth is obtained, and examines the similarities and differences between quantitative and qualitative research. Author believes that if nursing scholars limit themselves to one method of inquiry, restrictions will be placed on the development of nursing knowledge (CR 2.6, 2.29, 2.36).

2.9.6 Clarke, L. (1995) Nursing research: science, visions and telling stories. *Journal of Advanced Nursing*, 21 (3) 584–93   87 References

Examines aspects of quantitative and qualitative research in nursing. A critical assessment is made of qualitative approaches and their lack of generalizability. Grounded theory, reliability and validity are also explored (CR 2.24, 2.25, 2.28, 2.42).

2.9.7 Dzurec, L.C. & Abraham, I.L. (1993) The nature of inquiry: linking quantitative and qualitative research. *Advances in Nursing Science*, 16 (1) 73–9   30 References

Article proposes that inquiry, regardless of the chosen paradigm or method, is governed by six pursuits that integrate quantitative and qualitative research methods. These are: the pursuit of mastery over self and the world; understanding through recomposition; complexity reduction to enhance understanding;

innovation; meaningfulness; and truthfulness. Authors believe that distinctions serve little purpose and perhaps limit nursing knowledge (CR 2.6, 2.29, 2.36).

2.9.8 Ellis, L.B. (1996) Evaluating the effects of continuing nurse education on practice: researching for impact. *NT Research*, 1 (4) 296–306   46 References

Paper considers a shift from qualitative research designs in studying the effects of education on practice, to a small number which have adopted the classical experimental approach. This is discussed from both a epistemological and methodological viewpoint. Author believes that a quantitative approach can add other dimensions to the study of this area (CR 2.6, 2.29, 2.36).

2.9.9 Garcia, J.C. & Martinez, M.R. (1996) The debate on qualitative versus quantitative investigation [Spanish]. *Enfermería clínica*, 6 (5) 212–17   34 References

Covers the debate on using either or both qualitative and quantitative methodologies when studying aspects of nursing care. A synthesis of both is suggested where appropriate.

2.9.10 Hammick, M. (1995) Qualitative and quantitative research: adjuvants and alternates. *British Journal of Therapy and Rehabilitation*, 29 (7) 341–2 Editorial

Discusses quantitative and qualitative research in the context of the therapy professions and how these techniques may be used (CR 2.29, 2.36).

2.9.11 Harré, R. (1981) The positivist-empiricist approach and its alternative, in Reason, P. & Rowan J. (eds), *Human Inquiry: a Sourcebook of New Paradigm Research*. Chichester: Wiley. ISBN 0471279358 Chapter 1, 3–17   References

Author discusses the meaning and problems related to the posivitist-empiricist approach to research and suggests an alternative which acknowledges the humanity and contribution of those being used as research subjects (CR 2.11.9).

2.9.12 Krantz, D.L. (1995) Sustaining versus resolving the quantitative–qualitative debate. *Evaluation and Programme Planning*, 18 (1) 89–96   References

Article discusses the factors involved in the ongoing quantitative–qualitative debate in evaluation research (CR 2.43).

2.9.13 MacNair, R.H. (1996) A research methodology for community practice. *Journal of Community Practice*, 3 (2) 1–19   51 References

Article reviews the history of research methods in community practice organizations over the last three decades. A systematic description and analysis of nine specific methods, including their purpose, stage of knowledge development and feasibility, is provided (CR 2.6, 2.14, 2.46, 2.86, 2.87).

2.9.14 Milburn, K., Frascr, E., Secker, J. & Pavis, S. (1995) Combining methods in health promotion research: some considerations about appropriate use. *Health Education Journal*, 54 (3) 347–56   22 References

Critically assesses the use of combined methods in health promotion research, and invites reflection on the assumption that combining quantitative and qualitative approaches will produce the most valid and reliable results (CR 2.29, 2.36).

2.9.15 Newman, I. & Benz, C.R. (1998) *Qualitative–Quantitative Research Methodology: Exploring the Interactive.* Carbondale, IL: Southern Illinois University Press. ISBN 0809321505

2.9.16 Reichardt, C.S. & Rallis, S.F. (1994) *The Qualitative–Quantitative Debate.* San Francisco, CA: Jossey-Bass. ISBN 0787999679   Refcrences

2.9.17 Salmon, P. (1994) Research: a Kellyan perspective. *Changes*, 12 (3) 199–205   3 References

Discusses the contribution of George Kelly to research and examines the quantitative and qualitative debate in psychological research (CR 2.77).

2.9.18 Scheurich, J.J. (1997) *Research Method in the Postmodern.* London: Falmer Press. ISBN 0750706457   References

Provides a comprehensive introduction to research methods in the postmodern. The book shows how it can be used to critique a wide range of approaches to research. It describes and discusses the implications of

postmodernism for practice, going beyond the philosophical level.

2.9.19 Schultz, P.R. (1992) Attending to many voices: beyond the qualitative/quantitative dialectic, in *Communicating Nursing Research. Silver Threads – 25 Years of Nursing Excellence.* Volume 25 Boulder, CO: Western Institute of Nursing. No ISBN 73–83   23 References

Documents the development of the qualitative/quantitative debate from 1968 to 1991. The author believes that we need to move beyond this debate and suggests some methods, together with an epistemology (CR 2.6).

2.9.20 Shadish, W.R. (1995) Philosophy of science and the quantitative–qualitative debate: thirteen common errors. *Evaluation and Program Planning*, 18 (1) 63–75   References

Discusses 13 common errors about the philosophy of science in evaluation research and its consequences for the debate (CR 2.5, 2.8, 2.43).

2.9.21 Tullver, F., Bass, M.J., Dunn, E.V., Norton, P.G. & Stewart, M. (eds) (1992) *Assessing Interventions: Traditional and Innovative Methods.* Newbury Park, CA: Sage. ISBN 0803947704   References

Quantitative and qualitative methods in assessing interventions in primary care are explored (CR 2.29, 2.36).

2.9.22 Wakefield, J.C. (1995) When an irresistible epistemology meets an immovable ontology. *Social Work Research*, 19 (1) 9–17   15 References

Discusses the problems and advantages of both quantitative and qualitative research methods and reports that no solution has yet been found which will enable social work researchers to move forward in their search for knowledge (CR 2.5, 2.6, 2.29, 2.36).

2.9.23 Warner, S. (1996) The drive towards numbers for credible research in clinical psychology. *Changes: An International Journal of Psychology and Psychotherapy*, 14 (3) 187–91   12 References

Discusses the role of qualitative and quantitative research methods in clinical psychology (CR 2.29, 2.36).

2.10   FEMINIST RESEARCH

'Not only do men and women view a common world from different perspectives, they view different worlds as well.' (Bernard, 1973: 782)

Feminist research is multi-disciplinary in nature and is in the process of defining, gathering and making knowledge. It is rigorous because gender is taken into consideration and the experiences of women are deemed to be as important as those of men. As such, it has much to offer the predominantly female nursing profession.

Definition

Feminist research – involves an epistemological stance . . . that gives direction to the diversity of evolving research practices in the field. The goal is to entertain a critical dialogue that focuses on women's experiences in historical, cultural and socio-economic perspectives

Example

Reinharz, S. (1993) Neglected voices and excessive demands in feminist research. *Qualitative Sociology*, 16 (1) 69–76   References

Reports the analysis of a large set of examples of feminist research which aimed to answer the question: is there a distinctive feminist research method?

Annotations

2.10.1   Allan, H. (1997) Reflexivity: a comment on feminist ethnography. *NT Research*, 2 (6) 455–67   54 References

Paper comments on feminist research and the use of reflexivity in feminist ethnography. Using a specific study for illustration, the methodology of feminist approaches is questioned (CR 2.42).

2.10.2   Bungay, V. & Keddy, B.C. (1996) Pearls, pith and provocation. Experiential analysis as a feminist methodology for health professionals. *Qualitative Health Research*, 6 (3) 442–52   29 References

Authors discuss experiential analysis as a feminist methodology and the opportunity it provides in thinking about how knowledge is created, the power associated with it and how it can be deconstructed.

2.10.3   Campbell, R. (1995) Weaving a new tapestry of research: a bibliography of selected readings on feminist research methods. *Women's Studies International Forum*, 18 (2) 215–22   References

Provides material on various aspects of feminist research methods.

2.10.4   Cardwell, M.M. (1993) Family nursing research: a feminist critique, in Feetham, S.L., Meister, S.B., Bell, J.M. & Gilliss, C.L. (eds), *The Nursing of Families: Theory/Research/Education/Practice*. Newbury Park, CA: Sage. ISBN 080394716X Part VI, Chapter 21, 200–10   References

Chapter presents an overview of feminist critique of research, analyses some current family nursing research studies and discusses the issues raised.

2.10.5   Carryer, J. (1995) Feminist research: strengths and challenges. *Contemporary Nurse: A Journal for the Australian Nursing Profession*, 4 (4) 180–6   19 References

Discusses some methodological issues encountered when studying the experience of large body size for nine New Zealand women, medically deemed to be obese. The applicability of feminist research, its objectivity and the researcher's role are discussed.

2.10.6   Draper, J. (1997) Potential and problems: the value of feminist approaches. *British Journal of Midwifery*, 5 (10) 597–600 21 References

Article explores the meaning of feminist research, describes its distinguishing characteristics and examines its potential and associated problems.

2.10.7   Easterday, L., Papademas, D., Schorr, L. & Valentine, C. (1982) The making of a female researcher: role problems in field work, in Burgess, R.G. (ed.), *Field Research: a Sourcebook and Field Manual*. London: Allen & Unwin. ISBN 004312013X Chapter 9, 62-7   References

Specific problems of being a female field researcher are related to general methodological issues. Suggestions are made as to how they may be overcome (CR 2.16).

2.10.8   Eichler, M. (1988) *Non-sexist*

Research Methods: a Practical Guide. Boston: Allen & Unwin. ISBN 0044970455 References

Book, written for students in many disciplines, provides a systematic approach to identifying, eliminating and preventing sexist bias in social science research. Each chapter is illustrated from recent literature. A non-sexist research checklist, which may be used when evaluating or carrying out research, is included.

2.10.9 Fahy, K. (1997) Postmodern feminist emancipatory research: is it an oxymoron? *Nursing Inquiry*, 4 (1) 27–33   37 References

Presents arguments to help emancipator researchers defend their practices, both in relation to research participants and in the ways the subject is theorized. Postmodernism can be compatible with politically motivated, humanistically based inquiry.

2.10.10 Fine, M. (1992) *Disruptive Voices: the Possibilities of Feminist Research.* Ann Arbor, MI: University of Michigan Press. ISBN 0472094653

A collection of previously published articles which reflect the methods used and developed in feminist research.

2.10.11 Gelsthorpe, L. (1992) Response to Martyn Hammersley's paper 'On feminist methods'. *Sociology*, 26 (2) 213–18   19 References

Author responds to points made in Hammersley's article and believes he demolished a case that never was (CR 2.10.15).

2.10.12 Ginzberg, R. (1995) Feminism, science and nursing, in Omery, A., Kasper, C.E. & Page, G.G. (eds), *In Search of Nursing Science.* Thousand Oaks, CA: Sage. ISBN 0803950942 Chapter 8, 93–105   3 References

Chapter asks questions relating to the nature and scope of science and feminism and how they relate to nursing (CR 2.8.11).

2.10.13 Gould, A. (1995) A feminist perspective on the researcher–researched relationship. *British Journal of Therapy and Rehabilitation*, 2 (2) 93–7   21 References

Article demonstrates the value of a feminist approach to the relationship between researchers and the researched in facilitating

the validity of the subjective experience (CR 2.25).

2.10.14 Hall, J.M. & Stevens, P.E. (1991) Rigor in feminist research. *Advances in Nursing Science*, 13 (3) 16-29   80 References

Authors analyse the meaning of scientific adequacy in feminist research and propose standards by which nurse researchers can plan and evaluate their studies. Conventional criteria of reliability and validity are critiqued and those appropriate for feminist research are presented (CR 2.24, 2.25).

2.10.15 Hammersley, M. (1992) On feminist methodology. *Sociology*, 26 (2) 187–206   66 References

Article summarizes the features of feminist methodology: the ubiquitous social significance of gender, the validity of experience as against method, the rejection of hierarchy in the research relationship, and the adoption of the emancipation of women as the goal of research. Author concludes that while some of these arguments are convincing, the overall case for feminist methodology is not (CR 2.10.11).

2.10.16 Harding, S. (ed.) (1987) *Feminism and Methodology: Social Science Issues.* Milton Keynes: Open University Press. ISBN 033515560X   References

A collection of essays which provides an introduction to the crucial methodological and epistemological issues that feminist inquiry raises for scholars in all fields (CR 2.6).

2.10.17 Hedin, B.A. & Duffy, M.E. (1991) Researching: designing research from a feminist perspective, in Neil, R.M. & Watts, R. (eds), *Caring and Nursing: Explorations in Feminist Perspectives.* New York: National League for Nursing. ISBN 0887375014 Publication number 14–2369 Chapter 19, 227–35   16 References

Chapter examines what it means to design research studies with a feminist perspective. A reconceptualization of the research process is used with six phases: being, thinking, designing, encountering, making sense and communicating.

2.10.18 Henderson, D.J. (1995) Consciousness raising in participatory research: method and methodology for emancipatory nursing inquiry. *Advances in Nursing Science*, 17 (3) 58–69   43 References

Article presents participatory research as a methodology and consciousness raising as a method for nursing research that addresses the emancipatory goals of feminist and critical theories.

2.10.19 King, K.E. (1994) Method and methodology in feminist research: what is the difference? *Journal of Advanced Nursing*, 20 (1) 19–22   19 References

Paper explores the concepts of method and methodology and explains their interrelationship. Author believes that it is essential to differentiate between them before embarking on feminist research.

2.10.20 Maynard, M. (1999) *Feminist Social Research: Pragmatics, Politics and Power*. London: Taylor & Francis. ISBN 1857283090 References.

Book is a guide to feminist social research which combines an overview of the conflicts, tensions and lessons to be learned from feminist debates. A critical analysis of current practices is made and possible pitfalls highlighted. [from www.heffers.co.uk]

2.10.21 Maynard, M. & Purvis, J. (eds) (1994) *Researching Women's Lives from a Feminist Perspective*. London: Taylor & Francis. ISBN 0748401520

2.10.22 Millen, D. (1997) Some methodological and epistemological issues raised by doing feminist research on non-feminist women. *Sociological Research Online*, 2 (3). URL:<http://www.socresonline.org.uk/socres on line/2/3/3.html>

Two key concepts within feminist research – empowerment of women and the equality of the research relationship are examined in light of research conducted on a population of women unsympathetic to feminism and constructions of gender. Author suggests that while there is a need to conduct gender-sensitive work, a too rigid definition may lead to problems. A more appropriate strategy may be to site the conflict in epistemology, rather than methodology, and define feminist research in terms of values which it might uphold rather than techniques it may use (CR 2.6).

2.10.23 Miller, C. & Treitel, C. (eds) (1991) *Feminist Research Methods: an Annotated Bibliography*. Westport, CT: Greenwood Press. ISBN 031326029X

A compilation of English-language sources which help to answer the question 'what makes a research project feminist?'. Each item addresses some aspect of feminist research, including both general and specific literature. [from www.heffers.co.uk]

2.10.24 Nielson, J.McC. (ed.) (1990) *Feminist Research Methods: Exemplary Readings in the Social Sciences*. Boulder, CO: Westview Press. ISBN 0813305772   References

Book offers a practical guide to conducting research informed by feminist methods.

2.10.25 Perry, P.A. (1994) Feminist empiricism as a method for inquiry in nursing. *Western Journal of Nursing Research*, 16 (5) 480–94   55 References

Author believes that feminist empiricism may provide a valuable approach for the acquisition, evaluation and integration of biological knowledge in nursing epistemologies. Hypertension in women is used to illustrate how feminist empiricism could be used to modify the traditional scientific approach (CR 2.6).

2.10.26 Ramazanoglu, C. (1992) On feminist methodology: male reason versus female empowerment. *Sociology*, 26 (2) 207–12   14 References

Author acknowledges that Hammersley's criticism is useful in adding to the debate on problems of validity in feminist research, but believes the particular position adopted will stifle further discussion and disempower women (CR 2.10.15, 2.25).

2.10.27 Reinharz, S. (1993) *Social Research Methods: Feminist Perspectives*. New York: Oxford University Press. ISBN 008032794X References

Book reports a survey of experimental methodology undertaken by feminist researchers. This explains the relationship between feminism and methodology and challenges stereotypes about feminist research methods. A bibliography of 20 years of feminist scholarship is also included.

2.10.28 Ribbens, J. & Edwards, R. (eds) (1997) *Feminist Dilemmas in Qualitative Research*. London: Sage. ISBN 0761956646 References

Book explores the key dilemma of producing work relevant to theoretical and formal traditions and the requirements of academic knowledge while remaining faithful to the participants' experiences. The interplay between theory, epistemology and the detailed practice of research are all discussed (CR 2.6, 2.7, 2.36).

2.10.29 Ristock, J.L. & Pennell, J. (1997) *Research as Empowerment: Feminist Links, Postmodern Interruptions*. Don Mills, Ontario: Oxford University Press. ISBN 0195410807 References

Volume suggests ways of carrying out research for social action in order that power is both critically analysed and responsibly used at all stages of the research. Examples of research methods used by the author in various feminist situations are included (CR 2.2).

2.10.30 Roberts, H. (ed.) (1990) *Doing Feminist Research* 2nd edition. London: Routledge. ISBN 0415025478 References

Volume presents accounts of research where practical, methodological, theoretical and ethical issues are raised where the sociologist adopts or is aware of a feminist perspective.

2.10.31 Sigsworth, J. (1995) Feminist research: its relevance to nursing. *Journal of Advanced Nursing*, 22 (5) 896–9 18 References

Explores feminist research and its relevance to nursing practice.

2.10.32 Sollie, D.L. & Leslie, L.A. (eds) (1994) *Gender, Families and Close Relationships: Feminist Research Journeys*. London: Sage. ISBN 0803952074 References

Various authors discuss the incorporation of gender into a research programme informed by feminist ideas, methods and ethics.

2.10.33 Stanley, L. (ed.) (1990) *Feminist Praxis: Research, Theory and Epistemology in Feminist Sociology*. London: Routledge. ISBN 041504202X References

Text combines theoretical discussion of feminist methodology with detailed accounts of practical research processes (CR 2.6, 2.7).

2.10.34 Torkelson, D.J. (1996) Feminist research. *Journal of Neuroscience Nursing*, 28 (2) 121–4 31 References

Article defines feminism and feminist research and gives a brief developmental history. It is then compared with more traditional forms of research and examples are given of its use in clinical studies. Issues of rigour are also discussed.

2.10.35 Webb, C. (1993) Feminist research: definitions, methodology, methods and evaluation. *Journal of Advanced Nursing*, 18 (3) 416–23 32 References

Reviews feminist research from nursing and other literature. Methodological approaches are discussed with interviewing and ethnography being evaluated for possible use. Paradoxes and dilemmas facing feminist researchers are identified and ways forward suggested (CR 2.12, 2.42, 2.68).

2.10.36 Williams, A. (1995) The relationship between ethnography and feminist research. *Nurse Researcher*, 3 (2) 34–44 47 References

Explores the question of whether there can be a feminist ethnography together with how it may be defined and distinguished from other kinds of ethnography. Author believes there is a relationship, albeit an uneasy one (CR 2.42).

2.10.37 Williams, A. (1996) The politics of feminist ethnography. *Canadian Journal of Nursing Research*, 28 (1) 87–94 28 References

Author discusses the political aspects of issues that arise from putting feminist principles into practice. Feminist ethnographers do not necessarily adopt the same approaches, but by examining these, researchers can try to understand both themselves and their respondents (CR 2.42).

2.10.38 Wuest, J. (1994) A feminist approach to concept analysis. *Western Journal of Nursing Research*, 16 (5) 577–86 23 References

Exploration of traditional approaches to concept analysis shows their limitations for contextual analysis, but when conducted from a feminist perspective these weaknesses are overcome and become a powerful tool for the development of nursing knowledge (CR 2.6, 2.89).

2.11 NEW PARADIGM RESEARCH

'New paradigm research is another way of doing research. It puts forward alternatives to "orthodox" research methods and capitalizes on the contributions of those who are normally just subjects. It is an approach to inquiry which is a systematic, rigorous search for truth but which does not kill off all it touches. It is a synthesis of naive inquiry and orthodox research'. (Reason & Rowan, 1981: xiii)

Definition

New paradigm research – research which is done with people rather than on people. It involves working with people so that they may discover some truth about themselves.

Example

Smith, P., Masterson, A. & Lask, S. (1995) Health and the curriculum: an illuminative evaluation. Part 1: methodology. *Nurse Education Today*, 15 (4) 245–9   22 References. Part 2: findings and recommendations. *Nurse Education Today*, 15 (5) 317–22   10 References

Paper describes a six-month exploratory study which evaluated the integration of a philosophy of health within pre- and post-registration curricula in England. The principle of including such a philosophy is discussed together with the project's aims, methodology, relevant literature, findings and their implications.

Major text

Reason, P. & Rowan, J. (eds) (1981) *Human Inquiry: a Sourcebook of New Paradigm Research*. Chichester: Wiley. ISBN 0471279358   References (CR 2.11)

Annotations

2.11.1   Collin, A. (1981) Mid-career change: reflections upon the development of a piece of research and the part it played in the development of the researcher, in Reason, P. & Rowan, J. (eds), *Human Inquiry: a Sourcebook of New Paradigm Research*. Chichester: Wiley. ISBN 0471279358   References

Discusses the learning process of discovering a methodology while undertaking research on the changes various groups of men were experiencing in a new phase of their life or experience (CR 2.11.9).

2.11.2   Connors, D.D. (1988) A continuum of researcher–participant relationships: an analysis and critique. *Advances in Nursing Science*, 10 (4) 32–42   33 References

Explores the nature of researcher–participant relationships and discusses the importance of this as a central focus of nursing inquiry.

2.11.3   Hamilton, D., Jenkins, D., King, C., Macdonald, B. & Parlett, M. (eds) (1977) *Beyond the Numbers Game: a Reader in Educational Evaluation*. Basingstoke: Macmillan Education. ISBN 0333198727   References

This reader on illuminative evaluation covers innovation in the school context or 'learning milieu'. Its methodological strategies are described, together with techniques of data collection and analysis, problems versus potential, range of applicability, validity and generalizability of evidence and the skills and obligations of the research worker (CR 2.25, 2.28, 2.43).

2.11.4   Heron, J. (1981) Experiential research methodology, in Reason, P. & Rowan, J. (eds), *Human Inquiry: a Sourcebook of New Paradigm Research*. Chichester: Wiley. ISBN 0471279358 Chapter 12, 153–66 References

Traditional and experiential research methodologies are contrasted. Contributions of the latter to the body of knowledge are explored (CR 2.11.9).

2.11.5   Heron, J. (1996) *Co-operative Inquiry: Research into the Human Condition*. London: Sage. ISBN 0803976844   References

Book explores the philosophical and methodological grounds of co-operative inquiry and gives practical advice on doing this type of work. Topics include a critique of established research techniques, the underlying participative paradigm of co-operative inquiry, the epistemological and political aspects of participation, different types and range of inquiry studies, ways of setting up groups and encouraging their development and carrying out the necessary procedures used to enhance validity (CR 2.6, 2.25).

2.11.6 Parlett, M. (1981) Illuminative evaluation, in Reason, P. & Rowan, J. (eds), *Human Inquiry: a Sourcebook of New Paradigm Research*. Chichester: Wiley. ISBN 0471279358 Chapter 19, 219–26   References

Chapter summarizes this approach, largely, although not exclusively, used in education. Four perspectives are examined: definition of problems studied; its methodology; underlying conceptual framework; and the values embodied in this approach (CR 2.11.9).

2.11.7 Reason, P. (ed.) (1989) *Human Inquiry in Action: Development in New Paradigm Research*. London: Sage. ISBN 0803980892   References

Presents an up-to-date assessment on the theoretical and methodological debates in collaborative research. Problems are discussed and research is reported which helped to resolve them (CR 2.15).

2.11.8 Reason, P. (ed.) (1994) *Participation in Human Inquiry*. London: Sage. ISBN 080398832X   References

Book provides a theoretical perspective and set of examples to give would-be researchers a range of possible research approaches. It is not a text, but is about research as a participative process with, rather than on, people (CR 2.15).

2.11.9 Reason, P. & Rowan, J. (eds) (1981) *Human Inquiry: Sourcebook of New Paradigm Research*. Chichester: Wiley. ISBN 0471279358   References

Sourcebook suggests a new paradigm for the philosophy and practice of research which is collaborative and experiential. New paradigm research means doing research with people rather than on people, and seeks to develop new insights into the actions and behaviour of diverse groups. The book covers the philosophy, methodology, practice and prospects of new paradigm research. Many examples are included to illustrate these new approaches.

2.11.10 Reinhart, S. (1981) Implementing new paradigm research: a model for training and practice, in Reason, P. & Rowan, J. (eds), *Human Inquiry: a Sourcebook of New Paradigm Research*. Chichester: Wiley. ISBN 0471279358 Chapter 36, 415–35

Chapter presents a model of the process by which individuals may develop a commitment and the skills to carry out new paradigm research. An appendix suggests the elements needed in a training programme for researchers (CR 2.11.9).

2.11.11 van den Hoonaard, W.C. (1997) *Working with Sensitizing Concepts: Analytical Field Research*. Thousand Oaks, CA: Sage. ISBN 0761902074   References

Monograph explores the sensitizing concept which is a construct derived from the participants' perspective, uses their language or expression and sensitizes the researcher to possible lines of inquiry. It is examined from several overlapping angles, and critics' views of the concept, dealing with data, constructing concepts, cross-cultural settings and theoretical and analytical aspects are all explored (CR 2.53).

2.12   LITERATURE REVIEWS AND REVIEWING

Once preliminary ideas and working definitions have been developed for the proposed research, the next step is to examine current knowledge about the concept under study by means of a literature review. This should be carried out carefully and critically with special attention being given to identifying inconsistencies, incompleteness and subtle differences of meaning. The reviewer should include, but not be confined to, the nursing literature and should attempt to trace the development of the concept under study. Both recent and past literature should be examined.

Examples of literature reviews are included in this section, together with ways in which systematic reviews may be carried out.

Definitions

Literature review – a carefully designed, logically developed discussion that provides the rationale for the problem statement, significance of the problem, theoretical perspective, research design and methodology
Systematic review – the process of systematically locating, appraising and synthesizing evidence from scientific studies in order to obtain a reliable overview

Annotations

2.12.1 Arthur, V.A.M. (1995) Written patient information: a review of the literature. *Journal of Advanced Nursing*, 21 (6) 1081–6   46 References

Examines mainly British literature from 1944 to 1992 on written patient information. Areas covered are readability, recall, communication, compliance and patient satisfaction, especially in the context of those with rheumatoid arthritis.

2.12.2 Bassett, C. (1992) The integration of research in the clinical setting: obstacles and solutions. A review of the literature. *Nursing Practice*, 6 (1) 4–8   39 References

Review examines the relationship between nursing research and practice, concentrating on the areas of education, communication and constraints (CR 2.15, 2.98, 2.101, 2.102, 3.7, 3.8, 3.13, 3.14, 3.16, 3.17).

2.12.3 Beal, J.A. & Betz, C.L. (1992) Intervention studies in pediatric nursing research: a decade of review. *Pediatric Nursing*, 18 (6) 586–90   50 References

Article examines paediatric nursing research, published mainly in America, in seven research and paediatric practice journals over the past decade. Of 319 research articles, 16.6 per cent were intervention studies which evaluated the outcomes of care. Paediatric nurses are urged to develop research questions about the effectiveness of their practice (CR 2.43, 2.102, 3.8).

2.12.4 Bentley, H. (1996) The need for change in nurse education: a literature review. *Nurse Education Today*, 16 (2) 131–6   21 References

Reviews the literature suggesting the need for change in nurse education and why these were not made earlier. The Project 2000 proposals are explored with the benefit of hindsight and author urges ongoing research to evaluate the present courses (CR 3.17).

2.12.5 Beyea, S.C. & Nicoll, L.H. (1995) Administration of medications via the intramuscular route: an integrative review of literature and research-based protocol for the procedure. *Applied Nursing Research*, 8 (1) 23–33   57 References

Article reviews the extensive US research conducted in health-related disciplines during the last seven decades. A critique of this material forms the basis for a clinical practice protocol (CR 3.7).

2.12.6 Billings, D.M. & Bachmeier, B. (1994) Teaching and learning at a distance: a review of the nursing literature, in Allen, L.R. (ed.), *Review of Research in Nursing Education* Volume VI. New York: National League for Nursing. ISBN 0887375960 Chapter 1, 1–32   69 References

Review critically examines North American and the UK literature from 1984 to 1993 regarding distance education in order to assist nurse educators and administrators in making informed decisions about the use and effectiveness of distance education. Recommendations for further research are given (CR 3.17).

2.12.7 Billings, J.R. & Cowley, S. (1995) Approaches to community needs assessment: a literature review. *Journal of Advanced Nursing*, 22 (4) 721–30   106 References

Examines mainly British literature from 1967 to 1994 and covers definitions, the community health profile, validity of data sources and the consumer perspective.

2.12.8 Bowers, L. (1992) A preliminary description of the UK community psychiatric nursing literature 1960–1990. *Journal of Advanced Nursing*, 17 (6) 739–46   15 References

Article examined 502 items of the community psychiatric nursing (CPN) literature from 1960 to 1990 and established various categories. These are the clinical role of the CPN, descriptive/analytical research, management, administration and education. Much literature however cannot be classified by the specialism of community psychiatric nursing. Practising CPNs are the most prolific authors, followed by academics and managers. Originally, most articles were published in populist nursing journals but are now more likely to be found in academic publications.

2.12.9 Butterworth, T. (1996) Individualised nursing care: a cuckoo in the team's nest? *NT Research*, 1 (1) 34–7   13 References

Examines mainly British literature from 1977 to 1995 which has linked the idea that individualized patient care is synonymous with good quality care.

2.12.10 Chalmers, I. & Altman, D.G. (eds) (1995) *Systematic Reviews*. London: British Medical Journal Publishing Group. ISBN 0727909045   References

Book, based on papers given at a BMJ/UK Cochrane Centre meeting in 1993, discusses the processes involved in undertaking systematic reviews. The identification of relevant studies, obtaining data from randomized controlled trials and meta-analysis data are all discussed. Guidelines are given for assessing reviews, how they may be prepared, updated and disseminated. A bibliography on the science of reviewing research is included. Updated versions of this will be disseminated on disk as the Cochrane Database of Systematic Reviews and also through the Internet using the FTP servers at the Canadian and UK Cochrane Centres. Addresses, telephone, fax and e-mail addresses are included for the eight Cochrane Centres (CR 1.8, 2.29, 2.85, 2.92).

2.12.11 Cooper, H.M. (1998) *Synthesizing Research: a Guide for Literature Reviews* 3rd edition. Thousand Oaks, CA: Sage. ISBN 0761913483   References

Book gives guidance on conducting an integrative research review in a systematic, objective way. The process of reviewing is carried out in five phases: problem formulation, data collection, data evaluation, analysis, interpretation and public presentation. This enables more rigorous reviews to be carried out with greater potential for creating consensus among scholars and focusing debate in a constructive fashion. This new edition has been revised and updated, and includes the latest information on the use of electronic technology and the Internet to conduct literature searches. The American Psychological Association's most recent guidelines are also included (CR 1.8, 2.99).

2.12.12 Coyne, I.T. (1995) Parental participation in care: a critical review of the literature. *Journal of Advanced Nursing*, 21 (4) 716–22   70 References

Reviews US and UK literature from 1951 to 1993 on parents' expectations, roles in hospital care for their children and factors influencing their attitudes. Nurses' attitudes towards parental participation are also discussed. Author believes that the respective roles of both parents and nurses need to be more clearly defined.

2.12.13 Cullum, N. (1998) Getting to grips with the research evidence. *Nursing Times*, 27 May, 94 (21) 60–1   2 References

Author describes the best sources of information for finding out which systematic reviews of literature are currently available. Many can be found on the Internet and databases together with reports and journal articles. Website URLs ('addresses') are given.

2.12.14 Davies, S., Laker, S. & Ellis, L. (1997) Promoting autonomy and independence for older people within nursing practice: a literature review. *Journal of Advanced Nursing*, 26 (2) 408–17   89 References

Article reviews US, UK and Scandinavian literature from 1975 to 1995 which showed a number of indicators associated with attempts to promote patient autonomy and independence. These are systems of care delivery, attempts to encourage patients/clients to participate in decisions about their care, patterns of communication and ways of modifying the environment to make it safer.

2.12.15 Dickson, R. & Entwistle, V. (1996) Systematic reviews: keeping up with research evidence. *Nursing Standard*, 31 January, 10 (19) 32   2 References

Outlines the need for systematic reviews of the literature, how this may be done and lists key features of good-quality reviews.

2.12.16 Droogan, J. & Cullum, N. (1998) Systematic reviews in nursing. *International*

Journal of Nursing Studies, 35 (1/2) 13–22
22 References

Discusses the process of undertaking systematic literature reviews and their historical development. A particular strategy for identifying those relevant to nursing is outlined.

2.12.17 Droogan, J. & Song, F. (1996) The process and importance of systematic reviews. *Nurse Researcher*, 4 (1) 15–26
17 References

Article provides an outline of the key processes involved in carrying out a systematic review and examines the importance of these reviews for nurses, midwives and health visitors.

2.12.18 Dunn, L. (1997) Literature review of advanced clinical practice in the USA. *Journal of Advanced Nursing*, 25(4) 814–19
45 References

Reviews British and American literature from 1965 to 1993 on advanced nursing practice. Its historical development is described. Education for advanced practice and the role components required are also discussed (CR 3.15).

2.12.19 Dyson, J., Cobb, M. & Forman, D. (1997) The meaning of spirituality: a literature review. *Journal of Advanced Nursing*, 26 (6) 1183–8   57 References

Reviews American, British and Canadian literature from 1959 to 1996 on the meaning of spirituality. The authors suggest that the themes emerging could be used as a framework for future exploration of this concept.

2.12.20 Elliott, D. (1997) Costing intensive care services: a review of study methods, results and limitations. *Australian Critical Care*, 10 (2) 55–6, 58–63   35 References

Studies reviewed in this paper utilized various methodologies to capture different components of service and patient costs. These are reported but because of the variety of methods used only a limited comparative analysis was possible.

2.12.21 Fowler, J. (1996) The organisation of clinical supervision within the nursing profession: a review of the literature. *Journal of Advanced Nursing*, 23 (3) 471–8   44 References

Review includes mainly UK literature from 1966 to 1994. Areas examined are the need for supervision, how the concept is used in practice and the profession's perception of good practice. Various models of supervision are identified and the preparation and roles of supervisors are discussed (CR 3.18).

2.12.22 Francke, A.L., Garssen, B. & Abu-Saad, H.H. (1995) Determinants of change in nurses' behaviour after continuing education: a literature review. *Journal of Advanced Nursing*, 21 (2) 371–7   47 References

Discusses literature from the Netherlands, the USA and the UK from 1971 to 1994 which examined the characteristics of participants, programmes undertaken, teachers and social systems in continuing education. Expectations of change are outlined and further work is suggested.

2.12.23 Gillies, M.J. (1993) Post-operative pain in children: a review of the literature. *Journal of Clinical Nursing*, 2 (1) 5–10
70 References

Reviews British and American medical and nursing literature from 1968 to 1992 and examines post-operative pain, children and pain, misconceptions, assessment and management.

2.12.24 Gould, D. (1994) Writing literature reviews. *Nurse Researcher*, 2 (1) 13–23
10 References

Author offers advice to those writing literature reviews on how to undertake this difficult task successfully. A strategy is included for critiquing research reports (CR 2.95).

2.12.25 Gould, D. & Chamberlain, A. (1994) Gram-negative bacteria: the challenge of preventing cross-infection in hospital wards: a review of the literature. *Journal of Clinical Nursing*, 3 (6) 339–45   71 References

Reviews American and British literature from 1956 to 1993. Areas covered include the emergence of this infection, how it is spread, where it occurs and the work of nurses in relation to cross-infection.

2.12.26 Hanrahan, A. & Reutter, L. (1997) A critical review of the literature on sharps injuries: epidemiology, management of exposures and prevention. *Journal of*

Advanced Nursing, 25 (1) 144–54
130 References

Article reviews American, Canadian, Australian and British literature from 1974 to 1995 on workplace infections, the extent and consequences of sharps injuries, post-exposure management, prevention issues and implications for nursing research and practice (CR 2.41).

2.12.27 Hilton, P.A. (1997) Theoretical perspectives of nursing. *Journal of Advanced Nursing*, 26 (6) 1211–20   80 References

Paper presents British, American and Scandinavian literature from 1933 to 1993 on various theoretical perspectives derived from the literature. These are: nursing as an interpersonal process, a unique art, a science, a humanistic art and science, a therapeutic intervention and nursing as caring.

2.12.28 Hockey, J. (1993) Research methods: researching peers and familiar settings. *Research Papers in Education: Policy and Practice*, 8 (2) 199–225   121 References

Paper presents a review of research methods literature examining the benefits and pitfalls of doing research in familiar settings and among peers. Educational literature and material from anthropology and sociology are included. The problems of researching peers are discussed, including the blurring of roles of researcher and research education, and deciding which role to adopt. Being researched can be uncomfortable as one is under professional scrutiny. Issues of confidentiality are also discussed (CR 2.16, 2.22, 3.15).

2.12.29 Holmes, S. (1996) Systematic search offers a sound evidence base ... literature review. *Nursing Times*, 24-30 January, 92 (4) 37–9   5 References

Paper explains why literature reviews are necessary, how to gain access to information and review it, and how to write it up (CR 2.95, 2.97).

2.12.30 Hudacek, S. & Carpenter, D.M. (1994) Doctoral education in nursing: a comprehensive review of the research and theoretical literature, in Allen, L.R. (ed.), *Review of Research in Nursing Education* Volume VI New York: National League for

Nursing ISBN 0887375960 Chapter 3, 7–90
79 References

Reviews North American literature from 1960 to 1992 and examines the historical evolution of doctoral education, types of programme, the similarity and differences in programmes, their quality and excellence, the need for doctorally prepared nurses and future directions for research. A summary of conferences on doctoral education from 1977 to 1990 is also given (CR 3.17).

2.12.31 Jarrett, N. & Payne, S. (1995) A selective review of the literature on nurse–patient communication: has the patient's contribution been neglected? *Journal of Advanced Nursing*, 22 (1) 72–8   61 References

Examines mainly British literature from 1961 to 1994 on nurse–patient communication. Authors believe that the patients' contribution has received less emphasis and this should be taken into account in future research.

2.12.32 Kitson, A. (1994) Post-operative pain management: a literature review. *Journal of Clinical Nursing*, 3 (1) 7–18   77 References

Literature review formed part of a three-year, Department of Health-funded study called the ODySSSy project. British and American literature from 1952 to 1989 was examined and grouped under the following headings: environmental issues, nursing actions, patient outcomes and a review of a number of pain measures (CR 2.43).

2.12.33 Kyle, T.V. (1995) The concept of caring: a review of the literature. *Journal of Advanced Nursing*, 21 (3) 506–14   50 References

Examines literature from 1975 to 1993 from the USA and the UK on caring which is seen as the central focus of nursing care. Theoretical perspectives are examined, together with the quantitative and qualitative methods used in the studies. The strengths and limitations of each are discussed.

2.12.34 Lait, M.E. & Smith, L.N. (1998) Wound management: a literature review. *Journal of Clinical Nursing*, 7 (1) 11–17   34 References

Reviews British and American literature from 1984 to 1986 on wound management. Areas covered are wound assessment, wound care and their relationship to the healing process. Some problems found in the literature are discussed.

2.12.35 Land, L. (1995) A review of pressure damage prevention strategies. *Journal of Advanced Nursing*, 22 (2) 329–37 70 References

Review focuses on elements of care that are within the power of nurses to attain and suggests strategies for promoting quality by simple, economic and effective means.

2.12.36 Logan, V. (1995) Incidence and prevalence of lymphoedema: a literature review. *Journal of Clinical Nursing*, 4 (4) 213–19 26 References

Reviews international literature from 1987 to 1994 and covers the incidence and prevalence of lymphoedema. Factors influencing the development of the condition, and the controversy concerning axillary node sampling and dissection are discussed.

2.12.37 Maggs, C. & Laugharne, C. (1996) Relationship between elderly carers and the older adult with learning disabilities: an overview of the literature. *Journal of Advanced Nursing*, 23 (2) 243–51 56 References

Literature from the UK and the USA from 1979 to 1994 covers the changing needs and circumstances which occur between carers and the cared for. Authors believe that a lack of understanding and limited resources will make adequate provision unlikely but the needs of both groups should be addressed by the health and social services.

2.12.38 Maggs, C. & Snoxall, S. (1992) *A Critical Review of the Literature on Outcomes in Nursing Practice and Management: a Report to the Department of Health.* Bath: Maggs Research Associates. ISBN 0951922610 Bibliography

This literature review, commissioned by the Department of Health, provides an overview of the debate about nursing practice and management outcomes. North American and British literature was examined, together with similar debates from other public services. Sections include an introduction, the policy context, current developments in outcome use in nursing practice and management. The conclusion comments on future research in this field (CR 2.43).

2.12.39 Mallik, M. (1997) Advocacy in nursing: a review of the literature. *Journal of Advanced Nursing*, 25 (1) 130–8 94 References

Covers British and American literature from 1970 to 1995 on the need for, meanings and models of advocacy. Justifying a career in patient advocacy and the attendant risks are also discussed.

2.12.40 Martin, P.A. (1997) Writing a useful literature review for a qualitative project. *Applied Nursing Research*, 10 (3) 159–62 5 References

Author offers advice to those writing a literature review (CR 2.36).

2.12.41 Mason, G. & Webb, C. (1993) Nursing diagnoses: a review of the literature. *Journal of Clinical Nursing*, 2 (2) 67–74 60 References

Paper examines literature between 1966 and 1992 on nursing diagnoses. Topics covered are: what is nursing diagnosis?, defining the term, developing a diagnostic role for practice, the construction of a taxonomy, a critique of the categories and their applicability to nursing in the UK.

2.12.42 McKee, M. & Britton, A. (1997) Conducting a literature review on the effectiveness of health care interventions. *Health Policy and Planning*, 12 (3) 262–7 26 References

Article sets out the necessary steps when undertaking a literature review. These are: defining the question, locating relevant literature, assessing the quality of studies and deciding whether they should be included, synthesizing and re-analysing the results and presenting them in a clear and precise manner. The leading sources of information are identified, including electronic databases and Internet addresses. Guidance is given on conducting each stage. The strengths and weaknesses of the different approaches are discussed, together with ways in which bias may be introduced (CR 1.8, 2.27, 2.43).

2.12.43 O'Connor, S.E. (1992) Network

theory: a system method for literature review. *Nurse Education Today*, 12 (1) 44–50 13 References

Article discusses the nature and purpose of literature reviews and describes the 'standard' method for their construction. The author suggests this is non-systematic and time-consuming, and an alternative method entitled Network Theory is advocated and discussed.

2.12.44 Oxman, A.D. & Guyatt, G.H. (1988) Guidelines for reading literature reviews. *Canadian Medical Association Journal*, 15 April, 138 697–703 56 References

Eight guidelines, listed as a series of questions, are given which will assist readers in assessing the scientific quality of literature reviews. They focus on definition of the question, comprehensiveness of the search strategy, methods of choosing and assessing primary studies, methods of combining the results and reaching appropriate conclusions.

2.12.45 Parker, M.J. & Handoll, H.H.G. (1997) Extracapsular femoral fractures: replacement arthroplasty versus internal fixation, in Musculoskeletal injuries module of the Cochrane Database of Systematic Reviews (Gillespie, W.J. et al.) *The Cochrane Library. The Cochrane Collaboration Sep 1 Issue 4.* 1 Reference [software, disk or CD-ROM updated quarterly]

Provides an example of a systematic review undertaken at the Cochrane Library. Relevant, randomized, controlled trials were sought using various strategies with only one being identified in this instance (CR 2.29).

2.12.46 Pinch, W.J. (1995) Synthesis: implementing a complex process. *Nurse Educator*, 20 (1) 34–40 21 References

Describes in detail the process of synthesizing materials using a literature review as an example.

2.12.47 Pollock, V.E. (1993) Meta-analysis in literature reviews. *Biological Psychiatry*, 34 (6) 345–7 References

Discusses the processes involved in using this technique when undertaking literature reviews (CR 2.92).

2.12.48 Roe, B. (1993) Undertaking a critical review of the literature. *Nurse Researcher*, 1 (1) 31–42 20 References

Key points in literature reviewing are described which accumulate into a research method in itself. Examples are given of existing reviews, factors thought to limit the use of research, and a list of questions to be asked when evaluating papers (CR 2.92, 2.95, 2.102).

2.12.49 Sakzewski, L. & Ziviani, J. (1996) Factors affecting the length of hospital stay for children with acquired brain injuries: a review of the literature. *Australian Occupational Therapy Journal*, 43 (3/4) 113–24 55 References

Authors address the factors affecting the length of stay of brain-injured children which are severity of injury, complicating factors and the effects of intervention procedures.

2.12.50 Schlatter, S. & McNatt, G.E. (1995) Risk of community infections in transplant patients: a literature review. *ANNA Journal*, 22 (6) 590–5, 630 23 References

Covers American literature from 1985 to 1994 and examines nosocomial and ubiquitous infections, those associated with animals and travelling, and possible interventions.

2.12.51 Spence, J.E. & Olson, M.A. (1997) Quantitative research on therapeutic touch: an integrative review of the literature 1985–1995. *Scandinavian Journal of Caring Sciences*, 11 (3) 183–90 23 References

Authors examine what is and is not known about therapeutic touch in order to facilitate application in practice and make recommendations for future research. Eleven quantitative studies were analysed and evidence obtained to show the value of therapeutic touch for reduction of pain and anxiety. Problems encountered are discussed (CR 2.29).

2.12.52 Sweet, S.J. & Norman, I.J. (1995) The nurse–doctor relationship: a selective literature review. *Journal of Advanced Nursing*, 22 (1) 165–70 41 References

Mainly British literature from 1966 to 1993 is examined to explore this issue. Areas covered include a sociological perspective, the 'doctor–nurse game' and nurse–doctor interactions today.

2.12.53 Thomas, L.H. & Bond, S. (1995) The effectiveness of nursing: a review. *Journal of Clinical Nursing*, 4 (3) 143–51 52 References

Reviews literature published in three British journals from 1989 to 1994. Areas covered include intervention studies, different methods of nursing organization and grade-mix, and evaluation of different aspects of the nursing service. Authors also examined the studies' design and sample sizes. A lack of rigour was noted.

2.12.54 Tierney, A.J. (1995) HIV/AIDS knowledge, attitudes and education of nurses: a review of the research. *Journal of Clinical Nursing*, 4 (1) 13–21   56 References

Reports research from North America and the UK from 1985 to 1993. Areas covered include the review process, surveys of nurses' knowledge and attitudes, education provision, evaluation of educational approaches and initiatives.

2.12.55 Tierney, A.J. (1996) Under-nutrition and elderly hospital patients: a review. *Journal of Advanced Nursing*, 23 (2) 228–36 66 References

Paper includes literature from the UK and the USA from 1974 to 1994 and provides a résumé of the knowledge accumulated from research on detection of under-nutrition, together with what is known about its causes and effects. The principles of nutritional management are discussed and the implications for practice.

2.12.56 Wainwright, S.P. (1994) Recovery from liver transplantation: a literature review. *Journal of Advanced Nursing*, 20 (5) 861–9 67 References

Examines American and British literature from 1966 to 1993 and covers the state of the art in liver transplantation. Literature on psychiatric factors, functional status and quality-of-life aspects of patient recovery are discussed and suggestion made for further research.

2.12.57 Wainwright, S.P. & Gould, D. (1997) Non-adherence with medications in organ transplant patients: a literature review. *Journal of Advanced Nursing*, 26 (6) 968–77 108 References

Reviews British, American and Scandinavian literature from 1973 to 1996 on adherence in adult liver, kidney and heart transplantation. The problem of paediatric adherence is also discussed. The literature is then evaluated within the broader context of social science research on medication adherence.

2.12.58 Webb, C. & Koch, T. (1997) Women's experiences of non-invasive breast cancer: literature review and study report. *Journal of Advanced Nursing*, 25 (3) 514–25 62 References

Reviews the post-1990 literature on breast cancer which identified a large body of psychosocial research focusing on coping styles, quality of life and women's participation in choice of treatment. Some methodological problems were found, making comparisons difficult, because of a variety of diagnoses included in samples within and between studies. A small study was conducted to explore women's experience of ductal carcinoma *in situ*. Findings are discussed in relation to the literature on information-giving and the role of the nurse.

2.12.59 Wensing, M. & Grol, R. (1994) Single and combined strategies for implementing changes in primary care: a literature review. *International Journal for Quality in Health Care*, 6 (2) 115–32   100 References

Covers European and North American literature from 1976 to 1993. Reports an analysis of 75 studies which examined different strategies in primary health care for continuing medical education. The methods most frequently used were feedback, reminders and group education. Strategies which were most effective are reported.

2.12.60 Wilkins, H. (1993) Trans-cultural nursing: a selective view of the literature 1985–1991. *Journal of Advanced Nursing*, 18 (4) 602–12   118 References

Reviews selected work published in nursing journals between 1985 and 1991 under the following headings: theory and concepts, nurse education, health education and patient teaching, clinical counselling, sexuality, care of the child and research. Common themes and problems are discussed (CR 2.53).

2.12.61 Wilkinson, J. & Wilkinson, C. (1995) How to conduct a literature review.

Nursing Standard, 10 (9) 28–30   16 References

Article outlines the skills needed to review literature and discusses how this can be made relevant to practice.

2.13   REPLICATION RESEARCH

Replication of nursing research, particularly clinical studies, is an essential element of a sound empirically based body of knowledge which is fundamental to nursing practice. Replication studies are rarely found in the literature, but it is a vital step in the development of nursing science and should be supported and encouraged.

Definition

Replication – a study that repeats all aspects of an original study on another sample from the same population

Example

Schmieding, N.J. & Kokuyama, T. (1995) The need for and process of collaborative international research: a replication study of Japanese staff nurses' perceptions of head nurses' actions. *Journal of Advanced Nursing*, 21 (5) 820–6   35 References

Describes a replication study in a Japanese hospital, previously conducted in the USA. This compared the type of response staff nurses would prefer in a problem situation in contrast with that of a head nurse. The results of the two studies showed marked similarities (CR 2.15).

Annotations

2.13.1   Beck, C.T. (1994) Replication strategies for nursing research. *Image: Journal of Nursing Scholarship*, 26 (3) 191–4   35 References

Article compares and contrasts four of the most frequently cited classifications of replication research and reviews methods of such studies in nursing over the last 10 years. A list of replication studies is included.

2.13.2   Collins, H.M. (1992) *Changing Order: Replication and Induction in Scientific Practice* 2nd edition. Chicago: University of Chicago Press. ISBN 0226113760   References

Discusses the processes and outcomes of replication from a philosophical point of view and uses three field studies for illustration. These examined laser building, the detection of gravitational radiation and 'mind over matter'. The complexities involved are explored.

2.13.3   Connelly, C.E. (1986) Replication research in nursing. *International Journal of Nursing Studies*, 23 (1) 71–7   27 References

Discusses the importance and contribution of replication research to the development of nursing science. Factors which have deterred such studies are discussed, together with various types and examples of replication research. Criteria for replicating a study are outlined.

2.13.4   Gillett, R. (1990) Determining the sample size for a replication attempt: a short and simple microcomputer program *Current Psychology: Research and Reviews*, 9 (3) 304–7   References

Describes the computer programme EUREKA which will help determine the sample size in replication research (CR 2.22).

2.13.5   Hayes, P. (1993) Replicative studies. *Clinical Nursing Research*, 2 (3) 243–4 Editorial

Outlines the value of replication studies and suggests ways in which they may be encouraged. A function of this particular journal will be to report such studies.

2.13.6   Krueger, J.C., Fitzpatrick, J.J. & Kramer, M. (1981) Questions and answers: research replication. *Western Journal of Nursing Research*, 3 (1) 94–7   5 References

Various points related to research replication are posed: ethical issues, a change of site and additional tools. Each question is answered by three experts (CR 2.17).

2.13.7   Martin, P.A. (1995) More replication studies needed. *Applied Nursing Research*, 8 (2) 102–3   15 References

Author believes replication studies to be a legitimate form of scholarship and reports on a study by Connelly which reviewed 16 texts from 1978 to 1984 for information on replication. These were found to be uninformative. A more recent review shows that replication is missing from only one of the major nursing research texts reviewed.

2.13.8   Mulkay, M. & Gilbert, G.N. (1986) Replication and mere replication. *Philosophy of the Social Sciences*, 16 (1) 21–37   12 References

Documents some of the recurrent factors when scientists' talk of replication. It identifies how scientists' conceptions of research differ and ways in which these may be used to portray their own and others' reactions.

2.13.9   Neuliep, J.W. (1990) Editorial bias against replication research. *Journal of Social Behaviour and Personality*, 5 (4) 85–90 References

Author believes that existing editorial bias against replication research prevents the formation of cumulative knowledge and confirmation of existing findings.

2.13.10   Neuliep, J.W. (ed.) (1991) *Replication Research in the Social Sciences*. Newbury Park, CA: Sage. ISBN 0803940920 References

Discusses all aspects of replication research including the processes involved, its importance and editorial bias against it. Illustrative material is given from the literature of several disciplines (CR 2.27).

2.13.11   Ryland, R.K. (1989) A plea for replication studies. *Journal of Advanced Nursing*, 14 (9) 699 Guest Editorial

Author argues that we cannot afford the luxury of allowing students in centres of higher education always to produce original work. More co-operation is needed within universities and research centres to concentrate on key issues and undergraduates should be encouraged to replicate other studies. In this way the body of nursing knowledge would grow and students would also receive the research training required.

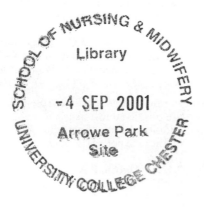

DESIGNING NURSING RESEARCH

2.14 RESEARCH PLANNING

Studies of previous research in nursing reveal that many have had both quantitative and qualitative components, and to understand the complexity of nursing, with its wide range of problems, a variety of approaches may be required.

Definitions

Gatekeeper – a person whose permission must be sought by the researcher in order to gain access to the respondents
Research protocol – the overall plan or recipe for procedures to be carried out in a particular study

---

Annotations

2.14.1 Abbott, P. & Sapsford, R. (eds) (1997) *Research into Practice: a Reader for Nurses and the Caring Professions* 2nd edition. Buckingham: Open University Press. ISBN 0335196950   References

This revised and updated edition contains papers relating to nursing, health and community care, showing the types of research which may be undertaken by a small team or single researcher. Papers show a variety of approaches, the limitations typical of small-scale projects and how research works out in practice. Three major sections are: observing and participating; talking to people and asking questions; controlled trials and comparisons (CR 2.16, 2.29, 2.68, 2.72, 3.16).

2.14.2 American Sociological Association. *Sociological Methodology.* URL:http://weber.u.washington.edu/ ~socmeth2/

An annual volume of methods of research in the social sciences. The website provides contents pages and abstracts of articles from 1994, along with subscription details and information for authors.

2.14.3 Arrington, M. & Byers, V.L. (1991) Anatomy of a nursing study: generation to implementation. *Journal of Neuroscience Nursing*, 23 (4) 261–3   No references

Article discusses the process and practical dilemmas of conducting a clinical nursing study (CR 2.16).

2.14.4 Ash, A. (1995) The design and analysis of hospital utilization studies. *International Journal for Quality in Health Care*, 7 (3) 245–52   18 References

Paper discusses general design strategy, the value of explicit protocols for sampling and data collection, analyses appropriate to the sampling, and generating reports that managers can use. More co-ordination is needed so that comparisons can be made across studies so that the value of each individual study and collectively can be raised (CR 2.22, 2.64).

2.14.5 Balogh, R. (1996) Exploring the links between audit and the research process. *Nurse Researcher*, 3 (3) 5–16   44 References

Explores the strong links between audit and research. The policy background is outlined, audit in the literature and research about audit are also discussed. The similarities, differences and mutual benefits are highlighted.

2.14.6 Beck, C.T. (1997) Developing a research program using qualitative and quantitative approaches. *Nursing Outlook*, 45 (6) 265–9   29 References

In this article a research study on post-partum depression is used to illustrate how both qualitative and quantitative approaches can be used to develop a programme that is knowledge directed and not method limited (CR 2.29, 2.36).

2.14.7   Belza, B. (1996) Conducting research in respondents' homes: benefits, problems and strategies. *Applied Nursing Research*, 9 (1) 37–44   16 References

Article describes the potential problems and strategies for conducting research in respondents' homes. Author believes that with adequate funding, attention to safety and a mechanism for making and confirming appointments, homes serve as valuable sites for obtaining data (CR 2.16).

2.14.8   Bickman, L. & Rog, D.J. (eds) (1997) *Handbook of Applied Social Research Methods*. Thousand Oaks, CA: Sage. ISBN 076190672X   References

Provides a practical guide to selecting the appropriate questions and procedures from among the diverse perspectives available for studying some of the highly complex areas within the real world (CR 2.16, 2.18, 2.20, 2.29, 2.36).

2.14.9   Blaikie, N. (1993) *Approaches to Social Enquiry*. Cambridge: Polity Press. ISBN 0745611737   References

Book is intended for experienced and novice researchers and covers science and social science, research strategies and some methodological issues.

2.14.10   Brewer, J. & Hunter, A. (1990) *Multi-method Research: a Synthesis of Styles*. Newbury Park, CA: Sage. ISBN 080393078X References

Book explores ways in which multi-method approaches can contribute to social science research. Aspects covered are formulation of problems, data collection, sampling, generalization, reliability and validity, hypothesis-testing and causal analysis, writing and publishing results (CR 2.18, 2.20, 2.22, 2.24, 2.25, 2.28, 2.97, 2.99).

2.14.11   Canadian Nurse Researcher Database. (1998)
URL:http: //142.104.153.202/index.asp

This interactive database, launched in 1998, designed by and for nurse researchers, aims to serve the cause of nursing research by improving the means of communication and co-ordination between researchers. The database maintains up-to-date records of demographic profiles and research fields of nurse researchers across Canada and around the world. The classification system initially adopted is directed towards research methodologies and covers research designs, data collection and analysis techniques, funding and grant experience and research domains. Populations of interest may also be identified.

2.14.12   Closs, S.J. & Cheater, F.M. (1996) Audit or research – what is the difference? *Journal of Clinical Nursing*, 5 (4) 249–56 24 References

Paper presents definitions of research and audit and examines their attributes and inter-relationships. Areas covered include their purpose, what type of process they are, their theoretical bases, methods used, sampling, confidentiality and the time-frame of each.

2.14.13   Copeland, A.P. & White, K.M. (1991) *Studying Families*. Newbury Park, CA: Sage. ISBN 0803932480   References

Book examines the inherent problems researchers face when studying families.

2.14.14   Cowley, S., Bergen, A., Young, K. & Kavanagh, A. (1996) Establishing a framework for research: the example of needs assessment. *Journal of Clinical Nursing*, 5 (1) 53–61   46 References

Paper explores the early planning stages of a study commissioned by the English National Board. This aimed to investigate the changing educational needs of community nurses with regard to needs assessment and quality of care in the context of the National Health Service and Community Care Act 1990. Findings are not discussed, but the process of establishing a confident base from which to launch a detailed study, when a standard literature search seemed insufficient, are explored (CR 2.69).

2.14.15   Doordan, A.M. (1998) *Research Survival Guide*. Philadelphia: Lippincott. ISBN 0781710405

Book is designed to serve as a reference to research and research terminology for novices and experienced researchers. It contains an overview of research, a glossary of over 1,000 terms and a compendium of supplementary resources (CR 2.2).

2.14.16 Douglas, S. (1993) The reporting of consent rates in nursing dissertations. *Western Journal of Nursing Research*, 15 (4) 495–505 19 References

Reports a study which analysed 203 nursing dissertations from 1980 to 1989 at five mid-western universities listed in *Dissertation Abstracts International*. Its purpose was to determine the reporting of consent rates which is needed to evaluate the external validity of the studies undertaken. Author stresses the importance of documenting consent rates which should lead to generalizability and less biased results (CR 2.17, 2.27, 2.28, 2.91).

2.14.17 Ford-Gilboe, M., Campbell, J. & Berman, H. (1995) Stories and numbers: coexistence without compromise. *Advances in Nursing Science*, 18 (1) 14–26 41 References

Attention to quality of data, process, investigator bias, and usefulness of the findings are necessary to produce valid research. Both quantitative and qualitative data or a combination of both may enhance the value of a study and result in new methodologies (CR 2.29, 2.36).

2.14.18 Fuller, R. & Petch, A. (1995) *Practitioner Research: the Reflexive Social Worker*. Buckingham: Open University Press. ISBN 0335193226 References

Discusses the relationships between practice and research and how these can be married together and what types of research can realistically be undertaken by busy practitioners. It also provides a conceptual framework for practitioner research.

2.14.19 Gibson, V. (1996) The problems of researching sensitive topics in health care. *Nurse Researcher*, 4 (2) 65–74 22 References

Some problems when researching sensitive topics are identified. These include 'blocking' by ethics committees, accessing and recruiting representative samples, the effects the research may have on themselves, their career, family, on participants and organizations (CR 2.16, 2.17, 2.22, 2.25).

2.14.20 Hart, E. (1995) Research challenges: issues in the management of research projects. *Journal of Nursing Management*, 3 (6) 313–18 21 References

Discusses the challenges posed by research in the volatile organizational context of the British National Health Service in two particular areas: the early stages of establishing a project and defining the roles and responsibilities of those involved in the research. Many of the problems can be traced back to lack of clarity about its aims and objectives and the lack of attention given to the respective relationships between managers, researchers and other team members. Ways forward are suggested (CR 3.16).

2.14.21 Herbert, M. (1990) *Planning a Research Project: a Guide for Practitioners and Trainees in the Helping Professions*. London: Cassell Educational. ISBN 0304318469 References

A practical text covering all aspects of planning and executing a research project from generating ideas to the final report.

2.14.22 Hockey, L. (1992) *Surviving the Research Process*. Geelong, Victoria, Australia: Deakin University Press. ISBN 0730013723 1 Reference

Monograph offers practical advice on planning, developing and carrying out research projects. Author shares some of the pitfalls and pleasures of research.

2.14.23 Hornsby-Smith, M. (1993) Gaining access, in Gilbert, N. (ed.), *Researching Social Life*. London: Sage. ISBN 0803986823 Chapter 4, 52—67 References

Chapter considers the problems of gaining access to informants and respondents and other sources of data. Ethical issues are discussed together with the multiple responsibilities of researchers (CR 2.1.25, 2.17).

2.14.24 Hundley, V. & Graham, W. (1997) Research and audit in midwifery: does the difference matter? *British Journal of Midwifery*, 5 (10) 597–600 21 References

Article aims to clarify the differences between research and audit, showing that there are implications for practice.

2.14.25 Hutchins, S.A. & Eckes, R. (1996)

Clinical research: considerations for prospective participants. *Nursing Clinics of North America*, 31 (1) 125–35   17 References

Article describes the purpose and process of clinical research, the patient perspective, ethical considerations and the role of the nurse (CR 2.3, 2.17, 2.22, 2.29, 3.16).

2.14.26   International Council of Nurses. (1998) A practical guide for nursing research. *International Nursing Review*, 45 (2) 40

Contains information on conceptualizing and implementing research. A large body of evidence exists to show that nursing care affects health outcomes and costs and contributes to improving the quality of people's lives (CR 2.43).

2.14.27   Kirk-Smith, M. (1996) How to design an effective research study. *Nursing Times*, 10–16 July, 92 (28) 40–1   3 References

Aspects of research design and procedures are considered.

2.14.28   Leddy, S.K. & Pepper, J.M. (1998) Research processes and utilization, in Authors, *Conceptual Bases of Professional Nursing* 4th edition. Philadelphia: Lippincott. ISBN 0397552777 Section 2, Chapter 7, 143–63   22 References

Chapter gives an overview of asking questions, qualitative and quantitative approaches and steps in the research process. Utilization of nursing research, barriers to it and strategies for facilitating its use are given. Roger's theory of diffusion of innovations and the Stetler-Marram Decision Making Model are discussed (CR 2.20, 2.29, 2.36, 2.102).

2.14.29   Lee, R.M. (ed.) (1993) *Doing Research on Sensitive Topics*. London: Sage. ISBN 0803988613   References

Book is a comprehensive guide to the methodological, ethical and practical issues involved in undertaking research on sensitive topics. Author explores the reasons why research may be politically sensitive or contentious; its relationship to power, its capacity to encroach on peoples' lives and potentially problematic nature for the researcher. Issues covered are the choice of methodologies, estimating the size of 'hidden' populations, sampling, surveying, interviewing and the handling of data. Political and ethical issues

and the dissemination of information are all discussed (CR 2.10, 2.17, 2.22, 2.52, 2.53, 2.68, 2.98, 3.11).

2.14.30   MacNair, R.H. (1996) A research methodology for community practice. *Journal of Community Practice*, 3 (2) 1–19   51 References

Article reviews the research methods used by community practice organizations over three decades. These are comparative analysis, quantitative analysis, qualitative study and historical research. A description is given of nine specific methods which should stimulate further work (CR 2.46, 2.87).

2.14.31   Mander, R. (1992) Seeking approval for research access: the gatekeeper's role in facilitating a study of the care of the relinquishing mother. *Journal of Advanced Nursing*, 17 (12) 1460–4   18 References

Explores issues relating to gaining research access. The experience with various gatekeepers is described (CR 2.17).

2.14.32   Maruyana, G. & Deno, S. (1992) *Research in Educational Settings*. Newbury Park, CA: Sage. ISBN 0803942087   References

Book is intended to help prospective and inexperienced researchers think carefully about a range of important issues in planning educational research. It complements existing methods texts by dealing with the types of practical problems encountered in the field. So little is written about these pitfalls that personal experiences are used to describe them. A sample research project is followed through the book and exercises given to stimulate discussion (CR 2.16, 2.36).

2.14.33   Mead, M. (1996) How to plan a project. *Practice Nurse*, 12 (1) 50, 52, 54–5   2 References

Some ground rules are set out to enable practice nurses to maximize the return of their investment in time and effort when undertaking a piece of research.

2.14.34   Milburn, K., Fraser, E., Secker, J. & Pavis, S. (1995) Combining methods in health promotion research: some considerations about appropriate use. *Health Education Journal*, 54 (3) 347–56   22 References

Paper assesses the value of using both qualitative and quantitative methods in health promotion research and suggestions are made for combining these approaches. Authors believe that more valid and reliable results will be obtained. A more critical approach is urged, based on consideration of epistemology, methodology and practical application. Reports should discuss and analyse the contradictions and compatibility in the production of data using combined methods (CR 2.6, 2.9, 2.29, 2.36).

2.14.35 Minnick, A., Kleinpell, R.M., Micek, W. & Dudley, D. (1996) The management of a multi-site study. *Journal of Professional Nursing*, 12 (1) 7–15   6 References

Article presents a framework, based on a study of patient-centred care at 17 hospitals, for multi-site studies involving many different personnel and patients. Five key areas of research are discussed: general systems design, public relations, human resource issues, data quality assurances and data management. Management of such a study is described (CR 2.15).

2.14.36 Moore, M., Beazley, S. & Maelzer, J. (1997) *Researching Disability Issues*. Buckingham: Open University Press. ISBN 0335198031   References

Book provides illustrations of how to carry out research which seeks to explore disability issues. Both quantitative and qualitative frameworks are considered and a variety of studies reviewed which examine different aspects of disabled people's lives. Substantive examples of dilemmas which face researchers in this field are highlighted (CR 2.16, 2.29, 2.36, 3.20).

2.14.37 Morse, J.M. (1994) Designing funded qualitative research, in Denzin, N.K. & Lincoln, Y.S. (eds), *Handbook of Qualitative Research*. Thousand Oaks, CA: Sage. ISBN 0803946791   Chapter 13, 220–35   62 References

Chapter describes major design issues in the planning stage of qualitative projects and suggests ways in which researchers may overcome the paradoxes inherent in this type of inquiry (CR 2.36.13, 2.96).

2.14.38 Mulhall, A. (1998) Nursing research, and the evidence. *Evidence-based Nursing*, 1 (1) 4–6   15 References

Outlines the nature of nursing, the type of evidence needed to improve practice, choosing the research design to fit the question and maximizing the potential of evidence-based nursing (CR 2.3, 2.20, 2.29, 2.36).

2.14.39 Murphy, E., Spiegal, N. & Kinmonth, A.L. (1992) Will you help me with my research?: Gaining access to primary care settings and subjects. *British Journal of General Practice*, 42 (357) 162–5   10 References

Describes the strategies adopted for obtaining access to research subjects. Steps in this process include gaining relevant background information, strategic planning, identifying gatekeepers and negotiating with individuals (CR 2.17, 2.22).

2.14.40 Owen, D. & Davis, M. (1991) *Help with your Project: a Guide for Students of Health Care*. London: Edward Arnold. ISBN 0340552700   References

A basic guide to undertaking a simple research project (CR 3.19).

2.14.41 Pranulis, M.F. & Koschnitzke, L. (1993) Establishing guidelines to determine whether a potential study is a qualitative assessment study or scientific research. *Western Journal of Nursing Research*, 15 (2) 258–62   4 References

Identifies the characteristics of a qualitative assessment project and scientific research to assist decision-makers in selecting and sanctioning appropriate work (CR 2.29, 2.36).

2.14.42 Rees, R.W. (1997) Audit or research? A personal view. *Complementary Therapies in Medicine*, 5 (4) 233–7   No references

Author identifies the main differences between research and audit to encourage practitioners to use the most appropriate type of investigation.

2.14.43 Robertson, J. (ed.) (1994) *Handbook of Clinical Nursing Research*. Melbourne: Churchill Livingstone. ISBN 0443048665   References

Book, written primarily for facilitating the conduct of nursing research in the clinical setting, is intended to complement other methodology texts. The steps involved in undertaking research are described and some common problems encountered in clinical settings are discussed. Book includes standards for nursing research compiled in 1990 by members of the Western Australian Nurse Researchers Network (CR 2.1, 2.101, 3.2).

2.14.44   Rolfe, G. (1995) Playing at research: methodological pluralism and the creative researcher. *Journal of Psychiatric and Mental Health Nursing*, 2 (2) 105–9   16 References

Paper draws on the work of several writers from the philosophy of science to argue that the focus in mental health nursing research on methodological rigour stifles individual creativity and excludes many of the brightest and most creative researchers. Author proposes a new approach, anarchistic epistemology, which temporarily abandons the accepted rules and methods of the research process. Journal editors are urged to consider publishing papers describing the early, exploratory stages of research, based on criteria of creativity and innovation (CR 2.6).

2.14.45   Shipman, M. (1997) *The Limitations of Social Research* 4th edition. London: Longman. ISBN 0582311039   References

Book examines the underlying assumptions of different traditions that justify different research methods; examines techniques for collecting evidence and preparing for publication, and the processes and restrictions in publication. Each chapter is preceded by a controversy illustrating problems in the following text. This new edition is fully updated to take account of new developments in methodology and a chapter is included on designing research.

2.14.46   Strasser, J.A. (1991) Qualitative clinical nursing research: when a community is the client, in Morse, J.M. (ed.), *Qualitative Nursing Research: a Contemporary Dialogue* Revised edition. Newbury Park, CA: Sage. ISBN 0803940793 Chapter 7, 106–25 19 References

Discusses justification for doing qualitative community studies and its cost benefits. An example illustrates the implementation of such a study and the challenges of field work.

2.14.47   Tierney, A. (1997) Planning and managing a research project to time. *Nurse Researcher*, 5 (1) 35–50   12 References

Article describes the importance of carefully planning the research proposal, the various stages of a project, how to timetable and manage time and deal with any problems or delays (CR 2.96, 3.18).

2.14.48   Usherwood, T. (1996) *Introduction to Project Management in Health Research: a Guide for New Researchers.* Buckingham: Open University Press. ISBN 0335197078 References

Offers advice to first-time researchers on a systematic and structured approach to research project management.

2.14.49   Vickers, A. (1995) A basic introduction to medical research. Part II: An overview of different research methods. *Complementary Therapies in Nursing and Midwifery*, 1 (4) 113–17   6 References

Discusses the advantages and relevance of both qualitative and quantitative research and suggests that the prospective researcher should choose a methodology which is appropriate to the question being asked (CR 2.9, 2.29, 2.36).

2.14.50   Walters, A.J. (1996) Nursing research methodology: transcending Cartesianism. *Nursing Inquiry*, 3 (2) 91–100 41 References

Paper explores the Cartesian debate which has polarized the discussion on nursing research methodology. Conventional methodologies do not provide nurses with adequate research foundations to understand the complex world of nursing practice. An alternative perspective is proposed – Gadamerian hermeneutics.

2.14.51   White, A. & Johnson, M. (1998) The complexities of nursing research with men. *International Journal of Nursing Studies*, 35 (1/2) 41–8   32 References

Paper explores issues that need to be considered when conducting research with (or on) men.

2.15   COLLABORATIVE RESEARCH

'In research partnerships ... individual personalities and interpersonal processes both play a crucial part. . . . The complex interplay between institutions and individuals, personal and professional agendas are important variables to consider. . . . [It is] through identifying . . . the principles of formal and informal processes impacting upon research, complementarity and reciprocity [that the important aspects of a research partnership are identified]. (Mackenzie, Husband & Gerrish, 1995: 88–9) [adapted]

Definition

Collaborative research – to labour or cooperate with another, especially in . . . scientific pursuits

Example

French, P., Anderson, J., Burnard, P., Holmes, C., Mashaba, G., Wong, T. & Binghua, Z. (1996) International comparison of baccalaureate nursing degrees: collaboration in qualitative analysis. *Journal of Advanced Nursing,* 23 (3) 594–602   28 References

Describes a study which examined the perceived similarities and differences of a selection of baccalaureate nursing degrees from different continents. Analyses were made of curricula aims, content, methods and assessment. A list of key issues was identified. Findings have implications for the development of credit transfer and international exchange schemes.

Annotations

2.15.1 Boyd, C.O. (1993) Towards a nursing practice research method. *Advances in Nursing Science,* 16 (2) 9–25   25 References

Article describes a structure for nursing research in which the primary feature is the nurse researcher-as-clinician in a collaborative relationship with client-as-subject. Elements of a theoretical rationale for blending the roles of clinician and researcher in a qualitative method are given. This method is not merely technical activity focusing on narrative data but is a recognition that research and knowledge development are taking place from this nurse/client relationship (CR 2.6, 2.15, 2.22, 2.89, 3.16).

2.15.2 Boyle, J.S. (1991) Field research: a

collaborative model for practice and research, in Morse, J.M. (ed.), *Qualitative Nursing Research: a Contemporary Dialogue* Revised edition. Newbury Park, CA: Sage. ISBN 0803940793. Chapter 16, 273–99   52 References

Describes the development of a collaborative research model using ethnographic field methods, and how their use can solve problems in nursing practice (2.36, 2.42).

2.15.3 Chenger, P.L. (1988) Collaborative nursing research: advantages and obstacles. *International Journal of Nursing Studies,* 25 (4) 295–300   12 References

Collaborative research in an academic and clinical setting is described. This provides one approach to developing the scientific base for nursing practice, but also recognizes economic realities. The advantages and obstacles of this type of research are highlighted.

2.15.4 Coeling, H.V.E. (1993) Limiting the indirect cost of research in health care institutions. *Applied Nursing Research,* 6 (2) 92–7   2 References

Describes how one guest researcher sought to reduce the institution's research expenses related to labour costs. Some benefits gained by inviting academics into clinical research projects are discussed (CR 3.13).

2.15.5 Crabtree, B.F., Addison, R.B., Gilchrist, V., Kuzel, A. & Miller, W.L. (eds) (1994) *Developing Collaborative Research in Primary Care.* London: Sage. ISBN 0803954891   References

Authors believe that multi-method research, moving beyond any particular discipline would enable more primary care research to be successful.

2.15.6 DePalma, J.A., O'Malley, J. & de Chesnay, M. (1996) A model for collaborative research. *Advanced Practice Nursing Quarterly,* 2 (3) 48–53   12 References

The design and implementation of a nursing research centre, based upon collaboration, can provide partners, practice and academia with essential services for conducting and disseminating research. This provides advantages for both settings, especially considering the current restraints on funding and emphasis on increased efficiency (CR 2.98, 3.14).

2.15.7 Fry, A., Mortimer, K. & Ramsay, L. (1994) Clinical research and the culture of collaboration. *Australian Journal of Advanced Nursing*, 11 (3) 18–25 14 References

Discusses some principles and strategies which facilitated the completion of an experimental research project in South West Sydney. The inter-dependence of academic and clinical nurse practitioners is shown and a collaborative approach to research is recommended (CR 2.29).

2.15.8 Hanson, S.M.H. (1988) Collaborative research and authorship credit: beginning guidelines. *Nursing Research*, 37 (1) 49–52 14 References

Article outlines the advantages of collaborative research and discusses the issues and problems which can arise, especially for inexperienced teams (CR 2.99).

2.15.9 Hinshaw, A.S., Chance, H.C. & Atwood, J. (1981) Research in practice: a process of collaboration and negotiation. *Journal of Nursing Administration*, 11 (2) 33–8 6 References

A discussion of the problems encountered by undertaking research in a practice setting, using an actual study for illustration. Collaboration and negotiation between researcher and clinicians were found to be most important. Other issues discussed are the rights of research subjects, interpretation and use of results, risk-taking, vested interests and contribution to scientific knowledge.

2.15.10 Lancaster, J. (1985) The perils and joys of collaborative research. *Nursing Outlook*, 33 (5) 231–2, 238 3 References

The advantages and disadvantages of collaborative research are described and summed up by the author as the six Cs: communication, commitment, consensus, compatibility, credit and contribution. The issues of project leadership, interpersonal relationships, organizational and funding difficulties and publication are discussed (CR 2.99, 3.13).

2.15.11 Ludington-Hoe, S.M. & Swinth, J. (1996) A successful long-distance research collaboration. *Applied Nursing Research*, 9 (4) 219–24 15 References

Article describes the application of Lancaster's criteria for close proximity collaborative success (communication, commitment, consensus, compatibility, contribution and credit) to a successful long-distance project that evolved over eight years.

2.15.12 Mackenzie, J., Husband, C. & Gerrish, K. (1995) Researching in collaboration: a guide to successful partnership. *Nurse Researcher*, 3 (1) 82–9 1 Reference

Article discusses the essential principles which support the research process through partnership involvement in collaborative research.

2.15.13 Pittman, L., Warmuth, C., Gardner, G. & King, J. (1991) Developing a model for collaborative research. *Australian Journal of Advanced Nursing*, 8 (2) 34–40 44 References

Describes a model, designed to foster collaborative research, which will guide research projects generated by clinical nurses from conceptualization to publication (CR 2.101, 2.102).

2.15.14 Reason, P. (1994) Three approaches to participative inquiry, in Denzin, N.K. & Lincoln, Y.S. (eds), *Handbook of Qualitative Research*. Thousand Oaks, CA: Sage. ISBN 0803946791 Chapter 20, 324–39 99 References

Chapter discusses three approaches to research: co-operative inquiry, participatory action research and action inquiry. Comparisons are made and ways in which they may be integrated are discussed (CR 2.11, 2.36.13).

2.15.15 Thiele, J.E. (1989) Guidelines for collaborative research. *Applied Nursing Research*, 2 (4) 150–3 5 References

Study examined guidelines for collaborative research together with the extent of agreement and disagreement within the research groups. Author suggests that written guidelines at the outset of a project may enable difficulties to be avoided.

2.15.16 Tierney, A.J. & Taylor, J. (1991) Research in practice: an 'experiment' in researcher–practitioner collaboration. *Journal of Advanced Nursing*, 16 (5) 506–10 6 References

Describes an 'experiment' in collaboration between academic researchers and practising nurses which aimed to minimize the research/practice gap. The positive benefits are highlighted and future developments outlined (CR 3.8).

2.15.17 Yonge, O., Skillen, D.L. & Henderson, D. (1996) Collaborative research by graduate students. *Image: Journal of Nursing Scholarship*, 28 (4) 365–7   19 References

Examines the assumptions and beliefs about collaborative research and offers a definition. Ethical considerations are also suggested (CR 2.17).

2.16   THE REALITIES OF DOING RESEARCH

The conventions within research require authors to present their work in a particular order and format. This may give the impression that research is more 'tidy' than it actually is, and the difficulties may not be mentioned. This section will highlight some of the problems which may be encountered.

Annotations

2.16.1 Bass, M.J., Dunn, E.V. & Norton, P.G. (eds) (1993) *Conducting Research in the Practice Setting*. London: Sage. ISBN 0803951264   References

Discusses some of the practical considerations necessary when conducting primary care research.

2.16.2 Bell, C. & Encel, S. (eds) (1978) *Inside the Whale: Ten Personal Accounts of Social Research*. Rushcutters Bay, New South Wales: Pergamon. ISBN 0080222447   References

A collection of papers which allow a view into a normally closed world. They discuss many of the activities and factors which take place behind and around the methodology of research. The political and social issues which lie behind much research are highlighted and a wide range of styles are included to illustrate the problems, issues and constraints.

2.16.3 Brannen, J. (1993) The effects of research on participants: findings from a study of mothers and employment. *Sociological Review*, 41 (2) 328–46   19 References

Article explores a neglected topic – the effects of research on participants. A three-year longitudinal study, concerning mothers' return to the labour market after maternity leave, was followed up by asking participants to assess their experiences of the research process. Aspects studied, with implications for the subjects, were the theoretical framework and research design, the data collection methods of interviews, self-completion questionnaires, child development tests and observations. The effects of these are described (CR 2.17, 2.22, 2.48).

2.16.4 Buckeldee, J. & McMahon, R. (eds) (1994) *The Research Experience in Nursing*. London: Chapman & Hall. ISBN 0412441101   References

Book explores many of the realities of doing research through the experience of 10 researchers. Examples of dilemmas, compromises, failure and solutions are all discussed. These bring the joys and sorrows of doing research alive (CR 2.20, 2.22, 2.23, 2.26, 2.29, 2.37, 2.54, 2.68, 2.86, 2.98, 2.102, 3.8).

2.16.5 Burr, G. (1996) Unfinished business: interviewing family members of critically ill patients. *Nursing Inquiry*, 3 (3) 172–7   14 References

Author discusses some of the difficulties when conducting a qualitative research study with relatives of patients admitted to intensive care. Intense emotions were generated, helpful for some relatives but not for others, and the effects on the researcher are described. Methodological and ethical issues are discussed (CR 2.17, 2.36, 2.68).

2.16.6 Crompton, J., Kipling, J. & Sutton, L. (1995) From novice to dissertation: an experiential learning curve. *British Journal of Midwifery*, 3 (11) 612–15   2 References

Describes the journey and frustrations experienced by a group of student midwives undertaking a simulated, secondary-data research project. The research skills gained are outlined (CR 2.91, 3.17).

2.16.7 Ervin, N.E. & Dawkins, C.E. (1996)

Agency and research team co-operation: an exploration of human territoriality. *Journal of Advanced Nursing*, 23 (4) 728–32 11 References

Paper discusses potential conflicts which may arise during research projects conducted in busy community-based agencies as both private and public arenas are involved (CR 2.15, 3.16).

2.16.8 Frost, P. & Stablein, R. (eds) (1992) *Doing Exemplary Research*. Newbury Park, CA: Sage. ISBN 0803939094 References

Book takes readers on seven 'journeys' using excerpts from selected articles. It focuses on research processes rather than content in order to understand phenomena relevant to organizational life. Contributions feature re-collections by researchers on the origins, experiences and outcomes of research. The accounts and commentaries aim to demystify the research process and provide inspiration for future research (CR 2.15).

2.16.9 Hanson, E.J. (1994) Issues concerning the familiarity of researchers with the research setting. *Journal of Advanced Nursing*, 20 (5) 940–2 13 References

Author states that familiarity with a research area is not such a black and white issue as commonly presented by qualitative researchers. There are merits in having subjective knowledge of a setting and the team who work there (CR 2.36).

2.16.10 Hardey, M. & Mulhall, A. (eds) (1994) *Nursing Research: Theory and Practice*. London: Chapman & Hall. ISBN 0412498502 References

Book gathers together material reflecting the diversity and richness of research in nursing. Opportunities and constraints of different approaches are discussed and illustrated by the authors' own experiences (CR 2.1, 2.12, 2.29, 2.36, 2.52, 2.91, 2.98, 2.102).

2.16.11 Hockey, L. (1985) *Nursing Research: Mistakes and Misconceptions*. Edinburgh: Churchill Livingstone. ISBN 0443028621 References

Discusses in a light-hearted way some of the pitfalls encountered by nurse researchers and how they might be avoided.

2.16.12 Hunt, J.C. (1989) *Psychoanalytic Aspects of Fieldwork*. Newbury Park, CA: Sage. ISBN 0803934734 References

Author discusses her own experiences when interviewing colleagues and reports on the unconscious strivings, aversions and emotional conflicts which arise. The roles that these factors play when selecting, studying and constructing hypotheses about target populations are examined (CR 2.20, 2.22, 2.68).

2.16.13 Huntington, A. (1996) Nursing research reframed by the inescapable reality of practice: a personal encounter. *Nursing Inquiry*, 3 (3) 167–71 19 References

While conducting research in academia, the author returned to the clinical field to improve her nursing skills. While deeply involved in the theoretical development of the thesis, the reality of nursing practice caused major disruption in all aspects of the research. The results of this experience are described.

2.16.14 Johnson, M. (1997) Observations on the neglected concept of intervention in nursing research. *Journal of Advanced Nursing*, 25 (1) 23–9 21 References

Discusses this neglected area which may affect both quantitative and qualitative nurse researchers. The redundancy of the more popular moral frameworks for dealing with problems raised by intervention are examined, and because nursing research can be 'messy', a more reflexive and contextual approach is required. Author suggests that action research, informed by feminist thinking, has the potential to be more creative and clinically relevant (CR 2.10, 2.29, 2.36, 2.37, 3.16).

2.16.15 Kauffman, K.S. (1994) The insider/outsider dilemma: field experience of a white researcher 'getting in' a poor black community. *Nursing Research*, 43 (3) 179–83 13 References

Discusses the various processes necessary to gain access and develop the trust of a group in a senior citizen centre from a poor inner city black ghetto. Five phases of 'getting in' are described to give researchers strategies for entering groups different from themselves (CR 2.22, 2.36).

2.16.16 King, A. (1995) Giving permission to embodied knowing to inform nursing research methodology: the poetics of voice(s). *Nursing Inquiry*, 2 (4) 227–34   31 References

Paper discusses some of the realities and personal changes resulting from trying to find an authentic way to research women's experience of premenstruum. Conflicts and insecurities resulted from the pressure of academia and other experiences. Integrating the roles of being a woman, nurse and researcher enabled the author to help participants disclose their embodied knowing.

2.16.17 Lee, R.M. (1995) *Dangerous Fieldwork*. London: Sage. ISBN 0803956614 References

Book explores the contexts, settings and situations which pose high physical risks to the field worker and presents strategies for maintaining personal safety (CR 2.36).

2.16.18 Mason, R. & Boutilier, M. (1996) The challenge of genuine power sharing in participatory research: the gap between theory and practice. *Canadian Journal of Community Mental Health*, 15 (2) 145–52   16 References

Discusses the dilemmas which may arise when a complex community service organization attempts to engage in participatory research. When working with multiple partners in a particular study, power imbalances arose which were not mentioned in the literature, showing that it is a complex and elusive factor in establishing equal relations (CR 2.15, 3.8).

2.16.19 Orna, E. & Stevens, G. (1995) *Managing Information for Research*. Buckingham: Open University Press. ISBN 0335193978 References

Text provides practical information for first-time researchers, which is often omitted from conventional books on research methods. Examples from real projects are used and students are encouraged to question their work, make their own decisions and move forward at each stage in the project (CR 2.1).

2.16.20 Punch, M. (1986) *The Politics and Ethics of Fieldwork*. Newbury Park, CA: Sage. ISBN 0803925174   References

Discusses many points relating to the practical, political and ethical aspects of field work

which are not often found or explored in conventional research texts (CR 2.11, 2.17, 3.11).

2.16.21 Reed, J. & Procter, S. (eds) (1995) *Practitioner Research in Health Care: the Inside Story*. London: Chapman & Hall. ISBN 0412498103   References

Explores important elements of research processes which face health care practitioners when conducting research into their own practice. A serious gap in methodological literature is identified. Basic issues are explored, including the nature of practitioner knowledge, how this may be used and the contribution of quantitative and qualitative approaches. Several studies are reported which illustrate some difficulties encountered. Evaluating and developing practitioner research forms the final chapter (CR 2.6, 2.9, 2.25, 2.27, 2.29, 2.36, 2.42, 2.72, 2.86, 2.87, 2.98).

2.16.22 Rosnow, R.L. & Rosenthal, R. (1997) *People Studying People: Artefacts and Ethics in Behavioural Research*. New York: W.H. Freeman & Co. ISBN 0761730715 References

Book discusses how unintended or uncontrolled factors, known as artefacts, can confound the outcome of behavioural research. Examples are given from actual experiments which show how things can go wrong when real people are involved. Ways of overcoming these difficulties are discussed (CR 2.17).

2.16.23 Roth, J. (1970) Hired hand research, in Denzin, N.K. *Sociological Methods: a Sourcebook*. London: Butterworths. ISBN 0408701250 Part XIII, Chapter 35, 540–57 References

Section discusses some of the disadvantages and problems relating to the use of additional researchers in a project. Using three case studies of his own, the author shows how observers may cheat in their record-keeping, coders can be inconsistent in analysing questionnaire responses and interviewers may fill in or fabricate answers for respondents (CR 2.17, 3.16).

2.16.24 Shakespeare, P., Atkinson, D. & French, S. (eds) (1993) *Reflecting on Research Practice: Issues in Health and Social Welfare*. Buckingham: Open University Press ISBN 0335190383   References

Book covers some of the 'hidden from view' aspects of social research and explores many of the complex processes involved. Specially written accounts by 10 researchers tell real stories about undertaking research.

2.16.25 Silverman, D. (1987) *Communication and Medical Practice: Social Relations in the Clinic*. London: Sage. ISBN 0803981090 References

An account of several research studies which examined doctor–patient interactions in hospital clinics. Author believes that many research reports are too 'polished' and do not necessarily reflect reality, so the book includes detailed accounts of his feelings as a researcher, and how apparently disparate work can be woven into a whole. Key themes are how doctor–patient talk varies according to the trajectory of the patient's medical career, the method of payment for treatment, the problems implicit in paediatric medicine with children and parents as actors, and the intrinsic difficulties in reforming medical practice and making it more patient-centred.

2.16.26 Steier, F. (ed.) (1991) *Research and Reflexivity*. Thousand Oaks, CA: Sage. ISBN 0803982399 References

Explores the implications of reflexivity and self-reference in social research, including issues of responsibility for researchers. Authors believe that researchers co-produce rather than discover the worlds of their research. Their assumptions and activities are as much part of the research as the data collected from subjects and it all contributes to the final outcome (CR 2.17).

2.16.27 Tarling, M. & Crofts, L. (1997*) The Essential Researcher's Handbook for Nurses and Health Care Professionals*. London: Baillière Tindall. ISBN 0702021156 References

Book provides guidance and 'real life' insights into the processes of doing research. It bridges the gap between theoretical explanations and practical aspects of undertaking studies which are not always included in standard texts (CR 2.12, 2.14, 2.17, 2.96, 2.99, 3.13).

2.16.28 Taylor, J.S. (1993) Resolving epistemological pluralism: a personal account of the research process. *Journal of Advanced Nursing*, 18(7) 1073–6 29 References

Issues of personal and professional development experienced during a research project are discussed.

2.16.29 Thompson, S. (ed.) (1997) *Nurse Teachers as Researchers: a Reflective Reader*. London: Arnold. ISBN 0340661933 References

Book includes the reflective experiences of many researchers, bringing home the realities and difficulties which were encountered in their own projects, conducted on courses leading to a degree. A description of the research process is given which will assist first-time researchers (CR 2.4, 2.14, 3.16).

2.16.30 Walford, G. (ed.) (1991) *Doing Educational Research*. London: Routledge. ISBN 0415052904 References

Thirteen educationalists give semi-autobiographical accounts of their own research focusing on the practical and personal realities.

2.16.31 Western Australian Nurse Researchers' Network. (1994) Common problems in the clinical setting, in Robertson, J. (ed.), *Handbook of Clinical Nursing Research*. Melbourne: Churchill Livingstone. ISBN 0443048665. Chapter 6, 105–17 1 Reference

Chapter discusses some realities of doing research. These include recruitment and retention of subjects, disruption of the research setting, problems with data collection, special groups, language, cultural differences and sensitive topics (CR 2.22).

2.16.32 Whyte, W.F. (1997) *Creative Problem Solving in the Field: Reflections on a Career*. Thousand Oaks, CA: AltaMira Press. ISBN 0761989218 References

This book guides researchers through the practical problems and conceptual complexities associated with field work and recounts how they were overcome (CR 2.36).

2.17 ETHICS, THE LAW AND RESEARCH

'Health care research is central to the quest for an increased understanding, improved knowledge and generalized explanation of the complexities of all health-related issues ... research and ethical considerations are inextricably linked. The researcher must consider the implications of the proposed research, primarily for the participating subjects, but also the resulting status of knowledge and its relevance to society as a whole' (Apps & Yeomans, 1995: 55).

Definitions

Anonymity – assurance that subjects' identities will not be disclosed in any way

Confidentiality – a subject's right to privacy ... anonymity and non-disclosure of information

Covert research – carrying out research without the knowledge or consent of those being studied or by misrepresenting the role of the researcher

Deception – involves the intentional misleading of prospective subjects or withholding information from them, so that subjects believe that the procedures or objectives of the research are different from what they actually are. Deception may include deliberate presentation of false information, suppression of material information, or selection of revealed truths in a way designed to mislead

Ethics – moral principles, which in the context of research, pertain to treating subjects fairly and responsibly throughout the research process

Informed consent – ... the extent to which prospective participants are aware of the exact nature of the research and their right to agree or decline to participate without fear of loss or reprisal

Institutional Review Boards – a group of individuals who convene to review proposed and ongoing studies with the respect to ethical considerations

Research misconduct – ... significant misbehaviour that improperly appropriates the intellectual property or contributions of others, that intentionally impedes the progress of research, or that risks corrupting the scientific record or compromising the integrity of scientific practices. Such behaviours are unethical and unacceptable in proposing, conducting or reporting research, or in reviewing the proposals or research reports of others

Annotations

2.17.1 to 2.17.17 Academic Medicine (1993) 68 (9). Supplement: Integrity in biomedical research. Edited by Friedman, P.J.

The following entry differs in format as it documents a special issue of the journal *Academic Medicine*. These articles have not been annotated.

Part 1: Responsibilities and responses of academic institutions

2.17.1 Bulger, R.E. & Reiser, S.J. Studying science in the context of ethics. S5–S9 18 References

2.17.2 Caelleigh, A.S. Role of the journal editor in sustaining integrity in research. S23–S29 11 References

2.17.3 Korenman, S.G. Conflicts of interest and commercialisation of research. S18–S22

2.17.4 Krulwich, T.A., & Friedman, P.J. Integrity in the education of researchers. S14–S18 3 References

2.17.5 Sieber, J.E. Ethical considerations in planning and conducting research on human subjects. S9–S13 3 References

Part 2: Dealing with misconduct in theory and practice

2.17.6 Dresser, R. Sanctions for research misconduct: a legal perspective. S39–S43 18 References

2.17.7 Gunsalas, C.K. Institutional structures to ensure research integrity. S33–S38 7 References

2.17.8 Shore, E.G. Sanction and remediation for research misconduct: differential diagnosis, treatment and prevention. S44–S48 6 References

Part 3: Government policies and practices

2.17.9 Fields, K.L. & Price, A.R. Problems in research integrity arising from misconceptions about the ownership of research. S60–S64 5 References

2.17.10   Klein, D.F. Should the government assume scientific integrity? S56–S59 1 Reference

2.17.11   Porter, J.P. & Dustira, A.K. Policy development lessons from two federal initiatives: protecting human research subjects and handling misconduct in science. S51–S55 4 References

Part 4:   Understanding scientific misconduct and research integrity

2.17.12   Douglas, J.D. Deviance in the practice of science. S77–S83   7 References

2.17.13   Goodman, K. Intellectual property and control. S88–S91   4 References

2.17.14   Hackett, E.J. A new perspective on scientific misconduct. S72–S76   21 References

2.17.15   Jasanoff, S. Innovation and integrity in biomedical research. S91–S95   9 References

2.17.16   Pritchard, I.A. Integrity versus misconduct: learning the difference between right and wrong. S67–S71   13 References

2.17.17   Reiser, S.J. Overlooking ethics in the search for objectivity and misconduct in science. S84–S87   8 References

2.17.18   Ackerman, T.F. (1994) Medical research, society and health care ethics, in Gillon, R. (ed.), *Principles of Health Care Ethics*. Chichester: John Wiley & Sons. ISBN 0417930334 Part IV, Chapter 75, 873–84 13 References

Chapter discusses moral issues and their resolution in medical research, specifies duties to subjects, social beneficence, and provides an assessment of alternative weighting strategies.

2.17.19   Alderson, P. (1995) Consent and social context. *Nursing Ethics: an International Journal for Health Care Professionals*, 2 (4) 347–50   1 Reference

Reports some of the main contributions from a series of eight multi-disciplinary conferences on consent to health care and research, held in London during the period 1992–95.

2.17.20   American   Medical   Association:
Council on Ethical and Judicial Affairs. (1994) Ethics committees in health care institutions, in Authors, *Code of Medical Ethics: Current Opinions with Annotations*. Chicago: American   Medical   Association.   ISBN 0899706231 9.11, 140–2   References

Gives guidelines to aid in the establishment and functioning of ethics committees in hospitals and other health care institutions.

2.17.21   Anderson, B. (1990) *Methodological Errors in Medical Research*. Oxford: Blackwell   Scientific.   ISBN   0632021373 References

Author states that many clinical research papers contain methodological flaws and errors and this book is a collection of over 200 examples. The majority are from well-known journals and relate to clinical trials. Each extract is followed by an explanation of why the conclusions may be flawed, together with other possible interpretations of the data. A final chapter lists textbooks and articles dealing with methodological problems in medical research (CR 2.29, 2.99).

2.17.22   Anonymous   (1997)   Research studies: subjects have no right to sue when project is discontinued. *Legal Eagle Eye Newsletter for the Nursing Profession*, 5 (1) 5

Reports a statement, made in the United States District Court, Texas in 1996, which said that 'Research is not treatment. No former or potential future patient/participant in a medical research project has the right to sue to stop a project's discontinuation or to compel a new project' (CR 2.22).

2.17.23   Apps, J. & Yeomans, M. (1995) Ethical issues in nursing research, in Henry, I.C. & Pashley, G. (eds), *Community Ethics and Health Care Research*. Dinton, Nr Salisbury: Mark Allen. ISBN 1856420868 Chapter 5, 53–60   24 References

Chapter addresses issues that arise through carrying out nursing research. Health care research is central to the expansion of knowledge and understanding but this brings with it questions of morality.

2.17.24   Bailey, C. (1996) Ethical issues in multi-centre   collaborative   research   on breathlessness in lung cancer. *International Journal of Palliative Nursing*, 2 (2) 95–6, 98–101   11 References

Article describes the ethical issues involved in developing a multi-centre collaborative project. The relationships between the researchers and participants are identified as the focus of attention. The principles of new paradigm and action research which provide foci on the quality of interaction between researcher and participant are explored (CR 2.11, 2.15, 2.37).

2.17.25 Baldwin, J. (1994) How to gain ethical committee approval. *Modern Midwife*, 4 (11) 27–9 2 References

Author guides readers through the process of submitting research proposals to a research ethics committee (CR 2.96).

2.17.26 Batchelor, J.A. & Briggs, C.M. (1994) Subject, project or self? Thoughts on ethical dilemmas for social and medical researchers. *Social Science and Medicine*, 39 (7) 949–54 8 References

Addresses the ethical issues arising for social and medical researchers in the course of undertaking studies. Few researchers have had sufficient training in the interactional aspects of their work and may be unprepared for the dilemmas and conflict of loyalties which may occur.

2.17.27 Baum, M. (1990) The ethics of clinical research, in Byrne, P. (ed.), *Ethics and Law in Health Care and Research*. Chichester: Wiley. ISBN 0471928062 1–7 3 References

Briefly discusses the difficulties of distinguishing between quackery and sound therapy. Section also points to the manner in which the criteria of proof demanded by scientific methodology places strains on the accepted ethics of doctor/patient relationships.

2.17.28 Beauchamp, T.L. & Childress, J.F. (1994) *Principles of Biomedical Ethics* 4th edition. New York: Oxford University Press. ISBN 019508537X References

A basic text on medical ethics which includes sections on morality and moral justification, types of ethical theory, respect for autonomy, non-maleficence, beneficence, justice, professional/patient relationships, virtues and ideals in professional life. Case histories are also included.

2.17.29 Behi, R. (1995) The individual's right to informed consent. *Nurse Researcher*, 3 (1) 14–23 15 References

Discusses the factors which need to be considered by nurse researchers when inviting potential subjects to participate in research (CR 2.22).

2.17.30 Behi, R. & Nolan, M. (1995) Ethical issues in research. *British Journal of Nursing*, 4 (12) 712–16 15 References

Discusses the important issues that researchers need to resolve in order to make research ethically acceptable.

2.17.31 Berry, D.L., Dodd, M.J., Hinds, P.S. & Ferrell, B.R. (1996) Ethical issues. Informed consent: process and clinical issues. *Oncology Nursing Forum*, 23 (3) 507–12 19 References

Reviews the issues related to informed consent in a clinical cancer care setting. Strategies are suggested to improve the process and researchers are reminded that maintaining consent throughout the whole project is just as important as the patient's initial signature.

2.17.32 Blancett, S.S. (1996) Integrity and misconduct in research. *Journal of Nursing Administration*, 26 (5) 7–8 10 References

Reports on recent cases of misconduct in research, including a professor of nursing, identified by a Federal Agency. The Commission on Research Integrity was set up under the National Institute of Health Revitalization Act of 1993 to make recommendations regarding the definition, investigation, prevention of research misconduct, the role of Federal Agencies in oversight and the protection of whistleblowers. A new definition is given.

2.17.33 British Medical Association's Ethics, Science and Information Division. (1993) *Medical Ethics Today: Its Practice and Philosophy*. London: British Medical Association. ISBN 0727908170 Chapter 8, 195–229 44 References

Chapter examines potential conflicts of interest arising in research, and how attempts are made to achieve balance between the rights of individuals and the needs of society. The work of local ethics committees is also discussed.

2.17.34 Broome, M.E. & Stieglitz, K.A. (1992) The consent process and children. *Research in Nursing and Health*, 15 (2) 147–52 26 References

Concepts of consent and assent are discussed relative to developmental characteristics of children and adolescents, and implications for these procedures are discussed.

2.17.35 Bulmer, M. (ed.) (1993) *Social Research Ethics*. London: Holmes & Meier. ISBN 0841907803   References

This anthology re-examines the responsibilities of social researchers to their subjects in terms of privacy, confidentiality and ethical practice. The merits of covert participant observation are evaluated by experienced researchers in studies relating to mental patients, policemen, extremist political groups, Pentecostal sects and homosexuals. The ethical and philosophical implications of covert research are discussed. Book contains a select bibliography (CR 2.72).

2.17.36   Butler, L. (1996) Consenting to participate in research for the treatment of cancer: the patient's perspective. *Canadian Oncology Nursing Journal*, 6 (3) 124–9   18 References

Study explored cancer patients' experience with the process of consenting to participate in experimental, randomized studies, with the aim of improving and facilitating discussions between researchers and patients. Implications for nursing practice and redefining the process from the subjects' point of view are all discussed (CR 2.22, 2.29).

2.17.37 to 2.17.44 Cambridge Quarterly of Healthcare Ethics (1996) 5 (3). Special section: Rejuvenating research ethics.

The following entry differs in format as it documents a special section within the journal. These articles have not been annotated.

2.17.37   Glass, K.C. & Speyer-Ofenberg, M. Incompetent persons as research subjects. 362–72   57 References

2.17.38   Guenin, L.M. Public science and norms of truthfulness. 325–33   23 References

2.17.39   Micetich, K.C. The ethical problems

of the open-label extension study. 410–14 3 References

2.17.40   Newman, A.M. Drug trials, doctors and developing countries: towards a legal definition of informed consent. 387–99 73 References

2.17.41   Schuklenk, U. & Hogan, C. Patient access to experimental drugs and AIDS clinical trial designs: ethical issues. 400–9 53 References

2.17.42   Shamoo, A.E. & Keay, T.J. Ethical concerns about relapse studies. 373–86 51 References

2.17.43   Shuster, E. For her own good: protecting (and) neglecting women in research. 346–61   55 References

2.17.44   Weijer, C. Evolving ethical issues in the selection of subjects for clinical research. 334–45   57 References

2.17.45   Chalmers, I. (1990) Under-reporting is scientific misconduct. *Journal of American Medical Association*, 9 March, 263 (10) 1405–8   38 References

Discusses some consequences of under-reporting clinical trials, difficulties in correcting the problem after the event, how it might be tackled, and the potential role of prospective registration of trials (CR 2.29).

2.17.46   de Raeve, L. (1996) *Nursing Research: an Ethical and Legal Appraisal*. London: Baillière Tindall. ISBN 0702018880 References

Using case studies, this book explores ethical issues, together with analysing and synthesizing material from various perspectives.

2.17.47   Demi, A.S. & Warren, N.A. (1995) Issues in conducting research with vulnerable families. *Western Journal of Nursing Research*, 17 (2) 188–202   39 References

Article explores methodological and ethical issues which may occur when conducting research with vulnerable families. Examples are given from several studies to illustrate these potential dilemmas (CR 2.14).

2.17.48   DeVito Dabbs, A. & Nolan, M.T. (1997) Nurses as members of Institutional

Review Boards. *Applied Nursing Research*, 10 (2) 101–7   21 References

Article provides a brief review of the literature concerning the role of Institutional Review Boards and nurses who serve on these committees. The responsibilities of the nurse as a board member is discussed (CR 2.12).

2.17.49   Dictionary of Medical Ethics. (1981) Edited by Duncan, A.S., Dunstan, G.R. & Welbourn, R.B. London: Darton, Longman & Todd. ISBN 0232514925

A source of information on all aspects of ethics.

2.17.50   Dowd, S.B. & Wilson, B. (1995) Informed patient consent: a historical perspective. *Radiologic Technology*, 67 (2) 119–24   21 References

Reviews the concept of informed consent by examining two long-term studies – the radiation experiments sponsored by the US government beginning in the 1940s and the Tuskegee Syphilis experiment conducted from 1932 to 1972. These experiments violated informed consent guidelines and research ethics. The implications for practice today are explored.

2.17.51   Drowatzky, J.N. (1995) Ethics in research. *Clinical Kinesiology: Journal of the American Kinesiotherapy Association*, 49 (3) 72–82   18 References

Because of heavy reliance on research to develop public policy, provide medical treatments and develop new products, many pressures are put on to researchers. Increased competition for funding, and the necessity for a successful track record may lead to some researchers pursuing unethical behaviours in their quest for funding and job security. Ethical decisions need to be made at many stages in a project and to maintain public confidence researchers must recognize these and behave accordingly (CR 3.11, 3.13).

2.17.52   Eby, M.A. (1995) Ethical issues in nursing research: the wider picture. *Nurse Researcher*, 3 (1) 5–13   18 References

Reviews the history of research and ethics, ethical codes and the principles found in nursing research.

2.17.53   Elliott, D. & Stern, J.E. (eds) (1997) *Research Ethics: a Reader*. Hanover, NH: University Press of New England. ISBN 0874517974

2.17.54   Firby, P. (1995) Critiquing the ethical aspects of a study. *Nurse Researcher*, 3 (1) 35–42   14 References

Discusses the ethical issues which need to be scrutinized when assessing a research proposal and at the later stage when a study has been completed (CR 2.95, 2.96).

2.17.55   Fryer, N. (1995) Informed consent: in therapeutic practice and research, in Henry, I.C. & Pashley, G. (eds), *Community Ethics and Health Care Research*. Dinton, Nr Salisbury: Mark Allen. ISBN 1856420868, Chapter 7, 75–87   12 References

Chapter deals with central ethical issues of informed consent and discusses aspects of therapeutic and non-therapeutic practice within the health care field.

2.17.56   Gavaghan, H. (1995) Commission redefines ethical practices. *Nature Medicine*, 1 (9) 859–60   No references

Discusses the US Commission on Research Integrity's new definition of research misconduct and includes a 'bill of rights' for whistle-blowers. The process of adopting this thinking is still ongoing.

2.17.57   Gillon, R. (1997) Clinical ethics committees – pros and cons. *Journal of Medical Ethics*, 23 (4) 203–4   14 References Editorial

Identifies the nature of clinical ethics committees and asks whether countries which do not have them at present should look seriously at the pros and cons of creating them.

2.17.58   Glenister, D. (1996) Nursing research ethics: some problems and recommended changes. *NT Research*, 1 (3) 184–90   7 References

The limits of current ethical codes and guidelines are shown together with the bias shown towards nursing research from medically dominated local research ethics committees. Two strategies adopted to scrutinize nursing research are explored – those in higher education and in trusts or hospitals. Their limitations are highlighted and alternatives discussed.

2.17.59   Grodin, M.A. & Glantz, L.E. (eds) (1994) *Children as Research Subjects: Science, Ethics and the Law.* New York: Oxford University Press. ISBN 0195071034   References

An inter-disciplinary text addresses the many questions and controversies which surround the use of children as research subjects. Issues are considered in terms of biomedical science, child psychology, ethics and the law.

2.17.60   Hammick, M. (1995) *Managing the Ethical Process in Research.* Dinton, Nr Salisbury: Mark Allen Publishing. ISBN 1856420639   References

Book covers patients' rights and the ethical and moral dilemmas that face those initiating research.

2.17.61   Harrison, L. (1993) Issues related to the protection of human research participants. *Journal of Neuroscience Nursing*, 25 (3) 51–5   41 References

Discusses difficulties related to the protection of human research participants and how the Belmont Report and federal regulations can provide useful frameworks. The ultimate responsibility however lies with the investigator.

2.17.62   Harth, S.C. & Thong, Y.H. (1995) Parental perceptions and attitudes about informed consent in clinical research involving children. *Social Science and Medicine*, 40 (11) 1573–7   50 References

Sixty-four parents were interviewed after their children had been involved in a clinical drug trial for their perceptions and attitudes about informed consent. The study findings showed a considerable variation in parents' knowledge about the purpose of drug trials, amount of risk involved, purpose of consent, and that they had the right to withdraw the child at any time. The implications are discussed (CR 2.29, 2.68).

2.17.63   Hayes, G.J. (1995) Ethics committees: group process concerns and the need for research. *Cambridge Quarterly of Health Care Ethics*, 4 (1) 83–91   48 References

Author examines the development of ethics committees and what is currently known about their functioning. Decision-making strategies are discussed together with what

research methods may be appropriate for evaluating their deliberations.

2.17.64   Henry, I.C. & Pashley, G. (eds) (1995) *Community Ethics and Health Care Research.* Dinton, Nr Salisbury: Mark Allen. ISBN 1856420868   References

Book, which is designed to complement other texts, comprises two major sections: one dealing with professional ethics, management and research issues, and the other debating important aspects of applied research relating to health and social care.

2.17.65   Hodges, L. (1993) Cheats are doing just nicely, thank you. *Times Higher Education Supplement*, 26 November, No. 1099 10

Reports on a large study which examined incidents of misconduct in laboratories ranging from plagiarism, falsifying research data and withholding findings from competitors.

2.17.66   Holloway, I. & Wheeler, S. (1995) Ethical issues in qualitative research. *Nursing Ethics: an International Journal for Health Care Professionals*, 29 (3) 223–32   21 References

Explores the specific ethical problems which may occur in qualitative research where researcher and subjects develop a close relationship and roles may become blurred. The subjective and objective elements of the research may also lead to tensions and need careful consideration (CR 2.36, 3.16).

2.17.67   Hunt, G. (ed.) (1994) *Ethical Issues in Nursing.* London: Routledge. ISBN 0415081459   References

Essays set out to make ethics less abstract and issues are related specifically to the concerns of nurses.

2.17.68   Illinois Institute of Technology. (1997) *Center for the Study of Ethics in the Professions: Codes of Ethics Online Project.* URL: http://csep.iit.edu/codes/index.html

This website is still under construction. A collection of 850 codes of ethics from professional societies, corporations, government and academic institutions have been assembled and all firms or organizations have given permission for their inclusion in the database. Earlier versions of some codes will be available so their development can be studied. A literature review, an introduction to the codes and a user guide will be available (CR 2.12).

2.17.69 International Council of Nurses. (1996) *Ethical Guidelines for Nursing Research.* Geneva: International Council of Nurses. No ISBN

Booklet provides guidelines to assist member associations in establishing ethical standards in nursing research.

2.17.70 Johnson, M. (1992) A silent conspiracy: some ethical issues of participant observation in nursing research. *International Journal of Nursing Studies*, 29 (2) 213–23 24 References

Article addresses some of the moral and ethical aspects confronting researchers in clinical areas. The use of deception in data collection is explored and a study which used covert observation is examined. The responsibilities of teachers and researchers are stressed (CR 2.72).

2.17.71 Lane, S.D. (1994) Research bioethics in Egypt, in Gillon, R. (ed.), *Principles of Health Care Ethics.* Chichester: John Wiley & Sons. ISBN 0471930334 Part IV, Chapter 76, 885–94 16 References

Chapter describes the initial stages in developing a code of research bioethics for Egypt. It includes an incident which showed the need for a code, discusses the social and cultural context of Egyptian research, and addresses how the four principles which guide such codes around the world might be applied in this country.

2.17.72 Lathlean, J. (1996) Ethical issues for nursing research: a methodological focus. *NT Research*, 1 (3) 175–83 26 References

Paper examines the shared and distinctive ethical features which are pertinent to qualitative and quantitative research approaches. It focuses on the implications of the medical model in research and its implications, and the challenge where the researcher needs to control the process, together with concerns about deception, anonymity and confidentiality (CR 2.29, 2.36).

2.17.73 Lock, S. & Wells, F. (eds) (1996) *Fraud and Misconduct in Medical Research* 2nd edition. London: British Medical Association. ISBN 0727909967 References

Book, which has been revised and updated, provides a comprehensive analysis of fraud in medical research both in academic work and in General Practitioner (GP)-based clinical trials. An historical approach is taken from 1975 when the first fraud became public knowledge. Problems are viewed from the perspectives of GPs, the head of an academic unit, a contract research company director, statistician, editor and a lawyer. Mechanisms for reporting suspicions are included together with suggested ways of combating fraud. A new chapter includes material from the USA and Europe.

2.17.74 Lowes, L. (1996) Paediatric nursing and research ethics: is there a conflict? *Journal of Clinical Nursing*, 5 (2) 91–7 39 References

Paper outlines the major ethical issues which need to be considered when conducting paediatric research. An overview of ethical theories and principles highlights the difficulties which can occur about the child's ability to consent to research. The potential conflict between being researcher and practitioner at the same time is discussed.

2.17.75 Madjar, I. & Higgins, I. (1996) Of ethics committees, protocols, and behaving ethically in the field: a case study of research with elderly residents in a nursing home. *Nursing Inquiry*, 3 (3) 130–7 12 References

Discusses differing discourses of research ethics committees and the clinical research field. Experience gained during a study in a nursing home is used to highlight the tensions and inconsistencies which arise from these discourses. While keeping to the guiding principles of ethical conduct, there was need to exercise judgement and discretion and consider the well-being of participants.

2.17.76 Mander, R. (1995) Practising and preaching: confidentiality, anonymity and the researcher. *British Journal of Midwifery*, 3 (5) 289–95 25 References

Article explores the principles of confidentiality in health care and the problems this may pose for researchers. Examples are given from the author's own research.

2.17.77 Martin, J. (1996) What ethical

principles should govern the conduct of research? *NT Research*, 1 (3) 193–7 15 References

Paper examines the rights of humans to autonomy, privacy and freedom from harm and discusses how they can be applied at all stages of the research process. Potential dilemmas which nurses may encounter are also discussed.

2.17.78 Martin, P.A. (1994) Responsibilities when a patient is a research subject. *Applied Nursing Research*, 7 (3) 158–61 12 References

Article outlines the specific knowledge needs of nurses when their patients become research subjects. These are to know the rights of the subject, the agency's research policies, what the patient has been told, the possible untoward effects and expectations of staff by the researcher (CR 2.22).

2.17.79 Mason, J.K. & McCall Smith, R.A. (1994) *Law and Medical Ethics* 4th edition. New Zealand: Butterworth. ISBN 0406024782 References

Book is intended as an analysis of ethical concepts based on positive legal principles and court decisions. Most of the difficult ethical problems encountered in practice today are included and come under the headings of reproductive medicine, medical practice, death, research and experimentation, psychiatry and the law. A list of statutes, cases, major oaths, codes and declarations are included.

2.17.80 Mason, T. (1997) Censorship of research in the health service setting. *Nurse Researcher*, 4 (4) 83–92   11 References

Provides an overview of the meaning of sensitive topics, the types of threat perceived or which may occur and their context. The types, technology and means of resisting censorship are all discussed (CR 2.14).

2.17.81 McHaffie, H. (1996) Ethics and midwifery. *Modern Midwife*, 6 (10) 34–5

Discusses the dilemmas researchers may face when tackling sensitive issues.

2.17.82 Merrell, J. (1995) Beneficence, respect for autonomy: principles in practice. *Nurse Researcher*, 3 (1) 24–34   35 References

Discusses the relationships between researcher and researched, together with the wider political context and outcomes of research.

2.17.83 Millar, B. (1997) Honesty on trial. *Nursing Times*, 27 August, 93 (35) 10–11   No references

Reports a recent case of clinical research fraud where a doctor falsified information during clinical trials. Action taken by a nurse to expose this is outlined (CR 2.29).

2.17.84 Miller, D.J. & Hersen, M. (eds) (1992) *Research Fraud in the Behavioural and Biomedical Sciences.* New York: Wiley. ISBN 0471520683   References

Book aims to fill a gap for students who have received little scholarly exposure to ethical issues in research. Its four parts cover general issues, the human investigator factor, system considerations and safeguards, and suggested directions for the future.

2.17.85 Mitchell, R.G. (1993) *Secrecy and Fieldwork.* Newbury Park, CA: Sage. ISBN 0803943849   References

Examines the methodological and ethical issues in covert field research (CR 2.16, 2.36).

2.17.86 Mitchell, T. & Fletcher, I. (1998) Stating the case for nursing research ethics committees: a discussion paper. *Nurse Education Today*, 18 (2) 133–7 15 References

Paper considers one centre's response to creating a nurse-led ethics committee to function in a symbiotic relationship with its medical counterpart. The arguments for and against are put forward and authors believe that nurse-led groups are more tolerant of the diversity of research proposals received from nurses. The viability of such groups is explored in light of the major changes in nurse education, and although regionally based multi-disciplinary groups are being created, authors believe that local groups should be retained.

2.17.87 Neuberger, J. (1992) *Ethics and Health Care: the Role of Research Ethics Committees in the UK.* London: King's Fund Institute. ISBN 1870607295 References Research report No. 13

Material based on research carried out by

postal questionnaire to members of research ethics committees, interviews with a sub-sample of chairpersons and observations of committees at work. The history, growth and past research on ethical committees are outlined together with their composition, functioning and policy issues. Specific issues are explored and recommendations included (CR 2.68, 2.72, 2.75).

2.17.88 Paddison, J. (1995) Ethical issues in qualitative studies. *Modern Midwife*, 5 (5) 23–5   12 References

Reports the moral dilemma which arose when collecting data in a unit where the researcher was known (CR 2.36).

2.17.89 Pence, T. (1986) *Ethics in Nursing: an Annotated Bibliography* 2nd edition. New York: National League for Nursing. ISBN 0887371922

Contains 1,324 citations from 1965 to 1985. References are mainly to American literature but some British sources are also included. Several citations refer to the ethics of nursing research.

2.17.90 Pinch, W.J. (1996) Research and nursing: ethical reflections. *N & H Perspectives on Community* 17 (1) 26–31   24 References

Discusses the ethical responsibility which needs to extend to the role of the dominant research paradigm, the research agenda and women as research subjects.

2.17.91 Rankin, M. & Esteves, M.D. (1997) Perceptions of scientific misconduct in nursing. *Nursing Research*, 46 (5) 270–6 26 References

Reports that attempts are being made to refine policies and procedures for handling allegations of scientific misconduct because of recent concerns.

2.17.92 Raudonis, B.M. (1992) Ethical considerations in qualitative research with hospice patients. *Qualitative Health Research*, 2 (2) 238–49   21 References

Article addresses three ethical issues in qualitative research with hospice patients. These are use of vulnerable populations, inherent role conflict in clinical research and informed versus process consent (CR 2.36).

2.17.93 Ringheim, K. (1995) Ethical issues in social science research with special reference to sexual behaviour research. *Social Science and Medicine*, 40 (12) 1691–7

Beginning with the philosophical origins of ethical principles, the paper discusses the key factors to be considered when conducting social science research. These are special precautions when adolescents are subjects, informed consent procedures and the formation and function of an ethical review committee.

2.17.94 Robinson, K. (1991) The layman's role in a research ethics committee. *Journal of the Royal College of Physicians* (London), 25 43   No references

The role and contribution of laypersons sitting on research ethics committees is discussed.

2.17.95 Robley, L.R. (1995) The ethics of qualitative research. *Journal of Professional Nursing*, 11 (1) 45–8   19 References

Discusses the many factors which need to be taken into account when undertaking qualitative research. Some of the less obvious, but very important, are highlighted (CR 2.36).

2.17.96 Rosenberg, S.A. & Barry, J.M. (1992) *The Transformed Cell: Unlocking the Mysteries of Cancer*. London: Chapmans. ISBN 1855926113 61–2

The Chief of Surgery at the US National Cancer Institute comments on the objectivity of scientific literature. He urges caution as some articles contain results which are wrong and not reproducible, while others stretch the results beyond that which their evidence supports. Judgements have to be made at many stages in the course of experimental research, and achievements depend as much on these as the actual techniques used (CR 2.29).

2.17.97 Royal College of Nursing of the United Kingdom. (1998) *Research Ethics: Guidance for Nurses Involved in Research or any Investigative Project Involving Human Subjects*. London: Baillière Tindall. No ISBN

This booklet provides guidelines for nurses undertaking research, those in positions of authority where research may be carried out, in clinical areas, commissioning, supervising and using research findings. It includes a bibliography of key texts and website addresses.

2.17.98   Royal College of Physicians. (1996) *Guidelines on the Practice of Ethics Committees in Medical Research involving Human Subjects* 3rd edition. London: RCP. ISBN 1860160425

A detailed and comprehensive guide to the role, functions and responsibilities of ethics committees is provided. The membership, terms of reference, scope, methods of working and of referral to the committee and its responsibilities in law are all examined. Issues of consent, therapeutic trials, research involving vulnerable groups, healthy volunteers and foetuses, payment for participation in trials and injuries due to clinical investigations are all fully explored.

2.17.99   Sadleir, G. & Robertson, J. (1994) Satisfying ethics committees, in Robertson, J. (ed.), *Handbook of Clinical Nursing Research.* Melbourne: Churchill Livingstone. ISBN 0443048665 Chapter 4, 49–66   2 References

Describes the composition of institutional ethics committees (IECs) in Australia, their roles, functions and expectations. Issues which may influence a decision to approve a research protocol are discussed from the perspective of a committee chairman and a research applicant.

2.17.100   Saunders, C.M., Baum, M. & Houghton, J. (1994) Consent, research and the doctor–patient relationship, in Gillon, R. (ed.), *Principles of Health Care Ethics.* Chichester: John Wiley & Sons. ISBN 0471930334 Part II, Chapter 40, 457–69 39 References

Chapter examines the ethical implications of undertaking clinical trials. Examples are given when particular difficulties arose and ways forward are suggested (CR 2.29).

2.17.101   Scharer, K. (1996) Researching sensitive issues in child psychiatric nursing: ethical concerns. *Journal of Child and Adolescent Psychiatric Nursing*, 9 (3) 17–27 38 References

Paper defines sensitive research and explores the ethical issues which need to be considered when undertaking research in the field of child psychiatric nursing.

2.17.102   Seedhouse, D. & Lovett, L. (1992) *Practical Medical Ethics.* Chichester: Wiley. ISBN 0471928437   References

Book, designed for students and practising doctors, aims to present a range of problems from clinical practice and teach decision-making methods. Reasons why doctors should study ethics are explored, and two instruments – the ethical grid and algorithm – are presented and applied through use of 15 cases.

2.17.103   Sharpe, G. & Weisstub, D.N. (1996) The ethics of deception in biomedical research. *Health Law in Canada*, 16 (4) 101–10 [ISBN 0433394897]   41 Notes and References

Discusses the exchange of information, the covetal bond, the legal dimension and relationship between researcher and subject. A definition of deception and a case study are given for illustration.

2.17.104   Siegler, M., Singer, P.A. & Schiedermayer, D.L. (1988) *Medical Ethics: an Annotated Bibliography.* London: British Medical Journal. ISBN 094312610X   References

190 articles are listed, organized by issues. Annotated articles with a clinical focus have been drawn from medical and ethics literature (CR 1.5).

2.17.105   Silva, M.C. (1995) *Ethical Guidelines in the Conduct, Dissemination and Implementation of Nursing Research.* Washington, DC: American Nurses Association. ISBN 1558101098

2.17.106   Sim, J. (1991) Nursing research: is there an obligation on subjects to participate? *Journal of Advanced Nursing*, 16 (11) 1284–9 21 References

Outlines the points which researchers need to consider about subjects' obligations to participate in any project. Three models of obligation are discussed: the notion of payment, the social contract, and establishing an unconditional contract. The conflicting relationship between obligation and consent is examined (CR 2.22).

2.17.107   Singleton, J. & McLaren, S. (1995) Ethical issues in health care research, in Authors, *Ethical Foundations of Health Care: Responsibilities in Decision Making.* London: Mosby. ISBN 072341873X. Chapter 13, 117–25   12 References

Chapter identifies the ethical principles inherent in health care research, discusses how research workers can act to promote the wellbeing of subjects and how their autonomy can be respected. The role of ethical committees is also discussed.

2.17.108 Smith, T., Moore, E.J.H. & Tunstall-Pedoe, H. (1997) Review by a local medical research ethics committee of the conduct of approved research projects by examination of patients' case notes, consent forms, research records and by interview. *British Medical Journal*, 31 May, 314 (7094) 1588–90 9 References

Reports a study which examined the conduct of 30 previously approved projects in Scotland. Some problems highlighted were obtaining/recording consent correctly, poor records and filing. Adverse events were reported, but there was a failure to notify the committee when projects were abandoned or not started, and in two instances the investigators failed to notify a change in the responsible researcher.

2.17.109 Springhouse Corporation. (1992) *Nurses Handbook of Law and Ethics.* Springhouse, PA: Springhouse Corporation. ISBN 0874343933 References

Covers nursing practice and the law in the USA, patients' rights, legal risks and responsibilities, legal risks off duty and malpractice liability. Legal aspects of documentation, nurses' rights as employees, ethical decision-making, and conflicts in clinical and professional practice are also explored. Appendices contain types of law, understanding the judicial process, information on how to interpret legal citations and a court case citation index.

2.17.110 Thompson, A. (1994) Towards a code of ethics ... International Confederation of Midwives. *Modern Midwife*, 4 (1) 27–8 2 References

Reports on the code of ethics adopted by the International Confederation of Midwives which aims to provide a position statement of midwives' beliefs and values.

2.17.111 Tierney, A. (1995) The role of research ethics committees. *Nurse Researcher*, 3 (1) 43–52 6 References

Examines the composition and function of local research ethics committees. Their future is also discussed as the ethics of research become more complex.

2.17.112 Titus, L.M. (1995) CNA ethics survey published ... 'Nursing ethics committees – where are they?' [June 1994 in *Nursing Management*] *Connecticut Nursing News*, 68 (4) 1

Reports the results of a survey which ascertained the number of nursing ethics committees which existed within the state. A resource pack has been developed to guide those setting up such a group. Although institutional ethics committees exist, author believes that specific nursing issues are not always appropriately addressed.

2.17.113 Tranter, J. (1997) The patient's rights in clinical research. *Professional Nurse*, 12 (5) 335–7 7 References

Author urges nurses taking part in research to become fully acquainted with the proper procedures, the pitfalls to watch out for, and the rights of the participants.

2.17.114 Tunna, K. (1997) Research and patient's rights. *Practice Nurse*, 13 (9) 531, 534–6 5 References

Outlines the ethical principles which must be considered when undertaking research.

2.17.115 Veatch, R.M. & Fry, S.T. (1995) *Case Studies in Nursing Ethics.* Sudbury, MA: Jones & Bartlett. ISBN 0867204818 References

Volume contains a collection of cases focusing on the ethical problems faced by nurses. It is divided into three parts: ethics and values in nursing; ethical principles; and special problem areas in nursing practice.

2.17.116 Verheggen, F.W.S., Jonkers, R. & Kok, G. (1996) Patients' perceptions on informed consent and the quality of information disclosure in clinical trials. *Patient Education and Counseling*, 29 (2) 137–53 13 References

Reports a survey on 26 clinical trials which studied how patients experience and evaluate the information disclosure on the clinical trials they are enrolled in, and which factors influence their perceptions. The objective was to obtain more insight into how informed consent is applied in the daily practice of clinical trials. Results are reported and authors have developed a patient motive classification based on criteria identified in the study. An informed decision checklist is suggested as a general outline for patient education (CR 2.29).

2.17.117 Vessey, J.A. & Campos, R.G. (1992) The role of the nursing research committee. *Nursing Research*, 41 (4) 247–9 4 References

Explores the role of, and problems with, nursing research committees and discusses ways in which they can facilitate clinical research.

2.17.118 Warren, R. & Allan, J. (1997) Clinical note: Getting through ethics committees: partnerships between researchers and clinicians working with mentally ill clients. *Australian and New Zealand Journal of Mental Health Nursing*, 6 (1) 37–43 11 References

Discusses the principles of ethics in nursing research when working with people suffering from mental illness. A set of protocols is offered which have been successful in gaining ethical approval to conduct research in this field.

2.17.119 Weiss, R.J. (1980) The use and abuse of deception. *American Journal of Public Health*, 70 (10) 1097–8 3 References

Paper refers to a research project where pseudo-patients are used to evaluate the quality of care. Author feels that such deception is unjustified and discusses some of the moral and ethical issues involved.

2.17.120 Weisstub, D.N. & Moorhouse, A. (1996) Advance directives for research: ethical guidelines. *Health Law in Canada*, 17 (1) 3–10 [ISBN 0433402458] 20 References

Discusses the ethical conflict between researchers and health care professionals which may occur when the subject is unable to give consent to research. With specific restrictions proposed, the use of advance research directives should provide a resolution to this difficulty.

2.17.121 Weymuller, E.A. Jr. (1996) A consideration of ethical issues in the design of clinical trials. *American Journal of Otolaryngology*, 17 (1) 2–11 26 References

Article discusses selected highlights of the modern history and current status of the application of ethical principles to the performance of clinical trials. It also shows that the dominant theme is the protection of subjects in an investigation where they may be coerced and unwittingly expose themselves to risk (CR 2.29).

2.17.122 Williams, A. (1997) Pitfalls on the road to ethical approval. *Nurse Researcher*, 5 (1) 15–22 6 References

Offers advice to those submitting research proposals to ethics committees. Four main points discussed are: the need to be well informed about local ethics committees; thoroughness in the attention to detail of submitted proposals; being prepared to speak knowledgeably about the proposal and surrounding issues; and making any amendments necessary (CR 2.96).

2.17.123 Zink, M.R. & Titus, L. (1997) Nursing ethics committees: do we need them?, in McCloskey, J.C. & Grace, H.K. (eds), *Current Issues in Nursing* 5th edition. St Louis: Mosby. ISBN 0815185944 Chapter 86, 640–6 27 References

Chapter discusses the need for, and functions of, nursing ethics committees. Authors believe they can empower nurses in their role as advocates as they prepare for more effective ethical deliberations with other health care professionals.

2.18 DEFINING THE PROBLEM

'The term problem may be a misnomer ... Rather than calling it the "problem statement", it might be clearer if we call it "the need for study" ... These needs may be based on personal experience with an issue, job-related problems, an adviser's research agenda, and/or the scholarly literature ... the strongest and most scholarly rationale for a study ... follows from a documented need in the literature for increased understanding and dialogue about an issue.' (Cresswell, 1998: 94) [adapted]

Definition

Problem statement – the statement of the research problem that identifies the key research variables, specifies the nature of the population, and suggests the possibility of empirical testing

---

Example

Moody, L., Vera, H., Blanks, C. & Visscher, M. (1989) Developing questions of substance for nursing science. *Western Journal of Nursing Research*, 11 (4) 393–404   15 References

Describes a study undertaken to establish, from leading nurse researchers, the sources and origins of their ideas, devices for finding and developing researchable questions or hypotheses, and how they decided which were significant for the discipline. Focused interviews were conducted by telephone and data analysed by computer. Data showed that significant questions are those aimed at nursing intervention and clinical research and that students need to be guided early to find those important to nursing (CR 2.20, 2.70, 2.84).

Annotations

2.18.1 Baldamus, W. (1979) Alienation, anomie and industrial accidents, in Wilson, M. (ed.), *Social and Educational Research in Action: a Book of Readings*. London: Longman, in association with the Open University Press. ISBN 058229004X Section 2, Reading 6, 104–40   References

This paper, by a social scientist, is rare in that it reports the very early stages of a major research project. It takes the reader to the position where an idea begins, before it is known whether there is a problem worth researching or what it might be. The focus is on the startling rise in industrial accidents reported to the Factory Inspectorate in the 1960s and the similarity between the variation by days of the week in the patterns of absenteeism and industrial accidents. More widely, methodological issues in studies on social change are explored and a preliminary assessment of the use and limitations of sociological time-series studies is made.

2.18.2 Butterworth, T. (1994) Developing research ideas: from theory to practice. *Nurse Researcher*, 1 (4) 78–86   24 References

Discusses the development of a research idea

which took place over many years. The subject of psychosocial intervention in schizophrenia is used to illustrate some of the processes involved in translating theory to practice.

2.18.3 Campbell, J.P., Daft, R.L. & Hulin, C.L. (1982) *What to Study: Generating and Developing Research Questions.* Beverly Hills, CA: Sage. ISBN 0803918720   References

A teaching device intended to examine what is being investigated, versus what should be. Book discusses how research questions are developed, gives a list of ideas for consideration, suggests ways of reformulating research questions and how difficulties may be avoided. Some resource materials are also included.

2.18.4 Cresswell, J.W. (1998) Introducing and focusing the study, in Author, *Qualitative Inquiry and Research Design: Choosing among Five Traditions*. Thousand Oaks, CA: Sage. ISBN 0761901442 Chapter 6, 93–107 References

Chapter discusses the problem and purpose statements and research questions (CR 2.36.11).

2.18.5 Fleming, J.W. (1984) Selecting a clinical nursing problem for research. *Image: Journal of Nursing Scholarship*, 16 (2) 62–4 5 References

A series of questions are identified which will assist in the appropriate selection of problems.

2.18.6 Hinds, P.S., Gattuso, J.S., Norville, R., Oakes, L. & Prichard, L. (1992) Bedside clinical research: a new category of research. *Clinical Nursing Research*, 1 (2) 169–79 12 References

Describes a type of clinical research which authors label 'bedside nursing research'. Features which characterize and separate it from the traditional view between research and practice are outlined. Examples and limitations are discussed together with issues that affect its conduct (CR 2.102).

2.18.7 Jorgensen, D.L. (1989) Defining a problem, in Author, *Participant Observation: a Methodology for Human Studies*. Newbury Park, CA: Sage. ISBN 0803928777 Chapter 2, 26–39

Chapter illustrates the logic and process of defining a problem. Procedures for formulating concepts and specifying indicators are outlined and exemplified. The process of problem definition is located within the human context of values, politics and ethics of research (CR 2.17, 2.72.12).

2.18.8 Liehr, P. (1992) Prelude to research. *Nursing Science Quarterly*, 5 (3) 102–3 6 References

Discusses where ideas may come from for subsequent research. Two examples show how some initial observations developed into researchable questions.

2.18.9 Martin, P.A. (1994) The utility of the research problem statement. *Applied Nursing Research*, 7 (1) 47–9 6 References

Discusses the value of a carefully formatted research problem statement and identifies the root of confusion which exists. Some helpful approaches are suggested.

2.18.10 Miles, J. (1994) Defining the research question, in Buckeldee, J. & McMahon, R. (eds), *The Research Experience in Nursing*. London: Chapman & Hall. ISBN 0412441101 Chapter 3, 31–46 12 References

Identifies some of the processes required when defining and developing appropriate, researchable questions in a project investigating creativity in nursing (CR 2.16.4).

2.18.11 Vaughan, B. (1991) Identifying clinical problems for research. *Surgical Nurse*, 4 (4) 10–12 10 References

Article examines sources of research questions, where to start, how to refine the question and clarify the purpose of a study.

2.19 IDENTIFICATION OF VARIABLES

Variables are those factors, events or behaviour about which information is desired, and which may be studied in isolation or in combination. They can be examined in their natural setting or be manipulated to see if a particular response is evoked. During a study unknown variables may arise which may affect the data collected.

Definitions

Construct – an hypothetical term designed to clarify and give meaning to behaviour. A construct cannot be observed but must be operationally defined by either an independent or dependent variable

Dependent variable – dependent upon or caused by another variable. It is *not* controlled by the researcher

Extraneous variable – when some factor produces error that becomes systematic and directional in nature

Independent variable – believed to cause or influence the dependent variable. In experimental studies it *is* manipulated by the researcher

Intervening variable – a third variable in a trivariate study that logically falls in a time sequence between the independent and dependent variables

Operational definition – links theoretical constructs with the real world by identifying what phenomena (empirical indicators/referents) will be observed and how they will be measured

Variable – factor within a situation which can change or be changed

Annotations

2.19.1 Beck, C.T. (1994) Achieving statistical power through research design sensitivity. *Journal of Advanced Nursing*, 20 (5) 912–16 9 References

Paper addresses a variety of factors and techniques, other than increasing sample size, that nurse researchers can use to enhance the sensitivity of a research design so that it can attain adequate statistical power (CR 2.87).

2.19.2 Burgess, R.G. (ed.) (1986) *Key Variables in Social Investigation*. London: Routledge & Kegan Paul. ISBN 0710099010 References

A series of papers which examine the relationship between theory and research, the identification of concepts and their translation into variables. Health and illness are two key variables explored.

2.19.3 Newell, N. (1994) Defining variables and hypotheses. *Nurse Researcher*, 1 (4) 37–47 4 References

The key features which govern the activities of researchers on the crucial steps of defining variables and hypotheses are outlined (CR 2.20).

2.20 FORMULATING HYPOTHESES OR RESEARCH QUESTIONS

A frequent goal in scientific research is to test an hypothesis which may be concerned with explaining relationships between observations or differences between groups. Some projects do not have hypotheses as they have different objectives. These may be guided by research questions and/or objectives.

Definitions

Alternative hypothesis – an hypothesis that is pitted against the null hypothesis. It usually emerges from theory and is the hypothesis that the investigator usually believes to be true prior to carrying out the research
Hypothesis – a conjecture about the relationships between two or more concepts
Null hypothesis – a logical assumption that there is no relationship between the two variables being studied in the population
Research objective – states the goal(s) of a study which is intended to describe rather than predict

Annotations

2.20.1 Harloe, L.J., Greenway, M.N., O'Connor, S., Fowle, T., Hayes, K., Pendall, D., Stewart, C., Squires, L., Bond, M. & White, K. (1995) Generating ideas for research: an Australian experience. *Gastroenterology Nursing*, 18 (4) 138–41 14 References

The nursing staff in an Australian gastroenterology unit describe their experience in defining a research project (CR 3.20).

2.20.2 La Schinger, H.K.S., Docherty, S. & Dennis, C. (1992) Helping students use nursing models to guide research. *Nurse Educator*, 17 (2) 36–8 8 References

Describes a strategy which enabled third-year undergraduate students to understand the importance of putting nursing research questions within a theoretical framework. Examples are given of questions before and after application of a model. Difficulties encountered are discussed.

2.20.3 Sutherland, H.J., Meslin, E.M., da Cunha, R. & Till, J.E. (1993) Judging clinical research questions: what criteria are used? *Social Science and Medicine*, 37 (12) 1427–30 13 References

Paper suggests that criteria for evaluating the merits of study questions or hypotheses have received little attention. A set of non-methodological criteria were generated from interviews with 40 researchers who were clinical investigators and laboratory scientists.

2.21 SELECTING A RESEARCH DESIGN

'The design is a blueprint for conducting research. It contains plans for collecting, organising and analysing the data. The choice of design depends on the purposes of the study but it is generally approached from a descriptive or experimental perspective. Research is never as perfect as we would like, every type of design involves compromise and error.' (Phillips, L.R.F., 1986: xiii).

Definition

Research design – the overall plan of research intended to yield specific, unambiguous answers to research questions or to allow useful hypotheses to emerge

Annotations

2.21.1 Hakim, C. (1993) *Research Design: Strategies and Choices in the Design of Social Research.* London: Routledge. ISBN 041507911X References

Text deals with all aspects of the design of social research covering both theoretical and policy research. The key features, strengths and limitations of nine main types of design are discussed. These are: literature reviews; secondary analysis and meta-analysis of existing data; qualitative research; analysis of administrative records; ad hoc sample surveys; regular surveys; case studies; longitudinal studies; and experimental social research. The focus is not on how to do any type of research, but when and why a particular design should be chosen. The second part of the book focuses on more general issues such as potential difficulties and possible solutions, obtaining research funding and designing and managing research programmes (CR 2.12, 2.29, 2.36, 2.39, 2.48, 2.52, 2.79, 2.91, 2.92, 3.13).

2.21.2 Lathlean, J. (1994) Choosing an appropriate methodology, in Buckeldee, J. & McMahon, R. (eds), *The Research Experience in Nursing*. London: Chapman & Hall. ISBN 0412441101 Chapter 3, 31–46   12 References

Chapter explores the issues faced when making decisions about methodology initially and during a research project. Two projects are used for illustration: one is an evaluation of an innovative training scheme for ward sisters; and the other an ongoing study of lecturer/practitioners in nursing (CR 2.16.4, 2.37, 2.42).

2.21.3 Leatt, P. (1986) Descriptive and experimental approaches to nursing problems: issues in design, in Stinson, S.M. & Kerr, J.C. (eds), *International Issues in Nursing Research*. Beckenham: Croom Helm. ISBN 0709944373 Part 1, Chapter 1, 1–27   References

Chapter discusses the purposes, types and complexity of research designs appropriate for studying a practice discipline. The major types of research design are discussed using the concept of a continuum of control and each is illustrated by existing studies (CR 3.22.12).

2.21.4 Steenbarger, B.N. & Manchester, R.A. (1996) Designing the study. *Journal of the American College of Health*, 44 (5) 201–5

2.22 POPULATIONS AND SAMPLES

Nursing research is usually concerned with people and the intention of researchers is to say something about them and their responses to a health care system. Careful identification and description of the population, together with appropriate sample selection techniques, are important steps in any research design.

Definitions

Populations

Population – the portion of the universe to which the researcher has access
Population element – a single member of a population
Population stratum – a population contained within another population
Target population – all the cases that meet a designated set of criteria
Subject – . . . the person who is being studied
Universe – all possible respondents or measures of a certain kind

Sampling

Sampling – the process of selecting a few elements from a population. These elements are expected to stand for all those within the population. The way in which this is done allows one to generalize the sample findings to a population, or does not allow one to do so. Sampling strategies are divided into two major groups:

Non-probability sampling techniques

Convenience (accidental) sample – sample obtained by accessing individuals who are easy to identify and contact
Purposive sample – cases to be included are hand-picked for their experience or knowledge or some other characteristic of interest to the researcher
Quota sample – sample aimed at ensuring adequate representation of underlying groups, e.g. age or ethnic groups
Snowball sample – selection is carried out by word of mouth. The first people contacted are asked to name others with similar characteristics

Probability sampling techniques

Cluster sample – groups of population elements with the same characteristics are chosen rather than individuals
Simple random sample – obtained using a

table of random numbers, or some other means, and each population element has an equal probability of being selected
Stratified random sample – population divided into sub-groups called strata, from which a simple random sample is obtained
Systematic random sample – obtained by taking every *N*th (selection interval) name on a population list

---

Annotations

2.22.1 Akers, J.A. & Bell, S.K. (1994) Should children be used as research subjects? *Nursing Forum*, 29 (3) 28–33   14 References

Authors explore the question of whether children should be used as research subjects (CR 2.17).

2.22.2 Annandale, E. & Lampard, R. (1993) Sampling in non-experimental research. *Nursing Standard*, 31 March 7 (28) 34–6   5 References

Decisions which have to be made about sampling in quantitative and qualitative research are discussed. Illustration is provided by an hypothetical study (CR 2.29, 2.36).

2.22.3 Arber, S. (1993) Designing samples, in Gilbert, N. (ed.), *Researching Social Life*. London: Sage. ISBN 0803986823 Chapter 5, 68–92   References

Chapter focuses on sampling for surveys although it is equally relevant for other types of research design (CR 2.1.25, 2.28, 2.52).

2.22.4 Bach, C.A. & McDaniel, R.W. (1995) Pearls, pith and provocation: techniques for conducting research with quadriplegic adults residing in the community. *Qualitative Health Research*, 5 (2) 250–5   4 References

Discusses techniques for recruitment of subjects and collection of data from people with quadriplegia. Strategies for increasing numbers and designing specific research tools are discussed together with suggestions for enhancing the effectiveness of group meetings. These strategies may also be useful with other client groups.

2.22.5 Barnett, V. (1994) *Sample Survey: Principles and Methods*. London: Edward Arnold. ISBN 0470233893

Text gives an overview of probability sampling and practical advice on carrying out a survey (CR 2.52).

2.22.6 Baron, S., Gilloran, A. & Schad, D. (1995) Researching with nurses and patients: from subjects to collaborators. *Social Sciences in Health: International Journal of Research and Practice*, 1 (3) 175–88   47 References

Reports on methodological aspects of research into new ways of assessing quality of care for those with special needs. Existing models are examined, but authors believe that those with special needs should themselves specify what quality of care means. This creates a new form of professional space for the nurses and different forms of researcher–researched relations (CR 3.16).

2.22.7 Blacktop, J. (1996) A discussion of different types of sampling techniques. *Nurse Researcher*, 3 (4) 5–15   11 References

Discusses the considerations which need to be made when selecting samples, together with methods of purposive probability and multistage sampling.

2.22.8 Blenner, J.L. (1992) Navigating the institutional labyrinth: clinical research strategies. *Applied Nursing Research*, 5 (3) 149–53   3 References

Article aims to help nurse researchers gain access and maintain their presence in large-scale institutions. Potential obstacles are discussed, and strategies developed by the author in hospital settings are described.

2.22.9 Faugier, J. & Sargeant, M. (1997) Sampling hard to reach populations. *Journal of Advanced Nursing*, 26 (4) 790–7   36 References

Paper examines the advantages and limitations of non-random methods of data collection such as snowball sampling. It reviews the literature on sampling hard-to-reach populations and highlights the dearth of research about the subject. The potential for using these methods in nursing research is discussed and a current example is used to illustrate the problems (CR 2.17).

2.22.10 Floyd, J.A. (1993) Systematic sampling: theory and clinical methods. *Nursing Research*, 42 (5) 290–3   14 References

Examines the systematic sampling procedure, its advantages, issues involved, the problem with variances, detection and management of departures with randomness.

2.22.11   Hague, P. & Harris, P. (1993) *Sampling and Statistics.* London: Kogan Page ISBN 0749409169   References

Book, intended for beginners and experienced market researchers, discusses how to make sense of figures and choose a sample. The subject of forecasting is introduced with the application of correlation and time series (CR 2.52, 2.75, 2.94).

2.22.12   Hautman, M.A. & Bomar, P. (1995) Interactional model for recruiting ethnically diverse research participants. *Journal of Multicultural Nursing and Health*, 1 (4) 8–15, 27   62 References

Paper explores the issues concerning the researcher, participants, site and community that promotes research sensitive to the needs of all. Specific recruitment and retention strategies are proposed to ensure diversity of ethnic and cultural backgrounds and encompass the assumptions that caring, reciprocity, trust, sensitivity and involvement influence all aspects of the research process (CR 3.16).

2.22.13   Hek, G. (1995) Sampling techniques in research. *Journal of Community Nursing*, 9 (3) 4–6   4 References

Article explains the complexities of sampling in research.

2.22.14   Henry, G.T. (1990) *Practical Sampling.* Newbury Park, CA: Sage. ISBN 0803929595   References

Book covers sample selection approaches, designs, frames, techniques, size and post-sampling choices.

2.22.15   Hill, P.D. & Humenick, S.S. (1995) Technical notes. Comparison of subjects who fully versus minimally participated in a breast feeding study. *Western Journal of Nursing Research*, 17 (3) 328–34   6 References

Sampling bias occurs when a large percentage of subjects who are eligible for a study refuse to participate. During the first phase of a multi-site Mother–Baby Feeding Project, approximately 50 per cent of the 235 potential participants declined to participate. The report

compares subjects who fully participated with those who minimally participated and explores factors which affected their refusal. Findings led to insight being gained into the problem of subject recruitment (CR 2.27).

2.22.16   Hillier, V. & Gibbs, A. (1996) Calculations to determine sample size. *Nurse Researcher*, 3 (4) 27–34   3 References

Article explains the process of estimating sample size as part of research study design.

2.22.17   Kelly, P.J. & Cordell, J.R. (1996) Recruitment of women into research studies: a nursing perspective. *Clinical Nurse Specialist*, 10 (1) 25–8   26 References

Article examines the barriers that exist to women participating in clinical trials and outlines strategies that nurses working in HIV research settings can develop to reduce them (CR 2.29).

2.22.18   Lancet. (1992) Volunteering for research. *Lancet*, 3 October, 340 (8823) 823–4 3 References Editorial

Discusses considerations necessary when selecting subjects for medical research, reasons why they may refuse and the responsibilities of doctors (CR 2.17).

2.22.19   Larson, E. (1994) Exclusion of certain groups from clinical research. *Image: Journal of Nursing Scholarship*, Fall, 26 (3) 185–90   20 References

Reports a review of 754 approved research protocols from one tertiary care centre in 1989/90 to examine demographic characteristics of subjects. Some groups had been excluded without identifiable justification from these protocols. The design implications of this are discussed.

2.22.20   Le Roux, B. (1996) The effect of statistical sampling error on reliability and validity. *Nurse Researcher*, 3 (4) 36–51   No references

Describes in detail how sampling error occurs and the effects it may have on results (CR 2.24, 2.25).

2.22.21   Maisel, R. & Hodges Purcell, C. (1996) *How Sampling Works.* Thousand Oaks, CA: Pine Forge Press. ISBN 0803990618   References

Book provides an elementary introduction to the theoretical and practical aspects of sampling for undergraduates.

2.22.22 Martin, P.A. (1993) Agency access to a targeted research population. *Applied Nursing Research*, 6 (4) 184–6   7 References

Gives guidance on selecting an agency or setting and suggests how researchers can improve their chances of gaining access (CR 2.17).

2.22.23 Martin, P.A. (1995) Recruitment of research subjects. *Applied Nursing Research*, 8 (1) 50–4   26 References

Discusses four major issues in the recruitment of research subjects: population characteristics that assist or deter recruitment efforts; population characteristics that contribute to an increased vulnerability of subjects; role conflict between practitioner and researcher; and participation motivation and time-frame barriers to recruitment plans (CR 3.16).

2.22.24 Minkes, J., Townsley, R., Weston, C. & Williams, C. (1995) Having a voice: involving people with learning difficulties in research. *Mental Handicap*, 23 (3) 94–7   10 References

Summarizes a symposium presented at the 1993 British Institute of Learning Disabilities Conference by researchers based at the Norah Fry Research Centre, University of Bristol. Article argues that the traditional model of research where detached observers set the agenda and findings are presented to colleagues should not be the only acceptable approach to research. Several pieces of work are cited where the involvement of people with learning difficulties were included at every stage of the research process. Authors believe that better research resulted which would be more beneficial to the subjects.

2.22.25 Morse, J.M. (1991) Strategies for sampling, in Morse, J.M. (ed.), *Qualitative Nursing Research: a Contemporary Dialogue* Revised edition. Newbury Park, CA: Sage. ISBN 0803940793. Chapter 8, 127–45   21 References

Discusses types of sample, the qualities of a good informant, methods for evaluating samples, researcher control over sampling and special problems which may arise.

2.22.26 Newell, R. (1993) Sampling and distribution issues. *Nurse Researcher*, 1 (2) 33–43   8 References

Article discusses different types of sample, sample size and three ways of distributing questionnaires – directly, by mail, or over the telephone. Steps to increase response rates are listed (CR 2.75).

2.22.27 Newell, R. (1996) The reliability and validity of samples. *Nurse Researcher*, 3 (4) 16–26   8 References

Discusses the importance of assessing the reliability and validity of a sample when conducting research (CR 2.24, 2.25).

2.22.28 Nolan, K. (1994) People with AIDS: finding and accessing a hidden sample, in Buckeldee, J. & McMahon, R. (eds), *The Research Experience in Nursing*. London: Chapman & Hall. ISBN 0412441101 Chapter 4, 47–62   12 References

Chapter looks at the realities of sampling, in particular accessing a hidden and vulnerable group of people with HIV and AIDS. Lessons to be learned are identified (CR 2.16.4, 2.23).

2.22.29 Pieper, B. (1996) Who is being missed in ostomy research? *Journal of WOCN*, 23 (4) 205–9   32 References

Article compares people who were or were not included in a research study about living with an ostomy. Those not included were too physically ill to be independent in care, were paralysed or mentally ill. Author believes that an ethnically diverse sample should be included together with special populations such as those in psychiatric units, rehabilitation units or long-term care facilities.

2.22.30 Pletsch, P.K., Howe, C. & Tenney, M. (1995) Recruitment of minority subjects for intervention research. *Image: Journal of Nursing Scholarship*, 27 (3) 211–15   23 References

Discusses use of a recruitment plan that consisted of a feasibility analysis, recruitment strategies and activities. Article reports on how an evaluation programme was developed and used for a smoking cessation study of pregnant Latinos. The success of this plan is discussed.

2.22.31 Polit, D.F. & Sherman, R.E. (1990)

Statistical power in nursing research. *Nursing Research*, 39 (6) 365–9   10 References

Sixty-two articles published in *Nursing Research* and *Research in Nursing and Health* in 1989 were analysed. Results showed that many had insufficient power to detect real effects, probably because of small samples (CR 2.87).

2.22.32   Reed, J., Procter, S. & Murray, S. (1996) A sampling strategy for qualitative research. *Nurse Researcher*, 3 (4) 52–68   8 References

Discusses the use of an explicit, systematic sampling strategy which can enhance the value of qualitative research (CR 2.36).

2.22.33   Rothenberg, R.B. (1995) Commentary: sampling in social networks. *Connections*, 18 (1) 105–11   References

Discusses the mathematical aspects of snowball, multiplicity and targeted sampling.

2.22.34   Rushforth, D. (1994) The adaptation of an experimental sampling procedure for application in naturalistic psychiatric nursing research settings. *Journal of Advanced Nursing*, 19 (5) 932–7   22 References

Discusses the value of the Buglass scale and minimization in the context of a quasi-experimental study which examined the management of deliberate self-harm by community psychiatric nurses. The scope for control of extraneous variables without sacrificing the naturalistic setting within which psychiatric nurses operate is explored and a worked example is given (CR 2.35).

2.22.35   Sandelowski, M. (1995) Sample size in qualitative research. *Research in Nursing and Health*, 18 (2) 179–83   22 References

Article discusses the adequacy of sample size in qualitative research, issues in purposive sampling, sampling sizes for different qualitative studies and in combined qualitative and quantitative work.

2.22.36   Sim, J. (1991) Nursing research: is there an obligation on subjects to participate? *Journal of Advanced Nursing*, 16 (11) 1284–9   21 References

Article discusses whether individuals are under any obligation at all to participate as subjects in nursing research. Three models of

such an obligation are explored: one based on payment, one on the social contract, and another which seeks to establish an unconditional obligation. Each is seen to be flawed. The conflicting relationships between obligations and consent are examined (CR 2.17).

2.22.37   Som, R.K. (1995) *Practical Sampling Techniques* 2nd edition. Basel: Marcel Dekker Inc. ISBN 0824796764

2.22.38   Spilker, B. & Cramer, J.A. (1992) *Patient Recruitment in Clinical Trials*. New York: Raven Press. ISBN 0881679313 References

Book focuses on clinical trials and developing strategies for successful recruitment. Parts cover the elements of recruitment, putting them together and consequences of the issues (CR 2.29).

2.22.39   Stewart, M.J. (1989) Target populations of nursing research on social support. *International Journal of Nursing Studies*, 26 (2) 115–29   136 References

Sixty-three empirical studies carried out over the last decade were examined to ascertain their target populations. Nurses have tended to study populations central to their professional activities and those examined related to surgical patients, the chronically ill, expectant couples, parents of infants, the bereaved and lay care-givers. Author believes there are several groups which have been overlooked, e.g. children, males, native peoples, the poor, unemployed and the victims of child and elderly abuse.

2.22.40   Sullivan, K. (1996) Experiences with a volunteer sample. *Nurse Researcher*, 3 (4) 69–76   5 References

Article discusses the pros and cons of volunteer samples, how to gain access, ethical considerations and the personal safety of the researcher (CR 2.17).

2.22.41   Williams, H.A. (1996) The silent ones: a review of sampling issues and biases pertinent to the area of pediatric oncology procedural pain. *Journal of Pediatric Oncology Nursing*, 13 (1) 31–9   76 References

Article presents a review of the past 10 years' literature on the phenomenon of pain in children. Author believes that the sociocultural influences of pain need to be studied and suggestions are made for improving sampling designs (CR 2.12, 2.27).

2.22.42 Wineman, N.M. & Durand, E. (1992) Incentives and rewards for subjects in nursing research. *Western Journal of Nursing Research*, 14 (4) 526–31   11 References

Discusses the use of incentives and rewards in recruiting research subjects together with potential administrative and ethical problems (CR 2.17).

2.22.43 Wray, J. & Gates, B. (1996) Problems of recruiting participants for nursing research: a case study. *NT Research*, 1 (5) 366–74   31 References

Authors believe that literature on recruiting subjects is a neglected area, but one which has profound effects on any research study. General guidelines are identified which will help researchers adopt effective strategies.

2.23   PILOT STUDIES

Pilot studies are undertaken to assess the feasibility of a planned study, adequacy of the instrumentation, and problems in data collection strategies and proposed methods. Other potential uses may be to answer a methodological question, or as part of the development of a research plan.

Definition

Pilot study – a small-scale preliminary study undertaken to test the feasibility of the proposed research and to improve the procedures and methods of measurement

Example

Glasson, J.E. (1995) A descriptive and exploratory pilot study into school reentrance for adolescents who have received treatment for cancer. *Journal of Advanced Nursing*, 22 (4) 753–8   29 References

Study examined problems encountered by adolescents on their return to school following treatment for cancer. Areas requiring further work were identified (CR 2.45, 2.68).

Annotations

2.23.1 Hinds, P. & Gattuso, J. (1991) From pilot work to a major study in cancer nursing research. *Cancer Nursing*, 14 (3) 132–5   17 References

The unique contributions and limitations of pilot studies are described. A study is used for illustration, and the impact made by the pilot study in the development of a three-year study is discussed.

2.23.2 Lackey, N.R. & Wingate, A.L. (1998) The pilot study: one key to research success, in Brink, P.J. & Wood, M.J.A. (eds), *Advanced Design in Nursing Research*. Newbury Park, CA: Sage. ISBN 0803958005 References

Chapter defines a pilot study, its philosophies and purposes. Discusses conducting the study and evaluating the results (CR 2.36.5).

2.23.3 Mason, D.J. & Zuercher, S.L. (1995) Pilot studies in clinical nursing research. *Journal of the New York State Nurses' Association*, 26 (2) 11–13   8 References

Describes the purposes of pilot studies, their potential positive and negative outcomes and gives three examples which had different outcomes. Issues relating to clinical nursing research are emphasized.

2.23.4 Ort, S.V. (1981) Research design: pilot study, in Krampitz, S.D. & Pavlovich, N. (eds), *Readings for Nursing Research*. St Louis: Mosby. ISBN 0801627478. Chapter 6, 49–53   References

Discusses the purposes and characteristics of a pilot study, its design and implementation. Ethical aspects are covered, reliability and validity of instruments, potential difficulties and guidelines are given for developing the study (CR 2.17, 2.24, 2.25).

2.23.5 Prescott, P.A. & Soeken, K.L. (1989) The potential uses of pilot work. *Nursing Research*, 38 (1) 60–2   3 References

Following a review of published studies and research texts, the authors reported that pilot studies are under-discussed, under-used and under-reported. Article focuses on the separate components within a main study, and highlights the contribution of pilot work to each. Although increasing the time spent in preparation for a study, it enables defects to be corrected which cannot be removed or remedied after the study has commenced.

2.23.6   Read, S., George, S., Westlake, L., Williams, B., Glasgow, J. & Potter, T. (1992) Piloting an evaluation of triage. *International Journal of Nursing Studies*, 29 (3) 275–88 78 References

Examines the problems facing accident and emergency departments, triage theory and research in the USA, and its introduction in the UK. A pilot study is discussed and the necessity for exhaustive work at this stage is examined.

2.23.7   Richardson, A. (1994) Piloting a study, in Buckeldee, J. & McMahon, R. (eds), *The Research Experience in Nursing*. London: Chapman & Hall. ISBN 0412441101. Chapter 5, 63–81   22 References

Chapter makes some general points about pilot studies from the literature. Author then describes some of the complexities and dilemmas encountered during a study which examined behaviour, initiated by patients, to control chemotherapy-induced nausea and vomiting (CR 2.16.4).

2.24   RELIABILITY

'Reliability and validity are two major characteristics which need to be considered when undertaking both quantitative and qualitative research. The criteria for these need to be differentiated as the purpose, goals and intent of each type of research are different. Many students are taught to use quantitative reliability and validity criteria for qualitative studies. This is inappropriate and results in confusion' (Leininger, 1985: 35).

The item below outlines the essential difference between the focus of reliability in quantitative and qualitative research:

Quantitative research
Focus is on measuring tool or its ability to assess the degree of consistency or accuracy with which it measures an attribute.

Qualitative research
Focus is on identifying and documenting features and phenomena in similar or different contexts.

Definitions

Inter-rater (inter-observer) reliability – the degree to which two raters or observers, operating independently, assign the same ratings or values for an attribute being measured or observed
Intra-observer (rater) reliability – . . . reproducibility of a set of observations on one variable made by the same observer at different times
Reliability – the extent to which a test would give consistent results if applied more than once to the same people under standard conditions
Split-half reliability – a set of items is divided in half and the two halves are correlated
Test–retest reliability – an approach to reliability that compares two administrations of the same measuring instrument

Annotations

2.24.1   Behi, R. & Nolan, M. (1995) Reliability: consistency and accuracy in measurement. *British Journal of Nursing*, 4 (8) 472–5   8 References

Explores the issue of reliability in measurement.

2.24.2   Brennan, P.F. & Hays, B.J. (1992) The Kappa statistic for establishing inter-rater reliability in the secondary analysis of qualitative clinical data. *Research in Nursing and Health*, 15 (2) 153–8   23 References

The nature and computation of Kappa and its application in analysis of clinical data are discussed (2.82, 2.89, 2.94).

2.24.3   Brink, P.J. (1991) Issues of reliability and validity, in Morse, J.M. (ed.), *Qualitative Nursing Research: a Contemporary Dialogue* Revised edition. Newbury Park, CA: Sage. ISBN 0803940793 Chapter 10, 164–86 51 References

Discusses many aspects of, and issues relating to, the reliability and validity of research (CR 2.25).

2.24.4   Carmines, E.G. & Zeller, R.A. (1979) *Reliability and Validity Assessment*. Beverly Hills, CA: Sage. ISBN 0803913710   References

A basic text which introduces the issues in

measurement theory. The concepts of reliability and validity are thoroughly discussed in light of current debate (CR 2.25).

2.24.5 Gates, B. (1996) Issues of reliability and validity in the measurement of challenging (behavioural difficulties) in learning disability: a discussion of the implications for nursing and practice. *Journal of Clinical Nursing*, 5 (1) 7–12 22 References

Article discusses a number of practical, theoretical and methodological issues relating to measuring challenging behaviour (CR 2.25, 2.57).

2.24.6 Gloth, F.M. III, Walston, J., Meyer, J. & Pearson, J. (1995) Reliability and validity of the Frail Elderly Functional Assessment Questionnaire. *American Journal of Physical Medicine and Rehabilitation*, 74 (1) 45–53 19 References

Reports a study which aimed to test the validity and reliability of an assessment questionnaire for the frail elderly. Initial data showed it to be valid and reliable (CR 2.25, 2.55).

2.24.7 Hinds, P.S., Scandrett-Hibden, S. & McAulay, L.S. (1990) Further assessment of a method to estimate reliability and validity of qualitative research findings. *Journal of Advanced Nursing*, 15 (4) 430–5 26 References

Discusses the use of an evaluative strategy with qualitative data in order to assess the reliability and validity of findings. Four qualitative studies are briefly outlined to illustrate the technique and ways of interpreting the results are explored (CR 2.25, 2.36).

2.24.8 Kirk, J. & Miller, M.L. (1986) *Reliability and Validity in Qualitative Research*. Beverly Hills, CA: Sage. ISBN 0803924704 References

Book concerns itself with the issues surrounding the scientific status of field data (CR 2.25, 2.36).

2.24.9 Knapp, T.R. (1985) Validity, reliability and neither. *Nursing Research*, 34 (3) 189–92 18 References

Explores the misuse of the terms reliability and validity. Author believes that too liberal a use is made of these technical terms (CR 2.25).

2.24.10 Laschinger, H.K.S. (1992) Intra-class correlations as estimates of inter-rater reliability in research. *Western Journal of Nursing Research*, 14 (2) 246–51 6 References

Article provides a brief description of the intra-class correlation coefficient, a lesser known measure of reliability.

2.24.11 Nolan, M. & Behi, R. (1995) Alternative approaches to establishing reliability and validity. *British Journal of Nursing*, 4 (10) 587–90 13 References

Article considers a variety of alternatives to the classic notions of reliability and validity. Authors believe there are no hard-and-fast rules that can be applied to all research studies and authentic research depends on the paradigm within which a study is conducted (CR 2.25).

2.24.12 Peräkyla, A. (1997) Reliability and validity in research based on transcripts, in Silverman, D. (ed.), *Qualitative Research: Theory, Method and Practice*. London: Sage. ISBN 0803976666 Part VI, Chapter 13, 201–20 68 References

Chapter deals with issues of reliability and validity in research based on tapes and transcripts and, in particular, in conversation analysis (CR 2.25, 2.28, 2.36.59, 2.89).

2.24.13 Ryan, J.W., Phillips, C.Y. & Prescott, P.A. (1988) Inter-rater reliability: the underdeveloped role of rater training. *Applied Nursing Research*, 1 (3) 148–50 No references

Discusses the process of establishing inter-rater reliability by developing a category scheme which has levels that are independent, mutually exclusive and exhaustive; training raters to use this scheme; evaluating them and then assuming reliability in the setting for which the measure was designed.

2.24.14 Traub, R.E. (1994) *Reliability for the Social Sciences: Theory and Applications*. Thousand Oaks, CA: Sage. ISBN 0803943253 References

Integrates theory and application of classic approaches to measurement reliability. Practical advice is given on the estimation of reliability and its statistics.

2.24.15. Yonge, O. & Stewin, L. (1988) Reliability and validity: misnomers for qualitative research. *Canadian Journal of Nursing Research* (Nursing Papers), (20) 2 61–7 21 References

Authors discuss their belief that the terms 'reliability' and 'validity' should not be applied to qualitative research methods. The essential differences, rigour in qualitative methods and the challenges are discussed (CR 2.25).

2.25 VALIDITY

The second major property required in any measuring instrument, in addition to reliability, is that of validity. The researcher should try to ensure that any existing tools that are used fulfil the required criteria and information on this should be sought prior to their use. The item below outlines the essential difference between the focus of validity in quantitative and qualitative research.

Quantitative research
Focus is on measurement.

Qualitative research
Focus is on gaining knowledge and understanding of the phenomena under study.

Definitions

Concurrent validity – a test or question is said to have concurrent validity if it correlates well with other measures of the same concept
Construct validity – the degree to which a test measures the desired characteristic or construct of interest. It is estimated by validating the theory underlying the instrument
Content validity – the degree to which the desired domain (content) is adequately sampled and represented in the instrument. Also considered is the adequacy of the operational definition of the domain being sampled
Convergent validity – a test or question has convergent validity when several dissimilar measures of the same concept correlate well with it
Criterion-related validity – the degree to which the instrument correlates with external variables or criteria believed to measure the concept under investigation. Concurrent and predictive validity are two types
External validity – the ability to generalize or frame a single study to other populations and conditions
Internal validity – the ability to believe in the conclusion that is drawn based on the design of the study. To assess this, one asks if the treatment did indeed make a difference
Member validation – an array of techniques that purport to validate findings by demonstrating a correspondence between the researcher's analysis and the collectivity members' descriptions of their social worlds
Predictive validity – the degree to which an instrument can predict a criterion observed at a future time
Qualitative validity – is concerned with confirming the truth or understandings associated with phenomena
Validity – the degree to which an instrument measures what it is intended to measure (in qualitative research validity refers to the extent to which the research findings represent reality)

Annotations

2.25.1 Andrews, M., Lyne, P. & Riley, E. (1996) Validity in qualitative health research: an exploration of the impact of individual researchers' perspectives within collaborative enquiry. *Journal of Advanced Nursing*, 23 (3) 441–7 19 References

Paper explores the problem of validity in qualitative inquiry and reports a review of published strategies for analysing interview data (CR 2.15, 2.36, 2.68).

2.25.2 Benfer, R.A., Brent, E.E. Jr. & Furbee, L. (1991) *Expert Systems*. Newbury Park, CA: Sage. ISBN 080394036X References

Discusses the process of expert systems development as a model for acquiring, representing and validating knowledge about relatively limited domains.

2.25.3 Bloor, M. (1997) Techniques of validation in qualitative research: a critical commentary, in Miller, G. & Dingwall, R. (eds), *Context and Method in Qualitative Research*. London: Sage. ISBN 0803976321 Part 1, Chapter 3, 37–50 References

Discusses the problems inherent in validating qualitative research, including triangulation and member validation. Examples are given examining these attempts to validate data and the difficulties which ensued. Author believes that neither technique can validate findings but both are relevant to the issue of validity (CR 2.26, 2.36.40).

2.25.4 Eby, M. (1993) Validation: choosing a test to fit the design. *Nurse Researcher*, 1 (2) 26–32   9 References

Discusses reliability and validity when developing questionnaires (CR 2.23, 2.24, 2.55, 2.75).

2.25.5 Ferketich, S.L., Figueredo, A.J. & Knapp, T.R. (1991) The multi-trait–multi-method approach to construct validity. *Research in Nursing and Health*, 14 (4) 315–20 7 References

Discusses the method and selected problems of this approach and proposes an alternative.

2.25.6 Goodwin, L.D. & Goodwin, W.L. (1991) Estimating construct validity *Research in Nursing and Health*, 14 (3) 235–43 56 References

Article discusses the meaning and estimation of construct validity. Authors urge cautious interpretation of construct validity evidence for many existing instruments.

2.25.7 Imle, M.A. & Atwood, J.R. (1988) Retaining qualitative validity while gaining quantitative reliability and validity: development of the Transition to Parenthood Concerns Scale. *Advances in Nursing Science*, 11 (1) 61–75   26 References

Discusses the nature of validity in qualitative research and suggests ways of developing the reliability and validity associated with quantitative research. A set of procedures for testing qualitative scales is described and these provide a base for item and scale revisions and formal quantitative testing (CR 2.24, 2.29, 2.36, 2.55).

2.25.8 Jayasuriya, R. & Caputi, P. (1996) Computer attitude and computer anxiety in nursing: validation of an instrument using an Australian sample . . . Nurses Computer Attitude Inventory (NCATT) Computer Attitude Scale (CATT). *Computers in Nursing*, 14 (6) 340–5   23 References

Reports a study which was designed to test and refine the reliability and validity of the above instrument. Results are reported and authors believe that the revised NCATT instrument may be of value in assessing nurses' attitudes prior to computer training (CR 2.24, 2.84).

2.25.9 Kahn, D.L. (1993) Ways of discussing validity in qualitative nursing research. *Western Journal of Nursing Research*, 15 (1) 122–6   17 References

Explores ways of establishing validity in qualitative research (CR 2.36).

2.25.10 Lowe, N.K. & Ryan-Wenger, N.M. (1992) Beyond Campbell and Fiske: assessment of convergence and discriminant validity. *Research in Nursing and Health*, 15 (1) 67–75   37 References

Article reviews this method of assessing convergent and discriminant validity, examines its applications in nursing literature, and describes limitations of the original method. The procedures, strengths and limitations of analysis of variance and confirmatory factor analysis approaches to the quantification of Campbell & Fiske's criteria are described.

2.25.11 McBride, S.H. & Nagle, L.M. (1996) Attitudes toward computers: a test of construct validity . . . Stronge and Brodt's Nurses' Attitudes Towards Computerization questionnaire. *Computers in Nursing*, 14 (3) 164–70   15 References

394 registered nurses and 299 baccalaureate students completed the Stronge and Brodt's questionnaire. Findings are reported and further work suggested.

2.25.12 McDaniel, C. (1988) Aspects of validity in clinical nursing research. *Applied Nursing Research*, 1 (2) 99–103   3 References

Discusses validity in field settings and the main interaction effects related to it.

2.25.13 Nolan, M. & Behi, R. (1995) Validity: a concept at the heart of research. *British Journal of Nursing*, 4 (9) 530–3   10 References

Discusses the nature and different forms of validity and explores the relationships between validity and reliability.

2.25.14   Reason, P. & Rowan, J. (eds) (1981) Issues of validity in new paradigm research, in Authors, *Human Inquiry: a Sourcebook of New Paradigm Research.* Chichester: Wiley. ISBN 0417279358 Chapter 21, 239–50   References

Chapter gathers together material from a number of sources in order to create a coherent statement about the principles and practices which lead to a more valid inquiry within new paradigm research (CR 2.11.9).

2.25.15   Rew, L., Stuppy, D. & Becker, H. (1988) Construct validity in instrument development: a vital link between nursing practice, research and theory. *Advances in Nursing Science*, 10 (4) 10–22   24 References

Author examined 17 articles published in *Advances in Nursing Science* for evidence of construct validity which provide links between practice, research and theory. Fourteen provided such evidence, with factor analysis being the most commonly used method. Findings indicated the need to develop further links between the three areas (CR 2.55).

2.25.16   Silverman, D. (1997) The logics of qualitative research, in Miller, G. & Dingwall, R. (eds), *Context and Method in Qualitative Research.* London: Sage. ISBN 0803976321 Part 1, Chapter 1, 12–25   References

Discusses the relationships between quantitative and qualitative methods and the problems of characterizing research using multiple techniques. Two examples are given which describe human–computer interaction and doctor–patient interviews in a cancer department to illustrate some of the dilemmas raised (CR 2.9, 2.24, 2.36.40, 2.68).

2.25.17   Thomas, S.D., Hathaway, D.K. & Arnheart, K.L. (1992) Face validity. *Western Journal of Nursing Research*, 14 (1) 109–12 13 References

Discusses the significance of measuring face validity in clinical research instrumentation and documents the measured dimensions of face validity.

2.26   TRIANGULATION

'The purpose of using triangulation is to provide a basis for convergence on truth. By using multiple methods and perspectives it is hoped that "true" information can be sorted from "error" information'. (Polit & Hungler, 1995: 362)

Definitions

Data triangulation – use of a variety of multiple data sources in a study (e.g. interviewing multiple key informants about the same topic)

Inter-disciplinary triangulation – . . . using other disciplines . . . to inform research processes . . . which may broaden . . . understanding of method and substance

Investigator triangulation – use of many individuals to collect and analyse a single set of data

Methodological triangulation – use of multiple methods to study a single problem (e.g. observation, interviews, inspection of documents)

Theory triangulation – use of multiple perspectives to interpret a single set of data

Triangulation – the use of different research methods or sources of data to examine the same problem

Example

Webb, C. & Pontin, D. (1996) Introducing primary care nursing: nurses' opinions. *Journal of Clinical Nursing*, 5 (6) 351–8 33 References

Reports one aspect of a research project which aimed to monitor and evaluate the introduction of primary nursing in one health authority. Multiple triangulation methods were used to obtain the data.

Annotations

2.26.1   Banik, B.J. (1993) Applying triangulation in nursing research. *Applied Nursing Research*, 6 (1) 47–52   19 References

Discusses four types of triangulation: theory; data; investigator and methodological. A study is used for illustration.

2.26.2   Begley, C.M. (1996a) Triangulation of communication skills in qualitative research instruments. *Journal of Advanced Nursing*, 24 (4) 688–93   27 References

Discusses the value of using triangulation as a method of conducting research. Using the concept within qualitative research instruments is highlighted and the benefits outlined. (CR 2.36).

2.26.3 Begley, C.M. (1996b) Using triangulation in nursing research. *Journal of Advanced Nursing*, 24 (1) 122–8   35 References

The five types of triangulation are described and their advantages and disadvantages discussed. The triangulation 'state of mind', consciously using multiple sources and methods to cross-check and validate findings, will increase the value of research.

2.26.4 Bergen, A. (1994) Experiences of method triangulation, in Buckeldee, J. & McMahon, R. (eds), *The Research Experience in Nursing*. London: Chapman & Hall. ISBN 0412441101. Chapter 8, 115–30   9 References

Chapter explores methodological issues with triangulation, the contradictions within a particular study, and offers some explanations (CR 2.16.4).

2.26.5 Bradley, S. (1995) Methodological triangulation in healthcare research. *Nurse Researcher*, 3 (2) 81–9   20 References

The value and problems of using triangulation in research studies are explored.

2.26.6 Breitmayer, B.J., Ayres, L. & Knafl, K.A. (1993) Triangulation in qualitative research: evaluation of completeness and confirmative process. *Image: Journal of Nursing Scholarship*, 25 (3) 237–43   34 References

Triangulated approaches are not always shown to have contributed to confirmation or completeness of a data set. Paper reviews these and describes how triangulation of qualitative and quantitative methods were built into a study to achieve them (CR 2.36, 2.86, 2.87).

2.26.7 Campbell, D.T. & Fiske, D.W. (1959) Convergent and discriminant validation by the multitrait–multimethod matrix. *Psychological Bulletin*, 56 (2) 81–105   References

A seminal paper advocating the use of cumulative evaluations rather than single methods of measurement.

2.26.8 Cowman, S. (1993) Triangulation: a means of reconciliation in nursing research. *Journal of Advanced Nursing*, 18 (5) 788–92   22 References

Discusses the use of triangulation as a research strategy in relation to the quantitative/qualitative debate. The types are outlined and their advantages and disadvantages are examined (CR 2.9, 2.29, 2.36).

2.26.9 Dootson, S. (1995) An in-depth study of triangulation. *Journal of Advanced Nursing*, 22 (1) 183–7   27 References

Article describes multiple triangulation methods and shows how care is needed to identify the paradigm underlying the work in order to avoid confusion.

2.26.10 Foster, R.J. (1997) Addressing epistemological and practical issues in multimethod research: a procedure for concept triangulation. *Advances in Nursing Science*, 20 (2) 1–12   47 References

Author states that little information exists on the combination of quantitative and qualitative methods. Conceptual triangulation offers one approach to multi-method research, addressing both epistemological and practical issues. This article offers some advice.

2.26.11 Hamilton, D. & Bechtel, G.A. (1996) Research implications for alternative health therapies. *Nursing Forum*, 31 (1) 6–10   18 References

Authors discuss the implications for triangulation techniques in nursing research related to non-traditional treatments. Six types of triangulation are defined and methods for using them are explained.

2.26.12 Jick, T.D. (1983) Mixing qualitative and quantitative methods: triangulation in action, in Van Maanen, J. (ed.), *Qualitative Methodology*. Newbury Park, CA: Sage. ISBN 0803921179 135–48   References

Chapter defines triangulation, provides an illustration of how it works, discusses whether there is convergence in the data, and outlines its advantages and disadvantages (CR 2.36).

2.26.13 Jones, W. (1996) Triangulation in clinical practice. *Journal of Clinical Nursing*, 5 (5) 319–23   3 References

Article clarifies the term triangulation. Examples are given to illustrate its use and strengths in both the design and analysis stages of a project.

2.26.14 Kimchi, J., Polivka, B. & Stevenson, J.S. (1991) Triangulation: operational definitions. *Nursing Research*, 40 (6) 364–6 11 References

Presents operational definitions for types of triangulation described by Denzin. An example of each type is given (CR 2.7.5).

2.26.15 Knafl, K.A. & Breitmayer, B.J. (1991) Triangulation in qualitative research: issues of conceptual clarity and purpose, in Morse J.M. (ed.), *Qualitative Nursing Research: a Contemporary Dialogue* Revised edition. Newbury Park, CA: Sage. ISBN 0803940793 Chapter 13, 226–39 32 References

Chapter discusses the origin, development and applications of triangulation.

2.26.16 Morse, J.M. (1991) Approaches to qualitative/quantitative methodological triangulation. *Nursing Research*, 40 (2) 120–3 16 References

Explores the principles underlying the use of methodological triangulation when combining qualitative and quantitative methods.

2.26.17 Nolan, M. & Behi, R. (1995) Triangulation: the best of all worlds. *British Journal of Nursing*, 4 (14) 829–32 18 References

Discusses the concept of triangulation, its meaning, types and purposes together with barriers to applying this approach.

2.26.18 Redfern, S.J. & Norman, I.J. (1994) Validity through triangulation. *Nurse Researcher*, 2 (2) 41–56 17 References

Discusses the purpose, types, limitations, strengths and challenges of triangulation. A recent study is used for illustration (CR 2.25, 2.72).

2.26.19 Sandelowski, M. (1995) Triangles and crystals: the geometry of qualitative research. *Research in Nursing and Health*, 18 (6) 569–74 43 References

Author believes that triangulation is being used inappropriately as a 'catch all' method,

which was not originally intended in the surveying context. 'The concept of triangulation should be reserved for designating a technique for confirmation, employed within paradigms, in which convergent and consensual validity are valued, and in which it is deemed appropriate to use information from one source to corroborate another' (Sandelowski 1995: 573) (CR 2.25, 2.36, 2.52).

2.26.20 Sim, J. & Sharp, K. (1998) A critical appraisal of the role of triangulation in nursing research. *International Journal of Nursing Studies*, 35 (1/2) 23–31 41 References

Triangulation raises a number of issues and some of these are discussed. Authors urge caution when using this approach.

2.27 BIAS

A major consideration at many stages in any research project is the possibility of bias. If this factor is not taken into account, then the results may be distorted.

Definition

Bias – any influence that produces a distortion in the results of a study

Example

Brick, J.M., Waksberg, J. & Kulp, D. (1995) Bias in list-assisted telephone samples. *Public Opinion Quarterly*, 59 (2) 218–35 References

Study examined the coverage bias for a particular method of list-assisted sampling as an alternative to random digit dialling. Results showed that although about 4 per cent of the population are excluded, the coverage bias differences were small (CR 2.22, 2.70).

Annotations

2.27.1 Cook, A.S. (1997) Investigator bias in bereavement research: ethical and methodological implications. *Canadian Journal of Nursing Research*, 29(4) 87–93 21 References

Article discusses types of investigator bias in bereavement research: emotional, normative, cultural and professional. Recognition of these factors will enable resulting research to be more credible (CR 2.17).

2.27.2 Dieckman, E.A. (1993) A procedural check for researcher bias in an ethnographic report. *Research in Education*, November, 50 1–4   6 References

Reports the use of a type of psychoanalysis as an alternative way of guarding against bias in data collection. Methodology, participants, materials and procedures are outlined (CR 2.42).

2.27.3 Hammersley, M. & Gomm, R. (1997) Bias in social research. *Sociological Research Online*, 2 (1)
URL: http://www.socresonline.org.uk/socresonline/2/1/2.html   73 References

Discusses the ambiguous nature of the term 'bias' and the problems which result from this. Authors see the growing threat of bias in the present state of social research (CR 2.27.7).

2.27.4 Haskins, A.R., Rose-St Prix, C. & Elbaum, L. (1997) Covert bias in evaluation of physical therapist students' clinical perform ance … including commentary by Simpson, S.D., Jensen, G.M., Brown, K. & Woodruff, L.D. with author response. *Physical Therapy*, 77 (2) 155–68   47 References

Study aimed to determine whether covert bias exists in the evaluative judgements of physical therapy practitioners. A convenience sample of 83 physical therapists (73 white, 3 black and 7 Hispanic) attending a conference were videotaped reading identical scripts about a patient's status. Ratings were given on a specially developed form. Results showed that the black students consistently received low ratings, indicating that racial or ethnic bias may influence the opinions of physical therapy practitioners.

2.27.5 Hughes, L.C. & Preski, S. (1997) Focus on qualitative methods. Using key informant methods in organizational survey research for informant bias. *Research in Nursing and Health*, 20 (1) 81–92   44 References

The major types of organizational bias are described and empirical approaches for assessment of rater-trait interaction bias in multiple informant data is demonstrated. Recognizing and addressing potential sources of bias should result in improved measurement of contextual variables (CR 2.19).

2.27.6 Resnick, B. (1996) The rough and ready jacknife. *Nursing Research*, 45 (3) 185–8 19 References

Describes the jacknife procedure which was introduced as a non-parametric device for estimating bias. Subsequent use has been to obtain approximate confidence intervals in problems where standard statistical procedures could not be done; to consider the stability of an analysis and to validate findings when a sample size is too small to do a positive validation (CR 2.25).

2.27.7 Romm, N. (1997) 'Becoming more accountable: a comment on Hammersley and Gomm' *Sociological Research Online*, 2 (3)
URL: http://www.socresonline.org.uk/socresonline/2/3/2.html>   33 References

Provides a response to Hammersley and Gomm's article entitled 'Bias in social research'. Their proposed conception of bias is rooted in a particular view of the pursuit of scientific knowledge – a view they call nonfoundationalist. The way in which they arrive at this view is challenged as author believes their account excludes a serious consideration of alternative epistemological orientations (CR 2.6, 2.27.3).

2.28   GENERALIZABILITY

An important research goal is to try to understand what is taking place in a general way during a series of events. One isolated event may have considerable importance, particularly in qualitative research, but the ability to extrapolate beyond the specifics is a characteristic of the scientific method.

Definition

Generalizability – the extent to which research findings are true for subjects or settings other than the ones which the researcher used

---

Annotations

2.28.1 Schofield, J.W. (1993) Increasing the generalizability of qualitative research, in Hammersley, M. (ed.), *Social Research: Philosophy, Politics and Practice*. London: Sage, in association with the Open University, ISBN 0803988052 Part 3, Chapter 16, 200–25 78 References

Explores traditional views of generalizability and the increasing interest in it. The process of reconceptualizing it is discussed together with three targets to be achieved (CR 2.36.25).

2.28.2 Shavelson, R.J. & Webb, N.M. (1991) *Generalizability Theory: a Primer*. Newbury Park, CA: Sage ISBN 0803937458 References

Discusses the underlying concepts and development of generalizability theory, and assists readers in applying measurement methods which will encourage consistency.

EXPERIMENTAL/QUANTITATIVE DESIGNS

2.29   EXPERIMENTAL DESIGNS – GENERAL

Experimental research involves the active manipulation of variables under the control of the researcher. This approach attempts to study how subjects will react to the manipulated conditions through monitoring one or more outcome measures. If an experiment is well designed, the experimenter may, in principle, detect causal relationships between variables. However, there are many threats to the satisfactory detection of such relationships.

Experimental studies involve the following steps:

* definition of the problem
* selection of the sample – this should be representative of the population
* assignment procedures – participants allocated to groups who should be as similar as possible

* treatment – researcher administers the intervention(s), i.e. the independent variables, in an unbiased way
* measurement of outcomes – this is measured via the dependent variable. It may be measured both before and after the treatment or only after

Definitions

Control group – the subjects who are not exposed to the experimental treatment
Double-blind trial – an experimental procedure, used particularly in drug trials, to guard against bias . . . neither the subjects nor the person gathering the data are aware which treatments are being given to which subjects
Experiment – . . . is characterized by randomization, manipulation and control
Multi-centre trials – the replication of an randomized clinical trial in several different settings to increase the level of confidence in research findings
Placebo effect – an effect whereby a completely inactive clinical treatment (placebo) causes a patient's condition to improve or seem to improve
Randomized clinical trial – . . . a form of experimental research in which the effects of one or more treatments (interventions) are compared with a control 'treatment' by randomly assigning study subjects to the groups and measuring the differences in effects (outcomes) of the alternative treatments over time

Annotations

2.29.1 Abrams, K.R. & Scragg, A.M. (1996) Quantitative methods in nursing research. *Journal of Advanced Nursing*, 23 (5) 1008–15 26 References

Considers some of the general principles common to quantitative research in nursing. The role of hypothesis testing is considered and the use of estimation is emphasized. Examples are given from the nursing literature (CR 2.20).

2.29.2 Alexander, J. (1995) Randomized controlled trials. *British Journal of Midwifery*, 3 (12) 656–9   4 References

Article outlines some principles of controlled trials and illustrates these from an ante-natal study.

2.29.3 Arrigo, C., Gall, H., Delogne, A. & Molin, C. (1994) The involvement of nurses in clinical trials: results of the EORTC Oncology Nurses Study Group survey (European Organization for Research and Treatment of Cancer). *Cancer Nursing*, 17 (5) 429–33 11 References

The Oncology Nurses Study Group surveyed 312 nurses in more than 15 European countries to discover their involvement in clinical trials. Results showed that they lacked training in oncology and research methods and were rarely involved in protocol preparation and review. There was considerable variation in the amount of information being circulated to nurses. Suggestions made to increase participation included summaries of nursing protocols in the local language, contact with colleagues involved in the trials and additional training (CR 3.16, 3.17).

2.29.4 Arvay, C.A. (1991) Clinical trials: bringing research to the bedside. *Journal of Neuroscience Nursing*, 23 (1) 64–7 9 References

Article aims to provide an understanding of investigative research studies through the use of clinical trials. The phases involved are discussed and steps to ensure the correct methodology and ethical aspects are also considered (CR 2.17).

2.29.5 Beck, S.L. (1989) The cross-over design in clinical nursing research. *Nursing Research*, 38 (5) 291–3 11 References

Discusses the use, advantages and disadvantages of cross-over designs.

2.29.6 Behi, R. & Nolan, M. (1996a) Research, causality and control: key to the experiment. *British Journal of Nursing*, 5 (4) 252–5 5 References

Article describes the concept of causality and outlines the four principles with which it is underpinned. Some methods of control are considered.

2.29.7 Behi, R. & Nolan, M. (1996b) Research: experimental designs. *British Journal of Nursing*, 5 (12) 754–6 3 References

Article discusses randomized clinical trials, double-blind and factorial designs and explains their main requirements (CR 2.19, 2.27).

2.29.8 Behi, R. & Nolan, M. (1996c) Research: the basic experimental design. *British Journal of Nursing*, 5 (9) 563–6 5 References

Considers the three essential characteristics of the basic experiment: random assignment of subjects, manipulation of relevant variables and control of irrelevant variables. Two of the most common, pre-test/post-test and post-test only, designs are described (CR 2.30, 2.31).

2.29.9 Black, T.R. (1998) *Doing Quantitative Research in the Social Sciences*. London: Sage. ISBN 0761953523 References

Book which offers a 'how to' approach is intended for students and researchers. It focuses on the design and execution of research so that planning, sampling, choice of statistical test and interpretation of results are all integrated within the research process (CR 2.22, 2.83, 2.95).

2.29.10 Bond, S. (1993) Experimental research in nursing: necessary but not sufficient, in Kitson, A. (ed.), *Nursing: Art and Science*. London: Chapman & Hall. ISBN 0412470705 Chapter 8, 94–112 53 References

Chapter discusses research styles, the limits of positivistic research, science, research and experiments, who gained from them and progress in explanation. Points for discussion are included.

2.29.11 Borenstein, M. (1997) Hypothesis testing and effect size estimation in clinical trials. *Annals of Allergy, Asthma and Immunology*, 78 (1) 5–16 49 References

Paper gives an overview of several key elements in planning and analysing a study, in particular highlighting the differences between significance tests (statistical significance) and effect size estimation (clinical significance). Advice is given on the way forward (CR 2.20).

2.29.12 Boruch, R.F., McSweeney, A.J. & Soderstrom, E.J. (1978) Randomized field experiments for programme planning, development and evaluation. *Evaluation Quarterly*, 2 655–95

A bibliography listing 300 randomized field experiments in ten different categories. These are: criminal and civil justice; mental health; training re-education; mass communications; information collection and retrieval; research utilization; commerce, industry and public utilities; social welfare; health services and medical treatment; and fertility control. It is suggested that randomized tests are numerous and have been used in many settings so the professional in one setting may learn from those conducted in another sphere.

2.29.13   Campbell, D.T. & Stanley, J.C. (1966) *Experimental and Quasi-experimental Designs for Research.* Chicago: Rand McNally College. ISBN 0395307872   References

Book examines 16 experimental/quasi-experimental designs with emphasis being given to factors affecting validity (CR 2.25, 2.35).

2.29.14   Chalmers, I., Dickersin, K. & Chalmers, T. (1992) Getting to grips with Archie Cochrane's agenda. *British Medical Journal*, 3 October, 305 (6857) 786–7 25 References

Discusses the problems associated with under-registering and reporting of randomized clinical trials (CR 2.17, 2.97).

2.29.15   Clinical Trials Dictionary: Terminology and Usage Recommendations. (1996) Edited by Meinert, C.L. Baltimore, MD: Meinert Curtis, L. ISBN 0964642409

This dictionary defines a large and complex vocabulary used to describe the methods and results of clinical trials. An index to the main entries facilitates the finding of terms associated with particular concepts and steps occurring during the trials. A section on usage provides illuminating discourse on nuances in the rhetoric of scientific speech and writing (CR 2.2).

2.29.16   Fahey, T., Hyde, C., Milne, R. & Thorogood, M. (1995) The type and quality of randomized controlled trials (RCTs) published in UK public health journals. *Journal of Public Health Medicine*, 17 (4) 469–74 28 References

Paper describes the type and methodological features of randomized controlled trials that appeared in five public health journals published in the UK. These trials will form the basis of a register of RCTs in public health.

2.29.17   Fall-Dickson, J.M. (1993) Clinical

trials and research in the community. *Seminars in Oncology Nursing*, 9 (1) 38–43 18 References

Explores the history of clinical trials, cancer research trials in the community, accrual to trials and the infrastructure of community-based clinical trial participation.

2.29.18   Fisher, P. (1995) The development of research methodology in homeopathy. *Complementary Therapies in Nursing and Midwifery*, 1 (6) 168–74   25 References

Reports the results of a systematic review of clinical trials in homeopathy. Various approaches to the problem of individualization in controlled trials are discussed and a method described to improve the auditing of the results (CR 2.12, 2.14).

2.29.19   Giffels, J.J. (1996) *Clinical Trials: What You Should Know Before Volunteering to Become a Research Subject.* New York: Demos Vermande. ISBN 1888799021

2.29.20   Good, M. & Schuler, L. (1997) Subject retention in a controlled clinical trial. *Journal of Advanced Nursing*, 26 (2) 351–5 9 References

Discusses strategies which encouraged continued participation of subjects in a controlled clinical trial, making sure that the interventions were acceptable to patients and compatible with other care activities. Qualities of research personnel and the patients' changing condition are also important factors, together with some individualization and keeping patients informed (CR 2.22, 3.16).

2.29.21   Hicks, C.M. (1990) *Research and Statistics: a Practical Introduction for Nurses.* New York: Prentice-Hall. ISBN 0138440778 References

Book concentrates on hypothesis testing and experimental design. A little statistical theory is included and worked examples are given for each test. Summaries of major points are given together with lists of keywords and exercises. Text relates research principles directly to nursing issues. Advice is also given on preparing research for publication (CR 2.20, 2.99).

2.29.22   Hicks, C.M. (1995) *Research for Physiotherapists: Project Design and Analysis* 2nd edition. Edinburgh: Churchill Livingstone. ISBN 0443049998   References

An introductory text for health care professionals approaching a research project for the first time. Self-assessment exercises are included.

2.29.23 Hill, M.N. & Schron, E.B. (1992) Opportunities for nurse researchers in clinical trials. *Nursing Research*, 41 (2) 114–15 No references

Article describes ancillary, data-based and sub-studies that can be conducted within clinical trials (CR 3.16).

2.29.24 Keeble, S. (1995a) *Experimental Research 1: an Introduction to Experimental Design*. Edinburgh: Churchill Livingstone. ISBN 0443052700 References

and

2.29.25 Keeble, S. (1995b) *Experimental Research 2: Conducting and Reporting Experimental Research*. Edinburgh: Churchill Livingstone. ISBN 0443052719 References

Books comprise part of an open learning series for health professionals. Each section includes an introduction, session objectives, text, activities, commentaries and summaries. Examples are included mainly from the nursing literature.

2.29.26 Kenkre, J. (1997) Running a clinical trial. *Practice Nurse*, 13 (7) 380, 382, 384 7 References

Outlines the different tasks involved in research and describes how nurses can balance their responsibilities to the investigation and the patients (CR 2.17, 3.16).

2.29.27 Kenyon, S. (1995) The Oracle trial. *Modern Midwife*, 5 (4) 26–8 5 References

Author gives a personal account of setting up a large multi-centre trial (CR 2.14, 2.16, 3.16).

2.29.28 Keppel, G., Saufley, W.H. Jr. & Tokunaga, H. (1992) *Introduction to Design and Analysis: a Students' Handbook* 2nd edition. Oxford: W.H. Freeman. ISBN 0716723212 References

Provides a practical introduction to the design and analysis of experiments, particularly in the social and behavioural sciences. Step-by-step descriptions, worked examples and exercises are included (CR 2.36, 2.79).

2.29.29 Lewis-Beck, M.S. (ed.) (1993) *Experimental Design and Methods*. Thousand Oaks, CA: Sage/Toppan. ISBN 0803954298 References

Book covers randomizing, experimental design and analysis, analysis of variance, covariance and multi-variate analysis of variance (CR 2.87).

2.29.30 Lipsey, M.W. (1990) *Design Sensitivity: Statistical Power for Experimental Research*. Newbury Park, CA: Sage. ISBN 0803930631 References

Book explores the concept of design sensitivity and explains the elements which determine statistical power. Examples are given.

2.29.31 Manly, B.J.F. (1992) *The Design and Analysis of Research Studies*. Cambridge: Cambridge University Press. ISBN 0521414539 References

Book aims to provide research workers in biological, health and social sciences with the information needed to collect and analyse data critically. Topics addressed are the potential for bias and misleading conclusions with observational studies, sample surveys, and counter-sampling methods, experimental and quasi-experimental designs, methods of analysis with random and non-random samples and ethical concerns (CR 2.17, 2.22, 2.27, 2.35, 2.36, 2.52, 2.72, 2.87).

2.29.32 McLaughlin, F.E. & Marascuilo, L.A. (1990) *Advanced Nursing and Health Care Research: Quantification Approaches*. Philadelphia: Saunders. ISBN 0721630987 References

Written for advanced-level students, graduates and experienced researchers, this book covers initial and advanced research techniques and statistical procedures. An extensive research example is used throughout the text and others illustrate special issues in nursing research. New techniques are introduced and the range and variety of quantification techniques useful for hypothesis testing is included (CR 2.20).

2.29.33 McMahon, R. (1994) Trial and error: an experiment in practice, in Buckeldee, J. & McMahon, R. (eds), *The Research Experience in Nursing*. London: Chapman & Hall. ISBN 0412441101 Chapter 6, 83–99 17 References

Describes some of the experiences of performing an experiment. Author stresses the importance of doing thorough exploratory work before embarking on the trial, and if difficulties arise which seem insurmountable, being prepared to abandon the project altogether (CR 2.16.4).

2.29.34 Oldham, J. (1994) Experimental and quasi-experimental research designs. *Nurse Researcher* 1(4) 26–36   11 References

Identifies and explores the characteristics of design in experimental and quasi-experimental research (CR 2.25, 2.35).

2.29.35 Orr, R.D. (1996) Guidelines for the use of placebo controls in clinical trials of psychopharmacologic agents. *Psychiatric Services*, 47 (11) 1262–4   10 References

Article presents guidelines, developed by a university's institutional review board, for the justifiable use of placebo controls in research with psychopharmacological agents. These are intended to assist planning and protect vulnerable subjects (CR 2.17).

2.29.36 Palmer, C.R. (1993) Ethics and statistical methodology in clinical trials. *Journal of Medical Ethics*, 19 (4) 219–22   10 References and Notes

Statisticians in medicine can disagree on appropriate methods and application of design and analysis in clinical trials. Two approaches, the Bayesian and Frequentists, are defined and author suggests when and where each may be appropriate (CR 2.17, 2.83).

2.29.37 Poole, K. & Jones, J. (1996) A re-examination of the experimental design for nursing research. *Journal of Advanced Nursing*, 24 (1) 108–14   63 References

Paper suggests there is a need to re-examine some of the erroneous assumptions regarding the philosophical origins of the experimental design. By ignoring its contribution some areas of nursing knowledge may be missed.

2.29.38 Portney, L.G. & Watkins, M.P. (1993) *Foundations of Clinical Research: Applications to Practice.* Norwalk, CT: Appleton & Lange. ISBN 0838510655 References

Book provides a comprehensive reference for clinicians and students in research design and statistical analysis. Although primarily written for physical and occupational therapists, a range of health-related applications should be understood by all health professionals. Both quantitative and qualitative approaches are included. Appendices contain statistical tables and other data (CR 2.36).

2.29.39 Raven, A. (1996) *Clinical Trials: an Introduction.* Abingdon, Oxon: Radcliffe Medical Press. ISBN 1857750357 References

2.29.40 Reaves, C.C. (1992) *Quantitative Research for the Behavioural Sciences.* New York: Wiley ISBN 0471573671   References

Covers a broad range of methods used by behavioural scientists. The practical importance of research is emphasized, many recent references are included and the theory behind the rules is discussed. Each chapter begins with a series of questions to focus upon and ends with exercises and detailed summaries. Sections include fundamentals, making and using measurements, experimental methods and dealing with results. A chapter is devoted to writing research reports (CR 2.97).

2.29.41 Robinson, I. (1990) Clinical encounters of the ethical kind. Clinical trials and the collective ethic: the case of hyperbaric oxygen therapy in the treatment of multiple sclerosis, in Weisz, G. (ed.), *Social Science Perspectives on Medical Ethics.* Dordrecht: Kluwer Academic Publishers. ISBN 0792305663 19–39 69 References

Chapter contends that the considerable effort vested in elucidating the ethical dilemmas and problems in the principles and practice of clinical trials has resulted in a partial and particular view of their ethical status. Author suggests that the ethical implications are more complex and embedded in a broader range of social and political forces than is usually assumed (CR 2.17).

2.29.42 Roe, B. (1994) Is there a place for the experiment in nursing research? *Nurse Researcher*, 1 (4) 4–12   17 References

Article presents an overview of quasi-experimental and true experimental research designs with an illustration of each. A case is made for wider use of both types of design. The Central Research and Development Committee's research priorities are listed. (CR 2.35, 3.20).

2.29.43 Rudy, E.B., Vaska, P.L., Daly, B.J., Happ, M.B. & Shiao, P. (1993) Permuted block design for randomization in a nursing clinical trial. *Nursing Research*, 42 (5) 287–9 6 References

Article examines some of the problems of randomization and suggests an approach which has been used successfully in a clinical trial (CR 2.22).

2.29.44 Shuldham, C. & Hiley, C. (1997) Randomized controlled trials in clinical practice: the continuing debate. *NT Research*, 2 (2) 128–34   21 References

Discusses the dilemmas which nurses face in the use of randomized controlled trials. Their apparent antipathy is explored and the authors believe that the main problem is a lack of experience, education and understanding of this method of research. Suggestions are made showing how nurses may become more informed and take up opportunities to become involved.

2.29.45 Skrutkowska, M. & Weijer, C. (1997) Do patients with breast cancer participating in clinical trials receive better nursing care? *Oncology Nursing Forum*, 24 (8) 1411–16   46 References

Reports a study which aimed to examine differences in nursing care received by patients in two groups, one enrolled in clinical trials and the others not. Results showed that there were differences in care received and authors believe that if this study is confirmed, measures must be taken to ensure all patients receive optimal care (CR 2.17).

2.29.46 Thornton, H. (1992) The luck of the draw. *Nursing Times*, 9 September, 88 (37) 58 References

Author discusses, from a personal point of view, the problems associated with large-scale trials which have been, and are being set up, to try to establish the most appropriate treatment regimes for breast cancer (CR 2.17).

2.29.47 Trilla, A. (1995) Components of a clinical trial: historical development, study personnel and nursing roles. *ANNA Journal* 22 (4) 375–9   7 References

Article examines the elements of a clinical trial, roles for nurses and historical influences

in the development of rules for conducting research (CR 3.16).

2.29.48 Wilson-Barnett, J. (1991) The experiment: is it worthwhile? *International Journal of Nursing Studies*, 28 (1) 77–87 30 References

Discusses how the experiment can be modified and interpreted to provide evidence for changes in nursing practice. A list of suggestions is given for improving the experimental approach with human subjects.

2.29.49 Wineman, N.M., Schwetz, K.M., Goodkin, D.E. & Rudick, R.A. (1996) Relationships among illness uncertainty, stress, coping, and emotional well-being at entry into a clinical drug trial. *Applied Nursing Research* 9(2) 53–60   19 References

Reports the findings of a cross-sectional study of 59 clients who were participating in a two-year trial using methotrexate for progressive multiple sclerosis. Results may be used to develop interventions so fostering emotional well-being at the time of entry into drug trials.

2.29.50 Zeller, R., Good, M., Anderson, G.C. & Zeller, D.L. (1997) Strengthening experimental design by balancing potentially confounding variables across treatment groups. *Nursing Research*, 46 (6) 345–9 29 References

Article written for nurses planning randomized clinical trials. A rationale is given for using minimization in intervention studies. Authors describe the development and testing of the Minimization & Computer Program for assigning subjects to as many as eight groups (2.22, 2.84).

EXPERIMENTAL DESIGNS

Sections 2.30–2.34 illustrate four types of experimental design. The use of standard notation is helpful in understanding alternative experimental designs.

R = Random assignment of subjects to experimental and control groups
O = Observation or measurement (O1 pre-test/O2 post-test)
X = Treatment or intervention

2.30   PRE-TEST/POST-TEST DESIGN

Measurements of the outcomes or dependent variables are taken both before and after the intervention. This allows the measurement of change in individual cases.

R	O1	X	O2	Experimental group
R	O3		O4	Control group

The measurement process may influence change, thereby introducing difficulties in attributing this to the intervention on its own.

Example

Wong, K.N., Hills, E.C. & Strax, T.E. (1994) Rotating stations: an innovative approach to third-year medical student education in physical medicine and rehabilitation. *American Journal of Physical Medicine and Rehabilitation*, 73 (1) 23–6   3 References

Reports a study where students were pre- and post-tested about their knowledge of physical medicine and rehabilitation. A one-day combined lecture/rotating stations conference was held as a way of introducing students to this field and testing showed it to be a cost-effective way.

Annotation

2.30.1   Dixon, J. (1984) Effects of nursing intervention on nutritional and performance status in cancer patients. *Nursing Research*, 33 (6) 330–5   30 References

Cancer patients were assigned to a control group or one of four intervention groups receiving (a) nutritional supplementation (b) relaxation training; (c) both (a) and (b); and (d) neither (a) nor (b). Findings suggested that the cachexia of cancer may be slowed or reversed through non-invasive interventions.

2.31   POST-TEST CONTROL DESIGN

This design may be useful in situations where it is not possible to pre-test the participants or where they have been randomly assigned.

R	X	O	Experimental group
R		O	Control group

Example

Kerr, S.M., Jowett, S.A. & Smith, L.N. (1996) Preventing sleep problems in infants: a randomized controlled trial. *Journal of Advanced Nursing*, 24 (5) 938–42   25 References

Research aimed to examine the efficacy of health education in reducing the incidence of sleep problems. Results showed that a preventative approach produced a significant improvement in infant sleep behaviour.

2.32   SOLOMON FOUR GROUP DESIGN

A complex design useful in studies of developmental phenomena which permits the investigator to differentiate between many effects. Two experimental and two control groups are used.

R	O1	X	O2	Experimental group 1
R	O3		O4	Control group 1
R		X	O5	Experimental group 2
R			O6	Control group 2

This design has potential for generating information about differential sources of effect of the dependent variable.

Example

Aschen, S.R. (1997) Assertion training therapy in psychiatric milieus. *Archives of Psychiatric Nursing*, 11 (1) 46–51   13 References

Using a Solomon Four Group design, author reports an attempt to develop a clinical procedure to decrease anxiety and increase responsiveness (assertion) of psychiatric in-patients of both sexes, in mixed diagnostic categories. The effectiveness of the procedure is reported.

Annotation

2.32.1 Malotte, C.K. & Morisky, D.E.
(1994) Using an unobtrusively monitored comparison study group in a longitudinal design. *Health Education Research*, 9 (1) 153–9 22 References

Study describes how a non-contact comparison group receiving treatment for tuberculosis, followed through medical records, can be used in combination with a randomized control design to assess pre-test and monitoring effects. Results and their implications are reported (CR 2.48).

2.33 FACTORIAL DESIGNS

Factorial designs allow the researcher to analyse the effects of two or more factors simultaneously. They also provide information on whether factors interact to produce differences in the outcome that would not have occurred if each factor was considered separately.

Example

Hicks, C. (1996) A study of nurses' attitudes towards research: a factor analytic approach. *Journal of Advanced Nursing*, 23 (2) 373–9 20 References

Study identified five coherent factors which underpinned the general attitude to research of a sample of 500 qualified nurses. These were subjective and organizational/structural barriers, doctors' and health care professionals' reactions to nursing research and its impact on practice. Author suggests that the tool which was developed could identify those needing specific attitude change programmes with a possible increase in nursing research activities.

Annotation

2.33.1 Gilmour, S.G. & Mead, R. (1995) Stopping rules for sequences of factorial designs. *Applied Statistics*, 44 (3) 343–55 References

Reports on stopping rules for sequentially designed factorial experiments used in Monte Carlo simulation.

2.34 SINGLE-CASE DESIGN

'Single-case experiments are scientific investigations in which the effects of a series of experimental manipulations on a single subject are examined . . . [This type of research] should not be confused with case studies – [they] are retrospectively written reports of observations on individuals, which may raise questions that initiate research; single-case experiments are, of course, prospectively planned' (Wilson in Breakwell, Hammond & Fife-Schaw, 1995: 69–70).

Examples of this design include the evaluation of behaviour modification and skill training programmes, assessment of the effects of drugs and the examination of treatments in physical rehabilitation.

Definition

Single-case design – an examination of a single subject in order to understand the specific causes of problems and the effectiveness of treatment applied to that individual

Example

Duff, A. (1996) Case study of a female client on a regional secure unit. *Journal of Advanced Nursing*, 23 (4) 771–5 4 References

Reports a single-case experiment design study which examined the maladaptive behaviour of a 32-year-old female in-patient.

Annotations

2.34.1 Barlow, D.H. & Hersen, M. (1992) *Single Case Experimental Designs*. New York: Pergamon. ISBN 0080301355 References

Book provides an historical overview of the single case in basic and applied research and discusses general issues, procedures and assessment strategies. Different designs are covered in depth and many examples are given. Methods of statistical analysis are included together with examples of direct, systematic and clinical replication (CR 2.13).

2.34.2 Behi, R. & Nolan, M. (1997) Single-case experimental designs 2: common examples. *British Journal of Nursing*, 6 (2) 116–19   7 References

Describes some commonly used single-case experimental designs, including reversal and non-reversal.

2.34.3 Elder, J.H. (1997) Single subject experiment for psychiatric nursing. *Archives of Psychiatric Nursing*, 11 (3) 133–8   17 References

Article describes single-subject experimentation, contrasts this approach with case study and group comparison designs, and discusses how this type of scientific inquiry can be incorporated into psychiatric nursing practice.

2.34.4 Galassi, J.P. & Gersh, T.L. (1993) Myths, conceptions and missed opportunity: single case designs and counseling psychology. *Journal of Counseling Psychology*, 40 (4) 525–31   56 References

Status of single-case designs is reviewed and reasons for their under-use are discussed. Potential contributions in research linking process and outcome, group counselling across a variety of theoretical approaches, evaluation and quality assurance are described.

2.34.5 Gray, M. (1998) Introducing single case research design: an overview. *Nurse Researcher*, 5 (4) 15–24   31 References

Author gives an overview of case-study research, its types, uses, and discusses the value of single-case studies. Advice is given on conducting a case study, and their strengths and weaknesses are outlined.

2.34.6 Kazdin, A.E. (1982) *Single Case Research Designs: Methods for Clinical and Applied Settings*. New York: Oxford University Press. ISBN 0195030214   References

Provides a concise description of single-case experimental designs and places this methodology in the context of applied research in general. Examples are given from clinical psychology, psychiatry, education, counselling and other disciplines. The methodology covers assessment, design and data analysis.

2.34.7 Newell, R. (1992) The single case

experimental design: a quantitative method for everyday use. *Nursing Practice*, 18 November, 24–8 6 (1)   10 References

Author urges further use of the single-case experimental case design. Its methodology is traced, the types of design are described, how they are handled statistically and the relevance of this approach to nursing.

2.34.8 Newell, R. (1998) Single case experimental design: controlling the study. *Nurse Researcher*, 5 (4) 25–39   12 References

Article explores some of the issues surrounding the introduction of experimental control in single-case research. A series of methods is examined which should increase the rigour with which the clinician can study everyday practice and apply research findings based on large group studies to the needs of the individual.

2.34.9 Ottenbacher, K.J. (1992) Analysis of data in ideographic research: issues and methods. *American Journal of Physical Medicine and Rehabilitation*, 71 (4) 202–8   34 References

The advantages and limitations of two procedures for data analysis, which will increase reliability and accuracy in single-case research, are examined. These are the split-middle method of trend estimation and the resistant trend line. Visual analysis of single-subject data is also described (CR 2.87).

2.34.10 Parry, A.W. (1995) Single subject research in clinical practice. *British Journal of Therapy and Rehabilitation*, 2 (1) 40–3   16 References

Discusses the value of single-subject research from an historical perspective together with its limitations and value to the therapy professions.

2.34.11 Proudfoot, L.M., Farmer, E.S. & McIntosh, J.B. (1994) Testing incontinence pads using single-case research designs. *British Journal of Nursing*, 3 (7) 316, 318–20, 322   25 References

Article discusses the value of single-case research designs for generating nursing knowledge (CR 2.6).

2.34.12 Ricketts, T. (1998) Single case research in mental health. *Nursing Times*, 10 June, 94 (23) 52–5   17 References

Article explores the rationale and requirements for single-case experimental designs and gives an example of this approach in mental health service development.

2.34.13 Robertson, V.J. & Lee, V.L. (1994) Some misconceptions about single subject designs in physiotherapy. *Physiotherapy*, 80 (11) 762–7   53 References

Paper discusses the relation between research and practice in physiotherapy and the role of baselines. Authors believe that replication-based designs have much to offer (CR 2.13).

2.34.14 Wilson, S.L. (1995) Single case experimental designs, in Breakwell, G.M., Hammond, S. & Fife-Schaw, C. (eds), *Research Methods in Psychology*. London: Sage. ISBN 0803977654 Part II, 69–84 References

Chapter discusses problems with the group comparison approach, general issues in single-case research, preparing and performing a single-case experiment and data analysis (CR 2.1.8).

2.35 QUASI-EXPERIMENTAL DESIGNS

Quasi-experimental designs are a compromise between a true experiment with random assignment and a pre-experiment. They also represent a compromise between maximizing internal and external validity.

Definitions

Interrupted time-series designs – effects of a treatment are inferred from comparing measures of performance taken at many time intervals
Non-equivalent control group – those in which responses of a treatment group and a comparison group are measured before and after the treatment
Quasi-experiment – a research design that has the features of manipulation and control, but in which participants are not randomly assigned to the treatment and control groups

---

Example

Girot, E.A. (1995) Preparing the practitioner for advanced academic study: the development of critical thinking. *Journal of Advanced Nursing*, 21 (2) 387–94   50 References

Explores the concept of critical thinking and its development in a study skills programme for academic post-registration courses in one college. Suggestions are made for developing these skills.

Annotations

2.35.1 Atwood, J.R. & Taylor, W. (1991) Regression discontinuity design: alternative design for nursing research. *Nursing Research*, 40 (5) 312–15   15 References

Identifies the regression discontinuity design as a scientifically advantageous approach. The relationship of this design to causal chains is also described.

2.35.2 Behi, R. & Nolan, M. (1996) Research: quasi experimental designs. *British Journal of Nursing*, 26 September–9 October, 5 (17) 1079–81   4 References

Article outlines the two main approaches to quasi-experimental designs, giving an example of each. Other related methods are also highlighted.

2.35.3 Caporaso, J.A. & Roos, L.L. Jr. (eds) (no date) *Quasi-experimental Approaches: Testing Theory and Evaluating Policy*. Ann Arbor: UMI Research Press. ISBN 0835794679

2.35.4 Cook, T.D. & Campbell, D.T. (1979) *Quasi-experimentation: Design and Analysis Issues for Field Settings*. Chicago: Rand McNally. ISBN 0528620533   References

Chapters cover some quasi-experimental designs which can be used in many social research settings. The literature on causation is reviewed, aspects of validity are explored and the two major categories of quasi-experimental designs, non-equivalent group and interrupted time-series, are covered in detail. Further chapters on inferring cause from passive observation and the conduct of randomized experiments are included. (CR 2.21, 2.25).

2.35.5 Fife-Schaw, C. (1995) Quasi-experimental designs, in Breakwell, G.M., Hammond, S. & Fife-Schaw, C. (eds), *Research Methods in Psychology*. London: Sage. ISBN 0803977654 Part II, Chapter 7, 85–98 References

Discusses pre- and quasi-experiments, non-equivalent control group, time-series and modifications to basic designs (CR 2.1.8).

2.35.6 Johnston, M.V., Ottenbacher, K.J. & Reichardt, C.S. (1995) Some quasi-experimental designs for research on the effectiveness of rehabilitation. *American Journal of Physical Medicine and Rehabilitation*, 74 (5) 383–92   50 References

Paper aims to improve the understanding of research design in medical rehabilitation. It describes two infrequently used but potentially rigorous designs – regression-discontinuity and multiple interrupted time-series design.

NON-EXPERIMENTAL/ QUALITATIVE DESIGNS

2.36   NON-EXPERIMENTAL DESIGNS – GENERAL

'. . . qualitative researchers seek to preserve the form and content of human behaviour and to analyze its qualities, rather than subject it to mathematical or other formal transformations.' (Lindlof, 1995: 21)
[This section includes texts on qualitative research. Those including both quantitative and qualitative research may be found in section 2.1].

Definitions

Field experiment – an experiment taking place in a real-world environment, where it is more difficult to impose controls
Field notes – notes taken by researchers regarding the unstructured observations they have made in the field, and their understanding of these observations
Field study – a study in which the data are collected 'in the field' from people in their normal roles with the aims of understanding the practices, behaviours and beliefs of individuals or groups as they normally function in real life
Field work – an anthropological research approach that traditionally involves prolonged residence with members of the culture that is being studied
Naturalistic inquiry – . . . the investigation of phenomena within and in relation to their naturally occurring contexts.
Qualitative research – is multi-method in focus, involving an interpretative, naturalistic approach to its subject matter

Annotations

2.36.1 Allen-Meares, P. (1995) Applications of qualitative research: let the work begin. *Social Work Research*, 19 (1) 5–7   13 References

The methodological debate about quantitative and qualitative research methods has largely levelled off and author argues that a third, integrated configuration may be needed to spur the exploration and application of qualitative research (CR 2.9).

2.36.2 Bailey, C.A. (1996) *A Guide to Field Research*. Thousand Oaks, CA: Pine Forge Press. ISBN 0803990588   References

Aims to give students clear and specific instructions on how to do field research. Examples are given to bring alive the abstract principles of this type of research.

2.36.3 Banister, P., Burman, E., Parker, I., Taylor, M. & Tindall, C. (1994) *Qualitative Methods in Psychology: a Research Guide*. Buckingham: Open University Press. ISBN 0335191819   References

Book is an introduction to qualitative methods giving practical advice on carrying out this type of research, and allowing evaluation skills to be developed (CR 2.95).

2.36.4 Beck, C.T. (1993) Qualitative research: the evaluation of its credibility, fittingness and auditability. *Western Journal of Nursing Research*, 15 (2) 263–6   6 References

Discusses how researchers have tried to use criteria from quantitative research to evaluate qualitative research. Because each method involves different assumptions, another set of criteria is required. Three terms are used, credibility, fittingness and auditability, and lists of questions are included.

2.36.5 Brink, P.J. & Wood, M.J. (eds) (1998) *Advanced Design in Nursing Research.* Thousand Oaks, CA: Sage. ISBN 0803958005 References

An advanced text focusing on research designs for students and teachers who have a basic knowledge of the research process. Three major designs – exploratory/descriptive, survey and experiential – are sub-divided into further levels and fully discussed. Each one is contrasted with experimental design, and its strengths and weaknesses are reviewed (CR 2.29, 2.52).

2.36.6 Britten, N. & Fisher, B. (1993) Qualitative research and general practice. *British Journal of General Practice*, 43 (372) 270–1 6 References

Authors suggest that qualitative research methods would be appropriate for general practitioners and suggests some areas which might be examined.

2.36.7 Cassell, C. & Symon, G. (eds) (1994) *Qualitative Methods in Organizational Research: a Practical Guide.* London: Sage. ISBN 0803987706 References

Book explores a variety of techniques and frameworks available for qualitative methods in organizational research. The role and distinctive features of qualitative methods are discussed and a number of different approaches are outlined. In addition to interviewing, participant observation and case studies, newer approaches such as stakeholder analysis and tracer studies are included (CR 2.39, 2.68, 2.72).

2.36.8 Cheek, J. (1996) Taking a view: qualitative research as representation. *Qualitative Health Research*, 6 (4) 492–505 34 References

Article discusses the frameworks, representations and discourses that have positioned and are positioning us as readers of qualitative research texts.

2.36.9 Crabtree, B.F. & Miller, W.L. (eds) (1992) *Doing Qualitative Research: Multiple*

Strategies 3rd edition. Newbury Park, CA: Sage. ISBN 0803943121 References

Overview of qualitative research methods is given together with data collection approaches and strategies for analysis. A step-by-step approach is used and two studies are cited to illustrate the process involved (CR 2.22, 2.64, 2.68, 2.72, 2.79, 2.86).

2.36.10 Craig, G. (1996) Qualitative research in an NHS setting: uses and dilemmas. *Changes: an International Journal of Psychology and Psychotherapy*, 14 (3) 180–6 20 References

With the increasing tendency in health care towards the rhetoric of evidence-based medicine, the author argues that this gives preference to quantitative research. Clinicians might regard qualitative methods as an easy option and in the process devalue them to the status of adjuncts to the supposedly more rigorous approach of positivism (CR 2.29).

2.36.11 Creswell, J.W. (1998) *Qualitative Inquiry and Research Design: Choosing among Five Traditions.* Thousand Oaks, CA: Sage. ISBN 0761901442 References

Book explores the philosophical underpinnings, history and key elements of each of five qualitative traditions: biography, phenomenology, grounded theory, ethnography and case study. Research designs are related to each tradition and each research strategy is compared for theoretical frameworks, writing introductions to studies, collecting and analysing data, writing the narrative, employing standards of quality and verifying results. Five articles in an appendix give examples of the five qualitative designs and a chapter shows how a case study can be re-interpreted using each of the other four traditions. Individual glossaries are given for each tradition (CR 2.2, 2.39, 2.42, 2.45, 2.49, 2.71).

2.36.12 Delamont, S. (1992) *Fieldwork in Educational Settings: Methods, Pitfalls and Perspectives.* London: Falmer Press. ISBN 1850009570 References

Book, based on author's own research, aims to fill some gaps in the methodological literature of qualitative research. Covering anthropological and sociological perspectives, in and beyond schools, it emphasizes writing up research and how to get a project finished (CR 2.42, 2.97).

2.36.13   Denzin, N.K. & Lincoln, Y.S. (eds) (1994) *Handbook of Qualitative Research.* Thousand Oaks, CA: Sage. ISBN 0803946791 References (extensive)

This major handbook attempts to synthesize the world of qualitative research. It progresses from the theoretical to the specific, examining the various paradigms for doing qualitative research. Strategies developed for studying people in their own settings and a variety of techniques for collecting, analysing, interpreting and reporting data are included. Contributors come from many disciplines and three continents (CR 2.64, 2.86, 2.97).

or

The following three entries constitute paperback versions of **Denzin, N.K. & Lincoln, Y.S.** (1994) *Handbook of Qualitative Research* (2.36.13).

2.36.14   Denzin, N.K. & Lincoln, Y.S. (eds) (1998) *The Landscape of Qualitative Research: Theories and Issues.* Thousand Oaks, CA: Sage. ISBN 0761914331

2.36.15   Denzin, N.K. & Lincoln, Y.S. (eds) (1998) *Strategies of Qualitative Inquiry.* Thousand Oaks, CA: Sage. ISBN 0761914358

2.36.16   Denzin, N.K. & Lincoln, Y.S. (eds) (1998) *Collecting and Interpreting Qualitative Materials.* Thousand Oaks, CA: Sage. ISBN 076191434X

2.36.17   Feetham, S.L., Meister, S.B., Bell, J.M. & Gilliss, C.L. (eds) (1993) *The Nursing of Families: Theory, Research, Education, Practice.* Newbury Park, CA: Sage. ISBN 080394716X Part III, Chapters 7–11   References

Sections examine the contributions of qualitative research to the study of families' experience with childhood illness, one approach to conceptualizing family response to illness, sampling issues, scoring family data and exploratory analysis (CR 2.22, 2.79).

2.36.18   Flick, U. (1998) *An Introduction to Qualitative Research.* London: Sage ISBN 0761955879 References

Book provides students with a systematic structure for comparing the various qualitative methods, designing the research process, ordering the claims and the evidence.

Practical examples are given together with summary boxes and further reading (CR 2.14).

2.36.19   Gardner, G. (1996) The nurse researcher: an added dimension to qualitative research methodology. *Nursing Inquiry*, 3 (3) 153–8   21 References

Author suggests that by integrating the characteristics of nursing practice with those of research, a 'nursing lens' approach to qualitative research can bring an added dimension to social methodologies in the nursing research context. Attention is drawn to the unique nature of the nurse–patient relationship and how this can enhance nursing research (CR 3.16).

2.36.20   Gilliss, C. & Davis, L.L. (1992) Family nursing research: precepts from paragons to peccadilloes. *Journal of Advanced Nursing*, 17 (1) 28–33   25 References

Author presents ten precepts that address the successes, as well complexities and shortcomings, found in family research over the last decade. Problems with methodology, data collection, aggregation, random variables and consistency with the unit of analysis all present challenges. Examples are given from literature in this developing field.

2.36.21   Graue, M.E. & Walsh, D.J. (1998) *Researching Children in Context: Theories, Methods and Ethics.* London: Sage. ISBN 0803972571   References

Book discusses the art and science of doing qualitative research involving children. The research process is covered and areas of particular difficulty when children are the subjects are highlighted.

2.36.22   Gubrium, J.F. & Sankar, A. (eds) (1994) *Qualitative Methods in Aging Research.* Thousand Oaks, CA: Sage. ISBN 0803949448   References

This volume of original articles explores the methodological possibilities and difficulties of doing qualitative work with elderly people. Using numerous examples, the strengths of qualitative strategies and techniques for uncovering meaning, dissecting processes and examining cultural and other differences between people and groups are discussed (CR 2.17, 2.43, 2.71).

2.36.23 Gummerson, E. (1991) *Qualitative Methods in Management Research.* Newbury Park, CA: Sage. ISBN 0803942044 References

Analyses the roles and methods used by academic researchers and management consultants when working with change processes in companies and organizations. The focus is on case-study research and the use of qualitative methods for data collection and analysis (CR 2.39, 2.64, 3.16).

2.36.24 Hammersley, M. (1989) *The Dilemma of Qualitative Method: Herbert Blumer and the Chicago Tradition.* London: Routledge. ISBN 0415017726 References

Examines the methodological ideas which underlie the Chicago tradition of qualitative research, focusing on the writings of Herbert Blumer.

2.36.25 Hammersley, M. (ed.) (1993) *Social Research: Philosophy, Politics and Practice.* London: Sage, in association with the Open University. ISBN 0803988052 References

Book addresses major issues including the relationship between qualitative and quantitative research, positivism, purposes of research, issues of race, gender and power, the politics and ethics of data collection, and the validity and relevance of research (CR 2.3, 2.5, 2.9, 2.10, 2.17, 2.25, 2.28, 2.29, 2.64).

2.36.26 Hill Bailey, P. (1997) Finding your way around qualitative methods in nursing research. *Journal of Advanced Nursing,* 25 (1) 18–22 21 References

Paper aims to assist new researchers to understand qualitative research literature. The language used and trustworthiness of this approach are discussed (CR 2.2).

2.36.27 Janesick, V.J. (1998) *Stretching Exercises for Qualitative Researchers.* Thousand Oaks, CA: Sage. ISBN 0761902554

Author believes that undertaking qualitative research needs more than simply learning about tools, rules and formats. She provides a series of exercises which can be used in or out of the classroom to enable researchers become more active observers, interviewers and learners.

2.36.28 King, G., Keohane, R.O. &

Verba, S. (1994) *Designing Social Inquiry: Scientific Inference in Qualitative Research.* Princeton, NJ: Princeton University Press. ISBN 0691034702

2.36.29 Koch, T. (1994) Establishing rigour in qualitative research: the decision trail. *Journal of Advanced Nursing,* 19 (5) 976–86 17 References

Article aims to show how the decision trail of qualitative research processes can be maintained by enabling the reader to audit the events, influences and actions of the researcher. A study is used for illustration (CR 2.49).

2.36.30 Layder, D. (1993) *New Strategies in Social Research.* Cambridge: Polity Press. ISBN 0745608817 References

Book aims to encourage the development of new strategies and is written for novices and experts. A bridge is suggested between recent theoretical debates in the social sciences and methodological issues. Theory generation, grounded theory, a resource map for research and multi-strategy research are all included, together with the historical dimension (CR 2.9, 2.45, 2.46).

2.36.31 Lindlof, T.R. (1995) *Qualitative Communication Research Methods.* Thousand Oaks, CA: Sage. ISBN 0803935188 References

Offers an up-to-date review of work being done in the communication field. Included are naturalistic inquiry, interpretative paradigm, ethnomethodology, symbolic interactionism, ethnography of communication, cultural studies, sampling and linearity. Many examples are included (CR 2.11, 2.22, 2.42).

2.36.32 Llewellyn, G. (1995) Qualitative research with people with intellectual disability. *Occupational Therapy International,* 2 (2) 108–27 55 References

Paper discusses the ethical concerns and issues of credibility in qualitative research with people who have an intellectual disability. An ethnographic study about the parenting experiences is used for illustration (CR 2.17, 2.42).

2.36.33 Lofland, J. & Lofland, L.H. (1995) *Analyzing Social Settings: a Guide to Qualitative Observation and Analysis* 3rd edition.

Belmont, CA: Wadsworth. ISBN 0534247806 References

This book teaches the techniques of gathering, focusing and analysing qualitative data in step-by-step discussions. Examples and applications are given throughout (CR 2.39, 2.42, 2.68, 2.72, 2.86).

2.36.34   Lowenberg, J.S. (1993) Interpretive research methodology: broadening the dialogue. *Advances in Nursing Science*, 16 (2) 57–69   89 References

Article sets the approaches of interpretative methodology within an historical and interdisciplinary context and discusses the shifts which have taken place to move research processes forward in nursing.

2.36.35   Lyon, E.S. & Busfield, J. (1996) *Methodological Imaginations*. Basingstoke: Macmillan Press. ISBN 0333630920   References

This collection of papers from the 1993 British Sociological Conference examines issues of research methodology in sociology.

2.36.36   Marrow, C. (1996) Using qualitative research methods in nursing. *Nursing Standard*, 11 (7) 43–5   10 References

Explores the problems and dilemmas encountered while conducting a longitudinal qualitative study in the clinical nursing environment. Strategies are highlighted to overcome the difficulties of using observation and interview techniques (CR 2.48, 2.68, 2.72).

2.36.37   Marshall, C. & Rossman, G.B. (1995) *Designing Qualitative Research* 2nd edition. Thousand Oaks, CA: Sage. ISBN 080395249X   References

Book discusses the critical traditions within qualitative inquiry, conceptualizations of researchers' roles and the possibilities for more collaborative ways of doing this type of research. Volume includes the important data collection methods, data management and analysis and resource allocation decisions. Vignettes are given which take readers through the complex processes of proposal development (CR 2.64, 2.79, 2.96).

2.36.38   May, C. (1996) More semi than structured? Some problems with qualitative research methods. *Nurse Education Today*, 16 (3) 189–92   16 References

Article advises caution when using qualitative techniques because of the limits on claims that can be made about their utility.

2.36.39   Mays, N. & Pope, C. (eds) (1996) *Qualitative Research in Health Care*. London: British Medical Journal Publishing. ISBN 0727910132   References

Book gives real-life examples of how the most commonly used qualitative research methods, such as interviews and focus groups, can be used in health care research. The benefits and pitfalls of each are discussed (CR 2.68, 2.69).

2.36.40   Miller, G. & Dingwall, R. (eds) (1997) *Context and Method in Qualitative Research*. London: Sage. ISBN 0803976321 References

Book addresses a range of methodological and practical issues central to the concerns of qualitative researchers. Major themes are validity and credibility, problems encountered using particular techniques in different social settings and moral issues raised in qualitative research (CR 2.17, 2.25).

2.36.41   Miller, S.I. (1994) *Qualitative Research Methods: Social Epistemology and Practical Inquiry*. New York: Lang. ISBN 0820423262   References

Provides an in-depth introduction to qualitative research methods for practising researchers. This type of inquiry is also put into the core of epistemological concerns (CR 2.6, 2.36).

2.36.42   Miller, W.L. & Crabtree, B.F. (1994) Clinical research, in Denzin, N.K. & Lincoln, Y.S. (eds), *Handbook of Qualitative Research*. Thousand Oaks, CA: Sage. ISBN 0803946791. Chapter 21, 340–52   99 References

Chapter discusses three goals: creating an open research space that celebrates qualitative and critical approaches to the clinical world, providing the tools and describing the means for sharing the stories and knowledge (CR 2.36.13).

2.36.43   Mitchell, M.L. (1998) *Employing Qualitative Methods in the Private Sector*. Thousand Oaks, CA: Sage. ISBN 0803959818 References

Book outlines some of the basic private-sector research settings and provides information on how to re-name skills and market most effectively to the business community.

2.36.44 Molzahn, A. & Sheilds, L. (1997) Qualitative research in nephrology nursing. *ANNA Journal,* 24 (1) 13–21   44 References

Some common forms of qualitative research are described: ethnography, grounded theory, feminist research, action research, historical research and evaluation research. Examples are given from nephrology nursing research literature when available and methods for critiquing and reviewing are suggested (CR 2.10, 2.37, 2.42, 2.43, 2.45, 2.46).

2.36.45 Morse, J.M. (ed.) (1994) *Critical Issues in Qualitative Research Methods.* Thousand Oaks, CA: Sage. ISBN 0803950438 References

Book addresses some lesser-known qualitative research methods, examines concepts of rigour and evaluation, discusses dilemmas of data collection and scientific misconduct. Ethical issues are explored, together with others which are not yet resolved or discussed in existing literature. Quality issues in qualitative research are also addressed (CR 2.17, 2.69).

2.36.46 Morse, J.M. (ed.) (1997) *Completing a Qualitative Project: Details and Dialogue.* Thousand Oaks, CA: Sage. ISBN 0761906010 References

With a contributor panel of 22 renowned qualitative research authors, this book addresses a wide range of topics from basics to the publishing process, and methodology to application. Each article is followed by dialogue resulting from brainstorming sessions between the contributors.

2.36.47 Morse, J.M. & Field, P.A. (1996) *Nursing Research: the Application of Qualitative Approaches* 2nd edition. London: Chapman & Hall. ISBN 0412605104 References

Book is intended as an introductory text on research methods for undergraduates and graduates. It presents a broad view of qualitative methodologies and discusses their history and subsequent development.

2.36.48 Munhall, P.L. & Boyd, C.O. (eds) (1993) *Nursing Research: a Qualitative Perspective* 2nd edition. New York: National League for Nursing Press. ISBN 0887375901 References

Text and reference book for nurse researchers and students. Parts contain a rationale for choice of qualitative method; selected qualitative approaches – phenomenology, grounded theory, ethnography, historical research and foundational inquiry; summary of the nature of qualitative nursing research and a framework for interpreting, writing about and evaluating this type of research (CR 2.42, 2.45, 2.46, 2.49, 2.86, 2.95).

2.36.49 Padgett, D.K. (1998) *Qualitative Methods in Social Work Research: Challenges and Rewards.* London: Sage. ISBN 0761902015 References

This introductory manual offers practical advice to students and researchers in social work on when and how to use qualitative research methods.

2.36.50 Platzer, H. & James, T. (1997) Methodological issues conducting sensitive research on lesbian and gay men's experience of nursing care. *Journal of Advanced Nursing,* 25 (3) 626–33 32 References

Discusses the nature of 'insider' status when conducting research, together with its advantages and problems. Using a particular study to examine the experience of lesbians and gay men, the authors describe conscious strategies to use this 'insider' status and explain how the ethical position taken was compromised (CR 2.16, 2.17).

2.36.51 QualPage. (1998) *Resources for Qualitative Researchers.* URL:http://www.ualberta.ca/~jrnorris/qual.html

This website lists information and resources of interest to qualitative researchers. Two new organizations, the Association for Qualitative Research (AQR) and The International Institute for Qualitative Methodology, are mentioned.

2.36.52 Rossman, G.B. & Rallis, S.F. (1998) *Learning in the Field: an Introduction to Qualitative Research.* Thousand Oaks, CA: Sage. ISBN 0761903534 References

Book provides an introduction to qualitative research in all its complexities.

2.36.53   Sandelowski, M. (1995) On the aesthetics of qualitative research. *Image: Journal of Nursing Scholarship*, 27 (3) 205–9 49 References

Discusses the efforts being made to show how qualitative data more closely resembles conventional science by the use of computerized systems for qualitative data analysis. Author considers the aesthetics of qualitative research which may reflect that of either or both the arts and sciences (CR 2.84).

2.36.54   Sandelowski, M. (1997) 'To be of use': enhancing the utility of qualitative research. *Nursing Outlook*, 45 (3) 125–32 58 References

Despite its popularity, qualitative research is inappropriately utilized, because it is often seen as useless. Author suggests ways in which its utility could be enhanced by improving the practice and criticism, mixing existing qualitative data by secondary analyses and synthesizing findings (CR 2.91, 2.92).

2.36.55   Sanders, P. & Liptrot, D. (1994) *An Incomplete Guide to Qualitative Research Methods for Counsellors.* Manchester: PCCS Books. ISBN 1898059047   References

Book provides an introduction to qualitative research for the uninitiated. Understanding and preparing to undertake qualitative research are discussed together with collecting, analysing and presenting data.

2.36.56   Schratz, M. & Walker, R. (1995) *Research as Social Change: New Opportunities for Qualitative Research.* London: Routledge. ISBN 0415118697   References

Authors believe that social research should become a part of the contemporary workplace. The book's main concern is to assist with the integration of different forms of qualitative action research and case-study methods within the ambit of professional practice (CR 2.37, 2.39).

2.36.57   Schutz, S.E. (1994) Exploring the benefits of a subjective approach in qualitative nursing research. *Journal of Advanced Nursing*, 20 (3) 412–17   27 References

Paper examines some issues of concern together with the benefits that may result from an openly subjective approach to qualitative nursing research.

2.36.58   Shaffir, W.B. & Stebbins, R.A. (eds) (1991) *Experiencing Field Work: an Inside View of Qualitative Research.* Newbury Park, CA: Sage. ISBN 0803936451   References

A group of experienced ethnographers address some practical questions involved in undertaking research. These are how you gain entry to a research setting, learn the rules of the study community without alienating them, how good relationships are maintained and what happens after you leave (CR 2.11, 2.14, 2.16, 2.42).

2.36.59   Silverman, D. (ed.) (1997) *Qualitative Research: Theory, Method and Practice.* London: Sage. ISBN 0803976666   References

Contains chapters written by an international team of researchers under the major headings of observation, texts, interviews, audio and video, validity and social problems (CR 2.25, 2.68, 2.72).

2.36.60   Stevenson, C. (1996) Taking the pith out of reality: a reflexive methodology for psychiatric nursing research. *Journal of Psychiatric and Mental Health Nursing*, 3 (2) 103–10   41 References

Discusses the problems in psychiatry relating to the use of existing research methods. A new methodology, which the author believes will enable the researcher to reflect on the research process in relation to the choice of method, gathering and interpreting the data, is discussed (CR 2.6).

2.36.61   Streubert, H.J. & Carpenter, D.R. (1995) *Qualitative Research in Nursing.* Philadelphia, PA: Lippincott. ISBN 039755091X

2.36.62   Symon, G. & Cassell, C. (eds) (1998) *Qualitative Methods and Analysis in Organizational Research: a Practical Guide.* London: Sage. ISBN 0761953515   References

Book describes a wide range of qualitative methods and shows how they can be used in practice. The development, position and value of qualitative approaches in organizations are discussed. Each chapter covers a particular method, describes how it has been used, gives a detailed example and instructions on how to use it and outlines its strengths and weaknesses.

2.36.63   Taylor, S.J. & Bogdan, R. (1998) *Introduction to Qualitative Research Methods: a Guidebook and Resource* 3rd edition. New York: John Wiley. ISBN 0471168688   References

Book is an up-to-date guide to qualitative study design, data collection, analysis and reporting. It reviews current theoretical development in feminist research and post-modernism. An extensive bibliography is included (CR 2.10).

2.36.64   Thompson, B. (ed.) (1998) *Advances in Social Science Methodology.* Hampton, Middlesex: JAI Press Inc. ISBN 0762302623

2.36.65   Thorne, S., Kirkham, S.R. & MacDonald-Emes, J. (1997) Focus on qualitative methods: interpretive description: a non-categorical qualitative alternative for developing nursing knowledge. *Research in Nursing and Health*, 20 (2) 169–77   51 References

Authors believe that nurses can develop and 'make their own' certain qualitative research approaches. General principles of an interpretative descriptive approach are discussed which reflect the unique mandate and epistemological foundations of nursing.

2.36.66   Too, S.-K. (1996) Issues in qualitative research: practical experiences in the field. *Nurse Researcher*, 3 (3) 80–91   19 References

Discusses how the theory behind qualitative research affected the process in a particular study relating to midwifery and birthplans (CR 2.16).

2.36.67   van den Hoonaard, W.C. (1997) *Working with Sensitizing Concepts: Analytical Field Research.* Thousand Oaks, CA: Sage. ISBN 0761902074   References

Author presents a history of the sensitizing concepts technique and gives practical applications for its use.

2.36.68   Weinholtz, D., Kacer, B. & Rocklin, T. (1995) Pearls, pith and provocation. Salvaging quantitative research with qualitative data. *Qualitative Health Research*, 5 (3) 388–97   12 References

Using two case studies, the authors show how ambiguous and misleading results from quantitative studies can be if not supplemented by qualitative data. This can also make them more cost-effective (CR 2.9, 2.29, 2.39).

2.36.69   Wilde, V. (1992) Controversial hypotheses on the relationship between researcher and informant in qualitative research. *Journal of Advanced Nursing*, 17 (2) 234–42   22 References

Paper examines some methodological issues which emerged during a qualitative study. These are interaction between researcher and informant; role conflict facing the nursing researcher; effect of the researcher's past experience on the interaction; use of counselling strategies and the principle of self-disclosure (CR 2.16, 2.65).

2.36.70   Wolcott, H.F. (1995) *The Art of Fieldwork.* Walnut Creek, CA: Alta Mira Press. ISBN 0761991018   References

Book covers the essential elements of field work. Sections include contexts, actual field work, field work as mind work and personal work. Its aim is to encourage field workers to reflect on how such work is an 'artistic' as well as scientific undertaking.

2.36.71   Wright, K.B. & Schmelzer, M. (1997) Qualitative research: exploring new frontiers. *Gastroenterology Nursing*, 20 (3) 74–8, 112   16 References

Article provides an introduction to qualitative research through comparing qualitative and quantitative perspectives, exploring qualitative designs and analysis. Examples are given using four methodological approaches and appropriate topics for research are suggested (CR 2.9).

NON-EXPERIMENTAL DESIGNS

2.37   ACTION RESEARCH

'. . . The participatory action research strategy has a double objective. One aim is to produce knowledge and action directly useful to a group of people . . . [A further] aim is to empower people at a second and deeper level through the process of constructing and using their own knowledge' (Denzin & Lincoln, 1994: 328).

Definition

Action research – research where, instead of minimizing the impact of the investigations on the subjects or individuals under study, changes are purposefully introduced in order to study what, if any, effects occur

Example

Gibbon, B. & Little, V. (1995) Improving stroke care through action research. *Journal of Clinical Nursing*, 4 (2) 93–100   19 References

Study attempts to bring about improvements in stroke care and rehabilitation in a general medical ward. Author states that the project led to increased knowledge, so reducing the theory/practice gap, improved care and more positive attitudes (CR 2.35).

Annotations

2.37.1   Birkett, M. (1995) Is audit action research? *Physiotherapy*, 81 (4) 190–4   22 References

Paper outlines the development of action research and examines its potential for use in physiotherapy. The similarities and differences between action research and audit are explored.

2.37.2   Cruickshank, D. (1996) The experience of action research in practice. *Contemporary Nurse: a Journal for the Australian Nursing Profession*, 5 (3) 127–32   31 References

Describes the process of using an action research approach within a surgical ward of a public hospital. At the end of the study, the nurses involved were able to recognize inconsistencies between what they said and did, and recognized their ability to bring about change in practice.

2.37.3   East, L. & Robinson, J. (1994) Change in process: bringing about change in

health care through action research. *Journal of Clinical Nursing*, 3(1) 57–61   16 References

Reports a study which aimed to facilitate management of change. Hospital managers and senior ward sisters had different views of the sources of challenges and problems within the organization, but results showed common ground between them (CR 2.101).

2.37.4   Fahy, K. (1996) Praxis methodology: action research without a group. *Contemporary Nurse: a Journal for the Australian Nursing Profession*, 5 (2) 54–8   23 References

Paper presents a modification of critical action research, praxis research, which is suitable for research projects which aim to empower individuals rather than groups. The steps in praxis research are described as an ongoing spiral of practice, self-reflection, scholarly inquiry and theorizing which leads to changed practice.

2.37.5   Greenwood, J. (1994) Action research: a few details, a caution and something new. *Journal of Advanced Nursing*, 20 (1) 13–18   34 References

The nature of action theories is explored together with the potential for development among practitioners who use these techniques. The costs of undertaking this kind of research are discussed together with a strategy for their reduction.

2.37.6   Hart, E. (1996) Action research as a professionalizing strategy: issues and dilemmas. *Journal of Advanced Nursing*, 23 (3) 454–61   58 References

Discusses the need for a debate about the appropriateness of using action research in nursing, incorporating literature from organizational culture and professionalization studies. Paper argues that in the managerialist context of the British National Health Service, action research may be used as a method of control and careful discussion needs to be undertaken so that its value does not become diminished.

2.37.7   Hart, E. & Bond, M. (1995) *Action Research for Health and Social Care: a Guide to Practice*. Buckingham: Open University Press. ISBN 0335192629   References

Book   is   designed   for   students   at

undergraduate and post-graduate level and others undertaking professional courses. It describes the processes of action research and how it may be used to solve problems and improve care. Five case studies of action research are described from the researchers' perspective. A tool kit is included which will assist in preparing research proposals, thinking about problems and formulating strategies (CR 2.14, 2.16, 2.20, 2.96).

2.37.8   Hart, E. & Bond, M. (1996) Making sense of action research through the use of a typology. *Journal of Advanced Nursing*, 23 (1) 152–9   14 References

Paper presents an original action research typology. The key criteria of re-education, problem focus, improvement and involvement are related to four broad types of action research. Three studies are used to illustrate these factors and the flexibility necessary when conducting action research is highlighted.

2.37.9   Hayes, P. (1996) Is there a place for action research? *Clinical Nursing Research*, 5 (1) 3–5   Editorial

Editor discusses the place of action research at a time of rapid change.

2.37.10   Hendry, C. & Farley, A. (1996) The nurse teacher as action researcher. *Nurse Education Today*, 16 (3) 193–8   40 References

Paper examines action research from the perspective of nurse teachers and authors believe it is an appropriate method for studying nurse education.

2.37.11   Johnson, M. (1997) Observations on the neglected concept of intervention in nursing research. *Journal of Advanced Nursing*, 25 (1) 23–9   21 References

Researcher intervention can be problematic for both positivist and qualitative researchers. Because nursing research is 'messy', a more reflexive and contextual approach is needed, applying both to moral justification and more pragmatic issues. Humanistic action research, informed by recent feminist thinking, has potential for more creative and clinically relevant work in nursing (CR 2.10, 2.29, 2.36).

2.37.12   McKibbin, E.C. & Castle, P.J. (1996) Nurses in action: an introduction to

action research in nursing. *Curationis: South African Journal of Nursing*, 19 (4) 35–9 29 References

Paper sets out a rationale for action research and describes its features, strengths and limitations.

2.37.13   Meyer, J. (1995) Stages in the process: a personal account. *Nurse Researcher*, 2 (3) 24–37   22 References

Describes the author's experience of carrying out an action research project in which the various stages are identified (CR 2.16).

2.37.14   Meyer, J. & Batehup, L. (1997) Action research in health care practice: nature, present concerns and future possibilities. *NT Research*, 2 (3) 175–84   44 References

Defines action research and locates it in the form of a new paradigm of research. Some current concerns are identified and suggestions are made as to how it may be used in future.

2.37.15   Newton, C.A. (1995) Action research: application in practice. *Nurse Researcher*, 2 (3) 60–71   16 References

Author gives some examples of action research projects and describes her own work which examined the effects of the care planning element of an integrated hospital information system (CR 2.15, 2.102).

2.37.16   Nichols, B.S. (1995) Action research: a method for practitioners. *Nursing Connections*, 8 (1) 5–11   26 References

Paper presents action research as a technique which combines grounded methods with organizational change to enhance clinical practice. The steps involved in action research are described and examples given. Techniques which enhance, maintain or increase rigour are discussed (CR 2.45).

2.37.17   Robinson, A. (1995) Transformative 'cultural shifts' in nursing: participatory action research and the 'project of possibility'. *Nursing Inquiry*, 2 (2) 65–74   55 References

Paper argues that through engaging with participatory action research, nurses can bring about transformative shifts in nursing culture. Examples from the author's own research are given.

2.37.18   Rolfe, G. (1996) Going to extremes: action research, grounded practice and the theory–practice gap in nursing. *Journal of Advanced Nursing*, 24 (6) 1315–20   29 References

Author believes that the full potential of action research methods is not fully used and there are also problems of definition. Paper suggests that this methodology goes beyond the confines of the scientific paradigm and can directly bring about improvements in practice.

2.37.19   Simmons, S. (1995) From paradigm to method in interpretive action research. *Journal of Advanced Nursing*, 21 (5) 837–44   37 References

Paper describes the often hidden process of moving from the researcher's world-view and perspective to decisions about which strategies are used for a particular research project. The process is illustrated by a study of community psychiatric nurses which examined the quality of life and social networks of clients with enduring mental health problems (CR 2.14).

2.37.20   Street, A. (1995) *Nursing Replay: Researching Nursing Culture Together.* Edinburgh: Churchill Livingstone. ISBN 0443047618   References

A guide to using participatory action research to explore the culture of nursing. The value of undertaking this type of research is discussed, techniques are explained and examples given.

2.37.21   Stringer, E.T. (1996) *Action Research: a Handbook for Practitioners.* Thousand Oaks, CA: Sage. ISBN 0761900659 References

Provides a series of tools for the novice practitioner when undertaking action research.

2.37.22   Titchen, A. (1995) Issues of validity in action research. *Nurse Researcher*, 2 (3) 38–48   18 References

Describes the stages necessary in establishing the validity of action research studies (CR 2.25).

2.37.23   Titchen, A. & Binnie, A. (1994) Action research: a strategy for theory generation and testing. *International Journal of Nursing Studies*, 31 (1) 1–12   24 References

Action research is defined and compared with other research strategies, together with its relationship to theory generation and testing, and their development. A set of criteria are presented for others engaged in this type of research (CR 2.7, 2.37).

2.37.24   Waterman, H. (1995) Distinguishing between 'traditional' and action research. *Nurse Researcher*, 2 (3) 15–23   17 References

The characteristics of action research and traditional research are discussed. Included are conceptual approaches, data collection methods, analyses, researchers and researched, ethical considerations, reliability and validity (CR 2.17, 2.24, 2.25).

2.37.25   Waterman, H. (1996) A comparison between quality assurance and action research. *Nurse Researcher*, 3 (3) 58–68 24 References

Evaluates the merits of audit and action research. Author believes that nurse researchers can benefit from both.

2.37.26   Waterman, H., Webb, C. & Williams, A. (1995) Parallels and contradictions in the theory and practice of action research and nursing. *Journal of Advanced Nursing*, 22 (4) 779–84   35 References

Paper argues that through a discussion of the core themes of action research, including 'knowledge in action' and 'self and group reflection', consideration should also be given to the symbiotic and complementary analysis of theory and practice. Many contradictions exist within action research and nursing and these need to be explored.

2.37.27   Williams, A. (1995) Ethics and action research. *Nurse Researcher*, 2 (3) 49–59 23 References

Article discusses how the agendas held by action researchers in their various roles affect the ethical component of research relationships (CR 2.17).

2.38   ATHEORETICAL RESEARCH

'Some purists may regard research which is not based on theoretical frameworks or conceptual orientations, as problem-solving rather than scientific research. However, early studies in clinical nursing research tended to be problem-solving endeavours rather than scientific research. More recently, emphasis has been put on the use of theory as the appropriate grounding, but there is still room for work to be done in nursing while a theoretical base is being discovered' (Phillips, L.R.F., 1986: 87).

Definition

Atheoretical research – research that is formulated without a theory base which involves problem-solving in specific situations

Example

Ritzer, G. (1981) The failure to integrate theory and practice: the case of the sociology of work. *Journal of Applied Behavioural Science*, 17 (3) 376–9   References

Article compares the work of theorists like Marx, Durkheim, and Weber with contemporary endeavours to apply theories to practical issues. These may fail because they are atheoretical or too abstract in character, or the theories may be misapplied or misinterpreted.

2.39   CASE STUDY RESEARCH

The term 'case study' does not denote a single specific technique, but rather a general strategy for research. Typically a case study involves one or several cases that are studied over time by multiple data gathering methods. They have a contemporary, rather than historical, focus, are naturalistic and conducted in a setting which is not controlled by the researcher.

Definition

Case study – a research method that involves a thorough, in-depth analysis of an individual, group, institution or other social unit

Example

Andrews, M. & Jones, P.R. (1996) Problem-based learning in an undergraduate nursing programme: a case study. *Journal of Advanced Nursing*, 23 (2) 357–65   46 References

Paper explores the use of a problem-based learning approach with a group of undergraduates. A case study design was used with observation as the main data collecting technique. Authors discuss its value as a motivating and educational tool (CR 2.72).

Annotations

2.39.1   Abramson, P.R. (1992) *A Case for Case Studies: an Immigrant's Journal.* Newbury Park, CA: Sage. ISBN 0803936966 References

Explores the question 'Can case studies be a relevant research tool in the social sciences?' Excerpts from the actual diary of a Jewish-Russian immigrant are used to demonstrate its appropriateness. Author describes how the technique is carried out and believes the results can increase our understanding of human behaviour (CR 2.67).

2.39.2   Fridlund, B. (1997) The case study as a research strategy. *Scandinavian Journal of Caring Sciences*, 11 (1) 3–4   11 References

Discusses some uses for case study research in nursing and its value in asking 'how' and 'why' questions.

2.39.3   Hamel, J., Dufour, S. & Fortin, D. (1993) *Case Study Methods.* Newbury Park, CA: Sage. ISBN 0803954166   References

Book places differing case study approaches into contrasting historical and societal contexts and makes suggestions about resolving some of the apparent contradictions and dilemmas associated with their use. A thematic bibliography for the case study is included.

2.39.4   Lane, H. (1979) *The Wild Boy of Aveyron.* Cambridge, MA: Harvard University Press. ISBN 0674953002   References

This classic case study shows the value of an in-depth study in the teaching of deaf children. The techniques developed are now used throughout the world in the education of deaf, handicapped and young normal children.

2.39.5   Muscari, M.E. (1994) Means, motive, and opportunity: case study research as praxis. *Journal of Pediatric Health Care*, 8 (5) 221–6   15 References

Article provides an overview and an example of research as praxis which will give pediatric nurses a research methodology alternative.

2.39.6   Scavenius, M. & Onland, J. (1996) Theoretical constraints in the first phase of a multi-site case study of health services. *Qualitative Health Research*, 6 (4) 506–25 18 References

Discusses the difficulties in conducting a multi-site case study of different health services. The considerable constraints of methodology and complexity of such research placed many theoretical constraints on the researchers. Constraints that were anticipated and experienced necessitated several reformulations of the research problem. These are discussed together with the general results of the pilot study (CR 2.14, 2.20, 2.23).

2.39.7   Woods, L.P. (1997) Designing and conducting case study research in nursing. *NT Research*, 2 (1) 48–56   27 References

Discusses use of this approach to study the phenomena of advanced nursing practice. Its appropriateness, rationale, use of multiple case studies, ethical issues, data collection and management are all considered (CR 2.17).

2.39.8   Yin, R.K. (1983) *The Case Study Method: an Annotated Bibliography 1983–1984 Edition*. Washington, DC: COSMOS Corporation. ISBN 0942570022

Cites publications dealing with the case study as a research method. The six sections include: general descriptions of the use of case studies; quality control issues; design and analysis; data collection; indirectly related topics; and coverage by traditional social science textbooks.

2.39.9   Yin, R.K. (1993) *Applications of Case Study Research*. Newbury Park, CA: Sage. ISBN 0803951191   References

Book augments earlier works and provides extensive applications of actual case study

research. Suggestions are made as to how it can be applied to broad areas of inquiry.

2.39.10   Yin, R.K. (1994) *Case Study Research: Design and Methods* 2nd edition. London: Sage. ISBN 0803956622 References

Textbook on case study design and analysis. The roles of theory and triangulation are discussed together with the debate in evaluation between qualitative and quantitative research.

2.40   CORRELATIONAL RESEARCH

Correlational research aims to describe the relationship between two naturally occurring events.

Definitions

Causal comparative – a type of correlational research in which two or more groups are compared with one another, either prospectively or retrospectively, to generate hypotheses regarding relationships between non-experimental variables
Correlational research – investigations that explore the interrelationships among variables of interest without any active intervention on the part of the researcher

Example

Taunton, R.L., Kleinbeck, S.V.M., Stafford, R., Woods, C.Q. & Bott, M.J. (1994) Patient outcomes: are they linked to registered nurse absenteeism, separation or workload? *Journal of Nursing Administration*, 24 (4S) 48–55   16 References

Authors explore the possible associations between patient outcomes, nurse absenteeism, separation from the work unit and work load. Clinical and methodological issues related to the findings are discussed.

Annotation

2.40.1   Fugleberg, B.B. (1986) Nursing research in the practice setting. *Nursing*

Administration Quarterly, Fall 38–42
12 References

A descriptive correlational study undertaken to investigate the attitudes of nursing administrators and staff nurses towards nursing research. Factors associated with a favourable environment and perceived level of competence in the research process were also examined.

2.41 EPIDEMIOLOGICAL RESEARCH

Epidemiological researchers have a special interest in data which may be retrospective in terms of diseases, epidemics or disasters, or prospective in trying to understand risk factors in the environment such as carcinogens or factors contributing to mental illness.

Definitions

Case control study – ... a retrospective epidemiological study in which subjects who have contracted a particular disease (the cases) are compared with similar subjects who did not contract the disease (the controls)
Epidemiological research – a strategy for trying to determine the causes, both necessary and sufficient, for the distribution and rates of occurrence of disease phenomena in human populations

---

Example

Ferguson, J.A., Goldacre, M.J. & Bulstrode, C.J.K. (1995) Workload in trauma and orthopaedic surgery: use of linked statistics to profile a specialty. *Health Services Management Research*, 8 (1) 55–63   22 References

Authors report use of linked hospital morbidity statistics to construct a profile of the epidemiological and demographic features of trauma and orthopaedic surgery in a defined population. Outcomes and implications are discussed.

Annotations

2.41.1 Abramson, J.H. (1990) *Survey Methods in Community Medicine* 4th edition. Edinburgh: Churchill Livingstone. ISBN 0443041962   References

Book provides a systematic guide to conducting investigations concerned with health and disease. It covers all aspects of design, execution and analysis, and would assist those planning many types of study (CR 2.52).

2.41.2 Breslow, N.E. & Day, N.E. (1980) *Statistical Methods in Cancer Research* Volume 1. Lyon: International Agency for Research on Cancer. ISBN 0197230326 References

Outlines the nature of case control studies, their objectives, strengths, limitations, planning, implementation and interpretation. Chapters 2–7 cover measuring techniques and analysis of case control studies.

2.41.3 Breslow, N.E. & Day, N.E. (1987) *Statistical Methods in Cancer Research* Volume 2. Lyon: International Agency for Research on Cancer. ISBN 9283211820 References

Book is an introduction to the design and execution of cohort studies. Chapter 1 gives a general overview of cohort studies, their historical role, significance and strengths, limitations, implementation and interpretation. Problems relating to proportional mortality studies are outlined. Chapters 2–7 discuss the statistical techniques and development applicable in this type of study. Appendices give statistical data and details of design and conduct of studies cited in the text.

2.41.4 Copp, L.A. (1987) Implications of epidemiological research. *Recent Advances in Nursing*, 17 94–107   References

Areas which have been studied in particular populations are discussed, together with special methods which may be required and the implications this could have for nursing.

2.41.5 Dean, K. (ed.) (1993) *Population Health Research: Linking Theory and Methods*. London: Sage. ISBN 0803987528 References

This compilation of papers focuses on quantitative research involving the collection and analysis of information about health issues from population groups. Evidence is given of the limitations of traditional approaches and the use of theory-guided multi-methods is discussed.

2.41.6 Dictionary of Epidemiology. (1988) 2nd edition. Edited by Last, J.M. New York: Oxford University Press. ISBN 0195054814

Contributions are included from over 100 epidemiologists worldwide in this dictionary. Clear and concise definitions are given for the discipline of epidemiology together with words from related fields, including statistics (CR 2.2, 2.84).

2.41.7 Esteve J., Benhamou, E. & Raymond, L. (1995) *Statistical Methods in Cancer Research. Volume 4: Descriptive Epidemiology.* Lyon: IARC Scientific Publications. ISBN 9283221281

2.41.8 Mulhall, A. (1996) *Epidemiology, Nursing and Health Care: a New Perspective.* London: Macmillan Press. ISBN 0333622529 References

Book explores epidemiology, its knowledge base, ideology and practice. Topics include principles, concepts and research designs, the developing relationship between epidemiology and nursing, and a critical appraisal of disease, illness, sickness and health.

2.41.9 Polivka, B.J. & Nickel, J.T. (1992) Case-control design: an appropriate strategy for nursing research. *Nursing Research,* 41 (4) 250–3   13 References

Article presents the structure of case control design and discusses points which need to be considered when using this technique. A study is used for illustration.

2.41.10 Teutsch, S.M. & Churchill, R.E. (eds) (1994) *Principles and Practice of Public Health Surveillance.* New York: Oxford University Press. ISBN 0195080211   References

An organized approach to planning, developing and implementing public health surveillance systems is given together with theoretical and practical tools for epidemiologists.

2.41.11 Unwin, N., Carr, S. & Leeson, J. (1997) *An Introductory Study Guide to Public Health and Epidemiology.* Buckingham:

Open University Press. ISBN 0335157858 References

Book covers some of the key issues in public health and epidemiology which are relevant to nursing. Also included are epidemiological study designs.

2.42   ETHNOMETHODS

'The growth of a new cultural movement, based on the anthropological tradition, developed in the USA in the 1960s focusing on how people know and understand their world. The term ethnomethods is used to describe a group of techniques which seek to explain human care and health attributes which are part of the social structure, world-views, language and different environmental contexts.' (Leininger, 1987: 13) [adapted]

Definitions

Emic – ... perspectives that are shared and understood by members of a particular culture, the 'insiders', in contrast to the perspective of the culture that observers, the 'outsiders', may have
Ethnography – ... the systematic process of observing, detailing, describing, documenting and analysing the life-ways or particular patterns of a culture (or sub-culture) in order to grasp the life-ways or patterns of the people in their familiar environment
Ethnology – the historical-geographical and comparative study of peoples or cultures
Ethnomethodology – a family of related approaches concerned with describing and portraying how people construct their own definitions of a social situation or, more broadly, with the social construction of knowledge
Ethnonursing – the study and analysis of the local or indigenous peoples' viewpoints, beliefs and practices about nursing care phenomena and processes of designated cultures
Ethnoscience – a formalized and systematic study of people from their viewpoint in order to obtain an accurate account of how people know, classify and interpret their life-ways and the universe
Ethology – a method of systematically

observing, analysing, and describing behaviours within the context in which they occur

Etic – . . . refers to the 'outsiders' view of the experiences of a cultural group

Reflexivity – . . . the process of critical self-reflection on one's biases, theoretical predispositions and preferences. The inquirer is part of the setting, context, and social phenomenon he or she seeks to understand

---

Annotations

2.42.1   Agar, M.H. (1996) *The Professional Stranger: an Informal Introduction to Ethnography* 2nd edition. New York: Academic Press. ISBN 0120444704   References

Book explores the nature of ethnographic research and discusses the key issues involved. It is contrasted with hypothesis-testing approaches and examples are given mainly from the author's own experience. Problems relating to ethnographic interviews and observation are discussed (CR 2.68, 2.72).

2.42.2   Altheide, D.L. & Johnson, J.M. (1997) Ethnography and justice, in Miller, G. & Dingwall, R. (eds), *Context and Method in Qualitative Research*. London: Sage. ISBN 0803976321 Part IV, Chapter 12, 172–84 References

Chapter addresses moral issues about contemporary institutions and organizations by analysing how ethnographers are 'justice workers', meaning that their studies are both the means of investigating ethical issues and of fostering greater justice in society (CR 2.17, 2.36.40).

2.42.3   Baillie, L. (1995) Ethnography and nursing research: a critical appraisal. *Nurse Researcher*, 3 (2) 5–21   43 References

Discusses the origins and development of ethnography as a research approach in nursing. Its uses, data collection methods, difficulties, ethical issues and its strengths and weaknesses are all explored (CR 2.12, 2.17).

2.42.4   Baszanger, I. & Dodier, N. (1997) Ethnography: relating the part to the whole, in Silverman, D. (ed.), *Qualitative Research: Theory, Method and Practice*. London: Sage. ISBN 0803976666 Part II, Chapter 2, 8–23 48 References

Chapter sums up the new developments in ethnography, particularly in terms of the concept of field work, the status this confers and the way the aggregation of cases is envisaged (CR 2.36.59).

2.42.5   Benson, D. & Hughes, J.A. (1983) *The Perspective of Ethnomethodology.* London: Longman. ISBN 058229584X References

Volume provides an introduction to ethnomethodology. Its intellectual background, in particular the work of Schutz, Garfinkel and Sacks, is examined and detailed discussions of research in the field are given.

2.42.6   Bernard, H.R. (1995) *Research Methods in Anthropology: Qualitative and Quantitative Approaches* 2nd edition. Walnut Creek, CA: Alta Mira Press. ISBN 0803952457   References

Revised edition of a major methods text intended also for social scientists. New sections include ethics, sampling, focus groups and the use of methods for theory development. There is increased emphasis on the use of computers (CR 2.1, 2.17, 2.29, 2.36, 2.69).

2.42.7   Bowers, L. (1992) Ethnomethodology I: an approach to nursing research. *International Journal of Nursing Studies*, 29 (1) 59–67   17 References

Paper introduce nurses to ethnomethodological approaches through examples mainly drawn from psychiatric nursing research. Suggestions are made as to where this approach may be appropriately used.

2.42.8   Bruni, N. (1995) Reshaping ethnography: contemporary postpositivistic possibilities. *Nursing Inquiry*, 2 (1) 44–52 42 References

Article discusses the 'new ethnography' which offers academics and others interested in generating knowledge, ways which open up possibilities in previously hidden areas of practice and one in which researchers are actively involved in taken-for-granted assumptions (CR 2.6).

2.42.9   Button, G. (ed.) (1991) *Ethnomethodology and the Human Sciences*. Cambridge: Cambridge University Press. ISBN 0521389526   References

Book re-examines the significance of ethnomethodology in sociology and the human sciences. Leading scholars discuss the various aspects involved in these approaches.

2.42.10 Clarke, L. (1992) Qualitative research: meaning and language. *Journal of Advanced Nursing*, 17 (2) 243–52 51 References

Discusses the problems relating to meaning and language in many ethnographic studies. Author believes there are also difficulties in sampling and reliability. Researchers are urged to acknowledge the tentative quality of their conclusions (CR 2.2, 2.22, 2.24, 2.45).

2.42.11 Coulon, A. (1995) *Ethnomethodology*. Thousand Oaks, CA: Sage. ISBN 0803947771 References

2.42.12 Davies, R.M. (1995) Introduction to ethnography in midwifery. *British Journal of Midwifery*, 3 (4) 223–7 26 References

Author introduces the principles underlying ethnographic research. It is suggested that greater use of the method may enable midwives to acquire cultural knowledge within the unique culture of midwifery.

2.42.13 Denzin, N.K. (1997) *Interpretive Ethnography: Ethnographic Practices for the 21st Century*. London: Sage. ISBN 0803972997 References

Author examines the changes, prospects, problems and forms of ethnographic interpretative writing in the 21st century. He believes that postmodern ethnography is the moral discourse of the contemporary world, and that ethnographers should explore new types of experimental texts to form a new ethics of inquiry.

2.42.14 Dingwall, R. & Strong, P.M. (1997) The interactional study of organizations: a critique and reformulation, in Miller, G. & Dingwall, R. (eds) *Context and Method in Qualitative Research*. London: Sage. ISBN 0803976321 Part III, Chapter 10, 139–54 References

Chapter focuses on ways in which qualitative research may simultaneously address micro and macro issues. The interactional literature on organizations is critically examined and an approach that focuses on language use and practical reasoning as features of

organizational and institutional settings is discussed (CR 2.36.40).

2.42.15 Ellis, C. & Bochner, A.P. (eds) (1996) *Composing Ethnography: Alternative Forms of Qualitative Writing*. Walnut Creek, CA: Alta Mira Press. ISBN 0761991646 References

Book comprises a collection of works which enlarge the space to practise ethnographic writing by telling stories through memoirs, poetry and other forms usually associated with the arts.

2.42.16 Erikson, K. & Stull, D. (1997) *Doing Team Ethnography: Warnings and Advice*. Thousand Oaks, CA: Sage. ISBN 0761906673 References

Authors examine the many challenges of doing team ethnography, including setting goals, creating a team, observing, sharing and collaborating on a finished product (CR 2.15).

2.42.17 Fetterman, D.M. (1998) *Ethnography: Step by Step* 2nd edition. Thousand Oaks, CA: Sage. ISBN 0761913858 References

Book guides readers in the steps necessary to conduct ethnographic research. This new edition includes ways of using the Internet for conducting searches and census data; conducting interviews by 'chatting' and videoconferencing; sharing information and debating issues with colleagues and downloading useful data and analysis software (CR 2.85).

2.42.18 Grills, S. (ed.) (1998) *Doing Ethnographic Research: Fieldwork Settings*. Thousand Oaks, CA: Sage. ISBN 0761908927 References

This collection of essays features the contributions of a wide range of researchers who consider the key research problems in their given field site.

2.42.19 Hammersley, M. (1997) *Reading Ethnographic Research: a Critical Guide* 2nd edition. London: Longman. ISBN 0582311047 References

Book provides an overview of ethnography and recent methodological developments. The process of undertaking and assessing ethnographic accounts is explored and illustrated by the author's own work.

2.42.20 Hammersley, M. & Atkinson, P. (1995) *Ethnography: Principles in Practice* 2nd edition. London: Routledge. ISBN 0415086647 References

Book provides an introduction to the principles and practice of ethnographic research, and is intended for students and experienced researchers. The principle of reflexivity is thoroughly explored as the authors believe this is the key to development of both theory and methodology in social science generally, and in ethnographic work in particular. Ethnographic research is put in the context of other qualitative methods, and each step in the process is examined using a wide range of examples. Book includes an annotated bibliography.

2.42.21 Hertz, R. (ed.) (1997) *Reflexivity and Voice.* Thousand Oaks, CA: Sage. ISBN 0761903844 References

This volume, which is an expanded version of a special issue of the journal *Qualitative Sociology*, presents an array of contemporary ethnographers grappling with the problems and new conventions of ethnographic writing (CR 2.97).

2.42.22 Hobbs, D. & May, T. (eds) (1993) *Interpreting the Field: Accounts of Ethnography.* Oxford: Clarendon Press. ISBN 0198258410 References

Book includes the field work experiences of eight ethnographers. The problems of the 'informal' and 'formal' worlds of research are discussed.

2.42.23 Johnson, J.C. (1991) *Selecting Ethnographic Informants.* Newbury Park, CA: Sage. ISBN 0803935870 References

Discusses how ethnographic informants can be selected systematically so maximizing the data collected. Techniques are included which determine the number and category of subjects, and guidance on how to select key people (CR 2.22).

2.42.24 Johnson, M. (1995) Coping with data in an ethnographic study. *Nurse Researcher*, 3 (2) 22–33 19 References

Article discusses data collection methods suitable for this type of study and how they may be developed into a useful research report.

2.42.25 Laugharne, C. (1995) Ethnography: research method or philosophy. *Nurse Researcher*, 3 (2) 45–54 19 References

Discusses ways in which ethnography has been used both as a method and an underlying philosophy. Author believes there should not be conflict between them, but its use as a method needs further exploration in nursing.

2.42.26 Leininger, M. (1997) Overview of the theory of culture care with the ethnonursing research method. *Journal of Trans-cultural Nursing*, 8 (2) 32–52 44 References

This classic and unique article represents a summative overview of substantive knowledge of the theory and method of ethnonursing, covering four decades of Leininger's work. Some aspects have been published elsewhere but are documented in the text, and referenced, to bring theory and method together in one article.

2.42.27 Lynch, M. & Peyrot, I. (1992) Introduction: a reader's guide to ethnomethodology. *Qualitative Sociology*, 15 (2) 113–22 References

Article introduces a special issue on ethnomethodology and its practical application.

2.42.28 Mackenzie, A.E. (1994) Evaluating ethnography: considerations for analysis. *Journal of Advanced Nursing*, 19 (4) 774–81 42 References

Discusses the factors which need to be considered when evaluating ethnographic studies, in particular issues of reliability and validity (CR 2.24, 2.25, 2.86).

2.42.29 Melia, K. (1993) The effects of nursing care: an ethnographic approach, in Kitson, A. (ed.), *Nursing: Art and Science.* London: Chapman & Hall. ISBN 0412470705 Chapter 8, 113–19 22 References

Reports a personal experience of illness and suggests that we need more ethnographic research on patients' experience of illness. Ethnography as a research method is discussed.

2.42.30 Miller, G. (1997a) Building bridges: the possibility of analytic dialogue between ethnography, conversation analysis and Foucault, in Silverman, D. (ed.), *Qualitative Research: Theory, Method and Practice.*

London: Sage. ISBN 0803976666 Part II, Chapter 3, 24–44   53 References

Chapter examines and elaborates the analytical potential of qualitative research by considering how it may be used to construct bridges between different theories of social life, particularly perspectives that focus on macro- and microscopic issues (CR 2.36.59, 2.89).

2.42.31   Miller, G. (1997b) Toward ethnographies of institutional discourse: proposal and suggestions, in Miller, G. & Dingwall, R. (eds), *Context and Method in Qualitative Research*. London: Sage. ISBN 0803976321 Part III, Chapter 11, 155–71   References

Chapter discusses how aspects of ethnomethodology, conversation analysis and Foucauldian discourse studies may be linked in qualitative research and discusses how this synthesis of perspectives may help in analysing power as a feature of organizational and institutional settings (CR 2.36.40, 2.89).

2.42.32   Morse, J.M. & Bottorff, J.L. (1990) The use of ethology in clinical nursing research. *Advances in Nursing Science*, 12 (3) 53–64   35 References

Discusses the historical development of ethology, its use in nursing, methods, the deductive and inductive phases and reliability/validity issues (CR 2.24, 2.25).

2.42.33   Parfitt, B.A. (1996) Using Spradley: an ethnosemantic approach. *Journal of Advanced Nursing*, 24 (2) 341–9   18 References

Study explored the common experience of expatriate nurses working in developing countries in primary health care. Spradley's Developmental Research Sequence was used as a data collection tool as well as for analysis. The results are reported.

2.42.34   Porter, S. (1993) Critical realist ethnography: the case of racism and professionalism in a medical setting. *Sociology*, 27 (4) 591–609   43 References

Paper demonstrates the possibility of using critical realism to overcome some of the epistemological weaknesses associated with ethnography. An ethnographic study which examines the effect of racism and professionalism on occupational relations between nurses and doctors is presented (CR 2.6).

2.42.35   Reid, B. (1991) Developing and documenting a qualitative methodology. *Journal of Advanced Nursing*, 16 (5) 544–51   55 References

Reports a study using an ethnographic approach to examine nursing observations. Each element of the research process is described and the problems encountered discussed (CR 2.16).

2.42.36   Rose, D. (1991) *Living the Ethnographic Life*. Newbury Park, CA: Sage. ISBN 080393999X   References

Author offers an alternative to the corporate mould of ethnography and reshapes it as a democratic form of thinking and being.

2.42.37   Schwartzman, H.B. (1993) *Ethnography in Organizations*. Newbury Park, CA: Sage. ISBN 0803943792   References

Book provides a methodological history of ethnography in organizations and guidelines for its conduct. The Hawthorne study is described and the role that anthropologists played in research arising from this. Recent studies are included to give pointers for other researchers.

2.42.38   Smith, S. (1996) Ethnographic inquiry in physiotherapy research. 2: The role of self in qualitative research. *Physiotherapy*, 82 (6) 349–52   13 References

Provides a reflective account of ethnographic research processes on the researcher and those studied. Ways in which the data may be influenced and some problems encountered during the observation and interview phases of a project are discussed (CR 2.16, 2.64, 2.68, 2.72).

2.42.39   Stewart, A. (1998) *The Ethnographer's Method*. Thousand Oaks, CA: Sage. ISBN 0761903941   References

Author helps ethnographers to devise a clearly articulated explanation of their methods. Also considered is what ought to be normative in methods discussions within ethnography from research design to the end product.

2.42.40   Thomas, J. (1993) *Doing Critical Ethnography*. Newbury Park, CA: Sage. ISBN 080393923X   References

Book offers a direct style of thinking about relationships between knowledge, society and political action. This type of ethnography can be scientific and csritical, and offers ways of going beyond conventional studies, without standing in opposition to it.

2.43 EVALUATION/OUTCOMES RESEARCH

'The practice of evaluation involves the systematic collection of information about the activities, characteristics and outcomes of programmes, personnel and products in order for judgements to be made about specific aspects of what these are doing or affecting.' (Patton, 1990: 18)

'[Recently] an important scientific methodology [outcomes research] has been developed to examine the end results of patient care. The strategies used in it are a departure from the traditional scientific endeavours. These include the incorporation of evaluation methods, epidemiology and economic theory perspectives.' (Burns & Grove, 1997: 569–611) [adapted]

Evidence-based nursing and medicine are becoming increasingly important in today's health services in order to ensure that the best possible care and treatments, based on research, are given. A new journal, *Evidence-based Nursing*, has recently been launched in the UK which may assist nurses in making appropriate decisions for patient care.

Definitions

Evaluation research – research that investigates how well a programme, practice or policy is working

Evidence-based medicine – . . . the conscientious, explicit and judicious use of current best-evidence in making decisions about the care of individual patients

Outcomes research – . . . any research that attempts to link either structure or process, or both, to the outcomes of medical care in the community, system, institution or patient level

---

Example

Wai-Han, C., Kit-Wai, C., French, P., Yim-Sheung, L. & Lai-Kwan, T. (1997) Which pressure sore risk calculator? A study of the effectiveness of the Norton Scale in Hong Kong. *International Journal of Nursing Studies*, 34 (2) 165–9   21 References

Reports a study which aimed to evaluate the effectiveness of the Norton Scale in predicting the likely occurrence of pressure sores compared to the Waterlow Scale in Hong Kong. The Norton score was found to be the better of the two and will continue to be used in elderly care wards until a better scoring system is found.

Annotations

2.43.1 Benjamin, K. (1995) Outcomes research and the allied health professional. *Journal of Allied Health*, 24 (1) 3–12   17 References

Article provides an overview of the history of the outcomes research movement with specific reference to federal government involvement. Differences between efficacy and effectiveness research are outlined and the problems in undertaking studies and strategies for increasing the use of outcomes research are all discussed (CR 3.11).

2.43.2 Boruch, R.F. (1997) *Randomized Experiments for Planning and Evaluation: a Practical Guide*. Thousand Oaks, CA: Sage. ISBN 0803935102   References

Book disentangles the complexities of randomized field experiments to enable researchers to evaluate better the impact of new programmes (CR 2.29).

2.43.3 Burns, N. & Grove, S.K. (1997) Outcomes research, in Authors, *The Practice of Nursing Research: Conduct, Critique and Utilization* 3rd edition. Philadelphia: W.B. Saunders. ISBN 0721630545 Chapter 21, 569–611

Chapter gives a brief history of endeavours to examine outcomes, outcomes research and nursing practice, its theoretical basis and the methodologies used. These are evaluation methods, epidemiology and economic theory perspectives (CR 2.1.13, 2.41).

2.43.4 Chelimsky, E. & Shadish, W.R. (eds) (1997) *Evaluation for the 21st Century: a Handbook.* London: Sage. ISBN 0761906118 References

A group of evaluators explain how evaluation has become what it is today and the likely outcomes in the future. Topics discussed include: what makes evaluation different from other disciplines, the links between the evaluation and auditing professions, which activities have priority in evaluation, new methodological approaches, the issues of advocacy versus truth and evaluating programmes versus empowering people to evaluate their own.

2.43.5 Colton, D. (1997) The design of evaluations for continuous quality improvement. *Evaluation and the Health Professions,* 20 (3) 265–85 27 References

Article examines the design of evaluations used for continuous quality improvement in health care and human service organizations. Using an example, the benefits of using alternative evaluation designs are explored.

2.43.6 Evaluation Thesaurus. (1991) 4th edition. Edited by Scriven, M.C. Newbury Park, CA: Sage. ISBN 0803943644 References

Covers major concepts, positions, acronyms, processes, techniques and checklists in the field of evaluation.

2.43.7 Fetterman, D.M., Kaftarian, S.J. & Wandersman, A. (eds) (1995) *Empowerment Evaluation: Knowledge and Tools for Self-assessment and Accountability.* Thousand Oaks, CA: Sage. ISBN 076190025X. References

The focus of this book, empowerment evaluation – a method for using evaluation concepts, techniques and findings to foster improvement and self-determination – is to examine the method as it has been adopted in academic and foundation settings.

2.43.8 Fink, A. (1995) *Evaluation for Education and Psychology.* Thousand Oaks, CA: Sage. ISBN 0803958544 References

Book provides information for those undertaking a programme evaluation within the context of a quantitative approach. Examples and exercises are given, do's and don'ts together with its advantages and disadvantages (CR 2.29).

2.43.9 Fitz-Gibbon, C.T. & Morris, L.L. (1988) *How to Design a Program Evaluation* 2nd edition. Newbury Park, CA: Sage. ISBN 080393128X References

Book covers evaluation designs in educational settings.

2.43.10 French, B. (1995) The role of outcomes in the measurement of nursing. *Nurse Researcher,* 2 (4) 5–13 19 References

Article describes the role and significance of outcomes measurement in nursing research. The difference between audit and research is outlined, together with the characteristics and sensitivity of measurements (CR 2.14, 2.54, 2.61).

2.43.11 French, B. (1997) British studies which measure patient outcome, 1990–1994. *Journal of Advanced Nursing,* 26 (2) 320–8 27 References

A total of 228 studies which measured patient outcome were retrieved and analysed in relation to the nursing specialty, intervention and outcome variables and the method of measurement used. Results are reported. Out of the total number of studies, 119 different outcome-measurement instruments were used, with only 20 tools used more than once. There was little coherence in definition and method of measurement between studies (CR 2.54, 2.61).

2.43.12 Goode, C.J. (1995) Evaluation of research-based nursing practice, in Titler, M.G. & Goode, C.J. (eds) *The Nursing Clinics of North America: Research Utilization.* 30 (3). Philadelphia: W.B. Saunders. ISSN 0029-6465 421–8 8 References

Article discusses the evaluation plan necessary to assess the value of research-based nursing practice. The steps, instruments, methods and feedback to clinicians are outlined. The difference between research utilization and replication is explained (CR 2.13).

2.43.13 Griffiths, P. (1995) Progress in measuring nursing outcomes. *Journal of Advanced Nursing,* 21 (6) 1092-100 73 References

Examines the progress made in measuring the outcomes of nursing over 30 years. Recent trends are examined which point the way forward and author suggests that this is dependent upon the use of a range of appropriate research methods and measurement techniques (CR 2.61).

2.43.14 Hall, J. (1996) The challenge of health outcomes . . . including commentary by McDonald, I. *Journal of Quality Care Practice*, 16 (1) 5–18   48 References

Author believes the health outcomes initiative can be seen either as another passing phase in health care management, or as a serious challenge to the planning, management and evaluation of health services. The article explores these challenges. Implementation will require the application of valid, reliable and sensitive measures, a broad approach to research, development of monitoring so that it becomes an integral part of the service, practice firmly based on evidence of outcomes and an approach that emphasizes generalizability (CR 2.24, 2.25, 2.28, 3.11).

2.43.15 Harrison, M.B., Juniper, E.F. & Mitchell-DiCenso, A. (1996) Quality of life as an outcome measure in nursing research: 'may you have a long and healthy life', *Canadian Journal of Nursing Research*, 28 (3) 49–68   63 References

Discusses the quality of life as a concept in health and health care, the problem of definition and the types of instrument which may be suitable for its measurement.

2.43.16 Ingersoll, G.L. (1996) Evaluation research. *Nursing Administration Quarterly*, 20 (4) 28–40   30 References

Common myths about evaluation are discussed and why these no longer fit with the current understanding of evaluation research. Aspects of the conduct of such studies are described and how they may be influenced by nursing executives.

2.43.17 Jenkinson, C. (ed.) (1997) *Assessment and Evaluation of Health and Medical Care: a Methods Text*. Buckingham: Open University Press. ISBN 0335197051   References

Text describes the variety of approaches available in the assessment and evaluation of health care. The principles of randomized controlled trials, case control studies, cohort studies and social surveys are described, together with qualitative methods which may

be used (CR 2.12, 2.29, 2.36, 2.41, 2.48, 2.52, 2.92).

2.43.18 Kelly, K.C., Huber, D.G., Johnson, M., McCLoskey, J.C. & Maas, M. (1994) The Medical Outcomes Study: a nursing perspective. *Journal of Professional Nursing*, 10(4) 209–16   30 References

Authors analyse the Medical Outcomes Study framework as a means of measuring the effectiveness of a multi-dimensional, inter-disciplinary health care delivery system. Its potential for measuring nursing outcomes is discussed and modifications are suggested which will assist in enhancing the functions of inter-disciplinary teams (CR 3.23).

2.43.19 Kirk-Smith, M. (1996) Clinical evaluation: deciding what questions to ask. *Nursing Times*, 8–14 May, 92 (19) 34–5 2 References

Discusses the processes involved in clinical evaluation, particularly how the necessary questions are formulated.

2.43.20 Koch, T. (1994) Beyond measurement: fourth generation evaluation in nursing. *Journal of Advanced Nursing*, 20 (6) 1148–55   39 References

Paper outlines the three generations of evaluation research and makes suggestions for the implementation of a fourth in health care settings.

2.43.21 Koyama, M., Holzemer, W.L., Kaharu, C., Watanabe, M., Yoshii, Y. & Otawa, K. (1996) Assessment of a continuing education evaluation framework. *Journal of Continuing Education in Nursing*, 27 (3) 115–19   8 References

Reports a study which analyses a systems model for evaluation research of continuing education. The results of a quasi-experimental study of a stoma care continuing education programme are described (CR 2.35).

2.43.22 Lin, C. (1996) Patient satisfaction with nursing care as an outcome variable: dilemmas for nursing evaluation researchers. *Journal of Professional Nursing*, 12 (4) 207–16 47 References

Article discusses the conceptualization and measurement of patient satisfaction with nursing care and the dilemmas which may arise. Implications for the future when using patient satisfaction instruments are outlined (CR 2.61).

2.43.23 Mark, B.A. (1995) The black box of patient outcomes research. *Image: Journal of Nursing Scholarship*, 27 (1) 42 6 References

Discusses the meaning of outcomes research and other terminology used in the field. Author believes that outcomes are but one stage in nursing care, with effectiveness and quality being equally important.

2.43.24 Miller, K.L. (1994) Assessing the context of care in patient outcomes research, in Fitzpatrick, J.J., Stevenson, J.S. & Polis, N.S. (eds), *Nursing Research and its Utilization*. New York: Springer. ISBN 0826180906 Chapter 9, 107–16 34 References

Presents an overview of conceptual and methodological issues related to the integration of contextual variables in patient outcomes research. A framework is suggested for analysing organizational contextual patterns in systems research. An example is given of research in progress that integrates variables in hospital sites (CR 2.102.17).

2.43.25 Mitchell, G.J. (1997) Questioning evidence-based practice for nursing. *Nursing Science Quarterly*, 10 (4) 154–5 1 Reference

Author lays bare some unexplained notions which may help nurses understand the opportunities and limitations of research and its usefulness for guiding practice.

2.43.26 Mohr, W.K. (1997) Interpretive interactionism: Denzin's potential contribution to intervention and outcomes research. *Qualitative Health Research*, 7 (2) 270–86 22 References

Describes Denzin's interpretative interactionism research method and its value to those studying interventions and outcomes. An example is used to demonstrate its potential.

2.43.27 Newman, D.L. & Brown, R.D. (1996) *Applied Ethics for Program Evaluation*. Thousand Oaks, CA: Sage. ISBN 0803951868 References

Book explores a set of principles which can serve as a guide to making ethical decisions in evaluation research. Using vignettes, the authors provide ethical dilemmas and questions to encourage discussion about the positive and negative consequences of each option. Suggestions are made about how evaluators can make informed ethical decisions (CR 2.17).

2.43.28 Nixon, C.T. & Northrup, D.A. (eds) (1997) *Evaluating Mental Health Services: How do Programs for Children 'Work' in the Real World?* Thousand Oaks, CA: Sage. ISBN 0761907955 References

Book addresses evaluation issues relating to community-based mental health services for children and young people with emotional and behavioural problems. Contributors discuss recent evaluations of the effectiveness of systems of care and specific intervention strategies. Their own research is described and issues facing researchers, limitations and the future are all discussed (CR 2.16).

2.43.29 Övretveit, J. (1997) *Evaluating Health Interventions: an Introduction to Evaluation of Health Treatments, Services Policies and Organisational Interventions*. Buckingham: Open University Press. ISBN 033519964X References

Book describes the strengths and weaknesses of different approaches to evaluation together with some of the practical pitfalls and politics associated with it.

2.43.30 Patton, M.Q. (1997) *Utilization-focused Evaluation: the New Century Text* 3rd edition. London: Sage. ISBN 0803952651 References

Book provides a comprehensive review of the literature on evaluation use and practice. Both practical and theoretical, the book gives advice on conducting programme evaluations (CR 2.12).

2.43.31 Pawson, R. & Tilley, N. (1997) *Realistic Evaluation*. London: Sage. ISBN 0761950095 References

Book shows how programme evaluation needs to be and can be improved. A new paradigm, called realistic evaluation, is described which promises greater validity and utility from the findings of evaluation studies. A complete blueprint for evaluation activities goes from design to data collection and analysis, the accumulation of findings across programmes and its development into policy (CR 2.25, 3.11).

2.43.32 Rossi, P.H. (1993) *Evaluation: a Systematic Approach* 5th edition. Beverly Hills, CA: Sage. ISBN 0803944586 References

A comprehensive text designed for practitioners in many disciplines which covers the role of evaluation research in the planning, design and implementation of programmes and projects. Examples of each stage are given throughout the text.

2.43.33 Sackett, D.L., Richardson, W.S., Rosenberg, W. & Hayes, R.B. (1997) *Evidence-based Medicine: How to Practise and Teach EBM.* Edinburgh: Churchill Livingstone. ISBN 0443056862 References

Book, written jointly by British and American physicians, discusses the areas to be considered in the development of evidence-based medicine. Authors give advice on questions which can be answered, searching for the best evidence, how it may best be evaluated and its validity for patient care (CR 2.25).

2.43.34 Sidani, S. & Braden, C.J. (1997) *Evaluating Nursing Interventions.* Thousand Oaks, CA: Sage. ISBN 0761903151 References

Book offers a comprehensive perspective on nursing intervention together with theory-driven guidelines for future study. The problems encountered in outcomes and intervention research are explained and authors then show via the Intervention Theory how such studies can be undertaken.

2.43.35 Slater, C.H. (1997) What is outcomes research and what can it tell us? *Evaluation and the Health Professions,* 20 (3) 243–64 38 References

Article provides a comprehensive and integrated view of outcomes research giving a definition, an integrated framework and several illustrative examples. The implications to be drawn are discussed and author recommends focusing efforts on building community health information systems.

2.43.36 Torres, R.T., Preskill, H.S. & Piontek, M.E. (1996) *Evaluation Strategies for Communicating and Reporting.* Thousand Oaks, CA: Sage. ISBN 0803959273 References

Book provides a model for doing evaluation

in a way that helps individuals and organizations to develop.

2.43.37 Waddell, D.L. (1991) Differentiating impact evaluation from evaluation research: one perspective of implications for continuing nursing education. *Journal of Continuing Education in Nursing,* 22 (6) 254–8 21 References

Two types of research, impact evaluation and evaluation research, are defined and compared across seven dimensions. Their strengths and weaknesses are also described.

2.44 EX-POST FACTO RESEARCH

In this type of research attempts are made to explain or describe events which have already occurred, and this has value when research problems cannot be studied by experimentation. Studies investigate cases where variables have been manipulated by life events, for example environmental pollution, the effects of thalidomide, and those which have taken place in natural settings, rather than in a laboratory.

Definition

Ex-post facto research – an after-only evaluation research design where pre-testing is not possible

---

Example

Dunn, S.A., Lewis, S.L., Bonner, P.N. & Meize-Grochowski, R. (1994) Quality of life for spouses of CAPD patients. *ANNA Journal,* 21 (5) 237–46, 257 34 References

Study describes the quality of life for spouses of Continuous Ambulatory Peritoneal Dialysis (CAPD) patients. Authors believe that nurses caring for the whole family can make a difference to the stability and well-being of the patient's spouse.

Annotation

2.44.1 Giuffre, M. (1997) Designing research: ex-post facto designs. *Journal of*

Perianesthesia Nursing, 12 (3) 191–5
4 References

Article discusses ex-post facto research.

2.45　GROUNDED THEORY RESEARCH

Grounded theory is a highly systematic research approach for the collection and analysis of qualitative data. Its purpose is to generate explanatory theory that furthers the understanding of social and psychological phenomena. It represents an advance in the technology for handling qualitative data gathered in the natural, everyday world. It has its roots in the social sciences, specifically in the symbolic interaction tradition of social psychology and sociology.

Definitions

Dimensional analysis – ... an alternative method of generating grounded theory conceived for the purpose of improving the articulation and communication of the discovery process in qualitative research
Grounded theory – an approach to collecting and analysing qualitative data with the aim of developing theories and theoretical propositions grounded in real-world observations
Heuristic research – a style of qualitative analysis in which research participants remain visible in the examination of data and continue to be portrayed as whole persons
Symbolic interaction – the study of how the self and the social environment mutually define and shape each other through symbolic communication

---

Example

Hamill, C. (1995) The phenomena of stress as perceived by Project 2000 students: a case study. *Journal of Advanced Nursing*, 21 (3) 528–36　56 References

Study identified stress-related factors in a group of students together with their coping strategies. Results showed that stress was directly related to non-integration with tertiary education and the ward team (CR 2.39).

Original text

Glaser, B.G. & Strauss, A.L. (1967) *The Discovery of Grounded Theory: Strategies for Qualitative Research*. Hawthorn, NY: Walter de Gruyter. ISBN 0202302601 (CR 2.45.6)

Annotations

2.45.1　Annells, M. (1996) Grounded theory method: philosophical perspectives, paradigm of inquiry, and postmodernism. *Qualitative Health Research*, 6(3)　379–93 27 References

Identification of the factors involved in understanding grounded theory is made and author believes that while it has traditionally been sited in a post-positivist inquiry paradigm, it is now evolving and moving towards the constructivist inquiry paradigm.

2.45.2　Barnes, D.M. (1996) An analysis of the grounded theory method and concept of culture. *Qualitative Health Research*, 6 (3) 429–41　44 References

Discusses the need to take account of the respondent's culture when conducting grounded theory analysis in order to enrich inductively derived material.

2.45.3　Beck, C.T. (1996) Grounded theory: overview and application in pediatric nursing. *Issues in Comprehensive Pediatric Nursing*, 19 (1) 1–15　27 References

Article describes the steps involved in the grounded theory approach which is illustrated by published work in paediatric nursing. Its application is then discussed. The results of a CD-ROM search of the Cumulative Index to Nursing and Allied Health Literature from 1983 to 1995 are summarized to identify grounded theory research in paediatric nursing.

2.45.4　Becker, P.H. (1993) Common pitfalls in published grounded theory. *Qualitative Health Research*, 3 (2) 254–60　7 References

Author reports that many grounded theory studies have in fact been descriptive with the underlying 'how and why' omitted. Some of the pitfalls for those using this method are highlighted.

2.45.5 Benoliel, J.Q. (1996) Grounded theory and nursing knowledge. *Qualitative Health Research*, 6 (3) 406–28 157 References

Paper examines the increasing use and development of grounded theory in studies since the 1960s. The focus of these included adaptations to illness, infertility, nurse adaptations and interventions, and status passages of vulnerable persons and groups.

2.45.6 Glaser, B.G. & Strauss, A.L. (1967) *The Discovery of Grounded Theory: Strategies for Qualitative Research*. Hawthorn, NY: Walter de Gruyter. ISBN 0202302601 References

A seminal work in the field of qualitative research which guides those planning such an approach.

2.45.7 Hickey, G. (1997) The use of literature in grounded theory. *NT Research*, 2 (5) 371–8 35 References

Paper discusses the disadvantages of undertaking a pre-study literature review which could lead to preconceived ideas about what issues need further investigation. There is little literature on how it may be used in grounded theory studies and the author makes some suggestions (CR 2.12).

2.45.8 Kearney, M.H. (1998) Ready-to-wear: discovering grounded formal theory. *Research in Nursing and Health*, 21 (2) 179–86 32 References

Discusses grounded formal theory analysis which can yield high-level, broadly applicable theory from analysis of situation-specific substantive theories. Although they may lack the cultural detail and context of similar smaller analyses, they have the potential to serve as 'ready-to-wear' models that fit the experiences of individuals in a variety of settings.

2.45.9 Keddy, B., Sims, S.L. & Stern, P.N. (1996) Grounded theory as a feminist research methodology. *Journal of Advanced Nursing*, 23 (3) 448–53 30 References

Discusses how grounded theory can be used in a creative and constantly evolving manner for feminist research (CR 2.10).

2.45.10 Kools, S., McCarthy, M., Durham, R. & Robrecht, L. (1996) Dimensional analysis: broadening the conception of grounded

theory. *Qualitative Health Research*, 6 (3) 312–30 15 References

Article traces the evolution of dimensional analysis, describes it in relation to traditional grounded theory and discusses its characteristics. An example is given to illustrate its application.

2.45.11 Melia, K.M. (1996) Rediscovering Glaser. *Qualitative Health Research*, 6 (3) 368–78 10 References

Article identifies the differences of opinion which have developed between the co-originators of the grounded theory approach and discusses the reasons for, and results of, this change.

2.45.12 Melia, K.M. (1997) Producing 'plausible stories': interviewing student nurses, in Miller, G. & Dingwall. R. (eds), *Context and Method in Qualitative Research*. London: Sage. ISBN 0803976321 Part 1, Chapter 2, 26–36 References

Reviews the recent disagreements between Glaser and Strauss about the nature of the research strategy they promoted in the 1960s. The author tries to establish where this leaves the followers of grounded theory. Interviews as text and as data are discussed, which raises questions about their appropriateness and limits (CR 2.36.40, 2.68).

2.45.13 Olshansky, E.F. (1996) Theoretical issues in building a grounded theory: application of an example of a program of research on infertility. *Qualitative Health Research*, 6 (3) 394–405 17 References

Article presents a research programme on infertility where a grounded theory of identity was developed and elaborated upon. Theoretical questions about methodology are raised in order to advance thinking.

2.45.14 Smith, K. & Biley, F. (1997) Understanding grounded theory: principles and evaluation. *Nurse Researcher*, 4 (3) 17–30 32 References

Outlines the steps which comprise the process of grounded theory and recommends criteria against which it can be measured.

2.45.15 Strauss, A. & Corbin, J. (1998) *Basics of Qualitative Research: Techniques and Procedures for Developing Grounded*

Theory 2nd edition. Thousand Oaks, CA: Sage. ISBN 0803959397   References

Book presents practical procedures and techniques for doing grounded theory studies and is intended for students and researchers in applied disciplines. A step-by-step approach to formulating the research question, various systems of coding and analysis, the process of writing or speaking on the topic are all covered. The final chapter provides criteria for evaluating a grounded theory research study (CR 2.36, 2.86, 2.97, 2.100).

2.45.16 Strauss, A.L. & Corbin, J. (eds) (1997) *Grounded Theory in Practice*. London: Sage. ISBN 0761907483   References

Volume presents a series of readings which emphasize different aspects of grounded theory and methodology. Selections are written by some of Strauss's former students and have been chosen for their accessibility and range. Commentaries by the editors are included for each paper.

2.45.17 Wiener, C.L. & Wysmans, W.M. (eds) (1990) *Grounded Theory in Medical Research: From Theory to Practice*. Amsterdam/Lisse: Swets & Zeitlinger, B.V. ISBN 9026511221   References

Papers covers theoretical issues in grounded theory, combining qualitative and quantitative methodologies, moving from theory to practice and analysing text (CR 2.29, 2.36).

2.45.18 Wilson, H.S. & Hutchinson, S.A. (1996) Methodological mistakes in grounded theory. *Nursing Research*, 45 (2) 122–4 19 References

Identifies the pitfalls of portraying descriptive studies as grounded theory and analyses additional methodological mistakes which detract from the credibility of authentic grounded theory approaches. The types of mistake discussed are muddling qualitative methods, generational erosion, premature closure, overly generic, importing concepts and methodological transgression.

2.45.19 Wuest, J. (1995) Feminist grounded theory: an exploration of the congruency and tensions between two traditions in knowledge discovery. *Qualitative Health Research*, 5 (1) 125–37   44 References

Author believes that feminist perspectives

and grounded theory offer approaches to discovering knowledge that can bring diversity and change. Tensions between the two are explored and reflexivity is seen as a way in which both may be respected (CR 2.10).

2.46   HISTORICAL RESEARCH (a) DOCUMENTARY

'Historiography provides one important route for researchers from nursing, midwifery and health visiting to interrogate "quality" in research practice and keep an evaluative eagle eye on intellectual standards more generally. We ignore the "lessons" of history . . . at our peril.' (Rafferty, 1997/98: 15).

Definitions

Historical research the critical investigation of events, developments and experiences of the past, the careful weighing of evidence of past sources of information and the interpretation of this evidence
Historiography – the writing of history
History – a recorded narrative of past events, especially those concerning a particular period, nation, individual

Example

Care, D., Gregory, D., English, J. & Venkatesh, P. (1996) A struggle for equality: resistance to commissioning of male nurses in the Canadian military, 1952–1967. *Canadian Journal of Nursing Research*, 28 (1) 103–17 6 References

This historical research study explored and described the forces of resistance that prevented male registered nurses from being employed and given officer status in the nursing division of the Canadian military. A 25-year struggle was needed to change this discriminatory policy.

Annotations

2.46.1 Burke, P. (ed.) (1992) *New Perspectives on Historical Writing*. Cambridge: Polity Press. ISBN 074560501X   References

A group of 'new' historians reflect on their practice, and more widely on those of the particular historical guild to which they belong (CR 2.16).

2.46.2 Carr, E.H. (1986) *What is History?* London: Macmillan Press. ISBN 0333389565 References

A classic text which explores historical theory, the origins of history, its relationship to science and morality, causation and how it expands the horizon of learning.

2.46.3 Christy, T.E. (1981) Can we learn from history? in McCloskey, J.C. & Grace, H.K. (eds), *Current Issues in Nursing.* Oxford: Blackwell Scientific. ISBN 086542005X Part 2, Chapter 13, 122-9 References

Author discusses the reasons for including the history of nursing in the curriculum and the value of undertaking historical research in preventing 'the rediscovery of the wheel'.

2.46.4 Church, O.M. (1990) New knowledge from old truths: problems and promises of historical enquiry in nursing, in McCloskey, J.C. & Grace, H.K. (eds) *Current Issues in Nursing* 3rd edition. St Louis: Mosby. ISBN 0801655250. Chapter 13, 94–8 20 References

Discusses the value of historical inquiry to the practice of nursing.

2.46.5 Cushing, A. (1996) Method and theory in the practice of nursing history . . . including commentary by Maggs, C. *International History of Nursing Journal,* 2 (2) 5–32 35 References

Paper examines two main issues connected to the writing of history: difficulties in writing an account of past events and the role of social theory in historical writing. The contributions of other historians, the diversity of views and underlying assumptions in methodological approaches are all discussed in relation to written documents.

2.46.6 Firby, P. (1993) Learning from the past. *Nursing Times,* 17 November, 89 (46) 32–3 9 References

Discusses the value and problems of historical research and suggestions are made on how to collect data in this type of study (CR 2.47, 2.86).

2.46.7 Hallett, C. (1997/1998) Historical texts: factors affecting their interpretation. *Nurse Researcher,* 5 (2) 61–71 25 References

Author discusses the types of historical text, medical treatises as a source for nursing history, difficulties with their interpretation and how they may be approached.

2.46.8 Hill, M.R. (1993) *Archival Strategies and Techniques.* Newbury Park, CA: Sage. ISBN 0803948255

2.46.9 Lusk, B. (1997) Historical methodology for nursing research. *Image: Journal of Nursing Scholarship,* 29 (4) 355–9 36 References

Describes the basic tenets of historical research methodology with emphasis on researching nursing history.

2.46.10 Mackinnon, M. (1997) What a difference a nurse makes: then and now. *Western Journal of Nursing Research,* 19 (6) 795–800 5 References

The historical biography method was used to study the practice of one nurse in Saskatchewan from 1929 to 1963. Interviews were held with the nurse and six former patients. The maternity portion of the data was analysed using the constant comparative method to identify themes. Findings showed that caring, being present and expert practice were of particular importance (CR 2.71).

2.46.11 Mansell, D. (1995) Sources in nursing historical research: a thorny methodological problem. *Canadian Journal of Nursing Research,* 27 (3) 83–6 9 Endnotes

Discusses some of the difficulties facing nurses when researching any historical subject. Limitations exist in available records which may give a skewed picture of particular groups of nurses and their activities. However, when these are combined with oral data, personal diaries and correspondence, a fuller picture may be gained (CR 2.28, 2.67, 2.71).

2.46.12 Marwick, A. (1989) *The Nature of History* 3rd edition. Basingstoke: Macmillan Press. ISBN 0333432355 References

Book explains the basic methods and principles of historical research, how sources are analysed and ways in which research may be written up.

2.46.13 Morris, R.J. (1991) History and computing: expansion and achievements. *Social Science Computer Review*, 9 (2) 215–30 References

Reports on developments in historical research using computers from 1980 to 1990. Included is information on large databases, developments in text analysis, information on associations, journals and data archives (CR 2.76, 2.89).

2.46.14 Rafferty, A.M. (1996) Historical research, in Cormack, D.F.S. (ed.), *The Research Process in Nursing* 3rd edition. Oxford: Blackwell Scientific Inc. ISBN 063204019X Chapter 16, 166–77 26 References

Chapter asks why we should study history, outlines the sources available for its study and asks whether it is a voyage of discovery or a journey without maps. The characteristic features of historical research in nursing are discussed (CR 2.1.18).

2.46.15 Rafferty, A.M. (1997/98) Writing, researching and reflexivity in nursing history. *Nurse Researcher*, 5 (2) 5–16 34 References

Author considers some of the questions which have 'exercised the minds and hearts of historians' since the 19th century. She believes that nurse researchers can learn from history, and particularly from that of other disciplines, to create building blocks for the development of further research in nursing.

2.46.16 Ruggles, S. & Menard, R.R. (1995) The Minnesota Historical Census Projects. *Historical Methods*, 28 (1) 6–10 References

Describes the potential and limitations of using census micro-data for historical research purposes.

2.46.17 Sarnecky, M.T. (1990) Historiography: a legitimate research methodology for nursing. *Advances in Nursing Science*, 12 (4) 1–10 36 References

Examines the historical approach, discusses its relevance to nursing and contrasts it with other epistemologies and ontologies (CR 2.5, 2.6).

2.46.18 Sorenson, E.S. (1988) Archives as sources of treasure in historical research. *Western Journal of Nursing Research*, 10 (5) 666–70 11 References

Discusses the use of historical archives and gives some of the sources available for the study of nursing history.

2.46.19 Stinson, S.M., Johnson, J.L. & Zilm, G. (1992) *History of Nursing Beginning Bibliography: a Proemial List with Special Reference to Canadian Sources*. Edmonton, Alberta, Canada: Faculty of Nursing, University of Alberta. ISBN 0888647727

4.4 Nursing research entry nos 828–67
5.2 Historical research methods entry nos 895–963

Bibliography is the first published list of references pertaining to the history of nursing with special reference to Canada. Sections cover the history of nursing research and historical research methods. The latter covers literature from 1952 to 1991 and includes both documentary and oral history (CR 1.5, 2.47).

2.46.20 Stryker, R. (1996) Beyond history versus theory: strategic narrative and sociological explanation. *Sociological Methods and Research*, 24 (3) 304–53 References

Explores the dialectic interaction between theory and data in historical research (CR 2.7).

2.46.21 Tuchman, G. (1994) Historical social science, in Denzin, N.K. & Lincoln, Y.S. (eds), *Handbook of Qualitative Research*. Thousand Oaks, CA: Sage. ISBN 0803946791 Chapter 19, 306–23 47 References

Chapter explores the methodologies, methods, and meanings of historical social science. Details of reference sources are given to access both primary and secondary materials (CR 2.36.13).

2.47 HISTORICAL RESEARCH (b) ORAL

The validity of oral history as a field of study has been questioned by some historians because of the difficulties of trying to reconstruct the past on minimal and perhaps biased evidence. Agreement can never be reached about what the past was really like, but oral history can assist in filling in some of the gaps about the more recent past.

Definition

Oral history – history based on verbal accounts instead of written records

Example

Nikkonen, M. (1994) Caring from the point of view of a Finnish mental health nurse: a life history approach. *Journal of Advanced Nursing,* 19 (6) 1185–95   46 References

Study described and analysed the work of one mental health nurse over a period of 30 years in the rehabilitation of long-term psychiatric patients for non-institutional care. Repeated interviews were held to ascertain her views of caring over many years (CR 2.42, 2.68, 2.71).

Annotations

2.47.1   Allen, B. (1984) Re-creating the past: the narrator's perspective in oral history. *Oral History Review,* 12 1–12   19 References

Article discusses the different perspectives of the narrator and interviewer and identifies the points of view from which each approaches the oral history interview. The differing emphases and the researcher's interest in reconstructing the past along chronological lines are outlined, whereas that of the client is one of association. Both angles are needed in order to create a composite picture.

2.47.2   Caunce, S. (1994) *Oral History and the Local Historian.* South Melbourne, Victoria: Longman. ISBN 0582072948

This book is 'a menu you can choose from, not an instruction manual'. The author sets out to demystify and broaden the basis of oral history.

2.47.3   Church, O.M. & Johnson, M.L. (1995) Worth remembering: the process and products of oral history. *International History of Nursing Journal,* 1 (1) 19–31   11 References

Paper describes oral history as a methodology, the process of data collection as it relates to working with a specific population of 18 women who graduated from the Illinois Training School near the turn of the century. The significance and implications of this technique are discussed.

2.47.4   Clifford, D. (1995) Methods in oral history and social work. *Oral History,* 23 (2) 65–70   28 References

Paper suggests ways in which useful connections can be made between social and health work practice and methods, and oral history.

2.47.5   Davis, C., Back, K. & Maclean, K. (1977) *Oral History: From Tape to Type.* Chicago: American Library Association. ISBN 0838902308   References

An instructional and operating manual designed to guide those beginning an oral history programme and a textbook for instructors. Illustrations and exercises are included to enable the novice to practise certain skills. Sample forms show how to do the paperwork which accompanies oral history interviewing and processing. A glossary and a list of additional sources are included (CR 2.2).

2.47.6   Dunaway, D.K. (1992) Method and theory in oral biography. *Oral History,* 20 (2) 40–4   14 References and Notes

Discusses oral biography and ethnography, the relative value of interviews to each other and the written record, memory and verbal performance (CR 2.42, 2.68).

2.47.7   Dunaway, D.K. & Baum, W.K. (eds) (1997) *Oral History: an Interdisciplinary Anthology* 2nd edition. Thousand Oaks: CA: Alta Mira Press. ISBN 0761991891   References

Book explains the basis of oral history and how to make use of it in research. It also includes a significant collection of classic readings by oral historians. Contributors come from France, Germany, Italy, Mexico and the UK.

2.47.8   Echevarria-Howe, L. (1995) Reflections from participants: the process and product of life history work. *Oral History,* 23 (2) 40–6   13 References

Reports the feelings and responses of two participants who were involved in a life history study (CR 2.22).

2.47.9   Elinor, G. (1992) Stolen or given: an issue in oral history. *Oral History*, 20 (1) 23 References and Notes

Discusses issues in editing and re-writing others' interview material and the ways in which it was obtained.

2.47.10   Finnegan, R. (1992) *Oral Traditions and the Verbal Arts: a Guide to Research Practices*. London: Routledge. ISBN 0415028419 References

Book is a guide to the practicalities of field work and the range of methods by which oral texts and performances can be observed, collected and analysed (CR 2.86).

2.47.11   Hagemaster, J.N. (1992) Life history: a qualitative method of research. *Journal of Advanced Nursing*, 17 (9) 1122–8 24 References

Paper describes this method of qualitative research for identifying and documenting health patterns of individuals and groups. Specific steps are identified for using this approach in nursing (CR 2.36, 2.71).

2.47.12   Humphries, S. (1984) *The Handbook of Oral History: Recording Life Stories*. London: Inter-Action   Inprint.   ISBN 0904571467   References

Book shows how a more accurate and authentic picture of the past may be created by talking to the people who were actually there. It includes sections on organizing a project, working with different groups, and all aspects of presentation and publication.

2.47.13   Hutching, M. (1993) *Talking History: a Short Guide to Oral History*. Wellington, NZ: Williams, Bridget Books/ Historical Department Branch, Department of Internal Affairs. ISBN 0908912463

Book is intended for those undertaking oral history for the first time. Oral history is defined and the processes involved, from preparation to interview and processing, are discussed. A list of questions and a short bibliography are included.

2.47.14   Kirby, S. (1997/98) The resurgence

of oral history and the new issues it raises. *Nurse Researcher*, 5 (2) 45–58   20 References

Author explores the nature and nurture of oral history and discusses ways of ensuring rigour when obtaining data from interviews. Its value to nursing is discussed (CR 2.68).

2.47.15   Maggs, C. & Rapport, F. (1995) Oral history and content analysis using Ethnograph. *International History of Nursing Journal*, 1 (2) 29–38   3 References

Paper presents a computer-based technique for analysing taped collections of material. An example is used to demonstrate how Ethnograph can assist in a more rapid but equally valid analysis of oral testimony (CR 2.84, 2.87, 2.88, Appendix A).

2.47.16   Martin, R.R. (1995) *Oral History in Social Work: Research, Assessment and Intervention*. Thousand Oaks, CA: Sage. ISBN 0803943830   References

Author defines oral history and introduces readers to its basic principles and methodologies. A step-by-step guide is given for using oral histories in various settings and with diverse populations. Examples are given.

2.47.17   Paterson, B. & Bramadat, I.J. (1992) Use of the pre-interview in oral history. *Qualitative Health Research*, 2 (1) 99–115 18 References

The use of pre-interviews is discussed, their content and structure identified and examples given highlighting their benefits and limitations (CR 2.68).

2.47.18   Perks, R. (ed.) (1990) *Oral History*. London: British Library. ISBN 071230505X

An annotated bibliography giving a wide range of health topics in over 2,100 entries. Sources of information on the processes involved in oral history are also included (CR 1.5).

2.47.19   Prins, G. (1992) Oral history, in Burke, P. (ed.), *New Perspectives on Historical Writing*. Cambridge: Polity Press. ISBN   074560501X   Chapter   6,   114–39 32 References

Discusses the reasons why the use of oral sources is controversial and asks what is oral evidence. The main problems of use and misuse and sources of primary data are included (CR 2.46.1, 2.90).

2.47.20 Seldon, A. & Pappworth, J. (1983) *By Word of Mouth: 'Elite Oral History'.* London: Methuen. ISBN 0416367402 References

A practical guide to the oral history of elite figures, i.e. from or about people eminent in their field. Book analyses the advantages of using oral history, offers advice on aspects of interviewing and gives information on the establishment and maintenance of an oral archive. A series of case studies showing the use of oral evidence by contemporary authors is included (CR 2.39, 2.68).

2.47.21 Thompson, P. (1988) *The Voice of the Past: Oral History* 2nd revised edition. Oxford: Oxford University Press. ISBN 0192892169 References

The accepted myths of the nature of historical scholarship are challenged. Author traces oral history through its past and into the future showing how the method could be developed. This new material can be evaluated alongside traditional sources to construct a more democratic record (CR 2.68).

2.47.22 Thompson, P. & Perks, R. (1993) *An Introduction to the Use of Oral History in the History of Medicine.* London: National Life Story Collection. ISBN 09521664[++]

2.47.23 Thomson, A., Frisch, M. & Hamilton, P. (1994) The memory and history debate: some international perspectives. *Oral History*, 22 (2) 33–43   25 References

Article attempts to take stock of the debates about memory and history and includes contributions from the USA, the UK and Australia. Areas covered are oral history's critics, ethical and political dilemmas, theory and practice, history and memory, memory as history, history as memory, authenticity of memory, memory and the national past, politics and popular culture.

2.47.24 Vaz, K.M. (ed.) (1997) *Oral Narrative Research with Black Women: Collecting Treasures.* Thousand Oaks, CA: Sage. ISBN 0803974299   References

Oral narrative researchers from a variety of disciplines present strategies they have used to examine the experiences of African and African-American women. Book explores in detail the strengths of oral narrative research for expanding and transforming knowledge and how carrying out this type of research has affected the researchers' personal and professional lives (CR 2.16, 2.78).

2.47.25 Yow, V.R. (1994) *Recording Oral History: a Practical Guide for Social Scientists.* Thousand Oaks, CA: Sage. ISBN 0803955790 References

Gives advice on all aspects of in-depth interviewing, handling tape recorders and asking probing questions. Ethical and legal issues are also covered (CR 2.17, 2.68).

2.48
LONGITUDINAL/DEVELOPMENTAL RESEARCH

This research strategy is useful for detecting change in individuals or groups over time, for example examining health maintenance or illness recovery.

Definitions

Cohort studies – studies based on a longitudinal design in which subjects are grouped by their ages for comparative purposes
Developmental research – research focusing on those aspects of human behaviour that change over time
Longitudinal designs – studies based on longitudinal data include *trend studies*, in which data are compared across time points on different subjects; *cohort studies* in which data from the same age cohort are compared at different points in time; and *panel studies*, in which the same subjects are compared across time points

Example

Lathlean, J. (1996) The challenges of longitudinal ethnographic research in nursing. *NT Research*, 1 (1) 38–43   16 References

Paper describes problems and strategies adopted during aspects of a project which examined the development of lecturer–practitioner roles in nursing. The long-term nature of the research and the challenges this posed for the researcher are discussed. The use of participant observation as a research method is highlighted (CR 2.42, 2.73).

Annotations

2.48.1 Armstrong-Stassen, M., Cameron, S.J. & Horsburgh, M.E. (1996) The impact of organizational downsizing on the job satisfaction of nurses. *Canadian Journal of Nursing Administration*, 9 (4) 8–32   36 References

This panel study examined the impact of health service restructuring in Canada on nurses' morale and job satisfaction. The organizational and management implications of the findings are discussed.

2.48.2 Donohue, L. (1995) Tracing lost research participants. *Australian Journal of Advanced Nursing*, 12 (3) 6–10   7 References

Discusses the strategies used to locate research participants with whom researchers had lost contact during a 13-year longitudinal study. The most useful information in tracing 'lost' participants was a record of correct names and next of kin. Contact was re-established most effectively by telephone (CR 2.22).

2.48.3 Donsbach, W. & Brosius, H.B. (1991) Panel surveys by telephone: how to improve response rates and sample quality. *Marketing and Research Today*, 19 (3) 143–50   References

Discusses methods for increasing responses in panel research by telephone interviews (CR 2.70).

2.48.4 Goldstein, H. (1979) *The Design and Analysis of Longitudinal Studies: Their Role in the Measurement of Change*. London: Academic Press. ISBN 0122895800   References

Provides comprehensive coverage of the theoretical background to this type of design together with a practical approach to the problems encountered in human field studies. Statistical aspects of longitudinal studies are thoroughly explored.

2.48.5 Huber, G.P. & Van De Ven, A.H. (eds) (1995) *Longitudinal Field Research Methods: Studying Processes of Organizational Change*. Thousand Oaks, CA: Sage. ISBN 0803970919   References

Book describes procedures on tabulating, coding and interpreting both qualitative and quantitative data collected in the field (CR 2.86, 2.87).

2.48.6 Ingersoll, G.L., Brooks, A.M., Fischer, M.S., Hoffere, D.A., Lodge, R.H., Wigsten, K.S., Costello, D., Hartung, D.A., Kiernan, M.E., Parrinello, K.M. & Schultz, A.W. (1995) Professional practice model research collaboration: issues in longitudinal, multi-site design. *Journal of Nursing Administration*, 25 (1) 39–46   References

Discusses issues associated with collaborating during the conduct of longitudinal studies. Factors which facilitated or hindered progress are explored and recommendations made for change (CR 2.15).

2.48.7 Jacobson, S.F. & Jordan, K.F. (1993) Nurses' response for participating in a longitudinal panel survey. *Western Journal of Nursing Research*, 15 (4) 509–15   8 References

Reports a study which examined 23 reasons why nurses chose to participate in a research study (CR 2.22, 2.49).

2.48.8 Magnusson, D. & Bergman, L. (eds) (1990) *Data Quality in Longitudinal Research*. Cambridge: Cambridge University Press. ISBN 052138091X   References

Book discusses data quality issues in different areas, drop-out and attrition, design and methods. The importance of ensuring reliability, validity and representativeness is stressed (CR 2.24, 2.25).

2.48.9 Magnusson, D., Bergman, L.R., Rudinger, G. & Torestad, B. (eds) (1991) *Problems and Methods in Longitudinal Research: Stability and Change*. Cambridge: Cambridge University Press. ISBN 052140195X   References

Covers many of the problems and difficulties which may be encountered in this type of research.

2.48.10 Marrow, C. (1996) Using qualitative research methods in nursing. *Nursing Standard*, 11 (7) 43–5   10 References

Discusses the problems and dilemmas encountered in a longitudinal qualitative study in the clinical field. Strategies used to overcome difficulties when interviewing and observing are reported (CR 2.16, 2.68, 2.72).

2.48.11 Robinson, S. & Marsland, I. (1994) Approaches to the problem of respondent attrition in a longitudinal panel study of nurses' careers. *Journal of Advanced Nursing*, 20 (4) 729–41 35 References

Paper discusses reasons for choosing a longitudinal panel design for a programme of research into the careers of nurses and midwives. Ways in which respondent attrition was approached is described.

2.48.12 Seed, A. (1995) Conducting a longitudinal study: an unsanitized account. *Journal of Advanced Nursing*, 21 (5) 845–52 22 References

Explores issues which emerged during a longitudinal study describing the experiences of 23 student nurses training for registration in the UK (CR 2.16, 2.45).

2.48.13 Watson, R. (1998) Longitudinal quantitative research designs. *Nurse Researcher*, 5 (4) 41–54 12 References

Author examines some of the designs, benefits and problems of longitudinal quantitative research (CR 2.29).

2.48.14 Wuerker, A.K. (1997) Longitudinal research using computerised clinical databases: caveats and constraints. *Nursing Research*, 46 (6) 353–5 19 References

Author believes that existing databases provide nurse researchers with opportunities to explore clinical questions, in particular those requiring information over time, without gathering new data. Some types of database are mentioned and issues relating to their use are discussed (CR 2.84, 2.91).

2.48.15 Young, C.H., Savola, K.L. & Phelps, E. (1991) *Inventory of Longitudinal Studies in the Social Sciences*. Newbury Park, CA: Sage. ISBN 0803943156 References

Inventory contains information on longitudinal studies conducted over the last 60 years in the USA and Canada. Each one is described in detail, including its purpose, names and addresses of principal investigators, how it

was conducted, its current status and a list of related references.

2.48.16 Youngblut, J.M., Loveland-Cherry, C.J. & Horan, M. (1990) Data management systems in longitudinal research. *Nursing Research*, 39 (3) 188–9 1 Reference

Issues relating to data management in a particular study are discussed in terms of integrity and structure.

2.49 PHENOMENOLOGICAL RESEARCH/APPROACHES

'Phenomenology is a 20th century philosophical movement dedicated to describing structures of experience as they present themselves to consciousness, without recourse to theory, deduction, or assumptions from other disciplines such as the natural sciences.' (Centre for Advanced Research in Phenomenology, 1997)
URL: http://www.connect.net/non/phenom. html

Definition

Phenomenology – a method of study that attempts to understand human experience through analysis of the participants' description of that experience

Example

Graham, I. (1994) How do registered nurses think and experience nursing: a phenomenological investigation. *Journal of Clinical Nursing*, 3 (4) 235–42 18 References

Study explores and describes the world-view of a group of registered nurses with particular emphasis on their practice. Findings show the dynamic nature of their thinking but also suggest that additional skills in change management are necessary.

Annotations

2.49.1 Baker, J.D. (1997) Phenomenography: an alternative approach to researching the clinical decision making of nurses. *Nursing Inquiry*, 4 (1) 41–7 39 References

Limitations to the study of clinical decision-making using current research approaches are reviewed. Research has failed to examine the development of decision-making skills and the learning that occurs in practice. Phenomenography, which aims to describe an individual's perception of a phenomenon, is seen as a relevant approach to the study of decision-making.

2.49.2   Beck, C.T. (1994) Phenomenology: its use in nursing research. *International Journal of Nursing Studies*, 31 (6) 499–510 54 References

Article reviews some philosophical and methodological issues and use of phenomenology in nursing research. Studies reviewed show the width of application of this type of approach for nursing.

2.49.3   Benner, P. (ed.) (1994) *Interpretive Phenomenology: Embodiment, Caring and Ethics in Health and Illness*. Thousand Oaks, CA: Sage. ISBN 0803957238   References

Book comprises a collection of theoretical materials offering an introduction to the subject, followed by chapters which illustrate interpretative phenomenology in research.

2.49.4   Bergum, V. (1991) Being a phenomenological researcher, in Morse, J.M. (ed.), *Qualitative Nursing Research: a Contemporary Dialogue* Revised edition. Newbury Park, CA: Sage. ISBN 0803940793 Chapter 4, 55–71 32 References

Discusses the importance in phenomenological research of the research question, method, writing and publishing the study, while being mindful of one's ethical commitments (CR 2.17).

2.49.5   Centre for Advanced Research in Phenomenology. (1997) *What is Phenomenology?*
URL: http://www.fau.edu/divdept/schmidt/carp/phenom.htm

Paper outlines aspects of phenomenology: seven widely accepted features of phenomenological research; its 100-year spread by nation and discipline; tendencies and stages within philosophical phenomenology so far and how it may develop in the 21st century.

2.49.6   Centre for Advanced Research in Phenomenology. (1997) *Collective Multidisciplinary Bibliography of the Phenomenological Movement.*
URL: http://www.fau.edu/divdept/schmidt/carp/biblio.htm

This resource is a complete list of all works by phenomenologists, both living and deceased beginning in the 1880s (CR 1.5).

2.49.7   Crotty, M.C. (1996) *Phenomenology and Nursing Research*. South Melbourne, Victoria: Churchill Livingstone. ISBN 0443054320   References

Author describes and discusses two phenomenologies and urges a return to 'the unadulterated phenomena'. Ways forward for nurse researchers are considered.

2.49.8   Drew, N. (1993) Re-enactment interviewing: a methodology for phenomenological research. *Image: Journal of Nursing Scholarship*, 25 (4) 345–51   22 References

Re-enactment is proposed as an alternative strategy for phenomenological research. Three techniques, borrowed from the psychodramatic method – warming-up, scene-setting and soliloquy – were used in a study of care-giver/patient relationship. The rationale for and implementation of these techniques are discussed (CR 2.68).

2.49.9   Green, A.J. & Holloway, D.G. (1997) Using a phenomenological research technique to examine student nurses' understanding of experiential teaching and learning: a critical review of methodological issues. *Journal of Advanced Nursing*, 26 (5) 1013–19 49 References

Reports use of a phenomenological research methodology to investigate student nurses' understanding of experiential learning in their educational programmes. Throughout the paper methodological concerns which arose are discussed.

2.49.10   Hallett, C. (1995) Understanding the phenomenological approach to research. *Nurse Researcher*, 3 (2) 55–65   25 References

Discusses Hursell's elements of phenomenology, examines whether it is a method or philosophical perspective and outlines how it may be used in nursing.

2.49.11 Hamill, C. (1994) Changing emphasis in nursing research. *British Journal of Nursing*, 3 (10) 510–12   21 References

Article outlines the methodology of phenomenology and discusses its contribution to nursing knowledge (CR 2.6).

2.49.12 Koch, T. (1995) Interpretive approaches in nursing research: the influence of Husserl and Heidegger. *Journal of Advanced Nursing*, 21 (5) 827–36   61 References

Paper discusses Husserlian phenomenology and Heidegger's hermeneutics with reference to some fundamental research issues. Author recommends that nurse researchers appraise the philosophical underpinnings in the methodologies they use (CR 2.5).

2.49.13 Moustakas, C. (1994) *Phenomenological Research Methods*. Thousand Oaks, CA: Sage. ISBN 0803957998   References

Author discusses the theoretical underpinnings of phenomenology and takes the reader step by step through the process of conducting a study. Numerous examples are given, together with form letters and other tools used in designing and conducting a study.

2.49.14 Mu, P. (1996) Phenomenology [Chinese], *Nursing Research (China)*, 4 (2) 195–202   12 References

Paper discusses the nature of lived experience, self-consciousness and the intentionalilty of phenomenological perspectives. The major concerns of data collection, reliability, validity and data analysis of the research procedure are also illustrated (CR 2.24, 2.25).

2.49.15 Paley, J. (1998) Misinterpretive phenomenology: Heidegger, ontology and nursing research. *Journal of Advanced Nursing*, 27 (4) 817–24   38 References

Author argues that Heidegger's phenomenology does not have the methodological implications usually ascribed to it in the nursing literature. The consequences of this are discussed.

2.49.16 Rose, P., Beeby, J. & Parker, D. (1995) Academic rigour in the lived experience of researchers using phenomenological methods in nursing. *Journal of Advanced Nursing*, 21 (6) 1123–9   48 References

Authors suggest that given appropriate attention to rigour, phenomenological methodology could become the basic instrument in the reform of nursing research as it moves from the positivist to the humanist paradigm.

2.49.17 Siddiqui, J. (1995) Midwifery research: a phenomenological approach, in Henry, I.C. & Pashley, G. (eds), *Community Ethics and Health Care Research*. Dinton, Nr Salisbury: Mark Allen. ISBN 1856420868 Chapter 11, 143–57   24 References

Chapter suggests adopting a phenomenological approach to midwifery, while acknowledging that it may be of value in all areas of nursing practice (CR 2.17.64).

2.49.18 Taylor, B. (1993) Phenomenology: one way to understand nursing practice. *International Journal of Nursing Studies*, 30 (2) 171–9   53 References

The relative merits of qualitative research are reviewed and some examples given of phenomenological inquiries in nursing (CR 2.9).

2.49.19 Taylor, B. (1995) Interpreting phenomenology for nursing research. *Nurse Researcher*, 3 (2) 66–79   28 References

Paper describes the search for a methodologically suitable way of examining peoples' experiences in health care settings. Some of the dilemmas faced are described.

2.49.20 Van Maanen, M. (1997) From meaning to method. *Qualitative Health Research*, 7 (3) 345–69   29 References

Article explores aspects of the relation between language, meaning and method in human science research. Phenomenology poses two distinct challenges: the thematic and expressive dimensions of inquiry which have implications for semantic, mantic, discursive and non-discursive understanding. Guiding principles of human science method are explored.

2.49.21 Walters, A.J. (1995) The phenomenological movement: implications for nursing research. *Journal of Advanced Nursing*, 22 (4) 791–9   23 References

Paper compares the phenomenologies of Edmund Husserl and Martin Heidegger to highlight some of the critical distinctions between these two schools. The implications for nursing research are discussed.

2.50 PRESCRIPTIVE THEORY RESEARCH

Empirical validation of prescriptive theory has lagged behind other methodologies, as multiple studies over a long period of time are essential for this process.

Definition

Prescriptive theory – theory whose aims include controlling, promoting and changing nursing phenomena. Its elements include the aim or goal, prescriptions to produce the goal, and a survey list

Example

Kogan, H. & Betrus, P. (1984) Self-management: a nursing mode of therapeutic influence. *Advances in Nursing Science*, 6 (4) 55–73   12 References

Study aimed to assess the reduction in stress following self-management training sessions. Results showed that it was successful in reducing symptoms.

2.51 SIMULATION AND GAMING

Role-playing has been used as a technique in educational research and the social sciences for assessing personality, in business training, and psychotherapy. Its value is in the possibility of using it for assessment, teaching, and as a therapeutic procedure.

Definitions

Role-play – a function performed in a particular situation, process or operation
Simulation – imitation, representation or feigning

Example

Wong, Y.Y., Nordin, M. & Suleiman, A.B. (1996) Preventive and promotive medicine in ambulatory clinical practice: a prospective simulated patient study. *International Journal for Quality in Health Care*, 7 (4) 333–41   17 References

Twenty-eight volunteers were trained to simulate five clinical conditions which required health advice. The aim was to assess the doctors' performance with the aid of a prepared checklist. Results showed that the extent of promoting health education in both public and private sectors in Malaysia is unacceptably low.

Annotations

2.51.1 Abbott, P. & Sapsford, R. (1993) Studying policy and practice: use of vignettes. *Nurse Researcher*, 1 (2) 81–91   9 References

Discusses the use of vignettes as a method of supplying systematic information on professional practice and underlying policies. Four vignettes are presented and the results of their use is discussed.

2.51.2 Cohen, L. & Manion, L. (1994) Role-playing, in Authors, *Research Methods in Education* 4th revised edition. London: Routledge. ISBN 0415102359. Chapter 12, 252–70 References

Chapter provides a brief introduction to role-playing; discussion of the argument about the technique and deception; its role and uses in educational settings; its strengths and weaknesses; and organizing and evaluating a session (CR 2.1.17).

2.51.3 Crookall, D.A. & Arai, K. (eds) (1995) *Simulations and Gaming across Disciplines and Cultures: ISAGA at a Watershed*. Thousand Oaks, CA: Sage. ISBN 0803971028   References

Discusses the 'state of play' in simulation and gaming techniques. Abstracts of all papers presented at the 25th ISAGA conference are also included.

2.51.4 Gredler, M. (1992) *Designing and Evaluating Games and Simulations: a Process Approach*. London: Kogan Page. ISBN 0749404787   References

Book contains an historical survey of games and simulations as learning tools and analyses of well-known simulations. It identifies a group of key categories and includes examples from both British and American sources.

2.51.5 Maerker, M., Lisper, H.-O. & Rickberg, S.-E. (1990) Role-playing as a method in nursing research. *Journal of Advanced Nursing*, 15 (2) 180–6   14 References

Describes a study which investigated the way in which patients were informed about their illness. Advantages are listed of commissioning research on certain problems and by role-playing studies with healthy people.

2.51.6 Mooney, C.Z. (1997) *Monte Carlo Simulation*. Thousand Oaks, CA: Sage. ISBN 0803959435   References

Monte Carlo simulation is a method of evaluating substantive hypotheses and statistical estimators by developing a computer algorithm to simulate a population, drawing multiple samples from this pseudo-population and evaluating estimates from these samples. The author explains the rationale behind the method and demonstrates its uses for social and behavioural research (CR 2.22).

2.51.7 Smith, H.W. (1991) Simulation and gaming, in Author, *Strategies of Social Research: the Methodological Imagination* 3rd revised edition. Austin, TX: Holt. ISBN 0030230772   References

Discusses the use of simulation as a research technique with its dimensions and properties outlined. Man, machine and man-machine simulation are discussed (CR 2.95.21).

2.51.8 Whicker, M.L. & Sigelman, L. (1991) *Computer Simulation and Applications: an Introduction*. Newbury Park, CA: Sage. ISBN 0803932464   References

Provides comprehensive coverage of computer simulations, discussing their strengths and weaknesses as a research method. The steps involved are identified as well as the purposes for which they may be used.

2.52   SURVEY RESEARCH

Surveys are a commonly used research design where information is sought from a group of people, usually by means of interviews or questionnaires. It is a flexible method, broad in scope and may be used in both quantitative and qualitative studies. There are several types and forms of survey depending on semantics. Writers and researchers may interchange the names of similar types of studies which may lead to confusion.

Definitions

Comparative survey – results from two groups or techniques are compared
Cross-cultural survey – study of more than one culture
Cross-sectional survey – several groups in various stages of development are studied simultaneously
Evaluation survey – researcher looks back at previous activities with a critical eye and evaluates results
Field survey – study conducted in the real world as opposed to in a laboratory
Long-term/longitudinal survey – a sequence of events is observed over more than five years but there is no control over the outcome. [Long-term/longitudinal surveys are given different names in the following disciplines: in psychology and education – longitudinal; in anthropology and sociology – historical; and in economics – time-series]
Short-term survey – sequence of events observed over less than five years
Survey – type of research plan undertaken to study a large population by systematically selecting samples from the group to discover the incidence, distribution, interrelationships and behaviour of variables

Example

Rhodes, P. (1995) Postal survey of continence advisers in England and Wales. *Journal of Advanced Nursing*, 21 (2) 286–94   24 References

Reports a study which surveyed all known continence advisers in England and Wales. Information obtained included the number in post, qualifications achieved, structures within which they worked, and the nature of their practice. Their roles as clinical nurse specialists are discussed together with some implications for current practice.

Annotations

2.52.1 Aday, L.A. (1996) *Designing and Conducting Health Surveys: a Comprehensive Guide.* San Francisco, CA: Jossey-Bass. ISBN 0787902942

2.52.2 CASS (no date)
URL: http://www.scpr.ac.uk/cass/

CASS is an ESRC (Economic and Social Research Council) Centre which provides short courses in survey methods and is developing a Survey Question Bank for use by social scientists and researchers in the academic world, government, market research, the independent and voluntary sectors. It also provides a reference source for question formats in major social surveys, including the Census and family expenditure.

2.52.3 Coomber, R. (1997) Using the Internet for survey research. *Sociological Research Online*, 2 (2)
URL: http://www.socresonline.org.uk/socresonline/2/2/2.html
21 References

Paper outlines some recent survey research using the Internet. The target group of illicit 'drug dealers' are normally difficult to access. A discussion of sampling issues concludes that the Internet can be a source of indicative, as opposed to easily generalizable, data. A practical guide to undertaking research on the Internet is included (CR 1.8, 2.22, 2.28, 2.85).

2.52.4 Czaja, R. & Blair, J. (1996) *Designing Surveys: a Guide to Decisions and Procedures.* Thousand Oaks, CA: Pine Forge Press. ISBN 0803990561 References

Describes how modern survey research is conducted with the novice in mind. Its emphasis is on the initial stages, through to completion of data collection.

2.52.5 de Vaus, D.A. (1996) *Surveys in Social Research* 4th edition. London: UCL Press. ISBN 1857285425 References

Gives advice on how to plan, conduct and analyse social surveys. This new edition includes a chapter on ethics and a detailed glossary (CR 2.2, 2.17, 2.75).

2.52.6 Edwards, J.E., Thomas, M.D., Rosenfeld, P. & Booth-Kewley, S. (1996) *How to Conduct Organizational Surveys: a Step-by-step Guide.* London: Sage. ISBN 0803955138 References

Provides a detailed and practical guide to planning organizational surveys. The issues involved, and the advantages and disadvantages of choices made are all discussed.

2.52.7 Ferketich, S., Phillips, L. & Verran, J. (1993) Development and administration of a survey instrument for cross-cultural research. *Research in Nursing and Health*, 16 (3) 227–30 7 References

Gives guidelines for development of culturally appropriate measures of phenomena. Discussion focuses on practical issues and is illustrated by a survey instrument used with a rural Mexican American and Euro-American population (CR 2.53).

2.52.8 to 2.52.17 Fink, A. (1995) *The Survey Kit.* Thousand Oaks, CA: Sage. ISBN 0803973888

The following entry differs in format as it documents a series of nine books. Each book is cross-referenced to the appropriate section within this book.

2.52.9 Fink, A. (1995) *The Survey Handbook.* (Volume 1) ISBN 0803959346 (CR 2.16, 2.22, 2.24, 2.25)

2.52.10 Fink, A. (1995) *How to Ask Survey Questions.* (Volume 2) ISBN 0803957459 (CR 2.20)

2.52.11 Bourque, L. & Fielder, E. (1995) (Volume 3) *How to Conduct Self-administered and Mail Surveys.* ISBN 0803971680 (CR 2.75)

2.52.12 Frey, J.H. & Oishi, S.M. (1995) (Volume 4) *How to Conduct Interviews by Telephone and in Person.* ISBN 080395719X (CR 2.68, 2.70, 2.75)

2.52.13 Fink, A. (1995) *How to Design Surveys.* (Volume 5) ISBN 080397387X (CR 2.29)

2.52.14 Fink, A. (1995) *How to Sample in*

Surveys. (Volume 6) ISBN 0803957548 (CR 2.2, 2.22)

2.52.15 Litwin, M.S. (1995) *How to Measure Survey Reliability and Validity.* (Voume 7) ISBN 0803957041 (CR 2.23, 2.24, 2.25)

2.52.16 Fink, A. (1995) *How to Analyze Survey Data.* (Volume 8) ISBN 0803973861 (CR 2.2, 2.81, 2.82, 2.86, 2.87).

2.52.17 Fink, A. (1995) *How to Report on Surveys.* (Volume 9) ISBN 0803973853 (CR 2.94, 2.97, 2.100)

The survey kit offers all the information necessary for conducting a state-of-the-art survey from the initial planning stages through to analysing and reporting the data. Its primary goal is to ensure that the data collected is accurate and useful. All books in the series contain instructional objectives, exercises and answers, examples of surveys in use, illustrations of survey questions, guidelines for action, checklists of dos and don'ts and annotated references.

2.52.18 Fink, A. & Kosecoff, J. (1998) *How to Conduct Surveys: a Step-by-step Guide* 2nd edition. Thousand Oaks: Sage. ISBN 0761914080 References

Text outlines the basic essentials required to organize a rigorous survey or evaluate the credibility of others using a step-by-step approach. New edition covers computer and interactive surveys and gives advice on informed consent procedures, sample size, ways to ask questions about ethnicity, reading computer printouts of survey results, preparing an abstract, new data analysis techniques and guidelines for presenting results (CR 2.17, 2.22, 2.86, 2.87, 2.94, 2.99).

2.52.19 Foddy, W. (1994) *Constructing Questions for Interviews and Questionnaires: Theory and Practice in Social Research.* Cambridge: Cambridge University Press. ISBN 0521467330 References

Book provides a theoretical basis for the construction of valid and reliable questions for interviews and questionnaires. Chapters address past problems of survey research, defining topics properly, formulating requests, providing response frameworks and using filters. Research literature is practically applied and each chapter is summarized (CR 2.24, 2.25, 2.56, 2.68, 2.75).

2.52.20 Folz, D.H. (1996) *Survey Research for Public Administration.* Thousand Oaks, CA: Sage. ISBN 0761901531 References

Book helps to clarify the basics of survey research as they apply to public administration. The fundamentals of the research process are covered together with practical illustrations. Data analysis using computers is covered and illustrations given of SPSS screens (CR 2.84, Appendix A).

2.52.21 Fowler, F.J. Jr. (1993) *Survey Research Methods* 2nd edition. Beverly Hills, CA: Sage. ISBN 0803950497 References

Book discusses the standards and practical procedures required for surveys designed to provide statistical descriptions of people by asking questions, usually of a sample. Surveys combine sampling, question design and interviewing techniques, and each of these is explored to show how precision, accuracy and credibility are achieved. This edition includes new methodological knowledge and more recent references on all aspects of survey research (CR 2.22, 2.68, 2.75).

2.52.22 Fowler, F.J. Jr. (1995) *Improving Survey Questions: Design and Evaluation.* Thousand Oaks, CA: Sage. ISBN 0803945833 References

Book shows how to write good questions, measure subjective phenomena, attack common measurement problems, evaluate the extent to which questions are consistently understood and administered, and gives advice on evaluating the resulting data.

2.52.23 Henry, R. (1992) Self-report measures: principles and approaches, in Tudiver, F., Bass, M.J., Dunn, E.V., Norton, P.G. & Stewart, M. (eds), *Assessing Interventions: Traditional and Innovative Methods.* Newbury Park, CA: Sage. ISBN 0803947704 Chapter 11, 109–17 9 References

Summarizes the characteristics of the survey as an instrument of measurement and discusses some principles for its use (CR 2.71).

2.52.24 Kangas, I., Topo, P. & Hemminki, E. (1995) Feedback for participants in a health survey: feasible and useful. *Women and Health*, 23 (4) 57–65 10 References

Reports use of a feedback leaflet sent to 1,713 respondents following a survey asking Finnish women about their climacterium. Authors believe that feedback gives fresh viewpoints and valuable critique for researchers as a result of being more in contact with respondents.

2.52.25 Mangione, T.W. (1995) *Mail Surveys: Improving the Quality*. London: Sage. ISBN 0803946627 References

Discusses ways in which data collection can be improved by careful question construction, sampling procedures and use of incentives. Management and processing of data are also considered.

2.52.26 McDonnell, A., Davies, S., Shewan, J. & Brown, J. (1998) In the field with practice nurses: practical lessons of survey research. *Nurse Researcher*, 5 (3) 65–76 11 References

Paper considers some of the methodological challenges of survey research with particular reference to a national study commissioned by the National Health Service Research and Development Executive. The survey formed part of a wider study investigating the role of practice nurses in the prevention of cardiovascular disease and stroke.

2.52.27 Moser, C.A. & Kalton, G. (1985) *Survey Methods in Social Investigation* 2nd revised edition. London: Gower. ISBN 0566050390 References

A classic text covering all aspects of social surveys.

2.52.28 Murphy, C.A. (1993) Increasing the response rates of reluctant professionals to mail surveys. *Applied Nursing Research*, 6 (3) 137–41 26 References

Discusses ways of increasing response rates to mail surveys, mechanical, perceptual, broad and specific motivational factors and response bias (CR 2.27).

2.52.29 Rea, L.M. & Parker, R.A. (1992) *Designing and Conducting Survey Research: a Comprehensive Guide*. San Francisco, CA: Jossey-Bass. ISBN 155542404X References

Covers all aspects of survey research, including developing and administering questionnaires, ensuring scientific accuracy, analysing and reporting results. Exercises are included in each chapter (CR 2.75).

2.52.30 Rees, C. (1995) Survey methods in midwifery. *British Journal of Midwifery*, 3 (12) 652–5 7 References

Discusses some of the skills required when using questionnaires and interviews as data collection methods (CR 2.68, 2.70, 2.75).

2.52.31 Schuman, H. & Presser, S. (1996) *Questions and Answers in Attitude Surveys: Experiments on Question Form, Wording and Context*. Thousand Oaks, CA: Sage. ISBN 0761903593 References

Covers all aspects of developing questions and analysing answers in attitude surveys (CR 2.56).

2.52.32 Weisberg, H.F., Krosnick, J.A. & Bowen, B.D. (1996) *An Introduction to Survey Research, Polling and Data Analysis* 3rd edition. Thousand Oaks, CA: Sage. ISBN 0803974027 References

Book covers the design of surveys, steps for sampling and question writing, interviewing, coding strategies, and analysing the data. Examples are given from large contemporary surveys and polls. The ethics of survey research are discussed and details given on how to read and write reports (CR 2.22, 2.75, 2.86, 2.87).

2.53 TRANS-CULTURAL/CROSS-CULTURAL RESEARCH

'Cross-cultural research seeks to investigate variables which exist in one or more communities. These include age, sexual division of labour, habits of cleanliness, religious ceremonies, courtship patterns, kinship terminology, birth and death rites and the prevention and cure of disease. The major difficulties associated with it are cost, communication difficulties and the maintenance of cultural meanings in an instruments language'. (Treece & Treece, 1986: 208)

The terms trans-cultural and cross-cultural are sometimes used interchangeably in the literature.

Definition

Cross-cultural research – nursing research within and across cultural contexts

Example

Molassiotis, A. & Newell, R. (1996) Nurses' awareness of restraint use with elderly people in Greece and the UK: a cross-cultural pilot study. *International Journal of Nursing Studies*, 33 (2) 201–11   33 References

Reports a small pilot study which examined British and Greek trained nurses' perceptions and experiences of the use of restraints on elderly people. Differences were found and the need for education, restraint policies and multi-disciplinary decision-making are discussed. Some principles of cross-cultural studies are outlined (CR 2.23).

Annotations

2.53.1   Alasuutari, P. (1995) *Researching Culture: Qualitative Method and Cultural Studies*. Thousand Oaks, CA: Sage. ISBN 0803978316   References

Book gives the range of approaches and methodological tools available for undertaking critical research, and shows how cultural studies transcend traditional divisions between qualitative and quantitative method and between social sciences and humanities. Ethnography, symbolic interactionism, semiotics, narrative analysis, conversation and discourse analysis, and quantitative analysis in terms of its relevance to data produced by research on culture are discussed (CR 2.42, 2.45, 2.88, 2.89).

2.53.2   Champion, V., Austin, J. & Tzeng, O.C.S. (1987) Cross-cultural comparison of images of nurses and physicians. *International Nursing Review*, 34 (2) (Issue 272) 43–8   23 References

Study investigated attitudes related to the image of nurses and physicians across 30 cultures using six concepts. Differences were found with respect to the power held by physicians and nurses, and the authors suggest that nurses' influence in health care decisions can be reduced unless they address this deficit. Physicians were highly correlated with knowledge and independence, nurses were correlated with kindness.

2.53.3   Chater, K. (1996) Dilemmas of difference and the politics of comparison: cross-cultural research on dementia. *Canadian Journal of Nursing Research*, 28 (1) 79–85   8 References

Examines some of the theoretical and methodological issues when undertaking cross-cultural research. The main concern is the difficulty of representation within cultural groups and ways forward are suggested.

2.53.4   Davis, D.K. & Cannava, E. (1992) Elements of trans-cultural and trans-linguistic research: a personal experience. *Nursing Science Quarterly*, 5 (4) 185–9   3 References

Authors discuss some elements which must be addressed when planning trans-cultural studies. These are: trans-cultural/trans-linguist literature review; protection of human subjects; trans-linguistics; maintaining contact with the research site; presenting research to the participants; structuring interviews; and post-session amenities. The study, not reported here, was a qualitative exploratory project on the phenomena of retirement in Italy (CR 2.17, 2.68).

2.53.5   Giger, J.N. & Davidhizar, R. (1990) Trans-cultural nursing assessment: a method for advancing nursing practice. *International Nursing Review*, 37(1) 199–202   12 References

Discusses a systematic method for comprehensive nursing assessment necessary for practitioners and researchers under the following headings: communication; space; social organization; time; environmental control; and biological variations.

2.53.6   Hockey, L. (1995) Implications for research: progress, problems and possibilities. *Asian Journal of Nursing Studies*, 2 (4) 17–25   12 References

Paper focuses on the possibilities and potential of nursing research in a multi-cultural world. The factors which may affect studies are identified as historical, linguistic, economic, social and political, but the author believes that the need for international collaboration is urgent (CR 2.15).

2.53.7   Jumbunathan, J. (1995) Doing trans-cultural nursing research. *Nursing Journal of India*, 86 (7) 149–55

2.53.8   Leininger, M. (1984) *Reference Sources for Trans-cultural Health and Nursing*. Thorofare, NJ: Slack Inc. ISBN 0913590932 Part II, D, 33–8

Contains selected references on many aspects of trans-cultural nursing, including theory and research methods.

2.53.9   Leininger, M. (1997a) Trans-cultural nursing research to transform nursing education and practice: 40 years. *Image: Journal of Nursing Scholarship*, 29 (4) 341–7 45 References

Article gives an overview of major trends, philosophical and theoretical perspectives alongside selected trans-cultural nursing research findings. Much knowledge has been launched since the 1950s and author believes that trans-cultural nursing knowledge is vital to meet health care needs in a multi-cultural world. Some misconceptions and reflections are offered to advance trans-cultural nursing research, and for 'newcomers' some basic readings are recommended.

2.53.10   Leininger, M. (1997b) Future directions in trans-cultural nursing in the 21st century. *International Nursing Review*, 44 (1) 19–23   18 References

Author documents some directions that trans-cultural nursing is taking and how it is becoming more meaningful to nurses and consumers.

2.53.11   Lipson, J.G. & Meleis, A.I. (1989) Methodological issues in research with immigrants, in Morse, J. (ed.), *Cross-cultural Nursing: Anthropological Approaches to Nursing Research*. Philadelphia: Gordon & Breach Science Publishers. ISBN 2881243835 103–15   References

Study addresses the following methodological issues: identifying the universe and sampling; access to information; distrust; interviewing style; providing a structure for reciprocity; non-termination; consent for participation; accuracy of data; and three strategies to improve data collection. Strategies for encouraging trust and the use of triangulation are also discussed (2.17, 2.22, 2.26, 2.68).

2.53.12   McGuigan, J. (ed.) (1997) *Cultural Methodologies*. London: Sage. ISBN 0803974841   References

Book illustrates the distinctiveness and coherence of cultural studies as a site of interaction between the humanities and social sciences. Major sections cover methodologies, research and reflections on the processes (CR 2.9, 2.10, 2.17, 2.42, 2.86, 2.89, 2.97).

2.53.13   Morse, J. (ed.) (1989) *Cross-cultural Nursing: Anthropological Approaches to Nursing Research*. Philadelphia: Gordon & Breach Science Publications. ISBN 2881243835   References

Comprises a series of studies illustrating anthropological approaches to nursing research.

2.53.14   Morse, J.M. (1986) Trans-cultural nursing research: process, problems and pitfalls, in Stinson, S.M. & Kerr, J.C. (eds), *International Issues in Nursing Research*. London: Croom Helm. ISBN 0709944373 Chapter 4, 61–75   References

Chapter explores the process, problems and pitfalls of clinical nursing research in different cultural settings. It aims to stimulate interest in this area and prepare those entering this field of research (CR 3.22.12).

2.53.15   Phillips, L.R., Luna, I., Russell, C.K., Baca, G., Lim, Y.M., Cromwell, S.L. & de Ardon, E.T. (1996) 'Towards a cross-cultural perspective of family caregiving'. Originally presented as a symposium at the Western Society for Research in Nursing (WSRN) Communicating Nursing Research Conference, Albuquerque, New Mexico, May 1991. *Western Journal of Nursing Research*, 18 (3) 236–51   32 References

Article gives the background to this symposium by introducing its theme: cross-cultural equivalence. The process described is based on experiences of the cross-cultural research team and Berry's model for developing equivalent research. Examples are given from the instrument development phase of an ongoing programme designed to generate and test a theory which explains the quality of family care for frail elders at home.

2.53.16   Sawyer, L., Regev, H., Proctor, S., Nelson, M., Messias, D., Barnes, D. & Meleis, A.I. (1995) Matching versus cultural competence in research: methodological considerations. *Research in Nursing and Health*, 18 (6) 557–67   51 References

Paper examines the complexities in using matching in research with diverse populations. Authors challenge the idea that matching of researchers and participants is the only strategy for generating valid knowledge. They argue that cultural competence could be used in the development of nursing knowledge.

2.53.17   van de Vijver, F. & Leung, K. (1997) *Methods and Data Analysis for Cross-cultural Research*. London: Sage.   076190106X References

Book covers methodological concepts in cross-cultural research, the theoretical background, methods, design and analysis. The analysis and design of four common kinds of cross-cultural studies are discussed.

2.53.18   Warwick, D.P. & Osherson, S. (eds) (1973) *Comparative Research Methods*. Englewood Cliffs, NJ: Prentice-Hall. ISBN 013153940X   References

Papers seek to show how the same problem may be studied in different societies and cultures using a combination of methods. The problems which may occur are included together with some successful outcomes. The five parts of the book cover an overview of comparative research methods, conceptual equivalence and cultural bias, equivalence of measurement and linguistics, translation and illustrative methods, survey research and participant observation (CR 2.52, 2.72).

MEASUREMENT

2.54 MEASUREMENT – GENERAL

The process of measurement involves the delineation of what needs to be measured in terms of the research problem, the development of an instrument to measure it and then analysis of the resulting data. Outcome measures are of particular importance in the current climate of health service development and some references to this literature are included here. Other material may be found in section 2.43.

Definitions

Criterion-referenced measures – techniques appropriate for determining whether or not an individual has acquired a set of behaviour or mastered a specific task
Measurement – the assignment of some numerical value to objects or events to represent the kind or amount of some characteristic of those objects or events. [Measurement as used in this context, includes qualitative data, in which objects are assigned to categories that represent the kinds of characteristic they possess and that are mutually exclusive and exhaustive]
Norm-referenced measures – techniques appropriate for evaluating the performance of an individual relative to some other individuals in a group
Outcome measures – . . . evaluate the efficacy of intervention: the extent to which a medication, procedure or program produced a desired effect

---

Annotations

2.54.1 Anthony, D. (1996) Receiver operating characteristic analysis: an overview. *Nurse Researcher*, 4 (2) 75–88   10 References

Reports use of receiver-operating characteristic analysis as a method of assessing classification systems, and it may be used to compare different classifiers quantitatively. Although used extensively in other disciplines, it has been overlooked in nursing research. Author believes it could be considered in audit and assessment tools that are numerical in nature with a clear output, but are imprecise in terms of diagnostic ability (CR 2.29).

2.54.2 Chance, K.S. (1997) The quest for quality: an exploration of attempts to define and measure quality patient care. *Image: Journal of Nursing Scholarship*, 29 (4) 326–9 48 References [Original article condensed in *Image* (1980) 12 (2) 41–5]

Author discusses attempts to define and measure quality nursing care. Definitions of quality are examined and variables which have or have not been associated with quality are cited. Conceptual models and frameworks are discussed, together with implications and recommendations for future research. Some nursing instruments are discussed (CR 2.61).

2.54.3 Fife-Schaw, C. (1995) Levels of measurement, in Breakwell, G.M., Hammond, S. & Fife-Schaw, C. (eds), *Research Methods in Psychology*. London: Sage. ISBN 0803977654 Part II, 38–49 References

Chapter discusses measurement issues that have been central to the pursuit of 'positivist' psychological science (CR 2.1.8, 2.29).

2.54.4 Gift, A.G. (1989) Visual analogue scales: measurement of subjective phenomena. *Nursing Research*, 38 (5) 286–8 24 References

Discusses use of visual analogue scales, associated issues, psychometric properties and questions of validity and reliability (CR 2.24, 2.25).

2.54.5 Griffiths, P. (1995) Progress in measuring outcomes. *Journal of Advanced Nursing,* 21 (6) 1092–100   72 References

Examines progress made in measuring the outcomes of nursing. The significance, the past, integrative review, scale development, nursing versus health outcomes, structural equation modelling and the limitations of scientific knowledge are all explored (CR 2.43).

2.54.6 Harrison, M.B., Juniper, E.F. & Mitchell-DiCenso, A. (1996) Quality of life as an outcome measure in nursing research: 'may you have a long and healthy life'. *Canadian Journal of Nursing Research,* 28 (3) 49–68   63 References

Discusses the nature, difficulties of definition, progress made in clarifying and operationalizing the concept of quality of life. Authors offer a viewpoint which separates what quality of life is from that which contributes to it. A definition of health arises from this and issues in its measurement are discussed.

2.54.7 Hyndman, S. (1994) Leaping to the right conclusions? The problems of confounding and measurement in a ward-based nursing research project, in Buckeldee, J. & McMahon, R. (eds), *The Research Experience in Nursing.* London: Chapman & Hall. ISBN 0412441101 Chapter 10, 147–63   22 References

Chapter describes many confounding factors or intervening variables, which may interfere with the measurement of outcome. The study involved used the Dynamic Standard Setting System to examine whether standard of pain management, in a surgical setting, could have an effect on the way patients recovered and the way they experienced care (CR 2.16.4, 2.61).

2.54.8 Jacoby, W.G. (1991) *Data Theory and Dimensional Analysis.* Newbury Park, CA: Sage. ISBN 0803941781   References

Examines basic scaling questions and discusses strategies for different research situations. Data theory and the study of how real-world observations can be transformed into data which can be analysed are all discussed.

2.54.9 Jacox, A. (1994) Nursing-sensitive patient outcomes, in Fitzpatrick, J.J., Steven-son, J.S. & Polis, N.S. (eds), *Nursing Research and its Utilization.* New York: Springer ISBN 0826180906 Chapter 8, 97–105   31 References

Chapter defines patient outcomes, gives a brief history of the concern that nurses have with such outcomes and describes recent events leading to the effectiveness initiative focused on them. Some work of nurse researchers in three related areas – selection of patient outcomes, modifications or development of measures and the incorporation of nursing-sensitive patient outcomes into inter-disciplinary programmes of research or evaluation of practice – are discussed (CR 2.43, 2.102.17).

2.54.10 Koch, T. (1992) A review of nursing quality assurance. *Journal of Advanced Nursing,* 17 (7) 785–94   51 References

Paper presents an overview of frameworks used in nursing quality assurance, an outline of the movement in nursing and its current concerns. The emphasis on measurement puts quality assurance within the quantitative paradigm but the author presents qualitative research as a complementary approach (CR 2.29, 2.36).

2.54.11 Lyne, P. (1994) The importance of measurement. *Nurse Researcher,* 1 (4) 13–25   4 References

Identifies the views of two cultural 'camps' in nursing relating to ways of measuring practice. What is to be measured and how are discussed, and points to look for to assess the accuracy and sensitivity of instruments are highlighted (CR 2.24, 2.25).

2.54.12 McCloskey, K.A. & Bulechek, G.M. (1994) Classification of nursing interventions: implications for nursing research, in Fitzpatrick, J.J., Stevenson, J.S. & Polis, N.S. (eds), *Nursing Research and its Utilization.* New York: Springer. ISBN 0826180906. Chapter 5, 65–81   38 References

Chapter summarizes research which aimed to develop a Nursing Interventions Classification System and presents the implications for research (CR 2.6, 2.102.17).

2.54.13 McCormick, K.A. (1994) Patient outcomes research: necessity and challenge, in Fitzpatrick, J.J., Stevenson, J.S. & Polis,

N.S. (eds), *Nursing Research and its Utilization*. New York: Springer. ISBN 0826180906
Chapter 7, 91–5   7 References

Outlines the spectrum of outcomes possible in nursing as not all patients are on the 'improvement curve'. Some effective tools are listed together with areas where outcomes research will need to be conducted (CR 2.102.17).

2.54.14 Miller, D.C. (1991) *Handbook of Research Design and Social Measurement* 5th edition. Newbury Park, CA: Sage. ISBN 0803942192   References

A reference guide to research design, sampling, collection of data, statistical analysis, selection of sociometric scales or indexes, research funding, costing and reporting. Contains extensive references to resource materials and includes examples of psychometric, social psychological, demographic and sociometric scales (CR 2.21, 2.22, 2.55, 2.64, 2.87, 3.13).

2.54.15 Nolan, M. & Behi, R. (1995) Measurement in research. *British Journal of Nursing*, 4 (7) 402–5   16 References

Discusses the importance of measurement in research and nursing generally. The process of operationalization is described and different levels of measurement are outlined.

2.54.16 Waltz, C.F., Strickland, O.L. & Lenz, E.R. (1991) *Measurement in Nursing Research* 2nd edition. Philadelphia: Davis. ISBN 0803690479   References

A comprehensive text for students and experienced researchers who are consumers or developers of nursing measures. The theories and principles of sound measurement practices are discussed together with the processes involved in designing, selecting and testing instruments. The appendix contains information on compilations of existing tools, a selection of nursing theories and their measurement implications, and guidance on resources useful for locating suitable tools (CR 2.17, 2.55, 2.65, 2.66, 2.68, 2.72. 2.73, 2.74, 2.75, 2.88).

2.55   DEVELOPING AND USING INSTRUMENTS

An issue that frequently faces nurses undertaking research is whether to use instruments developed by others or to develop new ones. It is generally less costly and time-consuming to use existing ones and this is beneficial from the knowledge-building perspective. Use of existing tools provides an increasing database for evaluating the properties of the instruments themselves.

Definition

Instrument – the device or technique that a researcher uses to collect data (e.g. questionnaires, tests, observation schedules)

Example

Autar, R. (1996) Nursing assessment of clients at risk of deep vein thrombosis: the Autar DVT Scale. *Journal of Advanced Nursing*, 23 (4) 763–77   42 References

Reports the development of a scale to predict the progress of deep vein thrombosis. Its limitations are outlined and further testing suggested (CR 2.61).

Annotations

2.55.1   Abu-Saad, H.H., Pool, H. & Tulkens, B. (1994) Further validity testing of the Abu-Saad Paediatric Pain Assessment Tool. *Journal of Advanced Nursing*, 19 (6) 1063–71   24 References

Reports the results of two studies conducted to further validate this Dutch-language pain assessment tool, designed for school-aged children. The results in relation to instrument development and multi-dimensional pain assessment in children are further discussed (CR 2.25).

2.55.2   Adams, A., Bond, S. & Arber, S. (1995) Development and validation of scales to measure organizational features of acute hospital wards. *International Journal of Nursing Studies*, 32 (6) 612–27   56 References

Research reports the development of The Ward Organizational Features Scales (WOFS) which aimed to create valid and reliable measures of the organizational features of acute hospital wards. Results are reported and implications for further research are discussed.

2.55.3 Arthur, D. (1995) Measurement of the professional self-concept of nurses: developing a measurement instrument. *Nurse Education Today*, 15 (5) 328–35 40 References

Describes the development of a 56-item instrument using Likert scales to measure the constructs of flexibility, creativity, knowledge, skills, competence, caring, communication, leadership and satisfaction with a pilot group of nurses in New South Wales. Results are reported and suggestions made for future use and development.

2.55.4 Arts, S., Kersten, H. & Kerkstra, A. (1996) The daily practice in home help services in the Netherlands: instrument development. *Health and Social Care in the Community*, 4 (5) 280–9 22 References

Article describes the development of several instruments to obtain a representative picture of the work of home helps. Details are given of a pilot study to establish the reliability and content validity of the main instrument, a registration form to record the activities performed. Results are reported ((CR 2.24, 2.25).

2.55.5 Baggs, J. (1994) Development of an instrument to measure collaboration and satisfaction about care decisions. *Journal of Advanced Nursing*, 20 (1) 176–82 24 References

The psychometric assessment of a new instrument for measuring the construct of nurse–physician collaboration in making specific care decisions is reported. Content and construct validity are discussed together with the need for further testing (CR 2.25).

2.55.6 Beland, D.K. & Froman, R.D. (1995) Preliminary validation of a measure of life support preferences. *Image: Journal of Nursing Scholarship*, 27 (4) 307–10 18 References

Reports the development of an instrument which provides illustrations of life support choices to discuss such measures with patients. Findings are reported (CR 2.25).

2.55.7 Bennett, S.J., Puntenney, P.J., Walker, N.L. & Ashley, N.D. (1996) Development of an instrument to measure threat related to cardiac events. *Nursing Research*, 45 (5) 266–70 11 References

Reports a study which evaluated the reliability and validity of the Cardiac Event Threat Questionnaire. Results showed initial support for construct validity (CR 2.24, 2.25).

2.55.8 Cheater, F. (1998) Quality of life measures for the health care environment. *Nurse Researcher*, 5 (3) 17–30 33 References

Author gives some definitions of quality of life within the context of the need to broaden measurements of outcome. The use of outcome measures in research, including issues of reliability and validity are also discussed. Some suggestions are made as to how quality-of-life measures will develop in the future (CR 2.24, 2.25).

2.55.9 Cheng, C.M. & Chapman, J.S. (1997) Assessment of reliability and validity of behavioural observation record for developmental care. *Nursing Research*, 46 (1) 40–5 21 References

Reports a study which evaluated the content and criterion validity and inter-rater reliability of the Modified Infant Behavioural Observation Record. Results are reported (CR 2.24, 2.25).

2.55.10 Clark, B.A. (1997) Development of the Conscious Sedation Scale: establishing content validity and reliability. *Gastroenterology Nursing*, 20 (1) 2–8 17 References

Describes a pilot study which aimed to determine content validity and reliability for a scale used to assess patient's response during intravenous conscious sedation. Findings showed that further refinement was required (CR 2.24, 2.25).

2.55.11 Cline, M.E., Herman, J., Shaw, E.R. & Morton, R.D. (1992) Standardization of the visual analogue scale. *Nursing Research*, 41 (6) 378–9 No references

Discusses the technical construction of the visual analogue scale and development of a scoring template.

2.55.12 Cromwell, S.L., Russell, C.K., Lim,

Y.M., Luna, I., de Ardon, E.T. & Phillips, L.R. (1996) 'Uncovering the cultural context for quality of family caregiving for elders'. Originally presented as a symposium at the Western Society for Research in Nursing (WSRN) Communicating Nursing Research Conference, Albuquerque, New Mexico, May 1991. *Western Journal of Nursing Research*, 18 (3) 284–98   28 References

This paper explored issues in developing cross-culturally equivalent conceptualizations and measures for a study of elder caregiving. An existing instrument, the Qualcare Scale, was examined and refined using Berry's model for cross-cultural research, which necessitated identification of appropriate cross-cultural indicators of quality. Examples of indicator clarification are given for several basic human rights based on the team's experience with Anglo and Mexican American care-givers (CR 2.53, 2.61).

2.55.13   Dai, Y.T., Schepp, K. & Lou, M.F. (1995) Psychometric assessment of Survey of Recent Life Experience scale on a Taiwanese sample [Chinese], *Nursing Research (China)*, 3 (3) 235–45   22 References

Discusses the reliability and validation of a translated English stress scale, Survey of Recent Life Experience, with a view to shortening and consolidating it on empirical data. Study provided adequate evidence supporting psychometric properties of the original and shorter versions. Information is given on methodological concerns when adapting scales from other cultures and written in different languages (CR 2.24, 2.25).

2.55.14   Davis, A.E. (1996) Instrument development: getting started. *Journal of Neuroscience Nursing*, 28 (3) 204–7   8 References

Article outlines the steps necessary to develop a valid and reliable instrument that will measure a phenomenon, characteristic or attribute demonstrated by a specific group. Steps include concept identification, item construction and testing to examine the issues of validity and reliability (CR 2.24, 2.25).

2.55.15   Demers, L., Weiss-Lambrou, R. & Ska, B. (1996) Development of the Quebec User Evaluation of Satisfaction with Assistive Technology (QUEST). *Assistive Technology*, 8 (1) 3–13   61 References

Paper describes the development of an instrument to evaluate user satisfaction with assistive technology devices. Preliminary versions were created and examined by a panel which were then pre-tested. The final French version which resulted is still undergoing testing.

2.55.16   Devellis, R.F. (1991) *Scale Development: Theories and Applications*. Newbury Park, CA: Sage. ISBN 080393775X   References

This book will enable researchers to develop reliable and valid instruments for measurement. Topics included are identification of the latent variable, generation of an item pool, the format for measurement, the application of scale length and factor analysis strategies. Exercises are included to illustrate each concept.

2.55.17   Dierckx de Casterle, B., Grypdonck, M. & Vuylsteke-Wauters, M. (1997) Development, reliability and validity testing of the Ethical Behaviour Test: a measure for nurses' ethical behaviour. *Journal of Nursing Measurement*, 5 (1) 87–112   50 References

Describes the development of the Ethical Behaviour Test which included two fundamental components of ethical behaviour: ethical reasoning (and the resulting decision) and the actual implementation of this decision (CR 2.17, 2.25).

2.55.18   Ellett, M.L. & Young, R.J. (1997) Development of the vulnerability scale. *Gastroenterology Nursing*, 20 (3) 82–6   7 References

Article describes the various complex processes necessary when developing a new data collection scale.

2.55.19   Gibbon, B. (1995) Validity and reliability of assessment tools. *Nurse Researcher*, 2 (4) 48–55   7 References

Discusses the importance of reliability and validity in assessment tools. The sensitivity, appropriateness and acceptability of tools should also be considered (CR 2.24, 2.25).

2.55.20   Gibbon, B. (1998) Selecting health care assessment tools: putting issues of validity and reliability into a wider context. *Nurse Researcher*, 5 (3) 5–15   21 References

Author discusses evaluating and selecting a health care assessment tool and emphasizes the importance of establishing reliability and validity (CR 2.24, 2.25).

2.55.21   Gotherstrom, C., Hamrin, E. & Gullberg, M. (1995) Development of a tool for measuring the concept of good care among patients and staff in relation to Swedish legislation. *International Journal of Nursing Studies*, 32 (3) 277–87   13 References

Reports on the development of an instrument to measure the concept of good care, in relation to the Swedish Health and Medical Services Act. Authors recommend that it be tested further in settings other than short-term care.

2.55.22   Hambleton, R.K., Swaminathan, H. & Rogers, H.J. (eds) (1991) *Fundamentals of Item Response Theory*. Newbury Park, CA: Sage. ISBN 0803936478   References

Using concepts from classical measurement methods and basic statistics, the book introduces the elements of item response theory. Its application to problems in test construction, identification of biased items, test-equating and computer-adaptation testing are all discussed. New directions are also explored.

2.55.23   Hilton, B.A. (1994) The Uncertainty Stress Scale: its development and psychometric properties. *Canadian Journal of Nursing Research*, 26 (3) 15–30   29 References

The development and testing of this new instrument is described together with its theoretical and empirical basis. Evidence of its use is given and suggestions for revisions are described (CR 2.24, 2.25).

2.55.24   Hodgkinson, K., Bear, M., Thorn, J. & van Blaricum, S. (1994) Measuring pain in neonates: evaluating an instrument and developing a common language. *Australian Journal of Advanced Nursing*, 12 (1) 17–22   15 References

Describes the development and evaluation of the pain assessment tool by a group of neonatal nurses. Recommendations for its future use are discussed.

2.55.25   Hoff, L.A. & Rosenbaum, L. (1994) A victimization assessment tool: instrument

development and clinical implications. *Journal of Advanced Nursing*, 20 (4) 627–734   44 References

Describes the development of a tool to assist nurses and other primary care providers with routine assessment of victimization in diverse health and mental health settings. Outcomes of preliminary validity and reliability studies are included (CR 2.24, 2.25).

2.55.26   Howe, T. (1995) Measurement scales in health care settings. *Nurse Researcher*, 2 (4) 30–7   15 References

Describes the types of measurement and measurement scale available to health care professionals.

2.55.27   Jacobson, S.F. (1992) Evaluating instruments for use in clinical research, in Frank-Stromborg, M. (ed.), *Instruments for Clinical Nursing Research*. Boston, MA: Jones & Bartlett. ISBN 0867203404 Chapter 1, 3–19   35 References

Chapter covers assessing the conceptual basis of instruments, measuring research frameworks, choosing a method of data collection, psychometric characteristics of instruments and item analysis. Also discussed are other procedures in instrument evaluation, state-of-the-art measurement in nursing research and ethical and legal aspects of tool use (CR 2.61.4).

2.55.28   Jayasuriya, R. & Caputi, P. (1996) Computer attitude and computer anxiety in nursing: validation of an instrument using an Australian sample. *Computers in Nursing*, 14 (6) 340–5   23 References

Reports a study which aimed to refine the instrument Nurses' Computer Attitudes Inventory and test its reliability and validity (CR 2.24, 2.25).

2.55.29   Jeffreys, M.R. & Smodlaka, I. (1996) Steps of the instrument design process: an illustrative approach for nurse educators. *Nurse Educator*, 21 (6) 47–52   23 References

Describes the development of a self-report instrument which measures and evaluates students' confidence for performing general trans-cultural nursing skills among diverse client populations (CR 2.24, 2.25, 2.53).

2.55.30   Jones, E.G. & Kay, M.C. (1992)

Instrumentation in cross-cultural research. *Nursing Research*, 41 (3) 186–8   16 References

Article proposes a systematic approach to preparing qualitative instruments for use in cross-cultural research (CR 2.36, 2.53).

2.55.31   Klakovich, M. (1995) Development and psychometric evaluation of the Reciprocal Empowerment Scale. *Journal of Nursing Measurement*, 3 (2) 127–43   48 References

Reports on the development and evaluation of a tool designed to measure empowerment in the context of the leader–follower relationship in institutional settings.

2.55.32   Lengacher, C.A. (1993) Development and study of an instrument to measure role strain. *Journal of Nursing Education*, 32 (2) 71–7   25 References

Describes the theoretical framework and processes involved in the design and development of an instrument to measure role strain in female nursing students. Criteria are given for writing items, the sample and procedure for testing, including its reliability and validity (CR 2.24, 2.25, 2.61).

2.55.33   Letts, L. & Marshall, L. (1995) Evaluating the validity and consistency of the SAFER Tool. *Physical & Occupational Therapy in Geriatrics*, 13 (4) 49–66   33 References

The Safety Assessment of Function and the Environment for Rehabilitation (SAFER Tool) was designed to evaluate the ability of seniors to manage safely in their homes. Results of testing are reported and authors recommend further testing.

2.55.34   Lin, L., Snyder, M. & Egan, E.C. (1996) The development of Taiwanese Elderly Stressor Inventory. *International Journal of Nursing Studies*, 33 (1) 29–36   24 References

Reports the development of a tool which allows the respondents to rate their degree of stress. Seventy-three stressors were identified and testing showed the need for some further refinement.

2.55.35   Lutjens, L.R.J. & Bostrom, A.C. (1995) Paving a middle road: point/counter-point … scales of measurement. *Michigan Nurse*, 68 (4) 10–11   8 References

Discusses the use of the ordinal level of measurement which may be used with self-report instruments such as attitude and psychological scales. The types of test used on these data is limited to non-parametric statistics. This is disputed by some researchers and the controversy is debated.

2.55.36   Mahoney, C.A., Thombs, D.L. & Howe, C.Z. (1995) The art and science of scale development in health education research. *Health Education Research*, 10 (1) 1–10   36 References

Describes a model for developing measurement scales using both quantitative and qualitative techniques. Open-ended interviews and focus groups were used to generate questionnaire items and quantitative methods were used to test and refine questionnaire sub-scales. Reliability and validity are discussed (CR 2.24, 2.25, 2.68, 2.69).

2.55.37   McCanse, R.P. (1995) The McCanse Readiness for Death Instrument (MRDI): a reliable and valid measure for hospice care. *Hospice Journal – Physical, Psychosocial, & Pastoral Care of the Dying*, 10 (1) 15–26   33 References

Reports a study which aimed to establish whether or not readiness for death, as an indicator of healthy dying, was a measurable concept. The MRDI was developed and tested and the results are reported.

2.55.38   Mead, D. (1996) Research-based tools in the audit process: issues of use, validity and reliability. *Nurse Researcher*, 3 (3) 17–34   8 References

Reports the use of a tool, the Magnitude Rating Scale, in the process of auditing care. Issues of reliability and validity are discussed (CR 2.24, 2.25).

2.55.39   Miller, D.C. (1991) Selected sociometric scales and indexes, in Author, *Handbook of Research Design and Social Measurement* 5th edition. Newbury Park, CA: Sage. ISBN 0803942192 Part 6, 323–581 References (extensive)

Section includes innumerable examples of scales and indices under the major headings of social status, group structure and dynamics, social indicators, measures of organizational structure, community and social participation. Also included are leadership in work organizations, morale and job status, attitudes, values and norms, family and marriage, personality measures, inventories of sociometric attitude scales, and evaluation of research continuity. Each scale is described and references to research applications are given, all of which have passed rigorous tests of reliability, validity and utility (CR 2.54.14, 2.56, 2.57, 2.63).

2.55.40 Morris, L.L., Fitz-Gibbon, C.T. & Lindheim, E. (1988) *How to Measure Performance and Use Tests* 2nd edition. Newbury Park, CA: Sage. ISBN 0803931328 References

Book includes many aspects of the development and use of performance tests: preliminary considerations, locating existing measures, its appropriateness for each programme, constructing tests, assessing validity and reliability and using the data (CR 2.24, 2.25).

2.55.41 Neelon, V.J., Champagne, M.T., Carlson, J.R. & Funk, S.G. (1996) The NEECHAM Confusion Scale: construction, validation and clinical testing. *Nursing Research*, 45 (6) 324–30 49 References

Reports the development of the NEECHAM scale for rapid and unobtrusive assessment and monitoring of acute confusion. Results showed it to be a valid and reliable bedside assessment, particularly at the onset of confusion and in patients with 'quiet' manifestations.

2.55.42 Neumann, J. (1996) Research corner. Certified neuroscience (sic) registered nurses' use of neuro-assessment tool(s) in their practice: perceived strengths and weaknesses of these tools. *Prairie Rose*, 64 (4) 4–6 21 References

Briefly reviews five neuro-assessment tools and examines their use by certified neuroscience registered nurses.

2.55.43 Norman, I.J. & Redfern, S.J. (1995) The validity of Qualpacs. *Journal of Advanced Nursing*, 22 (6) 1174–81 27 References

Discusses the validity of the quality assessment instrument, Qualpacs, which was

examined using a multiple triangulation design. The literature that is reviewed addresses the sensitivity, scoring and scope of the instrument, operational decisions, cost and policy implications. Results are compared with two other instruments, Monitor and Senior Monitor. Convergent and construct validity of the instrument are shown (CR 2.25, 2.26, 2.61).

2.55.44 Norman, I.J. & Redfern, S.J. (1996) The validity of two quality assessment instruments: Monitor and Senior Monitor. *International Journal of Nursing Studies*, 33 (6) 660–8 15 References

Study attempted to validate Monitor and Senior Monitor through a multiple triangulation research design. They were also compared to Qualpacs and other methods focusing on the quality of nursing care. Results did not give a clear picture (CR 2.25, 2.61).

2.55.45 Norman, I.J., Redfern, S.J., Oliver, S. & Tomalin, D.A. (1994) Evaluation of Kitson's Therapeutic Nursing Function Matrix in the assessment of quality of nursing in hospital. *International Journal of Nursing Studies*, 31 (4) 337–48 2 References

Paper describes authors' test of Kitson's structured observation and scoring technique (the Therapeutic Nursing Function Matrix – TNFM) and their development of her technique (referred to as the Quality Assessment Project scheme – QAP scheme) as methods of assessing the quality of patient care in hospital wards. Testing of both tools is reported and authors believe that their modifications make the QAP scheme a promising method for assessing the quality of care.

2.55.46 Oddi, L.F. & Cassidy, V.R. (1994) The JAND as a measure of nurses' perception of moral behaviour (Judgement About Nursing Decisions). *International Journal of Nursing Studies*, 31 (1) 37–47 32 References

A review of research which used the Judgement About Nursing Decisions (JAND) instrument as a measure of nurses' ethical decision-making. It raises numerous concerns about the conceptual basis, reliability and validity of this widely used instrument. Findings from studies which used this tool should be interpreted with caution until it is further refined (CR 2.17).

2.55.47   Pain, K., Hagler, P. & Warren, S. (1996) Development of an instrument to evaluate the research orientation of clinical professionals. *Canadian Journal of Rehabilitation*, 9 (2) 93–100   26 References

Outlines the development and validation of the Edmonton Research Orientation Survey (EROS) which was designed to assess professionals' research orientation. Preliminary analyses of the instrument show that the scale is reliable and has good content and construct validity (CR 2.24, 2.25, 3.7).

2.55.48   Poulton, B. (1998) Shaping care with patients and carers: user satisfaction tools. *Nurse Researcher*, 5 (3)   33–42   35 References

Author discusses what user satisfaction actually is and how it might be measured. She believes that any legitimate study of user evaluation of quality of care must involve the users themselves in setting the criteria and monitoring the outcomes.

2.55.49   Priest, J., McColl, E., Thomas, L. & Bond, S. (1995) Developing and refining a new measurement tool. *Nurse Researcher*, 2 (4) 69–81   13 References

Researchers from the University of Newcastle describe how they developed the Newcastle Satisfaction with Nursing Scales (NSNS). Part of the methodological work required is described in detail.

2.55.50   Rawlins, P.S., Rawlins, T.D. & Horner, M. (1990) Development of the family needs assessment tool. *Western Journal of Nursing Research*, 12 (2) 201–14   28 References

Discusses development of the family needs assessment tool, its conceptual framework and methods used to establish reliability and validity (CR 2.24, 2.25).

2.55.51   Redfern, S.J. & Norman, I.J. (1995) Quality assessment instruments in nursing: towards validation. *International Journal of Nursing Studies*, 32 (2) 115–25   24 References

Discusses the validity of three nursing quality assessment instruments: Monitor, Senior Monitor and Qualpacs. A multiple triangulation research design was used, and results reported focus on the experiences of using the

instruments, their inter-rater reliability and comparisons of scores within medical, surgical and elderly care wards (CR 2.24, 2.25, 2.26, 2.63).

2.55.52   Redfern, S., Norman, I.J., Tomalin, D.A. & Oliver, S. (1992) The reliability and validity of quality assessment measures in nursing. *Journal of Clinical Nursing*, 1 (1) 47–8   3 References

Outlines a Department of Health-funded project designed to test the reliability and validity of Monitor, Senior Monitor and Qualpacs. Methods used are listed and progress to date is reported (CR 2.24, 2.25, 2.61).

2.55.53   Rich, D. (1994) Measuring client satisfaction with psychiatric treatment: development of an objective, criterion referenced scale. *Australian New Zealand Journal of Mental Health Nursing*, 3 (3) 91–4   8 References

Paper describes development of the Patient Inpatient Satisfaction Survey and its range of uses is discussed.

2.55.54   Roberts, P. (1998) The service quality approach to developing user satisfaction tools. *Nurse Researcher*, 5 (3) 43–50   31 References

Author describes a step-by-step process for creating a user satisfaction tool, and suggests that there may be some value in health professionals considering adapting established generic instruments or developing contextual tools to measure the satisfaction of specific users.

2.55.55   Robinson, D., Reed, V. & Lange, A. (1996) Developing risk assessment scales in forensic psychiatric care. *Psychiatric Care*, 3 (4) 146–52   43 References

Paper gives preliminary details about a current research programme which seeks to develop and validate nursing assessments of potential danger. Authors wished to communicate their early ideas for such tools.

2.55.56   Salzberg, C.A., Byrne, D.W., Cayten, G., van Niewerburgh, P., Murphy, J.G. & Viehbeck, M. (1996) A new pressure ulcer risk assessment scale for individuals with spinal cord injury. *American Journal of Physical Medicine and Rehabilitation*, 75 (2) 96–104, 121–4, 140   18 References

Reports the development of a scale specifically for assessing risk in spinal-injured patients as no other method currently exists. Fifteen risk factors which met four pre-specified criteria were identified and a measurement tool was created.

2.55.57 Santamaria, N. (1995/96) The Difficult Patient Stress Scale: a new instrument to measure interpersonal stress in nursing. *Australian Journal of Advanced Nursing*, 13 (2) 22–9   29 References

Describes the development of a scale designed to investigate the stress which nurses experience when involved in interpersonal conflict with patients. Results of its use over a two-year period are discussed and the author believes it may be of value in the development of training programmes to help nurses deal with difficulties which may arise.

2.55.58 Scribante, J., Muller, M.E. & Lipman, J. (1996) Development and validation of a critical care patient classification system. *American Journal of Critical Care*, 4 (4) 282–8   7 References

Describes the research methodology used in the development and validation of a scientific patient classification instrument for South African critical care patients. Results are reported and authors believe that established systems can be adapted and validated for local use (CR 2.25).

2.55.59 Sheu, S. & Hwang, S. (1996) Validation of Chinese version of Mishel's Uncertainty in Illness Scale [Chinese]. *Nursing Research (China)*, 4 (1) 59–68   9 References

Study examined the usefulness of the Mishel Uncertainty in Illness Scale which had been translated into Chinese. Three items were deleted after item analysis and results showed that it was an acceptable instrument to measure uncertainty (CR 2.25).

2.55.60 Spector, P.E. (1992) *Summated Rating Scale Construction*. Newbury Park, CA: Sage. ISBN 0803943415   References

Aims to help researchers construct more effective scales. Information is given on how to estimate the number of items, choose good from bad, and how scales can be validated (CR 2.25).

2.55.61 Stewart, M., Tudiver, F., Bass, M.J.,

Dunn, E.V. & Norton, P.G. (1992) *Tools for Primary Care Research*. Newbury Park, CA: Sage. ISBN 0803944047   References

Covers basic concepts and tools for measurement and data collection.

2.55.62 Thomas, L.H. & Bons, S. (1996) Measuring patients' satisfaction with nursing: 1990–1994. *Journal of Advanced Nursing*, 23 (4) 747–56   48 References

Article reviews recent developments in measuring patient satisfaction with nursing. Studies published since 1990 show lack of clarity with regard to purpose or intent, together with a lack of conceptual and methodological rigour. Ways forward are suggested and a new scale, the Newcastle Satisfaction with Nursing Scale, is mentioned (CR 2.61).

2.55.63 Thomas, L.H., Macmillan, J., McColl, E., Priest, C., Hale, C. & Bond, S. (1995) Obtaining patients' views of nursing care to inform the development of a patient satisfaction scale. *International Journal for Quality in Health Care*, 7 (2) 153–63   39 References

This study aimed to develop a sensitive, valid and reliable measure of patient satisfaction. The paper describes the first phase of the study, the development of a multi-dimensional concept of satisfaction from the patient's perspective. Eleven main concepts were identified which provided the starting point for development of a scale. These were of importance to the patient rather than hospital personnel or research teams.

2.55.64 Tsai, S. & Chen, M. (1996) A test of reliability and validity of nurses' stress checklist [Chinese]. *Nursing Research (China)*, 4 (4) 355–62   16 References

Study aimed to build a reliable and valid instrument to measure nurse stress in Taiwan. A checklist was selected and translated into Chinese. Results showed it to be valid and reliable for use as a basis for designing stress management for nurses and further professional development (CR 2.24, 2.25).

2.55.65 Wang, J.F. & Paterson, J. (1996) Using factor analysis to explore nurses' fear of AIDS in the United States of America. *Journal of Advanced Nursing*, 24 (2) 287–95   36 References

Aim of study was to develop a reliable instrument to test the fear of AIDS (FOA) and explore the dimension of FOA among nurses. The processes of development are described and the use of factor analysis is discussed.

2.55.66   Ward, M.J. (1986) Nursing research instruments: some considerations and recommendations, in Stinson, S.M. & Kerr, J.C. (eds), *International Issues in Nursing Research*, Beckenham: Croom Helm. ISBN 0709944373 Part 1, Chapter 3, 41–60   References

Chapter lists the various approaches to data collection and then examines the properties of a research instrument. A series of questions which should be asked about an existing instrument to determine its appropriateness for the particular purpose is included, together with suggested steps for developing one's own. The Nursing Research Instruments Compilations Projects are outlined and nurses in other countries are urged to set up similar libraries of instruments (CR 3.22.12).

2.55.67   Watson, H. (1995) Psychometric analysis of assessment tools. *Nurse Researcher*, 2 (4) 56–68   14 References

Describes how the use of psychometric analysis assisted in the revision of a pre-established interview schedule to make it more appropriate for particular research needs (CR 2.68).

2.55.68   Watson, R. & Lea, A. (1997) The caring dimensions inventory (CDI): content validity, reliability and scaling. *Journal of Advanced Nursing*, 25 (1) 87–94   30 References

Reports on the content analysis of a questionnaire called the Caring Dimensions Inventory, its internal consistency and scalability. Possibilities for further analysis and development are discussed (CR 2.88).

2.55.69   Westbrook, J.I. (1993) Patient satisfaction: methodological issues and research findings. *Australian Health Review*, 16 (1) 75–88   57 References

Addresses some of the methodological issues related to measuring patient satisfaction and describes validated and reliable tools available in Australia.

2.55.70   Wilde, B., Larsson, G., Larsson, M.

& Starrin, B. (1994) Quality of care: development of a patient-centered questionnaire based on a grounded theory model. *Scandinavian Journal of Caring Sciences*, 8 (1) 39–48   26 References

Reports the development of a scale derived from a model of quality of care from the patient's perspective.

2.55.71   Willer, B., Ottenbacher, K.J. & Coad, M.L. (1994) The community integration questionnaire: a comparative examination. *American Journal of Physical Medicine and Rehabilitation*, 73 (2) 103–11   17 References

Study was designed to test the validity and other psychometric characteristics of the community integration questionnaire which aimed to assess home and social integration and productive activity in people with acquired brain injury. Areas for further work are identified.

2.55.72   Youngblut, J.M. & Casper, G.R. (1993) Single-item indicators in nursing research. *Research in Nursing and Health*, 16 (6) 459–65   28 References

Explores the use of single-item indicators, and discusses problems where these were used as part of a multi-item scale. A study is used for illustration.

SOURCES OF INSTRUMENTS

Sections 2.56 to 2.63 include compendia, books or articles which list or describe instruments of possible relevance to nursing. They are grouped under the following headings: 2.56 Attitudinal; 2.57 Behavioural; 2.58 Health related; 2.59 Medical; 2.60 Mental measures; 2.61 Nursing; 2.62 Physiological; and 2.63 Sociological/occupational.

The listing is not exhaustive and there is some overlap between compilations, but it illustrates the wide variety of tools already available. Before developing new tools, existing ones should be carefully examined to see if their validity for nursing practice can be further strengthened by repeated use. Please note that many compilations are 'old' but have not been superseded.

2.56 ATTITUDINAL

Annotations

2.56.1 Adams, A. (1998) Attitude scales: building a composite picture. *Nurse Researcher*, 5 (3) 51–62   11 References

Article explains what attitude scales are and why they are useful. Issues relating to developing and testing them are discussed and guidelines are given for using published scales (CR 2.24, 2.25).

2.56.2 Henerson, M.E., Morris, L.L. & Fitz-Gibbon, C.T. (1988) *How to Measure Attitudes* 2nd edition. Beverly Hills, CA: Sage. ISBN 080393131X   References

Book covers topics commonly confronted by evaluators of educational programmes. Its use should enable the development of basic skills in designing and using instruments for the assessment of attitudes. Included are preliminary questions, selecting from alternative approaches, finding and developing measures, validity and reliability of attitudinal instruments, analysing the data and its presentation (CR 2.24, 2.25, 2.86, 2.87, 2.94).

2.56.3 Procter, M. (1993) Measuring attitudes, in Gilbert, N. (ed.), *Researching Social Life.* London: Sage. ISBN 0803986823 Chapter 7, 116–34   References

Chapter examines attitudes, techniques of attitude scale construction, reliability, validity and factor analysis (CR 2.1.25, 2.24, 2.25, 2.55).

2.56.4 Robinson, J.P. & Shaver, P.R. (1973) *Measures of Social Psychological Attitudes.* Ann Arbor, MI: Institute for Social Research, University of Michigan. ISBN 0879440694

A compilation of 126 instruments measuring attitudes organized under the general headings of self-esteem and related constructs, locus of control, alienation, authoritarianism, socio-political attitudes, values, attitudes towards people, religious attitudes and social desirability scales. Bibliographical information is included for 30 additional self-concept measures. For each tool the following are described: variables, format, samples to whom it has been given, reliability and validity, bibliographical sources in which it has been described or used and the method of administration. An evaluation is also made.

2.56.5 Shaw, M.E. & Wright, J.M. (1967) *Scales for the Measurement of Attitudes.* New York: McGraw-Hill. No ISBN

A compilation of 176 attitude scales which fall into the general categories of social practices, social issues and problems, international issues, abstract concepts, political and religious attitudes, ethnic and national groups, significant others and social institutions. Each tool is described together with subjects used for testing, measurement properties of the response mode, reliability and validity data, together with an evaluation.

2.57 BEHAVIOURAL

Annotations

2.57.1 Andrulis, R.S. (1977) *A Source Book of Tests and Measures of Human Behaviour.* Springfield, IL: Charles Thomas. ISBN 0398036039   References

Volume contains descriptions of 155 commercially available tests to assess adult behaviour. Tests are categorized under intelligence and aptitude, achievement, cognitive style, general measures of personality, personality adjustment, vocational and interest inventories, attitude devices, personality performance, managerial and creativity tests. Each description includes variables measured, type of measure, where to obtain it, psychometric properties, its purpose, scoring, and groups used for testing. Some reliability and validity data are available for about 90 per cent of the tools.

2.57.2 Ciminero, A.R., Calhoun, K.S. & Adams, H.E. (eds) (1986) *Handbook of Behavioural Measurement* 2nd edition. New York: Wiley. ISBN 0471888494

A comprehensive review of general and specific issues in behavioural measurement. The book discusses: issues in assessment and a system to classify psychological responses that could be used as a framework for research. General approaches to behavioural assessment are included, with chapters on interviews, self-report tools, direct observation and psycho-physiological techniques, and descriptions are given on how these approaches may be used. A number of sources are included and some instruments are described (CR 2.68, 2.71, 2.72).

2.57.3 Lake, D.G., Miles, M.B. & Earle, R.B. Jr. (1973) *Measuring Human Behaviour: Tools for the Assessment of Social Functioning*. New York: Teachers College Press. ISBN 0807716480

Eighty-four behavioural instruments are described and critiqued and include personal, inter-personal, group or organizational variables. Each tool is described, variables tested and its scoring, administration, development, critique, and evaluation are discussed. Most have been tested for reliability and validity.

2.57.4 Pfeiffer, W.J., Heslen, R. & Jones, J.E. (1976) *Instrumentation in Human Relations Training* 2nd edition. LaJolk, CA: California University Associates Inc. ISBN 0883901161

Part 1 of this book deals with instrumentation issues such as administration, validity, reliability, instrument development and problems of instrumentation. Part 2 contains a guide to 92 instruments for use in the behavioural sciences. These are categorized as personal, inter-personal and organizational in focus. Although a variable amount of information is included for each instrument, length and time to complete, descriptions of scales and sub-scales and purchase information are given.

2.57.5 Sommer, B. & Sommer, R. (1997) *A Practical Guide to Behavioural Research: Tools and Techniques* 4th edition. India: Oxford University Press. ISBN 0195104188 References

Covers many of the tools and techniques required to conduct behavioural research.

2.58 HEALTH RELATED

Annotations

2.58.1 Bowling, A. (1991) Health care research: measuring health status. *Nursing Practice*, 4 (4) 2–8   23 References

Describes some of the most well-known and tested health status tools. These are the Sickness Impact Profile, Nottingham Health Profile, Rand Health Insurance Study Battery, The Social Health Battery (Rand Corporation), General Health Perceptions Battery, Spitzer's Quality of Life Index and the Linear Analogue Self-assessment Tool.

2.58.2 Bowling, A. (1995) *Measuring Disease*. Buckingham: Open University Press ISBN 0335192254   References

Book provides reviews of specific measures of the quality of life. Other scales are also included.

2.58.3 Bowling, A. (1997) *Measuring Health: a Review of Quality of Life Measurement Scales* 2nd edition. Buckingham: Open University Press. ISBN 033519754X   References

This revised and updated edition offers a comprehensive guide to measures of health and functioning, including psychological well-being, emotional well-being, social networks and support. A number of recently developed scales are included. New edition contains an index and a list of scale distributors.

2.58.4 Fitzpatrick, R. & Dunnell, K. (1992) Measuring outcomes in health care, in Beck, E., Lonsdale, S., Newman, S. & Patterson, D. (eds), *In the Best of Health?: the Status and Future of Health Care in the United Kingdom*. London: Chapman & Hall. ISBN 0412387107 Chapter 4, 60–86   References

Chapter makes reference to several instruments which have been developed to measure the different dimensions of health status and quality of life (CR 2.55).

2.58.5 Goldfield, N. (1996) The hubris of health status measurement; a clarification of its role in the assessment of medical care. *International Journal for Quality in Health Care*, 8 (2) 115–23   28 References

Paper outlines the difficulties of using health status measures as a means of evaluating outcomes of competing health plans. Suggestions are made for dealing with this important issue.

2.58.6 Karoly, P. (ed.) (1991) *Measurement Strategies in Health Psychology*. New York: Wiley. ISBN 0471554812   References

Book describes the current state of health psychology assessment and potential new directions. Many tests used have their applications discussed and references are given. In most instances the tests themselves are not included but research based on them is reported. Assessments that are given include quality of life, life-styles, risk factors, medical compliance, pain, illness cognition and life stress events. Methodological considerations are discussed.

2.58.7 Kelly, K.C., Huber, D.G., Johnson, M., McCloskey, J.C. & Maas, M. (1994) The Medical Outcomes Study: a nursing perspective. *Journal of Professional Nursing*, 10 (4) 209–16 30 References

Paper discusses the framework of the Medical Outcomes Study as a means of studying the effectiveness of health care delivery systems. Changes are suggested which would enable nursing and other professionals' input to contribute to enhanced patient care (CR 2.43, 2.59).

2.58.8 Lorig, K., Stewart, A., Ritter, P., González, V., Laurent, D. & Lynch, J. (1996) *Outcome Measures for Health Education and Other Health Care Interventions*. Thousand Oaks, CA: Sage. ISBN 0761900675 References

Book provides a compilation of more than 50 self-administered scales for measuring health behaviours, health status, self-efficacy and health care utilization (CR 2.43).

2.58.9 McDowell, I. & Newell, C. (1996) *Measuring Health: a Guide to Rating Scales and Questionnaires* 2nd edition. New York and Oxford: Oxford University Press. ISBN 0195103718

Book brings together scattered information on several types of health measurement techniques and aims to provide data necessary to choose, apply and score the chosen method. Fifty measures are reviewed and topics include physical disability and handicap, psychological well-being, depression, mental status testing, social health, pain, quality of life and general health. Descriptions cover the purpose of each test, its conceptual basis, reliability and validity and a copy of each is included. Alternative forms, a discussion of the method and the test developer's address are also given (CR 2.24, 2.25, 2.75).

2.58.10 to 2.58.31 Medical Care Supplement. (1989) Advances in health status assessment: conference proceedings. *Medical Care Supplement*, 27 (3) March

The following entry differs in format as it documents a special issue of the journal *Medical Care*. These articles have not been annotated.

2.58.10 Bergner, M. Quality of life, health status, and clinical research. S148–S156 37 References

2.58.11 Breslow, L. Health status measurement in the evaluation of health promotion. S205–S216 20 References

2.58.12 Connelly, J.E., Philbrick, J.T., Smith, G.R. Jr., Kaiser, D.L. & Wymer, A. Health perceptions of primary care patients and the influence on health care utilisation. S99–S109 18 References

2.58.13 Deyo, R.A. & Patrick, D.L. Barriers to the use of health status measures in clinical investigation, patient care and policy research. S254–S268 63 References

2.58.14 Epstein, A.M., Hall, J.A., Tognetti, J., Son, L.H. & Conant, L. Jr. Using proxies to evaluate quality of life: can they provide valid information about patients' health status and satisfaction with medical care? S91–S98 25 References

2.58.15 Erikson, P., Kendall, E.A., Anderson, J. & Kaplan, R.M. Using composite health status measures to assess the nation's health. S66–S76 36 References

2.58.16 Feeny, D.H. & Torrance, G.W. Incorporating utility-based quality-of-life assessment measures in clinical trials: two examples. S190–S204 73 References

2.58.17 Hall, J.A., Epstein, A.M. & McNeil, B.J. Multi-dimensionality of health status in an elderly population: construct validity of a measurement battery. S168–S177 23 References

2.58.18 Kaplan, R.M., Anderson, J.P., Wu, A.W., Matthews, C., Kozin, F. & Orenstein, D. The quality of well-being scale: applications in AIDS, cystic fibrosis and arthritis. S27–S43 36 References

2.58.19 Kaplan, S.H., Greenfield, S. & Ware, J.E. Assessing the effects of physician–patient interactions on the outcomes of chronic disease. S110–S127   69 References

2.58.20 Kazis, L.E., Anderson, J.J. & Meenan, R.F. Effect sizes for interpreting changes in health status. S178–S189 15 References

2.58.21 Lewis, C.C., Pantell, R.H. & Kieckhefer, G.M. Assessment of children's health status: field test of new approaches. S54–S65 14 References

2.58.22 Lipscomb, J. Time preference for health in cost-effectiveness analysis. S233–S253   39 References

2.58.23 Lohr, K.M. Advances in health status assessment: overview of the conference. S1–S11   47 References

2.58.24 Mosteller, F., Ware, J.E. Jr. & Levine, S. Finale panel: comments on the conference on advances in health status assessment. S282–S294   34 References

2.58.25 Mulley, A.G. Jr. Assessing patient's utilities: can the ends justify the means? S269–S281   56 References

2.58.26 Nelson, E.C. & Berwick, D.M. The measurement of health status in clinical practice. S77–S90   58 References

2.58.27 Patrick, D.L. & Deyo, R.A. Generic and disease specific measures in assessing health status and quality of life. S227–S232 95 References

2.58.28 Rothman, M.L., Hedrick, S. & Inui, T. The sickness impact profile as a measure of the health status of non-cognitively impaired nursing home residents. S157–S167 24 References

2.58.29 Steinwachs, D.M. Application of health status assessment measures in policy research. S12–S26   54 References

2.58.30 Temkin, N.R., Dikmen, S., Machamer, J. & McLean, A. General versus disease-specific measures: further work on the sickness impact profile for head injury. S44–S53   18 References

2.58.31 Verbrugge, L.M. & Balaban, D.J. Patterns of change in disability and well-being. S128–S147   37 References

2.58.32 Mukherjee, R. (1989) *The Quality of Life: Valuation in Social Research.* Newbury Park, CA: Sage. ISBN 0803995873   References

Examines the all-inclusive notion of the quality of life by using two perspectives, i.e. others' valuation of what people need and what the people involved actually want.

2.58.33 Reeder, L.G., Ramacher, L. & Gorelnik, S. (1976) *Handbook of Scales and Indices of Health Behaviour.* Pacific Palisades, CA: Goodyear. ISBN 0876203799

Seventy-eight studies are included and grouped under health behaviour, status, orientation, illness behaviour and use of health services. Information is presented using the steps of the research process. Approximately 85 per cent of studies used the survey method of data collection, and for about 25 per cent the tools, or sections of them, are included.

2.58.34 Streiner, D.L. & Norman, G.R. (1995) *Health Measurement Scales: a Practical Guide to their Development and Use.* Oxford: Oxford University Press. ISBN 0192626701 References

An explanatory text intended for medical researchers, it covers reliability, validity, response bias, telephone interviewing and other relevant topics (CR 2.24, 2.25, 2.27, 2.70).

2.58.35 Walker, S.R. & Rosser, R.M. (eds) (1992) *Quality of Life Assessment: Key Issues in the 1990s.* Dordrecht: Kluwer Academic Publishers. ISBN 0792389913   References

Book, based on presentations given at a workshop, comprises sections covering philosophies, concepts and key instruments involved in assessing the quality of life and in major disease areas. Viewpoints and perspectives from industry, regulatory authorities and health care purchasers, ethics, policy decisions and cost-effectiveness are all discussed. Appendices include shortened versions of some instruments (CR 2.17, 3.11).

2.59 MEDICAL

Annotations

2.59.1 Maistrello, I., Febbrari, M.D., Tramontini, M., Maistrello, M. & Natale, L. (1995) The multi-purpose surveillance-oriented medical record: a tool for quality care management. *International Journal for Quality in Health Care*, 7 (4) 399–405 15 References

Reports the use of the surveillance-orientated medical record which can be used to monitor the appropriateness of medical interventions. It can also identify risk areas and deduce outcome indicators which could lead to potential problems.

2.59.2 Read, J.D. (1990) The Read Classification for Primary Care, in *Royal College of General Practitioners 1990 Members Reference Handbook*. London: Royal College of General Practitioners. ISSN 0262-9275 253–4, 258, 260 11 References

Describes a comprehensive system of clinical classification coding covering diseases and symptoms for medical records. It contains 100,000 terms and 150,000 synonyms which may be used in primary, secondary and tertiary care by clinicians, technicians, paramedics, researchers, administrators and planners.

2.59.3 Smith, N., Wilson, A. & Weekes, T. (1995) Use of Read codes in the development of a standard data set. *British Medical Journal*, 29 July, 311 (7000) 313–15 12 References

Authors describe the experience and problems of developing and coding a standard data set.

2.60 MENTAL MEASURES

Annotations

2.60.1 Balogh, R., Bond, S. & Parker, K. (1992) Off-the-shelf audit: is it feasible? *Nursing Standard*, 23 September, 7(1) 35–8 6 References

Reviews the ways in which one instrument, the Central Nottinghamshire Psychiatric Nursing Audit, has been used in two settings. Value of the results is discussed and whether the exercise was cost-effective.

2.60.2 British Psychological Society. (1990) *Psychological Testing: a Guide*. Leicester: British Psychological Society. No ISBN References

Booklet, developed by the steering committee of the society, aims to give guidance mainly to non-psychologists and other prospective users on test standards. It includes an introduction to testing, different applications, quality control issues, details of what to look for in a test and further information.

2.60.3 Buros, O.K. (ed.) (1974) *Tests in Print II*. Highland Park, NJ: Gryphon Press. ISBN 0910674140

A guide to the tests of mental measurements in print up to 1974 and a cumulative index to the first seven *Mental Measurement Yearbooks*. Volume contains 2,467 entries and includes bibliographical sources, a cumulative index of all tests with references, publishers, author index, title index of tests both in and out of print, and an index stating populations for whom each test is intended. Editor recommends using *The Eighth Mental Measurements Yearbook* for a complete index to all tests.

2.60.4 Buros, O.K. (ed.) (1978) *The Eighth Mental Measurements Yearbook*. Highland Park, NJ: Gryphon Press. ISBN 0910674248

Compilation is divided into three sections: a list of 1,184 tests, 898 of which are critically reviewed. The remainder have reviews excerpted from journals. The second section contains 576 books on testing, with reviews of 229 books and also includes six indexes: author, title of test, book title, publishers, periodical and scanning index. Tests are organized into 13 categories: achievement tests; English; fine arts; foreign language; intelligence; mathematics; miscellaneous; reading; science; sensory and motor; social studies; speech and hearing; and vocations. Entries include title, population, variables, available forms and copyright information. This volume and *Tests in Print II* (2.60.3) provide a complete index to all tests of mental measurements. Tests of personality, intelligence, reading and vocational skills have been separated into individual volumes (2.60.5 to 2.60.10).

2.60.5   Buros, O.K. (ed.) (1968) *Reading Tests and Reviews* Volume 1. ISBN 0910674094

2.60.6   Buros, O.K. (ed.) (1975a) *Reading Tests and Reviews* Volume 2. ISBN 0910674205

2.60.7   Buros, O.K. (ed.) (1975b) *Intelligence Tests and Reviews.* ISBN 0910674175

2.60.8   Buros, O.K. (ed.) (1970) *Personality Tests and Reviews* Volume 1. ISBN 0910674108

2.60.9   Buros, O.K. (ed.) (1975c) *Personality Tests and Reviews* Volume 2. ISBN 0910674191

2.60.10   Buros, O.K. (ed.) (1975d) *Vocational Tests and Reviews.* ISBN 091067423X

All the above are published by Gryphon Press.

2.60.11   Chun, K.T., Cobb, S. & French, J.R.P. Jr. (1975) *Measures for Psychological Assessment: a Guide to 3,000 Original Sources and their Applications.* Ann Arbor, MI: University of Michigan, Institute for Social Research. ISBN 0879441682   References

A compilation of annotated references to the measures of mental health and related variables and their uses. A bibliography of all quantitative research which used these measures between 1960 and 1970 is included. Volume consists of two major sections, primary references, applications and two indexes. The section on primary sources lists approximately 3,000 references to articles or other publications in which the measures were first described. The section on application provides over 6,000 instances in which the measures are described. Details relating to each test are not included (CR 1.5).

2.60.12   Comrey, A.L., Backer, T.E. & Glaser, E.M. (1973) *A Sourcebook for Mental Health Measures.* Los Angeles, CA: Human Interaction Research Institute. No ISBN found

Contains abstracts of approximately 1,100

psychological and mental health-related tools. Topics of interest to nurses are alcoholism, drugs, family interaction, geriatrics, mental handicap and evaluation of professional service delivery. Abstracts include title, source, authors' names and addresses, purpose of the tool, a description, major applications and how it may be obtained. It also indicates for most tools where information on reliability and validity may be obtained.

2.60.13   Conoley, J.C. & Impara, J.C. (1995) *The Twelfth Mental Measurements Yearbook.* Lincoln, NB: University of Nebraska-Lincoln. ISBN 091067440X   References

Book contains reviews of new tests which have been significantly revised since *The Eleventh Mental Measurement Yearbook* in 1992. It includes a bibliography of 418 commercially available tests, 803 critical test reviews, bibliographies of references for specific tests related to the construction, validity or use in various settings, classified subject and names indexes, publishers' information, acronyms for easy reference and a score index.

2.60.14   Conoley, J.C., Kramer, J.J. & Mitchell, J.V. Jr. (eds) (1988) *The Supplement to the Ninth Mental Measurements Yearbook.* Lincoln, NB: University of Nebraska-Lincoln. ISBN 0910674302   References

Contains reviews of new or revised tests available since publication of *The Ninth Mental Measurements Yearbook.* This is not a comprehensive volume but contains 89 commercially available tests, 150 critical reviews, bibliography of references to the construction, validity or use of tests, title, subject and names indexes, acronyms for easy reference, publishers' information and a score index.
[From 1989 *Mental Measurements Yearbooks* and *Supplements* will be published in alternate years.]

2.60.15   Frank, S.H. (1992) Inventory of psychological measurement instruments useful in primary care, in Stewart, M., Tudiver, F., Bass, M.J., Dunn, E.V. & Norton, P.G. (eds), *Tools for Primary Research.* Newbury Park, CA: Sage. ISBN 0803944047 References Appendix 229–70

This inventory contains 179 tests under 30 topic headings. Information on each one includes the number of items, item format, original references and notes. Also, when available, a reference describing its use in the family practice setting (CR 2.55.61).

2.60.16 Goldman, B.A. & Mitchell, D.F. (eds) (1995) *Directory of Unpublished Experimental Mental Measures.* Volume 6 Washington, DC: American Psychological Association. ISBN 1557982899

and

2.60.17 Goldman, B.A., Osborne, W.L. & Mitchell, D.F. (eds) (1996) *Directory of Unpublished Experimental Mental Measures.* Volumes 4 to 5 Washington, DC: American Psychological Association. ISBN 1557983518

and

2.60.18 Goldman, B.A., Saunders, J.L. & Busch, J.C. (eds) (1995) *Directory of Unpublished Experimental Mental Measures.* Volumes 1 to 3 Washington, DC: American Psychological Association. ISBN 1557983364

Volumes provide information on over 1,000 mental measures which were identified by reviewing relevant psychology, sociology and educational journals. Information given includes: name; purpose; description; reliability; validity; bibliographical information and references.

2.60.19 Kramer, J.J. & Conoley, J.C. (eds) (1992) *The Eleventh Mental Measurements Yearbook.* Lincoln, NB: University of Nebraska-Lincoln. ISBN 0910674337 References

Contains reviews of tests which are new or significantly revised since the *Tenth Yearbook* was published in 1989. Contents include a bibliography of 477 commercially available tests, 703 critical test reviews, references to specific tests related to their construction, validity or use. Title, names and subject indexes are included.

2.60.20 Lyerly, S. (1973) *Handbook of Psychiatric Rating Scales* 2nd edition. Rockville, MD: National Institute of Mental Health. No ISBN found

Describes 61 rating scales which have been used in psychiatric settings, 38 of which include detailed descriptions. A table gives information on the population, type of rater, source of data, reliability and validity.

2.60.21 Mental Measurements Yearbook. (1994) University of Nebraska-Lincoln [Source: *Gale Directory of Databases.* Volume 1, *Online databases*, January 1994, No. 3438]

Contains descriptive information and reviews of English-language tests from the *Mental Measurements Yearbooks.* Covers more than 1,850 standardized educational, personality, vocational aptitude, psychological and related English-language tests. Information includes name and classification, author(s), publisher, publication data and price, time requirements, existence of validity and reliability data, score descriptions, levels, intended populations and critical reviews. Database covers from 1972 to date with some earlier materials and it is updated monthly. Online availability is from: BRS online, BRS after dark, BRS/COLLEAGUE (CR 1.8.6).

2.60.22 Mitchell, J.V. Jr. (1983) *Tests in Print III.* Lincoln, NB: University of Nebraska Press. ISBN 0910674523

Differs from other *Mental Measurements Yearbooks* as it contains no critical reviews or prices, but does includes a matrix index to *Yearbooks* 1–9 from 1938 to 1985. Tests are described by subject area, including those which are out of print.

2.60.23 Mittler, P.J. (ed.) (1974) *The Psychological Assessment of Mental and Physical Handicaps.* London: Tavistock. ISBN 0422756008 References

Text is designed to assist those who are concerned with systematic assessment of the handicapped. It does not cover the psychometric aspects of testing which may be found in other standard texts but covers comprehensively the diagnostic and assessment aspects. Individual tests are commented upon and extensive references given. Principles of psychological assessment, assessment of children and adults and experimental advances are included.

2.60.24 National Foundation for Educational Research – Nelson. *The Directory 1998: Tests, Assessments, Training and Information Services: Clinical Psychology, Educational Psychology, Child Development, Speech and Language Therapy and Occupational Therapy.*
URL: http: //www.nfer-nelson.co.uk

Company produces five separate, focused

directories for health and social care as listed above. They provide the professional user with information on the tests and relevant resource packs. Many tests included are relevant to nursing (CR 1.3).

2.60.25 Quinn, B. (1997) 'Hot' bibliographies. Internet resources for tests and measurements. *Internet Reference Services Quarterly*, 2 (4) 211–35   28 References

Study attempted to investigate what resources are now available on the Internet for tests and measurements. The emphasis is on those available for psychological testing with some educational psychological materials also included. Wherever possible evaluative summaries have been included (CR 2.64, 2.85).

2.61 NURSING

Annotations

2.61.1 Brettle, A. & Heaton, J. (1995) Outcome instruments for nurses: how to find out more about them. *Nurse Researcher*, 2 (4) 14–29   22 References

Article offers an overview of types of instrument available for measuring the outcomes of nursing practice. It also provides practical guidance on the action that can be taken to conduct customized searching for relevant information (CR 2.43, 2.55).

2.61.2 Brundage, D.J. & Swearengen, P.A. (1994) Chronic renal failure: evaluation and teaching tool. *ANNA Journal*, 21 (5) 265–70 6 References

Article describes the format, content and use of this tool which is used to assess and teach in-patients being treated medically with or without dialysis (CR 2.55).

2.61.3 Clayton, G.M. & Broome, M. (1989) *Instruments for Use in Nursing Education Research*. New York: National League for Nursing. ISBN 0887374247

Monograph categorizes, describes and evaluates instruments used in nursing education research during the 1980s. A wide range of topics is covered which shows a fragmented body of knowledge. The categories are:

prediction of success; student attitudes; student roles and socialization; curricula and methods of instruction; and faculty roles. The following are given for each instrument: an introduction; description and administrative details; psychometric properties; and research using the test. Qualitative studies are not included.

2.61.4 Frank-Stromborg, M. (ed.) (1992) *Instruments for Clinical Nursing Research* 2nd edition. Boston, MA: Jones & Bartlett. ISBN 0867203404   References

Book developed from a project undertaken by the Oncology Nursing Society which aimed to describe available instruments. It reviews the tools currently obtainable to measure a selected phenomenon. Their psychometric properties are described, details of the sample or studies which have utilized the tool are given and their strengths and weaknesses are identified. Their use in all areas of nursing is outlined. The evaluation of research instruments is discussed together with ways of identifying those assessing health, function and commonly occurring clinical problems. Most chapters are summarized and have extensive reference lists.

2.61.5 Frank-Stromborg, M. & Olsen, S.J. (eds) (1997) *Instruments for Clinical Health Care Research* 2nd edition. Sudbury, MA: Jones & Bartlett. ISBN 0763703168   References

The goals of this book together with *Instruments for Clinical Nursing Research* (2.61.4) are to provide reviews of clinical research instruments to measure selected clinical phenomena, describe their psychometric properties, review particular studies where they have been used, identify their strengths and weaknesses and discuss the relevance to nursing practice. The new title reflects the present emphasis on a team approach to health care. Major sections are an overview, including evaluating instruments for use in clinical research, instruments for assessing health and function, health promotion activities and clinical problems.

2.61.6 Holzemer, W.L. (1992) Measurement: a foundation of nursing science, in *Communicating Nursing Research Silver Threads – 25 Years of Nursing Excellence* Volume 25. Boulder, CO: Western Institute of Nursing.   No ISBN 45–54   46 References

Paper addresses the contribution made by compilations of instruments to the practice of nursing, centres of excellence, linking measurement and nursing research at the national level. Issues for the future are identified.

2.61.7 Kitson, A. & Harvey, G. (1991) *Bibliography of Nursing Quality Assurance and Standards of Care 1932–1987.* Harrow, Middlesex: Scutari. ISBN 1871364469

An annotated bibliography which cites literature on general theory, principles and methodological background issues related to quality and standards of care. It also includes philosophical aspects, a range of quality assurance measures available to nurses and articles relating quality of care to manpower studies (CR 1.5).

2.61.8 Martin, K. S. & Martin, D. L. (1997) How can the quality of nursing practice be measured, in McCloskey, J.C. & Grace, H.K. (eds), *Current Issues in Nursing* 5th edition. St Louis: Mosby. ISBN 0815185944 Chapter 42, 315–21 30 References

Chapter describes a practice, documentation and information management model that has been adopted by various service providers. This is congruent with the resources, regulations and contracts of the practice setting. It provides a way of integrating clinical, statistical and financial data and when considered in total, contains aspects of traditional and emerging indicators and client knowledge-behaviour status outcome measures (CR 2.43).

2.61.9 Redman, B.K. (1998) *Measurement Tools in Patient Education.* New York: Springer. ISBN 0826198600

Draws together instruments for measuring outcomes in patient education from a wide variety of sources. Book includes 52 tools, and each is accompanied by a descriptive review, critique, information on administration, scoring and psychometric properties.

2.61.10 Rinke, L.T. & Wilson, A.A. (eds) (1987a) *Outcome Measures in Home Care.* New York: National League for Nursing. ISBN 088737378X Volume 1, Publication No. 21–2194 References

Anthology provides a single reference to the classic and current literature addressing

outcomes in home care. Part 1 includes: basic issues in evaluating the quality of health care; the relationship of nursing process to nursing outcomes; criterion measures of nursing care quality and status of quality assurance in public health nursing. Parts 2–5 include two studies on maternal and child health; using records as a data source; a community-based demonstration project and instrument development.

2.61.11 Rinke, L.T. & Wilson. A.A. (eds) (1987b) *Outcome Measures in Home Care Service.* New York: National League for Nursing. ISBN 0887373798 Volume 2 Publication No. 21–2195 References

Volume covers a sample of both published and unpublished measurement outcome indicators for community-based nursing services. The six parts give an historical overview; examples of promulgated outcome standards; programmatic approaches; medical diagnosis approach; discipline specific indicators and a functional approach.

2.61.12 Ross, F.M. & Bower, P. (1995) Standardized assessment for elderly people (SAFE): a feasibility study in district nursing. *Journal of Clinical Nursing,* 4 (5) 303–10 28 References

Reports on the assessment measures developed by the Royal College of Physicians and the British Geriatric Society. Findings showed that SAFE comprises a practical and acceptable set of instruments, but some further refinement is necessary.

2.61.13 Royal College of Nursing Standards of Care Project. (1990) *Quality Patient Care: the Dynamic Standard System.* London: Royal College of Nursing. ISBN 1870687760 References

Describes a system developed by the Royal College of Nursing which aims to link the process of setting standards to patient outcome (CR 2.43).

2.61.14 Smith, L.N., Booth, N., Douglas, D., Robertson, W.R., Walker, A., Durie, M., Fraser, A., Hillan, E.H. & Swaffield, J. (1995) A critique of 'at risk' pressure sore assessment tools. *Journal of Clinical Nursing,* 4(3) 153–9 40 References

Paper critiques various pressure sore assessment tools. Criteria are suggested for an effective instrument, and reliability and validity studies are reviewed in relation to three tools: Norton, Barlow and Braden. Other issues discussed are threshold scores, research design and the need to view pressure sores as a clinical rather than just a nursing problem (CR 2.12, 2.24, 2.25).

2.61.15 Sparrow, S. & Robinson, J. (1992) The use and limitations of Phaneuf's nursing audit. *Journal of Advanced Nursing*, 17 (12) 1479–88   17 References

Reports use of the Phaneuf audit tool in an action research project involving quality assurance and peer review. Its historical background, development and the tool itself are described. Its reliability and validity are discussed together with its value and limitations (CR 2.37, 2.55).

2.61.16 Stewart, B.J. & Archbold, P.G. (1992) Nursing intervention studies require outcome measures that are sensitive to change: Part 1, *Research in Nursing and Health*, 15 (6) 477–81   15 References

and

2.61.17 Stewart, B.J. & Archbold, P.G. (1993) Nursing intervention studies require outcome measures that are sensitive to change: Part 2, *Research in Nursing and Health*, 16 (1) 77–81   24 References

A two-part article which discusses the importance of sensitivity to change in selecting an outcome measure for a study evaluating a nursing intervention. The relative lack in nursing and management literature is described, together with the conceptual link between intervention and outcome variable, the extent to which it is amenable to change and content validity. Other factors discussed are construct validity, distribution of scores on the outcome measure, reliability and correlational stability over time (CR 2.24, 2.25, 2.55).

2.61.18 Strickland, O.L. & Waltz, C.F. (eds) (1988) *Measurement of Nursing Outcomes. Volume II: Measuring Nursing Performance, Practice Education and Research*. New York: Springer. ISBN 0826152724

A collection of tools focusing on provider-centred outcomes. Some of the major topic areas include measuring professionalism, clinical performance, educational outcomes,

research and measurement and future directions. Measurement protocol for each tool includes: critical review and analysis of the literature; review and analysis of existing tools and procedures for measuring the variable; conceptual basis of the measure; purpose and/or objective of the measure; procedures for construction, revision or future development of the tool; procedures for administration and scoring; and a methodology for testing the reliability and validity of the measure, including the approach to data collection, protection of human subjects and statistical analysis procedures.

2.61.19 Strickland, O.L. & Waltz, C.F. (eds) (1990) *Measurement of Nursing Outcomes. Volume III: Measuring Clinical Skills and Professional Development in Education and Practice*. New York: Springer. ISBN 0826152732 References

Contains tools to measure clinical competence, performance in basic education and practice settings, attitudes and other factors affecting professional development. Each chapter includes detailed discussion of reliability and validity, administering, scoring and analysing results. A review of the literature and analysis of other tools is also included.

2.61.20 Strickland, O.L. & Waltz, C.F. (eds) (1990) *Measurement of Nursing Outcomes. Volume IV: Measuring Client Self-care and Coping Skills*. New York: Springer. ISBN 0826152740   References

Contains tools to measure caring behaviour, self-care ability, insulin management, radiation side-effect profile and parental coping with a chronically ill child. Each chapter includes detailed discussion of reliability and validity, administering, scoring and analysing results. A review of the literature and analysis of other tools are also included (CR 2.12).

2.61.21 Tomalin, D.A., Oliver, S., Redfern, S.J. & Norman, I.J. (1993) Inter-rater reliability of Monitor, Senior Monitor and Qualpacs. *Journal of Advanced Nursing*, 18 (7) 1152–8   16 References

Reports part of a Department of Health-funded study which is examining the reliability and validity of three quality assessment instruments: Monitor, Senior Monitor and Qualpacs. Two methods of analysis were used, percentage agreement and inter-class correlation coefficient. Acceptable levels of inter-rater reliability were reached with all three instruments (CR 2.24, 2.55).

2.61.22 Wainwright, P. (1992) Qualpacs: a practical guide, in Horne, E.M. & Cowan, T. (eds), *Ward Sisters' Survival Guide* 2nd edition. London: Wolfe Publishing. ISBN 0723418071 Chapter 23, 126–31 3 References

Discusses some of the practical problems involved in putting Qualpacs to work on the ward.

2.61.23 Waltz, C.F. & Strickland, O.L. (eds) (1988) *Measurement of Nursing Outcomes. Volume I: Measuring Client Outcomes.* New York: Springer. ISBN 0826152716

The aim of this publication is to disseminate information about the measurement of clinical and educational nursing outcomes. Included are measurement tools, protocols, their reliability and validity, results and conclusions. The instruments applicable to clinical settings are grouped under the following headings: illness-oriented measures, assessing the whole person, measuring wellness, factors in community-based care, quality of care and future directions.

2.61.24 Wandelt, M.A. & Ager, J. (1975) *Quality Patient Care Scale (Qualpacs).* New York: Appleton-Century-Crofts. No ISBN found

Qualpacs is a 68-item observation scale which assesses the quality of nursing care received by patients in any setting. It is sub divided into the following categories: psycho-social, group and individual, physical, general, communications and professional implications. Each category is defined and there is a 20-page cue sheet giving examples of activities. Qualpacs draws heavily from the Slater Nursing Competencies Rating Scale but the focus of measurement is care received by a patient rather than the competencies displayed by a nurse. Information is given about its development, format, application, administration, scoring, interpretation, reliability, validity, uses and some illustrations of its use.

2.61.25 Wandelt, M.A. & Stewart, D.S. (1975) *Slater Nursing Competencies Rating Scale.* New York: Appleton-Century-Crofts. No ISBN found

An 84-item scale intended for use by an observer-rater to assess the competencies displayed by a nurse while caring for a patient. The scale is divided into six categories: psycho-social, individual and group, physical, general, communication and professional implications. Tool is accompanied by a 20-page cue sheet listing examples of activities or behaviour illustrative of each item. Information is given about its development, application, administration, scoring, reliability, validity and uses. Some references illustrating its use are also included.

2.61.26 Ward, M.J. & Fetler, M.E. (1979) *Instruments for Use in Nursing Education Research.* Boulder, CO: Western Interstate Commission for Higher Education. No ISBN found

A major barrier to conducting research is the lack of appropriate data-collecting instruments, so this compilation aims to provide a collection relating specifically to nursing education research. It contains descriptions, critiques and reproductions of 78 instruments; brief descriptions and references to another 40; an annotated bibliography of other published compilations, a glossary; and appendices. Each tool is described with key concepts, title, author, variables measured, nature and content of the instrument, administration and scoring, rationale for development and sources of items. Data on reliability and validity are included together with studies where it has been used, selected comments, references, name and address of a contact person and name of the copyright owner.

2.61.27 Ward, M.J. & Lindeman, C.A. (1979) *Instruments for Measuring Nursing Practice and Other Health Care Variables.* Hyattsville, MD: Department of Health and Welfare. Publication Nos Volume 1 HRA 78-53; Volume 2 HRA 78-54. No ISBN found

Volumes contain descriptions, critiques, and reproductions of 138 psycho-social research instruments; descriptions of 19 instruments which measure physiological parameters; an annotated bibliography of other selected compilations; and a glossary of physiological instrument terms.

2.61.28 Werley, H.H. & Lang, N.M. (eds)

(1988) *Identification of the Nursing Minimum Data Set*. New York: Springer. ISBN 0826153402   References

Book describes the development of the nursing minimum data set. This information is unique to nursing practice and represents essential data. It enables nurses to use computers to assemble comparable nursing data across clinical populations, geographical areas and time through the use of consensually derived categories, variables and uniform definitions. Conceptual considerations, existing information about the data set, perspectives on data requirements across settings, multiple perspectives, effectiveness of nursing care, control of practice standards, quality assessment, health policy, work of the Task Force which generated the data set and future directions are all discussed.

2.62   PHYSIOLOGICAL

Physiological functions can often be measured very precisely by scientific instruments which yield numerical values and so allow a wide range of statistical procedures to be employed in their analysis.

Annotations

2.62.1   Oldham, J. (1995) Biophysiologic measures in nursing practice and research. *Nurse Researcher*, 2 (4) 38–47   8 References

Introduces and examines types of biophysiological measure, the principles involved and criteria for critiquing these tools.

2.62.2   Pagana, K.D. & Pagana, T.J. (1998) *Manual of Diagnostic and Laboratory Tests*. St Louis: Mosby. ISBN 0815155867

Book allows rapid access to clinically relevant laboratory and diagnostic tests. Information given includes: name of test; normal findings; critical values; indications; test explanation; contra-indications; potential complications; interfering factors; procedure and patient care; test results; clinical significance and related tests.

2.62.3   Pugh, L.C. & DeKeyser, F.G. (1995) Use of physiological variables in nursing

research. *Image: Journal of Nursing Scholarship*, 27 (4) 273–6   17 References

The National Institute of Nursing Research emphasizes the need for more physiologically-based nursing research. This study sets out to examine the use of physiological variables as described in research reports published between 1989 and 1993 in four broad-based research journals. Each report was evaluated for the population sampled, type of physiological variable, type of study, definitions and reporting of reliability and validity measures.

2.63
SOCIOLOGICAL/OCCUPATIONAL

Annotations

2.63.1   Beere, C.A. (1979) *Women and Women's Issues: a Handbook of Tests and Measures*. San Francisco: Jossey-Bass. ISBN 0875894186   References

Volume contains 235 instruments obtained from literature published since 1977. They are divided into the following categories: sex roles, stereotypes, role prescriptions, children's sex roles, gender knowledge, marital, parental, employee and multiple roles, attitudes towards women's issues, somatic and sexual issues. Each category constitutes a chapter and included for many of the instruments is the title, author, date, variables, type of instrument, item content, length, group for whom it is intended, sample items, scoring method, theoretical basis, reliability, validity, possible modifications, source and bibliographical information.

2.63.2   Bonjean, C.M., Hill, R.J. & McLemore, S.D. (1967) *Sociological Measurement: an Inventory of Scales and Indices*. San Francisco: Chandler. No ISBN found

Contains bibliographical information for 2,080 sociological scales and indices. Seventy-eight conceptual categories were used to classify the instruments and some of these were authoritarianism, family cohesion and attitudes towards medicine and health. The extent of the discussion varies but generally includes information on its development, use, administration, scoring and the sample used.

2.63.3 Miller, D.C. (1991) *Handbook of Research Design and Social Measurement* 5th edition. Newbury Park, CA: Sage. ISBN 0803942192 References

Contains sociological scales and indices under the general headings of social status, group structure and dynamics, social indicators, measures of organizational structure, evaluation research and organizational effectiveness, community, social participation, leadership in the workplace, morale and job satisfaction, scales of attitudes, norms and values. Descriptive information is given for most scales.

2.63.4 Murray, A., Strauss, M.A. & Brown, B.W. (1978) *Family Measurement Techniques: Abstracts of Published Instruments 1935–1974* Revised edition. Minneapolis: University of Minnesota Press. ISBN 0816607990

Includes abstracts of 813 instruments to measure the properties of the family or the behaviour of people in family roles. Four broad categories are husband/wife relationships, parent/child and sibling to sibling relationships, husband/wife and parent/child variables and sex and pre-marital relationships. Abstract includes author, test name, variables, test description, sample item, length, availability and references. Psychometric properties of the instruments are not included.

2.63.5 Price, J.L. (1986) *Handbook of Organizational Measurement.* London: Harper Business. ISBN 0685104966

Book is structured under 22 organizational concepts some of which are absenteeism, autonomy, centralization, communication, effectiveness, satisfaction and span of control. Each chapter contains a general discussion and definition of the concept, issues pertaining to its measurement and descriptions of relevant instruments. Other information includes a definition, data-collecting information, computation methods, reliability and validity of some instruments, evaluative comments and bibliographical sources.

2.63.6 Raynes, N.V. (1988) *Annotated Directory of Measures of Environmental Quality for Use in Residential Services for People with a Mental Handicap.* Manchester: Department of Social Policy and Social Work, University of Manchester. No ISBN found

Contains summaries of 62 instruments which can be used to evaluate aspects of the environment provided for mentally handicapped people, although some may be of relevance to other client groups. Each instrument is described using a standard format which includes title, authors, date of most recent edition, purpose, content, administration, scientific credibility focusing on standardization, reliability, validity and references. An appendix gives names and addresses of people to contact for further information.

2.63.7 Robinson, J.P., Athanasiou, R. & Head, K.B. (1969) *Measures of Occupational Attitudes and Occupational Characteristics.* Ann Arbor, MI: Institute for Social Research, University of Michigan. No ISBN found

Book cites 77 scales used to measure occupational-related variables. Ten general headings are used including: job attitudes for particular occupations, satisfaction with specific job features, concepts related to job satisfaction, occupational values, leadership styles, other work-related attitudes, vocational interests and occupational status. Information provided for most tests includes variables, description, sample, reliability, validity, source, results and comments. There is a wide variation in details of reliability and validity. Several chapters discuss topics such as status inconsistency, occupational similarity and social mobility. An overview of research and survey of literature related to job attitudes and performance is also included (CR 2.56).

2.63.8 Sawin, K.J., Harrigan, M. & Woog, P. (1994) *Measures of Family Functioning for Research and Practice.* New York: Springer. ISBN 0826176305

Book examines nearly 20 instruments for measuring family functioning. Information on each includes: a history of the instrument; an overview of the model and its conceptual framework; a description of the tool; information on scoring, reliability and validity; sample items; a description of its sensitivity to cross-cultural issues, gender and variant family structures. Also included are a summary of studies using the instrument and information on where it may be obtained.

DATA COLLECTION

2.64 DATA COLLECTION – GENERAL

Data collection refers to ways in which information can be obtained from the real world, recorded in a systematic way and quantified. There are many data collection techniques and sections 2.65 to 2.78 will guide the reader towards appropriate sources.

High-quality data will increase the value of research. Choices therefore need to be made in terms of the degree of structure which is possible or desirable, whether or how the data can be quantified, the obtrusiveness of the researcher which may lead to ethical problems, and how objective or subjective the data are, or need to be.

Definitions

Data – pieces of information obtained in the course of a study
Data collection – the gathering of information needed to address a research problem
Data set – a collection of related items
Database – a collection of data organized for rapid research and retrieval, usually by a computer; often a consolidation of many records previously stored separately
Primary source – a source of original data, such as documents, memorabilia or first-hand accounts
Secondary source – a source of data that consists of summarization of, or commentary about, primary data, such as writings or a life experience, by someone other than the person who produced the data or lived through the experience

---

Annotations

2.64.1 Ackroyd, S. & Hughes, J. (1992) *Data Collection in Context* 2nd edition. London: Longman. ISBN 0582053110 References

Book, which has been extensively revised and updated, covers many aspects of data collection.

2.64.2 Billings, J.R. (1996) Investigating the process of community profile compilation. *NT Research*, 1 (4) 270–83   82 References

Paper presents the methodological approach and findings of one facet of a larger study which had a health-visiting focus. It was concerned with examining the value of the community profile approach in needs assessment and contracting for family health care in one general practitioner fund-holding practice. The data collection processes are critically reviewed, including their identification, accessibility, practical use, reliability and validity (CR 2.24, 2.25).

2.64.3 Bostrom, J., Dibble, S. & Rizzuto, C. (1991) Data collection as an educational process. *Journal of Continuing Education in Nursing*, 22 (6) 248–53   7 References

Study describes the personal and professional characteristics of nurses who choose to work as data collectors. Their experience, perceptions of nursing research, the research environment and their plans for involvement are described. The implications of using this experience for educational purposes are outlined (CR 2.16, 3.16, 3.17).

2.64.4 Davis, L.L. (1992) Instrument review: getting the most from a panel of experts. *Applied Nursing Research*, 5 (4) 197–201 4 References

Discusses the use of a panel of experts for reviewing data collection instruments. Criteria for selecting experts and steps which may be taken in instrument review are suggested (CR 2.55).

2.64.5 Economic and Social Research Council. (1996) Qualitative data archival resource centre (QUALIDATA). *Sociological Research Online.*
URL: http://www.socresonline.org.uk/socresonline/1/3/qualidata.html#top

Describes the QUALIDATA Resource Centre located in the Department of Sociology at the University of Essex. Its aims are: locating, assessing and documenting qualitative data and arranging for their deposit in suitable public archives; disseminating information about these data; and raising archival consciousness among the social science research community. The QUALIDATA database is available on the Internet.
URL: http://www.essex.ac.uk/qualidata

2.64.6 Estabrooks, C.A. & Romyn, D.M. (1995) Data sharing in nursing research. advantages and challenges. *Canadian Journal of Nursing Research,* 27 (1) 77–88   35 References

Authors believe that research data should be shared and they address some of the issues which would be involved. Nurse researchers should seek to have data from all publicly funded projects in accessible repositories.

2.64.7 Freshwater, D. (1996) Complementary therapies and research in nursing practice. *Nursing Standard,* 12 (2) 73–84   24 References

Highlights research issues relating to complementary therapies and makes suggestions for collecting quantifiable data.

2.64.8 Hoffart, N. (1991) A member check procedure to enhance rigour in naturalistic research. *Western Journal of Nursing Research,* 13 (4) 522–34   19 References

Describes a study of joint appointments in nursing in which member checks were made to enhance rigour and the quality of data collected (CR 2.16, 2.36).

2.64 .9 Mallett, J. (1996) Sense of direction ... user's perspective, research methods. *Nursing Times,* 30 October–5 November, 92 (44) 40–2   3 References

Reports on research methods used to ascertain what patients want when receiving care.

2.64.10 Rodgers, B.L. & Cowells, K.V. (1993) The qualitative research audit trail: a complex collection of documentation. *Research in Nursing and Health,* 16 (3) 219–26   16 References

The types of data that contribute to credible investigations are discussed, together with strategies for maintaining records in qualitative studies (CR 2.36).

2.64.11 Sapsford, R. & Jupp, V. (eds) (1996) *Data Collection and Analysis.* London: Sage. ISBN 076195046X   References

Text covers both quantitative and qualitative approaches to data collection and analysis in social research. A wide range of academic and applied research studies illustrate the text and exercises are included to aid understanding (CR 2.79).

2.64.12 Sieber, J.E. (ed.) (1991) *Sharing Social Science Data: Advantages and Challenges.* Newbury Park, CA: Sage. ISBN 0803940831   References

Book highlights the advantages of data-sharing in the social sciences. The reasons for sharing practices in various disciplines, factors affecting the value of these data and concerns which may arise are discussed (CR 3.23).

2.64.13 Thomas, S.P. (1992) Storage of data: why, how, where? *Nursing Research,* 41 (5) 309–11   16 References

Reports a study which surveyed active biomedical and behavioural researchers to discover if institutions had policies on the storage of data. Questions asked were how long and where it was kept, the form of storage, and whether graduates were required to leave a file copy of their data upon graduation. Results of the study are reported and recommendations made (CR 2.17).

2.64.14 Thomas, S.P. (1993) Issues in data management and storage. *Journal of Neuroscience Nursing,* 25 (4) 243–5   7 References

Discusses use, storage and management of data to ensure that fabrication or alteration does not occur as scientific misconduct has been highlighted in several prestigious American institutions. The confidentiality of data is stressed. Guidelines are included and the value of a proposed national repository for data discussed (CR 2.17, 2.79).

METHODS OF DATA COLLECTION

2.65   CRITICAL INCIDENT TECHNIQUE

The critical incident technique employs a set of principles for collecting data on observable human activities. It provides a flexible way of examining interpersonal communication skills and has been used in many nursing studies, especially in the USA. Incidents are of particular value because it is reality which is being described rather than hypothetical situations.

Definitions

Critical incident – an observable type of human activity which is sufficiently complete in itself to permit inferences and predictions to be made about the person performing the act. To be critical it must be performed in a situation where the purpose or intent of the act seems fairly clear to the observer, and its consequences are sufficiently definite so there is little doubt concerning its effects
Critical incident technique – a set of procedures for collecting direct observations of human behaviour which have special significance and meet systematically defined criteria.

Example

Minghella, E. & Benson, A. (1995) Developing reflective practice in mental health nursing through critical incident analysis. *Journal of Advanced Nursing*, 21 (2) 205–13 31 References

Reports a study which evaluated the use of critical incident analysis as a teaching and learning strategy in a Project 2000 mental health nursing curriculum.

Original articles

Flanagan, J.C. (1947) *The Aviation Psychology Programme in the Army Air Forces. AAF Psychology Programme Research Report No. 1*. Washington, DC: Government Printing Office

Flanagan, J.C. (1954) The critical incident technique. *Psychological Bulletin*, 51 (4) 327–58   74 References

Annotations

2.65.1   Bermosk, L.S. & Corsini, R.J. (1973) *Critical Incidents in Nursing*. Philadelphia: W.B. Saunders. ISBN 0721616968

Book concentrates on 38 controversial issues documented in the form of critical incidents under the headings of: nurse and the patient, peers, doctors, the family, supervision and the system. The background to each incident is described. Opinions, reactions and some suggestions for resolution from experienced nurses who examined them, is described. The complex world in which nurses work, is portrayed.

2.65.2   Clamp, C.G.L. (1984) *Learning through Incidents: Studies in the Development and Use of Critical Incidents in the Teaching of Attitudes in Nursing*. M.Phil Thesis (unpublished). University of London, Institute of Education

Study aimed to develop a teaching method which could increase attitude awareness and develop interpersonal communication skills in nursing education. Critical incidents were used as triggers for in-depth discussions on the behaviour, attitudes and feelings reported by nurses. Many aspects of learning and areas of personal growth were highlighted.

2.65.3   Cormack, D.F.S. (ed.) (1996) The critical incident technique, in Author, *The Research Process in Nursing* 3rd edition. Oxford: Blackwell Science. ISBN 063204019X Chapter 24, 266–74   References

Describes the origins and applications of critical incidents in nursing (CR 2.1.18).

2.65.4   Cortazzi, D. & Roote, S. (1975) *Illuminative Incident Analysis*. London: McGraw-Hill. ISBN 0070844526

Using critical incidents as the focal point, authors describe the process of learning through illuminative incident analysis. The aim of the book is to encourage constructive team development by drawing on the incident, rather than discussing it. This method has been shown to develop understanding of attitudes, role perceptions and motivation. Solutions emerge which can become a 'health care plan' for the team.

2.65.5 Crouch, S. (1991) Critical incident analysis. *Nursing*, 27 June–10 July, 4 (37) 30–1 13 References

Outlines the use of the critical incident technique as a method of learning in an Enrolled Nurse conversion course.

2.65.6 Dunn, W.R. & Hamilton, D.D. (1986) The critical incident technique: a brief guide. *Medical Teacher*, 8 (3) 207–15 26 References

Authors maintain that the technique has stood the test of time as a means of identifying those activities essential to good practice in a profession, and as a tool to delineate the competencies needed by those members. Article reviews the technique and addresses the questions, what is the technique and when can it be applied in medical education?

2.65.7 Flanagan, J.C. (1954) The critical incident technique. *Psychological Bulletin*, 51 (4) 327–58 74 References

Article describes the development of critical incident methodology, its fundamental principles and status. Studies using this technique are reviewed and possible future use is identified.

2.65.8 Hayes, D.M., Fleury, R.A. & Jackson, T.B. (1979) Curriculum content from critical incidents. *Medical Education*, 13 (3) 175–82 6 References

Describes a study designed to create a medical school curriculum which would meet the needs of students, teachers and the community. Data were collected using the critical incident technique and ten major areas of behaviour identified. These areas of clinical activity were then sub-divided and subsequently formed the basis for the curriculum.

2.65.9 Norman, I.J., Redfern, S.J., Tomalin, D.A. & Oliver, S. (1992) Developing Flanagan's critical incident technique to elicit indicators of high and low quality nursing care from patients and their nurses. *Journal of Advanced Nursing*, 17 (5) 590–600 21 References

Discusses many aspects of using this technique in a study which examined care as seen by patients and nurses on medical, surgical and elderly care wards. Procedural stages are described, presuppositions held by most researchers who use this technique identified, and comments are made on its value as a method of data collection in nursing research.

2.65.10 Rich, A. & Parker, D.L. (1995) Reflection and critical incident analysis: ethical and moral implications of their use within nursing and midwifery. *Journal of Advanced Nursing*, 22 (6) 1050–7 52 References

Article suggests that reflection and critical incident analysis may be tools which can facilitate the integration of theory and practice (CR 2.17).

2.65.11 Rimon, D. (1979) Nurses' perception of their psychological role in treating rehabilitation patients: a study employing the critical incident technique. *Journal of Advanced Nursing*, 4 (4) 403–13 14 References

Study reports on the psychological role of nurses whose perceptions were explored using the critical incident technique. From these, the aims and objectives of psychological care were generated and found to support the limited available literature.

2.66 DELPHI TECHNIQUE

'The Delphi concept may be seen as a spin-off from defence research. Project Delphi was the name given to an Air Force-sponsored, Rand Corporation study in the early 1950s, concerning the use of expert opinion. The aim of this study was to select an optimal American industrial target system, and estimate the number of atom bombs required to reduce the munitions output by a prescribed amount. The study set out to obtain the most reliable consensus of opinion from a group of experts ... by a series of intensive questionnaires interspersed with controlled opinion feedback' (Linstone & Turoff, 1975: 10).

[Apollo became master of Delphi upon slaying the dragon Pythos, and he was renowned not only for his youth and perfect beauty but even more for his ability to see the future.]

Definitions

Consensus methods – provide a means of synthesizing information ... [using] a wider range of [material] than is common in statistical methods, and when published information is inadequate or non-existent

Delphi technique – ... a method for obtaining expert opinion on a topic ... it employs multiple rounds or waves of questionnaires, with each round utilizing information gathered during previous rounds, in an attempt to converge towards group consensus

Example

Sleep, J., Bullock, I. & Grayson, K. (1995) Establishing priorities for research in education within one college of nursing and midwifery. *Nurse Education Today*, 15 (6) 439–45 26 References

Reports a four-round Delphi survey used to develop an agenda for research priorities (CR 3.20).

Major text

Linstone, H.A. & Turoff, M. (eds) (1975) *The Delphi Method: Techniques and Applications.* Reading, MA: Addison-Wesley. ISBN 0201042940 References

Annotations

2.66.1 Beretta, R. (1996) A critical review of the Delphi technique. *Nurse Researcher*, 3 (4) 79–89 18 References

Reviews ways in which this technique has been used in the health service. Ways of using it, some advantages and disadvantages and ethical issues are all discussed (CR 2.17).

2.66.2 Chiou, S. & Tsai, S. (1996) Delphi technique: a nursing research method for expert's forecasting options [Chinese],

Nursing Research (China), 4 (1) 92–8 13 References

Describes the Delphi technique and makes suggestions about its use in China where, to date, it has been under-used.

2.66.3 Duffield, C. (1993) The Delphi technique: a comparison of results obtained using two expert panels. *International Journal of Nursing Studies*, 30 (3) 227–37 20 References

Describes a study in which two panels of experts involved in management or management education were asked to identify the competencies expected of first-line managers. Author believes the technique is worth considering for studying a wide range of topics on which consensus is required.

2.66.4 Jones, J. & Hunter, D. (1995) Nominal group technique (expert panel): consensus methods for medical and health services research. *British Medical Journal*, 5 August, 311 (7001) 376–80 46 References

Defines consensus and consensus methods, their application and methodological issues.

2.66.5 Linstone, H.A. & Turoff, M. (eds) (1975) *The Delphi Method: Techniques and Applications.* Reading, MA: Addison-Wesley. ISBN 0201042940 References

A major text covering the Delphi technique and its applications. It has been used in technological forecasting and in many other contexts. These include normative forecasts, the ascertainment of values and preferences, estimates concerning the quality of life, simulated and real decision-making and planning. Despite many uses, this technique lacks a completely sound theoretical basis. Book includes philosophy, general applications, evaluation, cross-impact analysis, specialized techniques, computers and the future of Delphi, a checklist of pitfalls and an extensive bibliography.

2.66.6 McKenna, H.P. (1994) The Delphi technique: a worthwhile research approach for nursing? *Journal of Advanced Nursing*, 19 (6) 1221–5 33 References

Provides an overview of what the Delphi technique is, criteria for selecting it as a research approach, studies where it has been used and its advantages and disadvantages.

2.66.7 Rudy, S.F. (1996) Research forum. A review of Delphi surveys conducted to establish research priorities by specialty nursing organizations from 1985 to 1995. *ORL – Head and Neck Nursing*, 14 (2) 16–24 26 References

Paper reviews various Delphi methods employed by specialty nursing organizations. The Delphi technique is introduced, described and methodological and practical aspects of conducting studies are discussed. Information is given on cost and the time required. Research priorities are not identified in order not to prejudice an ongoing study.

2.66.8 Walker, A.M. & Selfe, J. (1996) The Delphi method: a useful tool for the allied health researcher. *British Journal of Therapy and Rehabilitation*, 3 (12) 677–81 40 References

Provides a critical review of the Delphi technique, gives examples of its use and suggests other potential applications.

2.66.9 Williams, P.L. & Webb, C. (1994) The Delphi technique: a methodological discussion. *Journal of Advanced Nursing*, 19 (1) 180–6 23 References

The technique is outlined and applications, strengths, limitations, the meaning of consensus, panel selection and size are explored. A study which investigated the activities of supervising radiographers in support of the undergraduate curriculum is used for illustration, together with other nursing studies which used this technique.

2.67 DIARIES

Diaries can provide information which it is not possible to obtain in any other way. However skilful the questionnaire or interview schedule, inevitably the researcher imposes some structure. A diary may also be structured to a certain extent in that people can be asked to record particular things, but additional insights may be gained.

Definition

Diaries – a source of data which can provide an intimate descriptive comment on everyday life for an individual

Example

O'Brien, B., Relyea, J. & Lidstone, T. (1997) Diary reports of nausea and vomiting during pregnancy. *Clinical Nursing Research*, 6 (3) 239–52 21 References

As part of a larger study, participants who experienced nausea with or without vomiting/retching during pregnancy kept a diary recording activities and situations which exacerbated their symptoms. Data were categorized using content analysis. Results are reported and implications for nursing practice discussed (CR 2.88).

Annotations

2.67.1 Breakwell, G.M. & Wood, P. (1995) Diary techniques, in Breakwell, G.M., Hammond, S. & Fife-Schaw, C. (eds), *Research Methods in Psychology*. London: Sage. ISBN 0803977654 Part III, Chapter 19, 293–301 References

Chapter identifies the nature of diary techniques, the pros and cons of this approach, getting the best out of them and analysing diary data (CR 2.1.8).

2.67.2 Burman, M.E. (1995) Health diaries in nursing research and practice. *Image: Journal of Nursing Scholarship*, 27 (2) 147–52 46 References

Describes current uses of health diaries in nursing research and practice. Types of health diary, factors affecting the quality of data, the costs and analytic issues are all discussed. The implications for nursing research and practice are considered.

2.67.3 Elliott, H. (1997) The use of diaries in sociological research on health experience. *Sociological Research Online* 2 (2) URL: http://www.socresonline.org.uk/socresonline/2/2/7.html 34 References

Highlights the value of doing diary research, drawing on the literature of autobiographies and health service research, together with a qualitative study of need and demand for primary health care (CR 2.36, 2.71).

2.67.4 Gibson, V. (1995) An analysis of the use of diaries as a data collection method. *Nurse Researcher*, 3 (1) 66–73 18 References

Provides an overview of the diary as a data collection method and discusses its strengths and weaknesses (CR 2.86).

2.67.5   Malinowski, B. (1982) The diary of an anthropologist, in Burgess, R.G. (ed.), *Field Research: a Sourcebook and Field Manual*. London: Allen & Unwin. ISBN 004312013X Chapter 27, 200–5   References

An actual diary extract is reproduced.

2.67.6   Oleske, D.M., Heinze, S. & Otte, D.M. (1990) The diary as a means of understanding the quality of life of persons with cancer receiving home nursing care. *Cancer Nursing*, 13 (3) 158–66

Reports a study which discusses the rationale for using diaries as a data collection method with an ill population. Results are reported and the advantages of using diaries is discussed.

2.67.7   Phillips, R. & Davies, R. (1995) Using diaries in qualitative research. *British Journal of Midwifery*, 3 (9) 473–6, 493 15 References

Discusses the types and format of diaries together with key considerations in their use.

2.67.8   Richardson, A. (1994) The health diary: an examination of its use as a data collection method. *Journal of Advanced Nursing*, 19 (4) 782–91   53 References

Discusses the advantages and disadvantages associated with use of diaries as a data collection instrument in health care settings. Completion of the diary, respondent co-operation, format and issues surrounding analysis are all considered.

2.67.9   Ruffing-Rahal, M.A. (1986) Personal documents and nursing theory development. *Advances in Nursing Science*, 8 (3) 50–7 36 References

Discusses the use of personal documents as a means of providing insights into the nature of health and experiences of illness. Triangulated research strategies are advocated in order to incorporate these experiences into nursing research (CR 2.7, 2.26).

2.67.10   Tothill, C. (1992) Diary of a carer. *Nursing Times*, 18 November, 88 (47) 34–6 No references

Article gives extracts from a diary kept by a carer whose husband suffered with dementia. This identified her needs and enabled nurses to help more appropriately.

2.67.11   Verbrugge, L. (1980) Health diaries. *Medical Care*, 18 (1) 73–95   52 References

A review and methodological discussion of studies which used health diaries. Evidence is given on the following aspects: levels of reporting compared to retrospective interview; recall error; validity of health reports; value of diary data for a broad view of symptoms; and health behaviour. Also considered are individual-level analysis, studies of health dynamics, respondent co-operation, conditioning effects, quality of diary data, survey costs, complexity of data collection, processing and analysis (CR 2.25, 2.68).

2.67.12   Woods, N.F. (1981) The health diary as an instrument for nursing research: problems and promise. *Western Journal of Nursing Research*, 3 (1) 76–92   16 References

Discusses the use of a health diary as a means of obtaining valid data about symptoms. Its advantages and disadvantages are discussed together with reliability, validity and its purpose. Paper is illustrated by a study where 96 women completed a diary for three weeks. Results were weakly correlated with the Cornell Medical Index Health questionnaire, but the author believes the method should be further explored in nursing research (CR 2.24, 2.25).

2.67.13   Wykle, M.L. & Morris, D.L. (1988) The health diary. *Applied Nursing Research*, 1 (1) 47–8   3 References

Outlines the advantages and disadvantages of this technique and illustrates it with a study which aimed to identify the self-care practices of community-dwelling elders.

2.67.14   Zimmerman, D.H. & Wieder, D.L. (1977) The diary-interview method. *Urban Life*, 5 (4) 479–99   42 References

Describes a study of the counter-culture, i.e. freedom from a conventional schedule of activities, where participants were asked to record all their activities over one week in diary form and were subsequently interviewed in depth. The value of keeping diaries is discussed but authors believe that they need to be used in conjunction with interviews based around their content. This method is an adjunct to, or approximation of, the process of direct observation which is central to the ethnographic research tradition (CR 2.42, 2.68, 2.72).

2.68 INTERVIEW

'Research interviews require a very systematic approach to data collection which maximizes the chances of maintaining objectivity and achieving valid and reliable results. . . . Although biases may be introduced by the researcher and interviewee . . . it is a virtually infinitely flexible tool.' (Breakwell, Hammond & Fife-Schaw, 1995: 230–1) [adapted]

Definitions

Depth interview – an unstructured interview in which the aim is to probe deeply and obtain an exhaustive account of the subject's views and experiences
Exploratory interview – unstructured interview, intended to develop ideas and hypotheses, and to explore possible ways of gathering data
Interview – a data collection method employing a verbal questioning technique
Interview schedule – a set of questions with guided instructions for an interviewer to use in carrying out an interview
Pilot interview – mainly intended as an aid to the design of later research
Semi-structured interview – partly standardized but also allows the interviewer greater flexibility at the expense of possibly incurring greater bias
Standardized/structured interview – involves each subject being asked the same questions in exactly the same order
Transcript – the written form of a tape recording of an interview

Example

Dewar, A.L. & Morse, J.M. (1995) Unbearable incidents: failure to endure the experience of illness. *Journal of Advanced Nursing*, 22 (5) 957–64   21 References

Describes a study which aimed to identify the various physical and psychological assaults which may occur during illness, and which led patients to experience a breakdown of endurance. Authors suggest that this may be a useful phenomenon leading to adjustment in care plans.

Annotations

2.68.1 Baker, C. (1997) Membership categorization and interview accounts, in Silverman, D. (ed.), *Qualitative Research: Theory, Method and Practice*. London: Sage. ISBN 0803976666 Part IV, Chapter 9, 130–43 10 References

Chapter shows how interview data may be analysed in terms of categories that participants use and how these are attached to particular kinds of activity (CR 2.36.59).

2.68.2 Barriball, K.L. & While, A. (1994) Collecting data using a semi-structured interview: a discussion paper. *Journal of Advanced Nursing*, 19 (2) 328–35   36 References

Discusses some of the measures used to overcome threats to validity and reliability of a semi-structured interview exploring the perceptions and needs of continuing education among nurses in two health authorities (CR 2.24, 2.25).

2.68.3 Booth, T. & Booth, W. (1994) The use of depth interviewing with vulnerable subjects: lessons from a research study of parents with learning difficulties. *Social Science and Medicine*, 39 (3) 415–24 45 References

Paper explores the practicalities of using the techniques of depth interviewing to give people with learning difficulties a voice in the making of their own history (CR 2.71).

2.68.4 Bowler, I. (1997) Problems with interviewing: experiences with service providers and clients, in Miller, G. & Dingwall, R. (eds), *Context and Method in Qualitative Research*. London: Sage. ISBN 0803976321 Part II, Chapter 5, 66–76   References

Chapter describes a failure to obtain consent for formal field interviews as part of an ethnographic study of inequalities in health in Britain. The study focused on women of South Asian descent (mainly Pakistani) in a

British city and their experience of maternity services. Author suggests that interviewing may be a problematic method for obtaining the views of some groups, since it is a co-operative activity and relies upon a shared notion of the process of research (CR 2.17, 2.36.40, 2.42, 2.72).

2.68.5 Bray, J., Powell, J., Lovelock, R. & Philp, I. (1995) Using a softer approach: techniques for interviewing older people. *Professional Nurse*, 10 (6) 350–3   13 References

Article explores some of the issues and challenges involved in obtaining the views of older people on service quality and examines approaches to such research.

2.68.6 Britten, N. (1995) Qualitative interviews in medical research. *British Medical Journal*, 22 July, 311 (6999) 251–3   11 References

Discusses types of qualitative interview, how they may be conducted, researcher as research instrument, and recording and identifying interviewees (CR 2.22).

2.68.7 Buckeldee, J. (1994) Interviewing carers in their own homes, in Buckeldee, J. & McMahon, R. (eds), *The Research Experience in Nursing*. London: Chapman & Hall. ISBN 0412441101 Chapter 7, 101–13   17 References

Author discusses personal experiences when conducting unstructured interviews with carers in their own homes. She states that most research texts do not address the challenges and difficulties which may arise (CR 2.16.4).

2.68.8 Chapple, A. (1997/98) Personal recollections on interviewing GPs and consultants. *Nurse Researcher*, 5 (2) 82–90   17 References

Author discusses the problems associated with interviewing elite groups, gaining access, practical arrangements, conducting the interview, writing reports and giving feedback (CR 2.16, 2.36, 2.97).

2.68.9 Dunne, S. (1995) *Interviewing Techniques for Writers and Researchers*. London: A&C. Black ISBN 0713641924 References

Book covers methods and types of interview,

tools, finding subjects, preparing for and conducting the interview, transcribing and writing up the findings (CR 2.22).

2.68.10 Dzurec, L.C. & Coleman, P. (1997) A hermeneutic analysis of the process of conducting clinical interviews: 'what happens after you say hello?' *Journal of Psychosocial Nursing and Mental Health Services*, 35 (8) 31–6, 42–3   16 References

Although no right way to interview exists, author suggest that interviewers should develop a comfortable, personal style. Allowing an interview to take its own course, while remembering the overall agenda, will contribute to the quality of the data (CR 2.5).

2.68.11 Fielding, N. (1993) Qualitative interviewing, in Gilbert, N. (ed.), *Researching Social Life*. London: Sage. ISBN 0803986823 Chapter 8, 135–53   References

Chapter examines varieties of research interviews, communication in interviews, how to design an interview guide, interviewer effects, transcription and some problems of interview analysis (CR 2.1.25).

2.68.12 Fielding, N. (1994) Varieties of research interviews. *Nurse Researcher*, 1 (3) 4–13   9 References

Discusses different types of interview, their advantages and their limitations. Some problems of data analysis are also examined (CR 2.77).

2.68.13 Foddy, W. (1993) *Constructing Questions for Interviews and Questionnaires: Theory and Practice in Social Research*. Cambridge: Cambridge University Press. ISBN 0521467330   References

Book integrates the empirical findings on question design reported in the literature. The theoretical framework that is used leads to a set of principles that increases the validity and reliability of verbal data collected for research (CR 2.24, 2.25, 2.75).

2.68.14 Gordon, N. (1997/98) Critical reflection on the dynamics and processes of qualitative interviews. *Nurse Researcher*, 5 (2) 72–80   31 References

Paper focuses on the importance of methodological innovation when designing and implementing research which attempts to access lived experience. Three-stage serial interviewing, techniques, in-depth interviewing and psychotherapy are all discussed.

2.68.15 Gray, M. (1994) Personal experience of conducting unstructured interviews. *Nurse Researcher*, 1 (3) 65–71   5 References

Discusses some of the realities and practicalities of undertaking interviews (CR 2.16, 2.45).

2.68.16 Holstein, J.A. & Gubrium, J.F. (1995) *The Active Interview*. Thousand Oaks, CA: Sage. ISBN 0803958943   References

Examines the interview process and products. Authors believe that interviews are social productions with respondents best seen as narrators or story-tellers. Working together, interviewing is a collaboration but may be problematic.

2.68.17 Hutchinson, S. & Wilson, H.S. (1992) Validity threats in scheduled semi-structured research interviews. *Nursing Research*, 41 (2) 117–19   10 References

Discusses some problems in interviewing which may affect validity of the data. These are interview questions, timing, interviewer behaviour, problematic respondent behaviours and recording problems. Suggestions are made to minimize these effects (CR 2.25).

2.68.18 Kvale, S. (1996) *Interviews: an Introduction to Qualitative Research Interviewing*. Thousand Oaks, CA: Sage. ISBN 080395820X

Provides theoretical underpinnings and practical aspects of the interviewing process (CR 2.36).

2.68.19 Maple, F.F. (1998) *Goal Focused Interviewing*. Thousand Oaks, CA: Sage. ISBN 0761901809

Book presents Maple's model for categorizing information elicited from clients. Techniques for focusing on the competencies of clients rather than their deficiencies are discussed (CR 2.86).

2.68.20 Marshall, S.L. & While, A.E. (1994) Interviewing respondents who have English as a second language: challenges encountered and suggestions for other researchers. *Journal of Advanced Nursing*, 19 (3) 566–71   37 References

Outlines some challenges encountered in one study where respondents had English as a second language. Some strategies are suggested to ensure that respondents from ethnic minorities are included in research studies, and that the needs of both researcher and researched are met.

2.68.21 McCracken, G. (1988) *The Long Interview*. Newbury Park, CA: Sage. ISBN 0803933533   References

Provides a systematic guide to the theory and method of the long, qualitative interview. Key theoretical and methodological issues are identified. Research strategies and a simple four-step model of inquiry are described. Its value as a tool in scientific studies is outlined.

2.68.22 Miller, J. & Glassner, B. (1997) The 'inside' and the 'outside': finding realities in interviews, in Silverman, D. (ed.), *Qualitative Research: Theory, Method and Practice*. London: Sage. ISBN 0803976666 Part IV, Chapter 7, 99–112   26 References

Chapter addresses the issue of finding 'reality' in interview accounts. Authors believe that these accounts can be treated as situated elements in social worlds, drawing upon, revising and re-framing the cultural stories in those worlds (CR 2.36.59, 2.86).

2.68.23 Mishler, E.G. (1991) *Research Interviewing: Context and Narrative*. Cambridge, MA: Harvard University Press. ISBN 0674764617   References

Examines current views and practices of interviewing and concludes that they reflect a restricted conception of the interview process. Author makes the proposition that an interview is a form of discourse which is shaped and organized by asking and answering questions. He advocates using a family of methods as a framework for developing an alternative.

2.68.24 Mitchell, T.L. & Radford, J.L. (1996) Rethinking research relationships in qualitative research. *Canadian Journal of Community Mental Health*, 15 (1) 49–60   30 References

Re-examines the relationship between researcher and the research participant which takes place in qualitative studies. Using their own experience of working with high-risk individuals and vulnerable communities, authors discuss the interview process. They advocate social research protocols, expansion of the researchers' role, and patient advocacy (CR 2.16, 2.17, 2.36, 3.16).

2.68.25 Newell, R. (1994a) *Interviewing Skills for Nurses and Other Health Care Professionals: a Structured Approach.* London: Routledge. ISBN 041407794X References

This book, designed for students and qualified nurses, takes the reader through a series of interviews with a variety of clients in different settings. The emphasis is on gaining practical skills and readers are encouraged to adapt techniques to their own area of practice.

2.68.26 Newell, R. (1994b) The structured interview. *Nurse Researcher*, 1 (3) 14–22 4 References

Discusses the advantages and disadvantages of structured interviews, and the nature and development of interview schedules and techniques.

2.68.27 Phillips, R. & Davies, R.M. (1995) Using interviews in qualitative research. *British Journal of Midwifery*, 3 (12) 647–52 21 References

Article describes the variations of interview structure which may be used in qualitative research. Ethical issues are also discussed (CR 2.17, 2.36).

2.68.28 Platzer, H. & James, T. (1997) Methodological issues: conducting sensitive research on lesbian and gay men's experience of nursing care. *Journal of Advanced Nursing*, 25 (3) 626–33 32 References

Discusses the pros and cons of 'insider status' which can affect a study where sensitive information is sought. Methodological and ethical issues are discussed in relation to this particular study (CR 2.16, 2.17, 2.36).

2.68.29 Rose, K. (1994) Unstructured and semi-structured interviewing. *Nurse Researcher*, 1 (3) 23–32   10 References

Defines unstructured and semi-structured interviews and discusses when they may be appropriate. Planning and using them, and problems which can arise, are outlined.

2.68.30 Saris, W.E. (1991) *Computer-assisted Interviewing.* Newbury Park, CA: Sage. ISBN 0803940661   References

Book aims to help researchers improve the quality of their data. The possibilities and difficulties of computer-assisted interviewing are identified. Examples are annotated so that comparisons can be made with paper questionnaires. An overview is given of the important features to consider when purchasing a CADAC programme. Appendix lists computer programmes (CR 2.75, 2.84).

2.68.31 Smith, L. (1992) Ethical issues in interviewing. *Journal of Advanced Nursing*, 17 (1) 98–103   9 References

Article discusses unforeseen points which emerged during a study of help-seeking behaviour of alcohol-dependent and problem-drinking women. Areas highlighted are ethical dimensions of interviewing, prior considerations, revealing the research location, using interview data, the interviewer's role, publication of results and personal safety of interviewers (CR 2.16, 2.17, 2.99, 3.16).

2.68.32 Sohier, R. (1995) The dyadic interview as a tool for nursing research. *Applied Nursing Research*, 8 (2) 96–101   20 References

Reports the use of dyadic interviewing (interviews carried out with two people at a time) as a strategy for maintaining objectivity in qualitative interviews. This method may achieve criteria relating to evidence, credibility of data and ethical aspects of research. Their advantages, disadvantages and conflicts are all discussed (CR 2.36).

2.68.33 Sorrell, J.M. & Redmond, G.M. (1995) Interviews in qualitative nursing research: differing approaches for ethnographic and phenomenological studies. *Journal of Advanced Nursing*, 21 (6) 1117–22 17 References

Paper offers an overview of use of the researcher as an instrument in qualitative research. Also discussed are ways in which the differing purposes and styles of ethnographic and phenomenological approaches affect the format of an interview (CR 2.42, 2.49).

2.68.34 Spradley, J.P. (1979) *The Ethnographic Interview.* New York: Holt, Rinehart & Winston. ISBN 0030444969   References

This book, together with its companion

volume, *Participant Observation*, aims to provide a systematic handbook for doing ethnography and develops techniques initially used mainly by anthropologists. Ethnographic research is set in context and a series of steps, designed to develop skills in this type of interviewing, is discussed. The text is illustrated by many examples from the author's own and others' research (CR 2.42, 2.72.17).

2.68.35 Steeves, R.H. (1992) A typology of data collected in naturalistic interviews. *Western Journal of Nursing Research*, 14 (4) 532–6   9 References

Discusses three types of data generated in interviews – lexical maps, narratives and explanations which enable researchers to determine exactly what is present in the data. This is particularly important when these are being analysed (CR 2.71, 2.78).

2.68.36 Wibberley, C. & Kenny, C. (1994) The case for interactive interviewing. *Nurse Researcher*, 1 (3) 57–64   22 References

Examines the nature of interaction within data collection by interview and discusses why using this enhances the richness of the data.

2.68.37 Wiles, R. (1996) Quality questions: ... an alternative approach to discovering patients' views. *Nursing Times*, 30 October–5 November, 92 (44) 38–40   No References

Author believes that although questionnaires are the most commonly used method of data collection, other qualitative methods, such as focus groups and in-depth interviews, may be the best way of eliciting information about services (CR 2.69).

2.69 INTERVIEW – FOCUS GROUP

'Since 1988 there has been an exponential rise in the number of studies employing focus group methodology.... While its historical roots are in sociology ... its methodological evolution is attributable to market researchers ... providing a 'quick and dirty' means of fulfilling client needs, rather than as a sophisticated research tool.... Focus groups can enhance the ability of researchers

to answer specific questions but need to be rigorously conducted.' (Breakwell, Hammond & Fife-Schaw, 1995: 275–6) [adapted]

Definition

Focus group – a small group of individuals drawn together to express views on a specific set of questions in a group environment

Example

Land, L.M. (1994) The student nurse selection experience: a qualitative study. *Journal of Advanced Nursing*, 20 (6) 1030–7   34 References

Study explored the experience of student nurses recruited to three British colleges of nursing through the use of focus groups. Author believes that selection procedures should be updated using a range of objective, measurable criteria.

Annotations

2.69.1 Asbury, J. (1995) Overview of focus group research. *Qualitative Health Research*, 5 (4) 414–20   11 References

Provides a general introduction to the use of focus groups as a research tool.

2.69.2 Carey, M.A. (1995) Comment: concerns in the analysis of focus group data. *Qualitative Health Research*, 5 (4) 487–95   17 References

As there is little guidance of the processes involved in evaluating focus group data, this article discusses considerations in planning and implementing analyses of such material (CR 2.86).

2.69.3 Catterall, M. & Maclaren, P. (1997) Focus group data and qualitative analysis programs: coding the moving picture as well as snapshots. *Sociological Research Online*, 2 (1) URL: http://www.socresonline.org.uk/socresonline/2/1/6.html   63 References

Literature on analysis of focus group data is reviewed. This shows that important communication and learning also takes place during this method of data collection (CR 2.86).

2.69.4   Chamane, N.J. & Kortenbout, W. (1996) Focus group interview as a data gathering tool: its application to nurses' understanding of HIV infections and AIDS. *Curationis: South African Journal of Nursing,* 19 (4) 23–5   10 References

Discusses the appropriate and inappropriate uses of focus group interviews. A study which examined nurses' knowledge and understanding of HIV and AIDS is used for illustration.

2.69.5   Clark, J.M., Maben, J. & Jones, K. (1996) The use of focus group interviews in nursing research: issues and challenges. *NT Research,* 1 (2) 143–55   34 References

Drawing on the authors' experience of conducting focus group interviews, some of the main issues and challenges are highlighted. These include group size, access and sampling and group interactions. The role of the leader is also discussed, together with difficulties in analysing these data (CR 2.22, 3.16).

2.69.6   Greenbaum, T.L. (1998) *The Handbook for Focus Group Research* 2nd edition. Thousand Oaks, CA: Sage. ISBN 0761912533 References

Provides the latest information on conducting focus groups. New chapters discuss the technology revolution with particular reference to video-conferencing and the Internet, the need to understand the major differences between focus group research in different countries and how to make comparisons. Its weaknesses are also discussed.

2.69.7   Halloran, J.P. & Grimes, D.E. (1995) Application of focus group methodology to educational program development. *Qualitative Health Research,* 5 (4) 444–53   9 References

Describes the use of focus group methods to assess the perceived learning needs of nurses caring for people with HIV. The procedures used for formation, moderation, data collection and analysis, and the application of findings to programme development are all discussed.

2.69.8   Happell, B. (1996) Focus group interviews as a tool for psychiatric nursing research. *Australian and New Zealand Journal of Mental Health Nursing,* 5 (1) 40–4 12 References

Explores the potential of focus group interviews in psychiatric nursing. The advantages and disadvantages are discussed and the author's own experience is highlighted.

2.69.9   Henderson, N.R. (1995) A practical approach to analysing and reporting focus group studies: lessons from qualitative market research. *Qualitative Health Research,* 5 (4) 463–77   5 References

Article describes some ways in which a small qualitative research company analyses focus group data and prepares reports. Although the focus is different from health studies, other researchers can learn from their experience.

2.69.10   Kitzinger, J. (1994) The methodology of focus groups: the importance of interaction between researcher and participant. *Sociology of Health and Illness,* 16 (1) 103–21 41 References

Introduces focus group methodology, explores ways of conducting such groups and examines what this method of data collection can offer. Article concentrates on the interaction between research participants and argues for overt explanation and exploitation of such encounters.

2.69.11   Krueger, R.A. (1994) *Focus Groups: a Practical Guide to Applied Research* 2nd edition. Thousand Oaks, CA: Sage. ISBN 0803955669   References

Book provides a comprehensive and detailed analysis of focus group interviewing techniques. Part 1 presents an overview of focus groups and identifies the differences between this and other similar methodological procedures. Part 2 describes the processes used in conducting focus group interviews and Part 3 outlines the involvement of non-researchers, variations of focus groups and ways for contracting focus group assistance.

2.69.12   McShane, R.E. & Rantz, M.J. (1996) Focus group sessions: a research technique for nurses. *Journal of Nursing Science,* 1 (3/4) 71–6   18 References

Article summarizes the use of focus groups as a research technique for nurses. A definition is given, together with its uses, the method from conceptualization to analysis and reporting results. An illustration of an application to nursing practice is given.

2.69.13 Millar, B., Maggs, C., Warner, V. & Whale, Z. (1996) Creating consensus about nursing outcomes: I. an exploration of focus group methodology. *Journal of Clinical Nursing*, 5 (3) 193–7   19 References

and

2.69.14 Millar, B., Maggs, C., Warner, V. & Whale, Z. (1996) Creating consensus about nursing outcomes: II. nursing outcomes as agreed by patients, nurses and other health professionals. *Journal of Clinical Nursing*, 5 (4) 263–7   18 References

Articles describe a study which explored a method for achieving consensus about nursing outcomes. Focus group work as a research tool is described and reviewed and difficulties in recruitment and facilitation are discussed. Results are reported and areas where consensus was achieved are highlighted (CR 2.43).

2.69.15 Morgan, D.L. (1997) *Focus Groups as Qualitative Research* 2nd edition. Thousand Oaks, CA: Sage. ISBN 0761903437 References

Book gives an updated introduction to current social science approaches to focus groups. They are compared with interviews and their strengths and weaknesses described. Suggestions are made for planning, conducting and analysing these data.

2.69.16 to 2.69.22 Morgan, D.L. & Krueger, R.A. (1997) *Focus Group Kit.* Thousand Oaks, CA: Sage. ISBN 0761907602 Volume 1–6

The following entry differs in format as it documents a series of six books. The annotation includes the whole series.

2.69.17 Morgan, D.L. (1997) *The Focus Group Guidebook* Volume 1. ISBN 0761908188

2.69.18 Morgan, D.L. (1997) *Planning Focus Groups* Volume 2. ISBN 076190817X

2.69.19 Krueger, R.A. (1997) *Developing Questions for Focus Groups* Volume 3. ISBN 0761908196

2.69.20 Krueger, R.A. (1997) *Moderating Focus Groups* Volume 4. ISBN 0761908218

2.69.21 Krueger, R.A. (1997) *Involving Community Members in Focus Groups* Volume 5. ISBN 076190820X

2.69.22 Krueger, R.A. (1997) *Analyzing and Reporting Focus Group Results* Volume 6. ISBN 0761908161

This kit provides information on running successful focus groups, from the initial planning stages to asking questions, the final analysis of data to the reporting of findings.

2.69.23 Morris, R.I. (1996) Preparing for the 21st century: planning with focus groups. *Nurse Educator*, 21 (6) 38–42   6 References

Describes the process of using focus groups to facilitate dialogue between nurse administrators, clinicians, educators and students. Groups focused on adapting the curriculum to changing market conditions.

2.69.24 Reed, J. & Payton, V.R. (1997) Focus groups: issues of analysis and interpretation. *Journal of Advanced Nursing*, 26 (4) 765–71   15 References

Reports a study which aimed to understand the experiences of older people moving into nursing and residential homes. It brought into focus many issues relating to this method of data collection, its analysis and interpretation (CR 2.86).

2.69.25 Roberts, P. (1997) Planning and running a focus group. *Nurse Researcher*, 4 (4) 78–82   7 References

Outlines the advantages of focus groups and gives guidelines for planning and running a successful meeting.

2.69.26 Sim, J. & Snell, J. (1996) Focus groups in physiotherapy evaluation and research. *Physiotherapy*, 82 (3) 189–98 50 References

Paper explores the methodological characteristics of the focus group in relation to other methods of survey work and examines some of its strengths and weaknesses. The nature and quality of the data that are obtained is discussed as is the importance of developing good group dynamics. An example is given for illustration.

2.69.27 Smith, M.W. (1995) Ethics in focus groups: a few concerns. *Qualitative Health Research*, 5 (4) 478–86   28 References

Little has been written about ethical issues in

relation to focus groups. The author discusses ethical theories, concerns specific to focus groups, the role of the researcher and future considerations when using this method of data collection (CR 2.17, 3.16).

2.69.28 Straw, R.B. & Smith, M.W. (1995) Potential uses of focus groups in federal policy and program evaluation studies. *Qualitative Health Research*, 5 (4) 421–7   4 References

Discusses the potential uses of focus groups as a formal data collection method in studies which may affect policies and programme evaluation activities (CR 2.43, 3.11).

2.69.29 Vaughn, S., Schumm, J.S. & Sinagub, J.M. (1996) *Focus Group Interviews in Education and Psychology*. Thousand Oaks, CA: Sage. ISBN 0803958935   References

Book covers all aspects of conducting focus groups in educational and psychological settings. Areas covered are how to prepare for a focus group, creating a moderator's guide, selecting a setting and analysing results. A chapter is included on focus groups with children and adolescents.

2.69.30 White, G.E. & Thomson, A.N. (1995) Anonymized focus groups as a research tool for health professions. *Qualitative Health Research*, 5 (2) 256–61   4 References

Describes a study which used an anonymized telephone-based focus group methodology to examine family physicians' attitudes to sexual contact between them and their patients. This adapted use of traditional focus groups aimed to create a safe environment in which participants could be more honest about their feelings relating to a sensitive subject (CR 2.70).

2.70 INTERVIEW – TELEPHONE

Telephone interviews are one of the tools, used particularly in market research, to ascertain people's views on a wide range of topics, for example customer services provided by a particular company, or aspects of health care. New developments in this field include the use of computer-assisted and direct computer interviewing.

Definition

Telephone interview – questioning by telephone

Example

Bowman, G.S., Howden, J., Allen, S., Webster, R.A. & Thompson, D.R. (1994) A telephone survey of medical patients one week after discharge from hospital. *Journal of Clinical Nursing*, 3 (6) 369–73   18 References

Study investigated the feasibility of obtaining information about the patients' condition after discharge, monitoring their progress, offering advice and support.

Annotations

2.70.1 Barriball, K.L., Christian, S.L., While, A.E. & Bergen, A. (1996) The telephone survey method: a discussion paper. *Journal of Advanced Nursing* 24 (1) 115–21   36 References

Gives an account of strategies employed to recruit a study sample, minimize non-response and bias, and ensure sound practices during data collection. Suggestions are made for further work (CR 2.22, 2.27).

2.70.2 de Bortoli Cassiani, S.H., Zanett, M.L. & Pela, N.T.R. (1992) The telephone survey: a methodological strategy for obtaining information. *Journal of Advanced Nursing*, 17 (5) 576–81   7 References

Reports some methodological considerations in a study which aimed to assess the level of knowledge about existing nursing schools in Brazil.

2.70.3 de Leeuw, E.D. (1994) Computer-assisted data collection, data quality and costs: a taxonomy and annotated bibliography. *Bulletin de Méthodologie Sociologique*, 44 60–72   References

Includes a taxonomy on different forms of computerized interviewing. The influence on data quality and costs are discussed.

2.70.4 Frey, J.H. (1989) *Survey Research by*

Telephone 2nd edition. Beverly Hills, CA: Sage. ISBN 0803929854   References

The history of telephone interviewing is outlined and comparisons are made with mail and face-to-face methods. Sampling procedures and question-wording are discussed and methods are suggested for administering and implementing this method of data collection. Ethical issues are discussed together with the future of telephone surveys (CR 2.17, 2.22, 2.52, 2.68).

2.70.5   Glasper, A. (1993) Telephone triage: a step forward for nursing practice. *British Journal of Nursing*, 2 (2) 108–9   6 References Guest editorial

Discusses the possible use and abuse of this method for obtaining information.

2.70.6   Groves, R.M., Biemer, P., Lars, L., Massey, J., Nicholls, W. & Waksberg, J. (1988) *Telephone Survey Methodology*. New York: Wiley. ISBN 0471622184   References

Book provides a wide-ranging description of telephone interviewing applications.

2.70.7 Korner-Bitensky, N. & Wood-Dauphinee, S. (1995) Barthel Index information elicited over the telephone: is it reliable? *American Journal of Physical Medicine and Rehabilitation*, 74 (1) 9–18 20 References

Reports a study which examined the comparability of estimates of functional status elicited through both telephone and face-to-face interviews. The index, a commonly used instrument for assessing the activities of daily living, was administered to 366 individuals over the telephone and at home with both health professionals and trained lay interviewers being used. Results showed that, with the exception of a small sub-group of patients, functional status can be elicited reliably over the telephone by both laypeople and health professionals (CR 2.69).

2.70.8   Lavrakas, P.J. (1993) *Telephone Survey Methods: Sampling, Selection and Supervision* 2nd revised edition. Beverly Hills, CA: Sage. ISBN 0803953062   References

Three major elements of telephone survey techniques are explored in depth: generating and processing telephone survey sampling pools; selecting a respondent and securing co-operation; and structuring the work of interviewers and supervisors. Book contains a glossary of terms relevant to this method (CR 2.2).

2.70.9   Minnick, A., Roberts, M.J., Young, W.B., Kleinpell, R.M. & Micek, W. (1995) An analysis of post-hospitalization telephone survey data. *Nursing Research*, 44 (6) 371–5 9 References

Reports on some methodological aspects of a study in which 4,600 adults were interviewed by telephone after hospitalization. Response-rate differences, reasons for non-participation by gender, age, ethnicity and race are highlighted. Other issues discussed are understanding and reporting response rates, reducing losses due to ineligibility, dealing with refusals and tailoring approaches to special populations (CR 2.22).

2.71   LIFE HISTORY/BIOGRAPHY

Life histories may provide nurses with valuable 'inside' information about an individual for whom they may be caring, or wish to invite to co-operate in a research programme. Although the information gained will be 'subjective' in nature, it will nevertheless give valuable insights into the views of the patient or client about their experiences. Perhaps too often researchers impose structure upon their data gathering which can 'hide' the realities which respondents need to express.

Definitions

Biographical method – that combination of research approaches which draws upon life stories, life histories, case studies, oral histories, personal narrations and self-stories
Interpretative biography – . . . a form of biography that is based on the author being present in the study and open recognition that biographical writing is, in part, autobiographical of the author
Life history – a narrative self-report about a person's life experiences regarding some theme of interest to the researcher
Self-report – an indirect method for assessing health status

Example

Garro, L.C. (1994) Narrative representations of chronic illness experience: cultural models of illness, mind and body in stories concerning the temporo-mandibular joint. *Social Science and Medicine*, 38 (6) 775–88   53 Notes and References

Narratives report how people made sense of a perplexing set of symptoms which are not easily categorized and treated. While describing the effect of illness on individual lives, the narratives also illustrate how shared understanding shapes the interpretation and construction of individual experience.

Annotations

2.71.1   Atkinson, R. (1998) *The Life Story Interview.* Thousand Oaks, CA: Sage. ISBN 076190428X   References

Volume provides guidelines and suggestions for carrying out a life-story interview. In addition to putting it into context, advice is given on planning, conducting the interview, dealing with issues of transcribing and interpreting the data. A sample life-story interview is included (CR 2.68).

2.71.2   Denzin, N.K. (1989) *Interpretive Biography.* Newbury Park, CA: Sage. ISBN 0803933592   References

Book links postmodernism and interpretative social science to re-examine the biographical and autobiographical genres and shows a new way in which biographies can be conceptualized and shaped (CR 2.42).

2.71.3   Dex, S. (ed.) (1991) *Life and Work History Analyses: Qualitative and Quantitative Developments.* London: Routledge. ISBN 0415053382   References

Book examines a growing interest in the collection of life and work histories and discusses methods of analysing these data. Each paper takes a specific research topic and many common questions are answered. New concepts and methods of handling these data are reported (CR 2.9).

2.71.4   Giele, J.Z. & Elder, G.H. Jr. (eds) (1998) *Methods of Life Course Research: Qualitative and Quantitative Approaches.*

Thousand Oaks, CA: Sage. ISBN 0761914374 References

The field's founders and leaders answer the question: What are the most suitable methods for doing life-course research? Tips are given on the art and method of appropriate research designs, the collection of life-history data and the search for meaningful patterns to be found in the results (CR 2.29, 2.36).

2.71.5   Grady, K.E. & Wallston, B.S. (1988) *Research in Health Care Settings.* Newbury Park, CA: Sage. ISBN 0803928742 Chapter 7, 101–16   References

Chapter explores where self-report may be appropriate, gives examples and discusses possible biases (CR 2.27).

2.71.6   Harrison, B. & Lyon, E.S. (1993) A note on ethical issues in the use of autobiography in sociological research. *Sociology,* 27 (1) 101–9   References

Discusses the relative neglect of ethical aspects when using autobiographies in sociological research. The public and private worlds, together with potential for conflicts for both subject and researcher are considered (CR 2.17, 2.22).

2.71.7   Josselson, R. (ed.) (1996) *Ethics and Process in the Narrative Study of Lives.* London: Sage. ISBN 0761902376   References

The emphasis in this book is studying what happens after narratives have been obtained, how experts try to understand the material, re-narrate it for their own ends and assess the impact this may have on those involved. The 18 essays are addressed mainly from a psychological perspective (CR 2.17).

2.71.8   Lipson, J.G. (1991) The use of self in ethnographic research, in Morse, J.M. (ed.), *Qualitative Nursing Research: a Contemporary Dialogue.* Newbury Park, CA: Sage. ISBN 0803940793

Discusses the contribution researchers can make when conducting research. The background and assumptions inherent in this are discussed, together with influences on the use of self. Advice is given on how this technique may be improved.

2.71.9   Maruyama, M. (1981) Endogenous

research: the prison project, in Reason, P. & Rowan, J. (eds), *Human Inquiry: a Sourcebook of New Paradigm Research*. Chichester: Wiley. ISBN 0471279358 Chapter 23, 267–81 References

Endogenous research is where a culture is studied by its insiders. Chapter describes a project undertaken to investigate prison violence where the researchers were largely the inmates themselves. The ability of endogenous researchers to conceptualize, record, code and analyse data are discussed. A list of criteria for selecting such researchers is given (CR 2.11.9).

2.71.10 May, C. & Foxcroft, D. (1995) Minimizing bias in self-reports of health beliefs and behaviours. *Health Education Research*, 10 (1) 107–12   17 References

Paper discusses the problems of bias associated with using conventional qualitative methods and suggests ways of avoiding them (CR 2.27).

2.71.11 Plummer, K. (1983) *Documents of Life: an Introduction to the Problems and Literature of a Humanistic Method*. London: Allen & Unwin. ISBN 0043210295 References

Book is concerned with the use of life histories and other types of personal document which give first-hand accounts of social experience from the participants' point of view. Sections include in pursuit of a subject, the diversity of life documents, the making of a method, some uses of life documents, doing life histories and the personal face of private documents (CR 2.22).

2.71.12 Rew, L., Bechteld, D. & Sapp, A. (1993) Self-as-instrument in qualitative research. *Nursing Research*, 42 (5) 300–1 20 References

Discusses various issues associated with this method of data collection, including appropriateness, authenticity, credibility, intuitiveness, receptivity, reciprocity and sensitivity.

2.71.13 to 2.71.27 Sociology. (1993) 27 (1). Biography and autobiography in sociology.

The following entry differs in format as it documents a special issue of the journal *Sociology*. These articles have not been annotated.

Writing/reading selves

2.71.13 Erben, M. The problem of other lives: social perspectives on written biography. 15–25   28 References

2.71.14 Evans, M. Reading lives: how the personal might be social. 5–13   15 References

2.71.15 Sheridan, D. Writing to the archive: mass observation as autobiography. 27–40 28 References

2.71.16 Stanley, L. On autobiography in sociology. 41–52   22 References

Researching, teaching and writing

2.71.17 Aldridge, J. The textual disembodiment of knowledge in research account writing. 53–66   27 References

2.71.18 Cotterrill, P. & Letherby, G. Weaving stories: personal autobiographies in feminist research. 67–79   21 References

2.71.19 Harrison, B. & Stina Lyon, E. A note on ethical issues in the use of autobiography in sociological research. 101–9 44 References

2.71.20 Ribbens, J. Facts or fiction? Aspects of the use of autobiographical writing in undergraduate sociology. 81–92   56 References

2.71.21 Wilkins, R. Taking it personally: a note on emotions and autobiography. 93–100 40 References

Texts, intertexts and selves

2.71.22 Davies, M.L. Healing Sylvia: accounting for the textual 'discovery' of unconscious knowledge. 110–20   37 References

2.71.23 Dickinson, H. Accounting for Augustus Lamb: theoretical and methodological issues in biography and historical sociology. 121–32   22 References

2.71.24 Miller, N. & Morgan, D. Called to account: the CV as an autobiographical practice. 133–43   10 References

Life histories as accounts

2.71.25   Bytheway, B. Ageing and biography: the letters of Bernard and Mary Berenson. 153–65   16 References

2.71.26   Humphrey, R. Life stories and social careers: ageing and social life in an ex-mining town. 166–78   27 References

2.71.27   Rosie, A. He's a liar, I'm afraid: truth and lies in a narrative account. 144–52 5 References

2.71.28   Walmsley, J. (1995) Life history interviews with people with learning difficulties. *Oral History*, 23 (1) 71–7   45 References

Paper describes a project which aimed to discover what experiences people with learning difficulties have, and have had, of caring and being cared for. The challenges of this work are discussed, including the adaptations necessary, problematic issues such as explaining the research, giving the participants a voice, offering feedback and giving them the final say (CR 2.68).

2.72   OBSERVATION

'Observation is one of the major methods by which data are gathered and is particularly appropriate for complex research situations. These may be viewed as complete entities and would be difficult to measure either as a whole or separately' (Fox, 1982: 197).

Definitions

Non-participant observation – observer watches and records but does not participate as a member of the group of study subjects being observed
Observation – a method of collecting data in which the researcher scientifically watches and records pertinent information
Participant observation – observer watches, collects and records data while interacting with the group of study subjects as a member of the group

Example

Clarke, L. (1996) Participant observation in a secure unit: care, conflict and control. *NT Research*, 1 (6) 431–41   57 References

Reports a study which investigated the reality of a therapeutic community in a secure (forensic) unit. The relative weighting of custody and care was examined using strategies designed to minimize subjects' perceptions about the research, in order to present an 'uncontaminated' picture of the unit.

Annotations

2.72.1   Ashworth, P.D. (1995) The meaning of 'participation' in participant observation. *Qualitative Health Research*, 5 (3) 366–87 43 References

The technique of participant observation, as a process of social interaction, is viewed in the context of a phenomenology of participation and its various constituents are described (CR 2.49).

2.72.2   Barlow, S. (1994) Drawing up a schedule for observation. *Nurse Researcher*, 2 (2) 22–9   11 References

Paper discusses recording observational data, constructing and defining schedules and rating scales.

2.72.3   Buckingham, R., Kack, S.A., Mount, B.M., Maclean, L.D. & Collins, J.T. (1976) Living with the dying: use of the technique of participant observation. *Canadian Medical Association Journal*, 18 December, 115 1211–15   19 References

Describes the experience of an anthropologist who assumed the role of a terminally ill patient when admitted first to a surgical ward and then to a palliative care unit. Both units are compared and contrasted with particular reference to treatment, attitudes and interactions of staff, terminally ill patients and their families. Of particular note was the effect of this hospitalization on the researcher (CR 2.16, 2.17).

2.72.4   Dingwall, R. (1997) Accounts, interviews and observations, in Miller, G. & Dingall, R. (eds), *Context and Method in Qualitative Research*. London: Sage. ISBN

0803976321 Part II, Chapter 4, 51–65   References

Chapter discusses the decline of participant observation, relative to interviewing, in qualitative research. A case is made for reviving participant observation studies by focusing on the ways in which social realities are constructed and acted upon in the course of everyday life (CR 2.36.40, 2.68).

2.72.5   Endacott, R. (1994) Objectivity in observation. *Nurse Researcher*, 2 (2) 30–40   18 References

Article lists the potential sources of distortion in observation and examines how each may be overcome.

2.72.6   Fine, G.A. & Sandstrom, K.L. (1988) *Knowing Children: Participation with Minors.* London: Sage. ISBN 0803933649   References

Discusses some methodological aspects of participant observation in field research with children (CR 2.36).

2.72.7   Gerrish, K. (1997) Being a 'marginal native': dilemmas of the participant observer. *Nurse Researcher*, 5 (1) 25–34   15 References

Discusses some of the issues raised when being a participant observer in a study. This examined the extent to which district nurses achieved their intentions of providing individualized care to patients from different ethnic backgrounds. Difficulties that were highlighted include the role of the researcher, the effects of being directly involved, and relationships with participants. Ethical dilemmas are also discussed (CR 2.17, 2.42, 3.16).

2.72.8   Gould, D. (1996) Using vignettes to collect data for nursing research studies: how valid are the findings? *Journal of Clinical Nursing*, 5 (4) 207–12   22 References

Paper considers the advantages and disadvantages associated with the use of vignettes as data-collection tools and includes a checklist to help critique vignette studies (CR 2.24, 2.25, 2.95).

2.72.9   Gross, D. (1991) Issues related to validity of videotaped observational data. *Western Journal of Nursing Research*, 13 (5) 658–63   13 References

Discusses the external validity of this method, together with estimating the sample size, coding the data and its limitations (CR 2.25).

2.72.10   Gross, D. & Conrad, B. (1991) Issues related to the reliability of videotaped observational data. *Western Journal of Nursing Research*, 13 (6) 798–803   15 References

Discusses the reliability of videotaped observational material and includes points relating to training study personnel (CR 2.24).

2.72.11   Hagedorn, M. (1994) Hermeneutic photography: an innovative esthetic technique for generating data in nursing research. *Advances in Nursing Science*, 17 (1) 44–50   18 References

Outlines the use of hermeneutic photography as an aesthetic technique. The value of photography as a research method and suggestions for its use in nursing research are discussed.

2.72.12   Hunt, S.A. & Benford, R.D. (1997) Dramaturgy and methodology, in Miller, G. & Dingwall, R. (eds), *Context and Method in Qualitative Research.* London: Sage. ISBN 0803976321 Part II, Chapter 8, 106–18   References

Dramaturgy is a perspective that uses a theatrical metaphor to understand social interaction. Chapter considers how the dramaturgical perspective can be used to analyse research on organizations and institutions (CR 2.16, 2.36.40, 2.86).

2.72.13   Jorgensen, D.L. (1989) *Participant Observation: a Methodology for Human Studies.* Newbury Park, CA: Sage. ISBN 0803928777

Book is an introduction to the basic principles and strategies of participant observation for students and the more experienced researcher. Sections cover methodology, the process of defining a problem, gaining entry to a setting, participating in everyday life, developing and sustaining relationships. Observing and gathering information, keeping notes, records and files, analysing and theorizing, leaving the field and communicating the results are also discussed (CR 2.18).

2.72.14   Phillips, J.R. (1993) Virtual reality: a new vista for nurse researchers? *Nursing Science Quarterly*, 6 (1) 5–7   24 References

Article discusses the potential of virtual reality as a tool for nurse researchers.

2.72.15 Pretzlik, U. (1994) Observational methods and strategies. *Nurse Researcher*, 2 (2) 13–21   7 References

Examines and compares unstructured and structured observation strategies, together with participant and non-participant approaches. Event and time sampling are briefly covered.

2.72.16 Prosser, J. (ed.) (1998) *Image-based Research: a Source Book for Qualitative Researchers*. London: Falmer Press. ISBN 075070649X   References

Book gives a theoretical overview of image-based research, images in the research process and in practice.

2.72.17 Spradley, J.P. (1980) *Participant Observation*. New York: Holt, Rinehart & Winston. ISBN 0030445019   References

Book describes the techniques of participant observation when carrying out ethnographic research. Part 1 defines ethnography, identifies assumptions and distinguishes it from other approaches. Part 2 discusses the 'Developmental Research Sequence' which is a series of 12 tasks designed to guide the reader through each stage of observations in ethnographic research (CR 2.42, 2.68.34).

2.72.18 Swanwick, M. (1994) Observation as research method. *Nurse Researcher*, 2 (2) 4–12   24 References

Describes the value of observation in nursing research. Its history, relationship to empiricism, objectivity, reliability, roles of the observer and strategies are all discussed (CR 2.25, 3.16).

2.73   PROJECTIVE TECHNIQUES

'Projective techniques encompass many different measurement tools, devices, and strategies which may be used to examine fundamental aspects of psychological functioning' (Waltz, Strickland & Lenz, 1984: 255).

Definition

Projective techniques – personality tests which are distinctive in that the subject has to respond to an ambiguous stimulus. In doing so the subject is supposed to reveal aspects of his or her personality, such as needs, attitudes and unconscious desires

Example

Wood, S.P. (1983) School-aged children's perceptions of the causes of illness. *Pediatric Nursing*, March/April 9 101–4   12 References

Study examined the perceptions of causes of illness in a group of 65 children. Pictures were used with brief sentences attached to explore their ideas. Two major theories emerged as causes, illness as punishment and the germ theory.

Annotations

2.73.1 Bellak, L. (1992) Projective techniques in the computer age. *Journal of Personality Assessment*, 58 (3) 445–53 References

Reviews the history of projective techniques since 1940.

2.73.2 Finch, A.J. (1993) Projective techniques, in Finch, A.J. & Belter, R.W. (eds), *Handbook of Child and Adolescent Assessment*. Boston, MA: Allyn & Bacon. ISBN 0205145922   224–36   References

Describes the processes necessary when undertaking projective techniques.

2.73.3 Rabin, A.I. (1981) *Assessment with Projective Techniques: a Concise Introduction*. New York: Springer. ISBN 0826135501

Provides an introductory text to this range of techniques.

2.73.4 Semeonoff, B. (1976) *Projective Techniques*. New York: Wiley. No ISBN found   References and Bibliography

Describes the history of projective psychology and classifies the techniques.

2.74 Q Methodology

'Q methodology . . . is most often associated with quantitative analysis . . . but it is designed to examine elements which frequently engage the attention of the qualitative researcher interested in more than just life measured by the pound. It combines the strengths of both quantitative and qualitative research traditions' (Brown, 1996: 561–2).

Definition

Q sort – a research method consisting of rank ordering objects by sorting, and then assigning them to the sub-sets for statistical purposes

Example

Puntillo, K. & Weiss, S.J. (1994) Pain: its mediators and associated morbidity in critically ill cardiovascular surgical patients. *Nursing Research*, 43 (1) 31–6   54 References

Reports a study which determined the effects of age, sex, personality adjustment and analgesic administration on the magnitude of pain experienced by a group of cardiac and vascular surgical patients during their first few post-operative days. The McGill Pain Questionnaire and California Q-Set were used to obtain the data and results are reported.

Original text

Stephenson, W. (1953) *The Study of Behaviour: Q technique and its Methodology.* Chicago: University of Chicago Press. No ISBN found

Annotations

2.74.1   Brown, S.R. (1986) Q technique and method: principles and procedures, in Berry, W.D. & Lewis-Beck, M.S. (eds), *New Tools for Social Scientists: Advances and Applications in Research Methods.* Beverly Hills, CA: Sage. ISBN 0803926251 Chapter 3, 57–76 References

Although an old technique, having been introduced in the 1930s, author feels it is a neglected tool which has considerable value. Much of the chapter is devoted to discussion of two studies where the technique was used, and it closes with some methodological pointers.

2.74.2   Brown, S.R. (1996) Q methodology and qualitative research. *Qualitative Health Research*, 6 (4) 561–7   14 References

Q methodology is illustrated in a single case study of the subjective experience of health care. The data generated are used to illustrate the Q method package. This freeware program facilitates Q sort data entry, correlation and factor analysis, theoretical rotation and calculation of scores. Instructions are given for obtaining the Q method package, subscribing to a journal devoted to Q methodology, *Operant Subjectivity*, and for joining the Q method electronic discussion group (CR 2.34, 2.84).

2.74.3   Cordingley, L., Webb, C. & Hillier, V. (1997) Q methodology. *Nurse Researcher*, 4 (3) 31–45   27 References

Some important and influential examples of the use of Q methodology in health and nursing are discussed. There are still misunderstandings about its purpose so researchers using this method need to study its theoretical origins.

2.74.4   Dennis, K.E. (1986) Q methodology: relevance and application to nursing research. *Advances in Nursing Science*, 8 (3) 6–17 16 References

Explores the value of Q methodology, which is much more than the Q sort data-collection method, for the expansion of nursing knowledge. An overview of the technique is given and suggestions are made as to how it may be used.

2.74.5   McKeown, B. & Thomas, D. (1988) *Q Methodology.* Newbury Park, CA: Sage. ISBN 0803927533   References

Covers the principles, techniques and procedures of the Q method.

2.74.6   Q method page. (1997) URL: http://www.rz.unibw-muenchen.de/ ~p41bsmk/qmethod/

Provides information on Q methodology, Q method software, other software packages for analysis of Q sort data, Q studies data set archive and other resources on the World Wide Web.

2.74.7 Stainton Rogers, R. (1995) Q methodology, in Smith, J.A., Harré, R. & Van Langenhove, L. (eds), *Rethinking Methods in Psychology*. Thousand Oaks, CA: Sage. ISBN 0803977336 178–92

2.75 QUESTIONNAIRE

'The humble questionnaire is probably the single most common research tool in the social sciences . . . with the principle advantages being its apparent simplicity, versatility and low cost as a method of data gathering. . . . Designing the perfect questionnaire is, however, probably impossible . . . too many . . . produced over the years have contained simple errors that have seriously undermined the value of the data collected.' (Breakwell, Hammond & Fife-Schaw, 1995: 174–5)

Definition

Questionnaire – a data-collection technique consisting of a set of written items requesting a response from subjects

Example

Persson, L., Hallberg, I.R. & Ohlsson, O. (1997) Survivors of acute leukaemia and highly malignant lymphoma: retrospective views of daily life during treatment and when in remission. *Journal of Advanced Nursing*, 25 (1) 68–78   32 References

Study investigated, retrospectively, the experiences of treatment and nursing care provided to patients in remission. A questionnaire was used which had been developed from a previous interview study (CR 2.68).

Annotations

2.75.1 Butterfield, P.G., Lindeman, C.A., Valanis, B.G. & Spencer, P.S. (1995) Design of a questionnaire: occupational and environmental risks for Parkinson's disease. *AAOHN Journal*, 43 (4) 197–202   12 References

Discusses the process of questionnaire development, including establishing the conceptual background of the research, assuring integrity of the questions, specifying the content domain, wording, level, and formatting decisions. Also considered are establishing evidence for questionnaire validity, reliability, final editing and polishing. Authors believe that attention to detail will ensure accurate information on exposure from people affected with Parkinson's disease (CR 2.24, 2.25).

2.75.2 Carter, Y. (1996) Asking the questions. *Practice Nurse*, 11 (10) 717–18, 720–1   1 Reference

Author urges nurses to give careful thought to the design of questionnaires as it is easy to make costly mistakes.

2.75.3 Champion, P.J. & Sear, A.M. (1973) Questionnaire response rates: a methodological analysis, in Cochrane, R. (ed.), *Advances in Social Research: a Reader*. London: Constable. ISBN 0094581908 Chapter 15, 263–71 References

Report of a study which aimed to investigate the differential effects of three important variables on response rates of a mailed questionnaire. The variables examined were length of the questionnaire, type of postage used and the incentives given to respondents.

2.75.4 Coleman, M. & Mead, D. (1993) Simulation in training questionnaire design. *Nurse Researcher*, 1 (2) 52–61   4 References

Article explores some of the ethical and practical issues associated with research training. The value of simulation to develop quantitative research skills is described using computer software called EPI INFO (CR 2.17, 2.29, 2.51, 2.84, 3.17, Appendix A).

2.75.5 Dunning, T. & Martin, M. (1996/97) Developing a questionnaire: some methodological issues. *Australian Journal of Advanced Nursing*, 14 (2) 31–8   10 References

Reports the development of a questionnaire to be used in a survey of people with non-insulin dependent diabetes and those without the disease. The pre-test and pilot testing to establish the reliability, validity and stability of the tool are described (CR 2.24, 2.25, 2.55).

2.75.6 Hague, P. (1993) *Questionnaire Design.* London: Kogan Page. ISBN 0749409177 References

A comprehensive and practical guide to questionnaire design. Rules and principles are set out and numerous examples are included. The use of questionnaires, types, framing and examples of questions, layout and interviewer instructions are all discussed (CR 2.68).

2.75.7 Harris, H. & Inayat, Q. (1997) Semi-structured interview schedules for gathering psycho-social data. *Nurse Researcher*, 5 (1) 73–85 23 References

Gives guidelines on constructing questionnaires and their use in the context of an interview (CR 2.68).

2.75.8 Hicks, C. & Hennessy, D. (1996) Applying psychometric principles to the development of a training needs analysis questionnaire for use with health visitors, district and practice nurses. *NT Research*, 1 (6) 442–55 28 References

Paper reports the development of a training needs analysis questionnaire where the formal principles of psychometrics were included to increase its reliability (CR 2.24).

2.75.9 Jowett, S. & Shanley, E. (1993) Approaches to analysis and interpretation. *Nurse Researcher*, 1 (2) 44–51 16 References

Authors examine some common methods of identifying important information from questionnaire data, pointing out some of the possible pitfalls.

2.75.10 Kirk-Smith, M. & McKenna, H. (1998) Psychological concerns in questionnaire research. *NT Research*, 3 (3) 203–11 37 References

Paper examines many psychologically related issues and limitations in the use of questionnaires. These are theory building, validity of self-report, measurement and analysis. Authors suggest seeking expert advice during the development stages (CR 2.7, 2.71).

2.75.11 McColl, E. (1993) Questionnaire design and construction. *Nurse Researcher*, 1 (2) 16–25 3 References

Article focuses on practical issues in questionnaire construction, with emphasis on question content, format, wording, sequencing and layout.

2.75.12 McGibbon, G. (1997) How to avoid the pitfalls of questionnaire design. *Nursing Times*, 7 May 93 (19) 49–51 6 References

Author offers advice on the difficult task of designing good questionnaires.

2.75.13 Mead, D. (1993) Personal experiences of designing questionnaires. *Nurse Researcher*, 1 (2) 62–70 4 References

Discusses some of the problems of questionnaire design which usually remain undisclosed. Using her own research, creating, implementing and evaluating the questionnaire are discussed (CR 2.16, 2.66).

2.75.14 Meehan, T. (1994) Questionnaire construction and design for surveys in mental health. *Australian and New Zealand Journal of Mental Health Nursing*, 3 (2) 59–62 9 References

Provides a guide for nurses who need to develop questionnaires. Using questions that relate to issues in mental health, the problems which may be encountered are discussed (CR 2.52).

2.75.15 Newell, R. (1993) Questionnaires, in Gilbert, N. (ed.), *Researching Social Life*. London: Sage. ISBN 0803986823 Chapter 6, 94–115 References

Chapter provides guidelines and practical assistance so that most of the difficulties of preparing questionnaires can be avoided. The distinction is made between questionnaires and interview schedules (CR 2.1.25, 2.68).

2.75.16 Oppenheim, A.N. (1992) *Questionnaire Design, Interviewing and Attitude Measurement* 2nd edition. London: Pinter. ISBN 1855670445 References

This classic text has been considerably expanded and revised and is now a general survey research handbook. New chapters are included on survey, analytic and descriptive design, sampling, interviewing, questionnaire development, statistical analysis and pilot work (CR 2.22, 2.23, 2.52, 2.56, 2.68, 2.69, 2.70, 2.73).

2.75.17 Parahoo, K. (1993) Questionnaires:

use, value and limitations. *Nurse Researcher*, 1 (2) 4–15   16 References

Author defines questionnaires, discusses their purpose and the type of data collected. Their value to nursing practice, the strengths, weaknesses, use and abuse of this tool are also discussed.

2.75.18 Rees, C. (1995) Questionnaire design in midwifery. *British Journal of Midwifery*, 3 (10) 549–52   7 References

Discusses the principles of questionnaire design.

2.75.19 Robichaud-Ekstrand, S., Haccoun, R.R. & Milette, D. (1994) One method of validating the translation of a questionnaire [French], *Canadian Journal of Nursing Research* 26 (3) 77–87   7 References

Paper describes Haccoun's technique for validating a translated questionnaire. The method is based on the idea that if a questionnaire is well translated, bilingual subjects will provide equivalent responses to questions in either language (CR 2.25).

2.75.20 Robin, S.S. (1973) A procedure for securing returns to mail questionnaires, in Cochrane, R. (ed.), *Advances in Social Research: a Reader*. London: Constable. ISBN 0094581908 Chapter 16, 272–84 References

Describes a technique which has resulted in high returns of questionnaires in ten independent samples.

2.75.21 Simpson, M.A. (1984) How to design and use a questionnaire in evaluation and educational research. *Medical Teacher*, 16 (4) 122–7   24 References

Article discusses the points which contribute to a well-designed questionnaire and takes the reader step by step through the process.

2.75.22 Verran, J.A., Mark, B.A. & Lamb, G. (1992) Psychometric examination of instruments using aggregated data. *Research in Nursing and Health*, 15 (3) 237–40 9 References

Provides information on selecting and evaluating questionnaires which obtain responses from individuals, but are to be used as measures of group-level variables (CR 2.24, 2.55).

2.76   RECORDS/ARCHIVAL DATA

Records are a readily available and valuable source of data and may be found everywhere. Sources include government records, those kept by institutions and individuals.

Definitions

Archival research – a method of studying organizations or societies, based on the collected records they have produced
Records – compilations of writing, photographs and figures that individuals have collected

Example

Wright, D. (1996) The dregs of society? Occupational patterns of male asylum attendants in Victorian England. *International History of Nursing Journal*, 1 (4) 5–19 27 References

Paper presents the results of a database study of male attendants hired at Surrey asylums between 1868 and 1881. It challenges the widely held assumption that attending was an 'occupation of last resort' and places asylum work within the wider context of a rapidly changing labour market in Victorian England.

Annotations

2.76.1 Burgess, R.G. (ed.) (1982a) Keeping field notes, in Author, *Field Research: a Sourcebook and Field Manual*. London: Allen & Unwin. ISBN 0043120148 Chapter 25, 191–4   References

Covers aspects of keeping field notes and outlines the three types which may be kept: substantive, methodological and analytic.

2.76.2 Burgess, R.G. (ed.) (1982b) Personal documents, oral sources and life histories, in Author, *Field Research: a Sourcebook and Field Manual*. London: Allen & Unwin. ISBN 0043120148 Chapter 18, 131–5   References

Discusses the value of different data sources in field research (CR 2.47, 2.71).

2.76.3 Hill, M.R. (1993) *Archival Strategies*

and Techniques. Newbury Park, CA: Sage. ISBN 0803948255   References

Book aims to improve and increase the use of historical records in social research, in particular the use of records found in special collections. Practical and detailed advice is given in the form of contextual description together with methodological advice.

2.76.4   Krowchuk, H.K., Moore, M.L. & Richardson, I. (1995) Using health care records as sources of data for research. *Journal of Nursing Measurement,* 3 (1) 3–12 21 References

Examines the advantages and disadvantages of using health care records as data sources and discusses the issues relating to appropriate research methods.

2.76.5   Macdonald, K. & Tipton, C. (1993) Using documents, in Gilbert, N. (ed.), *Researching Social Life.* London: Sage. ISBN 0803986823 Chapter 10, 187–200 References

Examines types of document, and the evaluation, interpretation and the need for triangulation (CR 2.1.25, 2.26).

2.76.6   McGann, S. (1997/98) Archival sources for research into the history of nursing. *Nurse Researcher,* 5 (2) 19–29 2 References

Author gives a guide to the sources available for research into the history of nursing.

2.76.7   Nail, L.M. & Lange, L.L. (1996) Using computerized clinical data bases for nursing research. *Journal of Professional Nursing,* 12 (4) 197–206   28 References

Article identifies strategies for using computerized clinical databases in nursing research. The phases that are necessary are detailed, and procedures are discussed (CR 2.84).

2.76.8   Scott, J. (1992) *A Matter of Record: Documentary Sources in Social Research.* Cambridge: Polity Press. ISBN 0745600700 References

Book illustrates the diversity of documentary sources available for social research and discusses ways in which they may be used. Chapters cover social research and documentary sources, assessing sources, the official realm,

public and private, administrative routines and decisions. Explorations in official documents, the public sphere, mass communications and personal documents are all discussed.

2.76.9   Webb, B. (1982) The art of note taking, in Burgess, R.G. (ed.), *Field Research: a Sourcebook and Field Manual.* London: Allen & Unwin. ISBN 0043120148 Chapter 26, 195–9   References

Chapter discusses the processes involved in note-taking, which are essential for the creation of accurate records.

2.76.10   While, A.E. (1987) Records as a data source: the case for health visitor records. *Journal of Advanced Nursing,* 12 (6) 757–63   26 References

It is suggested that health records are a useful source of research data, and a case-study approach was used to evaluate health visitor records. Consideration must however also be given to their limitations (CR 2.39).

2.77   REPERTORY GRID TECHNIQUE

Personal construct theory, which forms the basis of the repertory grid technique, stresses the importance of eliciting constructs of the subject, rather than those supplied by a researcher. A construct is a way of viewing elements as alike or different, where these objects of study are provided by the researcher. These elements are then developed into a grid, the construct is examined and scores are generated.

Definitions

Personal construct – a cover term for each of the ways in which a person attempts to perceive, understand, predict and control the world
Repertory grid – a series of judgements made by a person, using his or her constructs, on some aspect of the world

---

Example

Hicks, C., Hennessy, D., Cooper, J. & Barwell, F. (1996) Investigating attitudes research in primary health care teams. *Journal of Advanced Nursing*, 24 (5) 1033–41 19 References

This study, which formed part of a larger project, aimed to develop a diagnostic tool for identifying training needs within health care groups.

Original texts

Kelly, G.E. (1955) *The Psychology of Personal Constructs* 2 volumes. New York: Norton. No ISBN

Kelly, G.E. (1963) *Theory of Personality*. New York: Norton. ISBN 0393001520

Major text

Fransella, F. & Bannister, D. (1977) *A Manual for Repertory Grid Technique*. London: Academic Press. ISBN 0122654560 References

Annotations

2.77.1 Bannister, D. (1970) Concepts of personality: Kelly & Osgood, in Mittler, P.J. (ed.), *The Psychological Assessment of Mental and Physical Handicaps*. London: Methuen. ISBN 0416045707 Chapter 26, 761–79 References

Outlines two techniques for exploring interpretive man: the repertory grid and the semantic differential. The semantic differential is a technique used to measure attitudes that ask the respondent to rate a concept of interest on a series of seven-point bipolar scales (CR 2.60).

2.77.2 Bannister, D. (1981) Personal construct theory and research method, in Reason, P. & Rowan, J. (eds), *Human Inquiry: a Sourcebook of New Paradigm Research*. Chichester: Wiley. ISBN 0471279358 Chapter 16, 191–9 References

Outlines the personal construct theory developed by Kelly in the 1950s and discusses the use of the repertory grid technique as a tool in various psychological fields (CR 2.11.9).

2.77.3 Bannister, D. & Fransella, F. (1990) *Inquiring Man: Theory of Personal Constructs* New edition of 3rd revised edition. London: Routledge. ISBN 0415034604 References

Book summarizes personal construct theory and reviews the research it has generated. It examines its value for psychologists and psychotherapists and challenges orthodox thinking.

2.77.4 Beail, N. (ed.) (1985) *Repertory Grid Technique and Personal Constructs: Applications in Clinical Settings*. London: Croom Helm. ISBN 0709932642 References

A collection of readings which explore various applications of the repertory grid technique. Included are a brief introduction to the technique and sections covering construct systems, constructs and disability, evaluation of change, exploring relationships through grids, practical applications in education, constructs of handicap and a caveat on some aspects of validity (CR 2.25).

2.77.5 Cohen, L. & Manion, L. (1994) *Research Methods in Education* 4th revised edition. London: Routledge. ISBN 0415102359 Chapter 14, 299–321 References

Outlines the personal construct theory of George Kelly and discusses the structure and development of repertory grids. Its strengths and weaknesses are identified and some examples of its use in education are given (CR 2.1.17).

2.77.6 Fransella, F. & Bannister, D. (1977) *A Manual for Repertory Grid Technique*. London: Academic Press. ISBN 0122654560 References

Manual describes a technique developed from George Kelly's personal construct theory which aimed to 'look beyond words'. A variety of commonly used grid formats are discussed and the many difficulties which may be encountered are outlined. The reader is given guidance on designing grids while also becoming aware of their limitations. Appendices contain an example of the use of grids and the first published annotated bibliography on grid usage.

2.77.7 Mazhindu, G.N. (1992) Using repertory grid research: methodology in nurse education and practice: a critique. *Journal of Advanced Nursing*, 17 (5) 604–8 28 References

Paper defines and describes the repertory grid technique and evaluates its potential as a research tool in nurse education and practice. Its merits and limitations are discussed and suggestions are made for developing the technique.

2.77.8 O'Connor, K.P. & Blowers, G.H. (1996) *Personal Construct Psychology in the Clinical Context*. Ottawa, Canada: University of Ottawa Press. ISBN 0776604228

2.77.9 Pollock, L.C. (1986) An introduction to the use of repertory grid technique as a research method and clinical tool for psychiatric nurses. *Journal of Advanced Nursing*, 11 (4) 439–45 24 References

Provides a summary of the repertory grid technique as a research method.

2.77.10 Rawlinson, J.W. (1995) Some reflections on the use of repertory grid techniques in studies of nurses and social workers. *Journal of Advanced Nursing*, 21 (2) 334–9 33 References

Outlines the history of the repertory grid technique together with its use in nursing and social work. Caution is urged in future studies as the author believes it is sometimes used inappropriately.

2.77.11 Scholes, J. & Freeman, M. (1994) The reflective dialogue and repertory grid: a research approach to identify the unique contribution of nursing, midwifery or health visiting to the therapeutic milieu. *Journal of Advanced Nursing*, 20 (5) 885–93 27 References

Discusses the use of two complementary methods within the interpretative paradigm, the reflective dialogue and repertory grid. The issues of reciprocity, equality of researcher and participant, and the fact that research can empower and educate are all explored (CR 2.11).

2.77.12 Winter, D.A. (1992) *Personal Construct Psychology in Clinical Practice: Theory, Research and Application*. London: Routledge. ISBN 0415005272 References

Book is intended for psychologists but contains many examples of clinical applications which would be of interest to nurses.

2.78
TALK/CONVERSATION/NARRATIVE

Talk is increasingly being recognized and used as a technique for obtaining information from subjects. Conversations are complex to analyse, but may yield data which can be of considerable value to researchers.

Definitions

Conversation – an informal spoken exchange of thoughts and feelings
Narrative – an orderly, continuous account of an event or series of events
Talk – to converse by means of spoken language

Example

Running, A. (1997) Snapshots of experience: vignettes from a nursing home. *Journal of Advanced Nursing*, 25 (1) 117–22 10 References

Study examined the experience of living in a nursing home using 'Visit', a relational research method, as a means of developing nursing knowledge (CR 2.6).

Annotations

2.78.1 Adelman, C. (ed.) (1981) *Uttering, Muttering: Collecting, Using and Reporting Talk for Social and Educational Research*. London: Grant McIntyre. ISBN 0862160421 References

Compilation of studies written by leading researchers which brings together the theory and practice of using talk in research. Details on how to gather, interpret and make use of talk in educational and cultural settings are given.

2.78.2 Berger, A.A. (1996) *Narratives in Popular Culture, Media, and Everyday Life*.

London: Sage. ISBN 0761903453 References

Book explores important narrative theorists and techniques. Key terms and concepts are discussed. Readers will be enabled to interpret narratives and make their analyses accessible (CR 2.2, 2.86).

2.78.3 Brock, S.C. (1995) Narrative and medical genetics: on ethics and therapeutics. *Qualitative Health Research*, 5 (2) 150–68 65 References

Discusses use of narrative as a lived experience and its value in phenomenological investigations relating to genetic counselling. By understanding the client's experience more clearly, counselling practice and ethical considerations can be altered (CR 2.17, 2.49).

2.78.4 Czarniawska, B. (1998) *A Narrative Approach to Organization Studies*. London: Sage. ISBN 0761906630   References

Book guides readers through the narrative approach to qualitative research, from setting up the field work to writing the research (CR 2.36).

2.78.5 Jones, J.A. (1989) The verbal protocol: a research technique for nursing. *Journal of Advanced Nursing*, 14 (12) 1062–70 20 References

Reports a pilot study undertaken to investigate use of the verbal protocol. It aimed to discover how nurses reach decisions about a patient's problems and how a nursing diagnosis is made. The theoretical background to the technique, its use in medical contexts and the analysis of such data are discussed.

2.78.6 Josselson, R., Lieblich, A., Sharabany, R. & Wiseman, H. (1997) *Conversation as Method: Analyzing the Relational World of People who were Raised Communally*. Thousand Oaks, CA: Sage. ISBN 0761905138 References

Book explores a methodology evolving from people coming together to talk, listen and learn from one another. Four feminist scholars discuss different ways of knowing from both quantitative and qualitative perspectives (CR 2.6, 2.10, 2.29, 2.36).

2.78.7 Lieblich, A. & Josselson, R. (1997)

The Narrative Study of Lives. Thousand Oaks, CA: Sage. ISBN 0761903259   References

Book explores the challenges of performing narrative work in an academic setting. Specific topics are given for illustration and the use of narrative as an additional approach within a larger quantitative project is discussed (CR 2.29).

2.78.8 Poirier, S. & Ayres, L.C. (1997) Endings, secrets and silences: overreading in narrative inquiry. *Research in Nursing and Health*, 20 (6) 551–7   18 References

Narrative inquiry is used to find meaning in stories told by research participants. It entails developing sensitivity to unspoken or indirect statements which are central to interpretation. Some of the tools are applied to two research interviews as they direct readers to inconsistencies, endings, repetition and silences (CR 2.68).

2.78.9 Sandelowski, M. (1991) Telling stories: narrative approaches in qualitative research. *Image: Journal of Nursing Scholarship*, 23 (3) 161–6   59 References

Narrative is presented as a framework for understanding the subject and interview data in qualitative research. Examples of approaches are given, the truth in narratives is considered, and narrative analysis is contrasted with other types of qualitative data (CR 2.36, 2.86).

2.78.10 Walker, K. (1995) Nursing, narrativity and research: towards a poetics and politics of orality. *Contemporary Nurse: a Journal for the Australian Nursing Profession*, 4 (4) 156–63   43 References

Author believes that clinical nursing culture is poorly understood and little theorized. It is suggested that we could articulate and critique the complexity and diversity of clinical practice through postmodern poetics and politics of orality.

2.78.11 Wardhaugh, R. (1990) *How Conversation Works*. Oxford: Blackwell. ISBN 0631139397   References

Book discusses the structure of conversation and describes what happens when people talk to each other.

DATA ANALYSIS, INTERPRETATION AND PRESENTATION

2.79 DATA MANAGEMENT AND ANALYSIS – GENERAL

'Data analysis consists of examining, categorizing, tabulating or otherwise re-combining the evidence, to address the initial propositions of a study' (Yin, 1984: 99).

Definitions

Data analysis – application of one or more techniques to a set of data for the purpose of discovering trends, differences or similarities. The type of technique used is guided by the subject matter of the problem
Non-parametric statistics – a set of statistical procedures that are not based on assumptions about population parameters, or the shape of the underlying population distribution. They are most often used when data are measures on the nominal or ordinal scales
Parametric statistics – statistical procedures for estimating population parameters, with assumptions about the distribution of variables and for use with interval or ratio measures
Raw data – observations as originally recorded, i.e. with no operations, transformations or re-categorization performed on the numbers or values

---

Annotations

2.79.1 Aaronson, L.S. (1990) Needed: a national data repository of nursing research data. *Nursing Research*, 39 (5) 311–13 15 References

Discusses the value of developing a national

data repository to maximize funding. Much existing data is already available which could be used for secondary analysis (CR 2.64, 2.91).

2.79.2 Anthony, D. (1996) A review of the statistical methods in the *Journal of Advanced Nursing*. *Journal of Advanced Nursing*, 24 (5) 1089–94   10 References

Paper examines articles from an academic journal for statistical errors and the misunderstanding of concepts. These are compared with similar studies in medical journals.

2.79.3 Ashworth, P. (1994) Analysis of observed data. *Nurse Researcher*, 2 (2) 57–66 10 References

Outlines the different methods of analysing quantitative and qualitative observational data (CR 2.29, 2.36, 2.72, 2.86, 2.87).

2.79.4 Bauer, I. (1995) Rank-ordering: a suitable method for nursing research. *Australian Journal of Advanced Nursing*, 13 (1) 32–6   11 References

Author presents a guide to the technique of rank-ordering data using a study on patients' perception of their privacy in hospital to illustrate the procedure.

2.79.5 Chow, S.L. (1996) *Statistical Significance: Rationale, Validity and Utility*. Thousand Oaks, CA: Sage. ISBN 0761952055 References

Book gives an overview of the most fundamental methodological issue for empirical researchers – how should statistical significance be interpreted? An introduction to null hypothesis testing and statistical significance is given, together with arguments for and against current interpretations and the use of significance testing in research. The book contributes to the debate on the proper role of significance testing in empirical research (CR 2.20, 2.25, 2.87).

2.79.6 Eaton, N. (1997) Parametric data analysis. *Nurse Researcher*, 4 (4) 17–27 13 References

Describes the nature of parametric statistics, outlines some of the information required to decide whether and when they should be used. Examples are given (CR 2.81, 2.82).

2.79.7 Erickson, B.H. & Nosanchuk, T.A. (1992) *Understanding Data* 2nd edition. Buckingham: Open University Press. ISBN 033509662X References

Book is intended for professional sociologists and students who have always feared numbers. It utilizes the techniques of exploratory data analysis. Students are fully involved in the data and its analysis. It draws on their strengths and enables development of their own ideas. Suggestions for examination questions and homework are included.

2.79.8 Fielding, J. (1993) Coding and managing data, in Gilbert, N. (ed.), *Researching Social Life*. London: Sage. ISBN 0803986823 Chapter 11, 218–38

Chapter examines the coding process, qualitative coding, creation of a code book, data cleaning and computer analysis of qualitative data (CR 2.1.25, 2.84).

2.79.9 Fox, J. & Long, J.S. (eds) (1990) *Modern Methods of Data Analysis*. Newbury Park, CA: Sage. ISBN 0803933665 References

Volume aims to raise the standard of statistical analysis and presentation of data in the social sciences. It focuses on four themes: graphical data analysis, use of computers, regression analysis and sampling characteristics of data (CR 2.84, 2.94).

2.79.10 Horn, R.V. (1993) *Statistical Indicators for the Economic and Social Sciences*. Cambridge: Cambridge University Press. ISBN 0521423996 References

Gives comprehensive coverage of indicators in a wide range of disciplines, explores their limitations and reviews many alternatives.

2.79.11 Hutchinson, T.P. (1993) Kappa muddles together two sources of disagreement: tetrachoric correlation is preferable. *Research in Nursing and Health*, 16 (4) 313–16 8 References

Difficulties of assessing agreement between experts is explored in relation to Cohen's Kappa statistic.

2.79.12 Jowett, S. & Shanley, B.A. (1993) Approaches to analysis and interpretation. *Nurse Researcher*, 1 (2) 44–51 16 References

Examines some common methods of identifying the important information from questionnaire data. Some pitfalls are also highlighted (CR 2.75, 2.93).

2.79.13 Keren, G. & Lewis, C. (1993) *A Handbook for Data Analysis in the Behavioural Sciences: Methodological Issues*. Hillsdale, NJ: Erlbaum. ISBN 0805810366 References

Covers many methodological issues of data analysis in the social sciences.

2.79.14 Knapp, T.R. (1993) Treating ordinal scales as ordinal scales. *Nursing Research*, 42 (3) 184–6 9 References

Paper discusses a variation of one strategy for analysing ordinal/ordinal relationships. Two examples are used for illustrative purposes.

2.79.15 Lane, V. (1996) Typists' influences on transcription: aspects of feminist nursing epistemic rigour. *Nursing Inquiry*, 3 (3) 159–66 17 References

Describes the process by which female typists became participants 'of sorts' while transcribing audiotaped interviews. The primary data included sensitive information on sexual matters and the typists had the tendency to interpolate and even normalize the data. In so doing they became unexpected participants as commentators, validators, analysts and normalizers of the data. The processes involved and effects are all discussed (CR 2.17, 2.90, 3.16).

2.79.16 Lauver, D. & Knapp, T.R. (1993) Sum-of-products variables: a methodological critique. *Research in Nursing and Health*, 16 (5) 385–91 23 References

Discusses methodological issues associated

with the use of sum-of-product variables in health-related research.

2.79.17 Lobo, M.L. (1993) Code books: a critical link in the research process. *Western Journal of Nursing Research*, 15 (3) 377–85 5 References

A major step in collecting and organizing raw data is described by the use of a code book. The components required to enhance its value are listed, and ways in which the book may be developed to enable complex data to be analysed are discussed.

2.79.18 Maisel, R. & Persell, C.H. (1995) *How Sampling Works: a Guide to Decisions and Procedures.* Thousand Oaks, CA: Sage. ISBN 0803990618 References

Book explains the principles of statistical sampling and inference. Software included with the book helps to clarify these concepts in a visual and non-mathematical way.

2.79.19 Martin, P.A. (1993) Data management for surveys. *Applied Nursing Research*, 6 (3) 142–4 No references

Discusses ways in which data may be handled and the importance of pre-planning (CR 2.52).

2.79.20 Miller, D.C. (1991) Guides to statistical analysis and computer resources, in Author, *Handbook of Research Design and Social Measurement* 5th edition. Newbury Park, CA: Sage. ISBN 0803942192. Part 5, 231–322 References

Book guides researchers to statistical tools and computer resources (CR 2.54.14, 2.84).

2.79.21 Moseley, L.G. & Mead, D.M. (1993) Good relations: the use of a relational data base for large-scale data analysis. *Journal of Advanced Nursing*, 18 (11) 1795–805 7 References

Reports on the method of analysis used in a study commissioned by the Department of Health entitled 'Innovations in nursing care: the development of primary nursing in Wales'. Both quantitative and qualitative data were obtained. The limitations of statistical packages are discussed and the use of relational databases is explored. Its strengths and weaknesses are examined, together with its potential value in nursing research (CR 2.9, 2.29, 2.36, 2.64, 2.66, 2.86, 2.87).

2.79.22 Phillips, J.L. Jr. (1995) *How to Think about Statistics* 5th edition. Oxford: W.H. Freeman. ISBN 0716722879 References

Book is intended to focus on statistical ideas rather than on mathematics and computations. The underlying logic of statistical analysis and problem-solving provide a framework for understanding how they are used, mis-reported and manipulated.

2.79.23 Ratcliffe, P. (1998) Using the new statistics in nursing research. *Journal of Advanced Nursing*, 27 (1) 132–9 36 References

Author argues that quantitative methods are under-used in nursing research. This may be because researchers are not always aware of modern, sophisticated data analysis techniques. Paper discusses probability and survival modelling techniques suitable for use in complex nursing situations. One dedicated computer programme, GLIM 4, is described (CR 2.29, Appendix A).

2.79.24 Roberts, B.L., Anthony, M.K., Madigan, E.A. & Chen, Y. (1997) Data management: cleaning and checking. *Nursing Research*, 46 (6) 350–2 4 References

Discusses some of the problems which have occurred in data management and suggestions are made about coding, entry and clearing strategies.

2.79.25 Watson, H. & McFadyen, A. (1997) Non-parametric data analysis. *Nurse Researcher*, 4 (4) 28–40 12 References

Article explains the appropriate use of non-parametric statistical tests and gives examples of their use.

2.80 STATISTICAL AND OTHER TEXTS

There are many statistical texts on the market. Some are suitable for use in any discipline, and a few have been written with nurses in mind. A selection of books is included here, several of which were written to develop the student's ability to understand statistics.

Annotations

2.80.1 Bradford Hill, A. & Hill, I.D. (1991) *Principles of Medical Statistics* 12th edition. London: Edward Arnold. ISBN 0340537396 References

Written for medical practitioners and describes in non-mathematical terms the principles and practice of statistics applied to medicine. Real examples and data are used to illustrate the text.

2.80.2 Castle, W.M. & North, P.M. (1995) *Statistics in Small Doses* 3rd edition. Edinburgh: Churchill Livingstone. ISBN 0443045429

A programmed learning text covering topics in statistics needed by medical students and those in related professions. Learning is progressively assessed by questions with answers. Each chapter is illustrated with a practical example and concludes with a short summary.

2.80.3 Caulcott, E. (1992) *Statistics for Nurses*. London: Scutari. ISBN 187136471X

Intended as a basic text for nursing degree students and others in the health care field. No assumptions are made about previous knowledge and examples are given from health care.

2.80.4 Chatfield, C. (1988) *Problem Solving: a Statisticians' Guide*. London: Chapman & Hall. ISBN 0412286807 References

Written for students and statisticians who feel unsure how to tackle a real problem where the data is 'messy' or the objectives unclear. General principles are given and a series of exercises to illustrate the practical problems of analysing real data is presented. A digest of statistical techniques with brief notes on two packages – MINITAB and GLIM – is included, together with useful addresses and statistical tables. Advice is given on choosing computer software and the role of statisticians (CR 2.83, 2.84, Appendix A).

2.80.5 Coggan, D. (1995) *Statistics in Clinical Practice*. London: British Medical Journal Publishing. ISBN 072790907X References

Book explains the principles of statistics using clinical examples.

2.80.6 Frankfort-Nachmias, C. (1997) *Social Statistics for a Diverse Society*. Thousand Oaks, CA: Pine Forge Press. ISBN 080399026X References

An introductory text which relates statistics to social science research. The use of graphics, real data, exercises and SPSS (Statistical Package for the Social Sciences) demonstrations will assist students' understanding. An Instructor's Manual includes sample examination questions, quizzes and step-by-step solutions for all exercises in the book (CR Appendix A).

2.80.7 Gibbons, J.D. (1993) *Nonparametric Statistics: an Introduction*. Newbury Park, CA: Sage. ISBN 0803939515 References

Book provides the specific methodology and logical rationale for many of the most frequently used non-parametric statistics, applicable for both small and large sample sizes.

2.80.8 Hinton, P.R. (1995) *Statistics Explained: a Guide for Social Science Students*. London: Routledge. ISBN 0415102863

Book outlines the major statistical tests used by undergraduates in psychology and the social sciences. Easy-to-understand explanations of how and why they are used are given. Book also helps students to understand the results of statistical analysis by computer.

2.80.9 Hooke, R. (1983) *How to Tell the Liars from the Statisticians*. New York: Marcel Dekker. ISBN 0824718178

Without using any mathematical calculations, this guide spotlights the effects of statistical reasoning and its misuse. It highlights the fascination of statistics and their value in decision-making. Seventy-six mini-essays, on a very wide range of topics, point out statistically incorrect arguments and dubious inferences. Illustrations are included which feature key points.

2.80.10 Huff, D. (1991) *How to Lie with Statistics*. Harmondsworth, Middlesex: Penguin. ISBN 0140136290 No references

Discusses ways in which statistics are used to deceive. Everyday examples are used to expose 'the preposterous religion of our time'.

2.80.11 Jaeger, R.M. (1990) *Statistics* 2nd edition. Beverly Hills, CA: Sage. ISBN 0803934211 References

Designed for those who want to understand rather than compute statistics. No equations, which can sometimes obscure the meaning of the subject, are included. Illustrations are provided from educational research and evaluation studies. Each chapter is summarized and contains example problems (CR 2.2, 2.20, 2.54, 2.81, 2.82).

2.80.12 Knapp, B.G. (1989) *Basic Statistics for Nurses* 2nd edition. New York: Delmar. ISBN 0827342713 References

Book is intended for undergraduate nursing students as an introductory statistics text. The emphasis is on teaching students to be consumers of research and not statisticians. Each chapter includes an overview, detailed objectives, worked examples and solutions taken from many nursing settings, exercises and a summary. A new chapter in this edition enables students to select the most appropriate statistical test in relation to the research question being asked.

2.80.13 Knapp, T.R. (1996) *Learning Statistics through Playing Cards*. Thousand Oaks, CA: Sage. ISBN 0761901094

Book aims to teach statistics in a non-threatening way using a deck of cards.

2.80.14 Lewis, J.P. (1998) *Statistics Explained*. Don Mills, Ontario: Addison-Wesley Longman Inc. ISBN 0201178028

2.80.15 Moore, D.S. (1996) *Statistics, Concepts and Controversies* 4th edition. New York: W.H. Freeman. ISBN 071672863X References

Book gives insights and ideas rather than statistical techniques. Its aim is to give non-mathematical readers an aid to clear thinking when collecting data, organizing it and drawing conclusions. One hundred and fifty new exercises are included, together with reviews at the end of each chapter. Examples have been updated and an expanded section on data analysis is included (CR 2.79).

2.80.16 Moroney, M.J. (1990) *Facts from Figures*. Harmondsworth, Middlesex: Penguin. ISBN 0140135405 References

Provides a 'tool-kit' of essential statistical techniques. Limitations and dangers of misuse are discussed and examples given.

2.80.17 Munro, B.H. (1997) *Statistical Methods for Health Care Research* 3rd edition. Philadelphia: Lippincott-Raven. ISBN 039755365X

Book demonstrates the best way to read, analyse and write up nursing research results. Practical solutions address real challenges and computer printouts are used for illustration. Exercises are given to enhance learning and a free disk with data sets will help with the application of statistical approaches (CR 2.2).

2.80.18 Pett, M.A. (1997) *Non-parametric Statistics in Health Care Research: Statistics for Small Samples and Unusual Distributions*. Thousand Oaks, CA: Sage. ISBN 0803970390 References

Gives a comprehensive overview of the uses of non-parametric tests, the process of hypothesis testing, the character of data, assumptions and violations of parametric tests. Practical examples are given from the fields of health and social care research and tables enable students to select the most appropriate test.

2.80.19 Phillips, J.L. Jr. (1995) *How to Think about Statistics* 5th edition. New York: Freeman. ISBN 0716722879 References

Book is intended for those without prior statistical knowledge and may be suitable for use in courses with a broad content. It may also be useful as a self-teaching tool for a course which focuses on statistics. The emphasis is on the logical structure of statistical thinking, rather than techniques of data manipulation. Fundamental concepts are introduced using concrete examples. Sample applications and their solutions are also included.

2.80.20 Rowntree, D. (1991) *Statistics without Tears: a Primer for Non-mathematicians*. Harmondsworth, Middlesex: Penguin. ISBN 0140136320 References

Intended for the non-mathematical reader and is a 'tutorial in print'. The basic concepts of statistics are illustrated by means of words and diagrams rather than by figures, formulae and equations. Questions are included at frequent intervals so that students can test their understanding of the concepts.

2.80.21   Sirkin, R.M. (1994) *Statistics for the Social Sciences*. Thousand Oaks, CA: Sage. ISBN 0803951450   References

A book on statistical analysis at an elementary level. Topics include the scientific method, levels of measurement and the interpretation of tables. Discusses how statistics relate to the larger field of research methodology (CR 2.8).

2.80.22   Swinscow, T.D.V. (Revised by Campbell, M.J.) (1996) *Statistics at Square One* 9th edition. London: British Medical Journal Publishing. ISBN 0727909169 References

Provides step-by-step instruction on the basic tools of the statistician. This new edition includes methods adapted for pocket calculators together with commonly asked questions with answers.

2.80.23   Wright, D.B. (1996) *Understanding Statistics: an Introduction for the Social Sciences*. London: Sage. ISBN 0803979185

Book describes the most popular statistical techniques, explains their principles and use in a wide range of social research. The theoretical relationship between statistics and research is explained, t-tests are described in detail, together with the three main families of tests – regression, analysis of variance and two-variable tests. A guide is also given to more advanced techniques.

2.81   Descriptive Statistics

The aim of descriptive statistics is to summarize in precise, standard ways, the characteristics and measurements of a sample.

Definition

Descriptive statistics – methods of summarizing large quantities of data so that patterns and relationships within the data may be seen, as distinct from statistical methods of hypothesis testing

Annotations

2.81.1   Clark, E. (1990) Making sense of descriptive statistics. *Nursing Standard*, 8 August, 4 (44) 36–41   8 References

Discusses use of descriptive statistics and covers some of the tests which may be used.

2.81.2   Hallett, C. (1997) The use of descriptive statistics in nursing research. *Nurse Researcher*, 4 (4) 4–16   18 References

Discusses the value of using descriptive statistics for analysing and presenting large and complex sets of data. They fulfil some purposes of both quantitative and qualitative research, offering techniques for handling figures generated in quantitative studies and means for expressing data in a descriptive, diagrammatic or pictorial manner (CR 2.29, 2.36, 2.94).

2.81.3   Miller, H. (1995) *Descriptive Statistics*. Edinburgh: Churchill Livingstone. ISBN 0443053413

Book forms part of an open learning series. Each section contains an introduction, objectives, text, activities, commentaries, examples and a summary.

2.82   Inferential Statistics

In many instances in research there is a need to do more than just describe data, and inferential statistics provide a means for drawing conclusions about a sample drawn from the population. Researchers are then able to make judgements, or generalize, about a large class of individuals based on the information gained from a limited number.

Definition

Inferential statistics – statistics used for hypothesis testing and prediction

Annotation

2.82.1   Brown, J.K., Porter, L.A. & Knapp, T.R. (1993) The applicability of sequential analysis to nursing research. *Nursing Research*, 42 (5) 280–2   17 References

Summarizes the basic principles of sequential hypothesis testing, its applications and disadvantages (CR 2.20).

and fluctuations that occur in nurses' work and personal lives, and can help explore conceptions and attitudes about work (CR 2.25).

2.83 CHOOSING A STATISTICAL TEST

Many research textbooks listed in section 2.1 include sections on statistics, but few actually give direct guidance on how to select an appropriate test. Because of the increasingly easy access to computer software, students need more advice about which test to use, rather than how to undertake the calculations. Several texts included in section 2.80 also give some guidance.

Annotations

2.83.1   Knapp, B.G. (1989) Selection of an appropriate statistical test, in Author, *Basic Statistics for Nurses* 2nd edition. New York: Delmar. ISBN 0827342713   References

Chapter gives advice on choosing suitable statistical tests. Several examples with their solutions are provided, together with a flow chart (CR 2.80.12).

2.83.2   Riegelman, R.K. (1996) *Studying a Study and Testing a Test: How to Read the Health Science Literature.* Philadelphia: Lippincott-Raven. ISBN 0316745219 Part 4, Selecting a statistic, 203–53 References

A framework for selecting a statistic is suggested and three questions are used to provide this: What question is being asked by the statistical test being used? Is the method appropriate to the type of data being collected? Are the conclusions drawn from the statistical procedure appropriate? A summary is included in the form of flow charts.

2.83.3   Williams, C., Soothill, K. & Barry, J. (1991) Nursing: just a job? Do statistics tell us what we think? *Journal of Advanced Nursing*, 16 (8) 910–19   5 References

Article examines a particular statistical technique called latent class analysis, and considers its validity and possible use in classifying elements in the complex world of nursing. Authors believe that it can allow for fluidity

2.84 USING COMPUTERS IN RESEARCH

Now that computer software is readily available researchers have the opportunity to assemble, correlate and present large amounts of both qualitative and quantitative data in sophisticated ways. Some programs are included here and further information may be found in Appendix A.

Annotations

2.84.1   Aljunid, S. (1996) Computer analysis of qualitative data: the use of Ethnograph. *Health Policy and Planning*, 11 (1) 107–11 4 References

Discusses the use of Ethnograph in analysing qualitative data. Author states that it is easy to use and needs little computer equipment. Weaknesses are that documents have to be rigorously prepared to meet its format and the printing option is limited. The absence of an online document when coding and some degree of incompatibility with word processors in quoting the retrieved section is also noted (CR 2.36, 2.86, Appendix A).

2.84.2   Brown, R.A. & Beck, J.S. (1996) *Medical Statistics on Personal Computers* 2nd edition. London: British Medical Journal Publishing. ISBN 0727907719   References

Authors show how to get the best out of software available for analysing statistical data. New chapters include survival analysis, statistical power calculations, writing up medical papers and notes on available packages.

2.84.3   Bryman, A. & Cramer, D. (1996) *Quantitative Data Analysis with Minitab: a Guide for Social Scientists.* London: Routledge. ISBN 0415123240   References

Using a non-technical approach, this book explains statistical tests for Minitab users (CR Appendix A).

2.84.4   Burnard, P. (1992) The free form

database programme as a research tool. *Nurse Education Today*, 12 (1) 51–6 20 References

Describes two types of database programme for IBM-compatible personal computers – the fixed and free form. Uses for the latter are described for compiling bibliographical databases, content analysis of interview transcripts and other materials (CR 1.5, 2.68, 2.88).

2.84.5 Burnard, P. (1993) *Personal Computing for Health Professionals.* London: Chapman & Hall. ISBN 0412496704 References

An introductory text for health professionals which will encourage the development of personal computing skills. Advice is given on selecting and purchasing a computer, the organization of a hard disk, software, word processing, databases and spreadsheets in the health care context. The use of a personal computer for writing essays, projects, reports or books is discussed, together with its value in the organization, analysis and reporting of research. Appendices provide further information (CR 2.2).

2.84.6 Burnard, P. (1994) Using a database program to handle qualitative data. *Nurse Education Today*, 14 (3) 228–31 6 References

Paper describes use of the program File Express to store and organize qualitative research data. The advantages and disadvantages of this approach to data organization are discussed (CR 2.86).

2.84.7 Burnard, P. (1995) Tips and traps in using computers for research, in Author, *Health Care Computing: a Survival Guide for PC Users*. London: Chapman & Hall. ISBN 0412605309 Chapter 10, 173–97 References

Author offers advice on the value and problems inherent in using computers at various stages of the research process. Information is given on using a word processor to analyse textual data (CR 2.88, 2.89).

2.84.8 Buston, K. (1997) NUD*IST in action: its use and usefulness in a study of chronic illness in young people. *Sociological Research Online*, 2 (3) URL: <http://www.socresonline.org.uk/socresonline/2/3/6.html>

Paper describes the use of NUD*IST when studying the experiences of chronically ill children and assesses the epistemological effect of its use. Practical information is given on some of its functions and issues are raised in the CAQDAS debate (CR 2.86, Appendix A).

2.84.9 Davidson, F. (1996) *Principles of Statistical Data Handling*. Thousand Oaks, CA: Sage. ISBN 0761901035 References

Book explores the principles of data handling and how to make better use of computer data in research or study. It shows how to input, manipulate and debug data to make analysis easier and more accurate. Using a series of principles, problems or situations are presented and the author suggests how they might be resolved. The implementation of each principle is demonstrated as it appears in the command language of SAS and SPSS (Statistical Package for the Social Sciences) (CR Appendix A).

2.84.10 Davis, C., Davis, B.D. & Burnard, P. (1997) Use of the QSR NUD*IST computer programme to identify how clinical midwife mentors view their work. *Journal of Advanced Nursing*, 26 (4) 833–9 30 References

Examines ways in which computer program QSR NUD*IST (Non-numerical unstrutured data indexing, searching and theory building) can be used to analyse qualitative data. Data from a study where clinical midwife mentors were interviewed is used for illustration. An account is given of analysing the data with reference to the literature, and how the programme was used to analyse it a second time. A description is given of how it functions, using the textual data as an example. The use of computers in general for analysing qualitative data is discussed together with their advantages and disadvantages (CR 2.86, 2.88, Appendix A).

2.84.11 Durkin, T. (1997) Using computers in strategic qualitative research, in Miller, G. & Dingwall, R. (eds), *Context and Method in Qualitative Research*. London: Sage. ISBN 0803976321 Part II, Chapter 7, 92–105 References

Author considers how qualitative researchers may incorporate computer-based analyses into their studies. The opportunities and pitfalls of using computer software in qualitative research are critically examined and practical advice is given on how to choose the most appropriate packages (CR 2.36.40, 2.86).

2.84.12 Einspruch, E.L. (1998) *An Introductory Guide to SPSS for Windows*. Thousand Oaks, CA: Sage. ISBN 0761900012 References

Book aims to enable readers to become proficient in using SPSS. All aspects of creating, running, using, manipulating and analysing data are covered (CR Appendix A).

2.84.13 Fielding, N.G. & Lee, R.M. (eds) (1991) *Using Computers in Qualitative Research*. Newbury Park, CA: Sage. ISBN 0803984251 References

Profiles and compares the principal programmes available for analysing qualitative data, identifying their strengths and limitations. Ways are suggested as to how computer-based techniques may be incorporated into research methods training (CR 2.36, 2.42, 3.17).

2.84.14 Fielding, N.G. & Lee, R.M. (1998) *Qualitative Research on Computers*. Thousand Oaks, CA: Sage. ISBN 0803974833

2.84.15 Francis, I. *Statistical Software: a Comparative Review*. Reprint. Ann Arbor, MI: Books on Demand ISBN 0608174734

Book presents a taxonomy of statistical software with broad comparisons being made rather than in-depth evaluations. Packages are grouped under the following programme headings: data management, editing, tabulation, survey variance estimation, survey analysis, general statistics, specific purpose interactive batch, multiway contingency table analysis, econometric and time series and mathematical sub-routine libraries. Each package is introduced and its capabilities are listed. Its extensibility, proposed improvements, sample job, developers' names and addresses, computer makes, interfaced language, source language, cost and documentation are all identified. [Annotation refers to 1981 edition.]

2.84.16 Gahan, C. & Hannibal, M. (1997) *Doing Qualitative Research Using QSR NUD*IST*. London: Sage. ISBN 0761953906

Book provides a practical guide to the latest version of QSR NUD*IST (Version 4.0), a software package for development, support and management of qualitative data analysis. Taking the users' perspective, the software is presented as a set of tools for approaching a range of research issues. The key stages in carrying out qualitative data analysis are described, together with how to code, index and search the data. Practical exercises are included (CR 2.86, Appendix A).

2.84.17 Healey, J.F., Babbie, E.R. & Halley, F. (1997) *Exploring Social Issues Using SPSS for Windows*. Thousand Oaks, CA: Pine Forge Press. ISBN 0761985263 References

Book includes information on using SPSS (Statistical Package for the Social Sciences) in its Windows version. A self-contained package guides students step by step through all exercises, and research reports follow a standardized, fill-in-the-blank format for presenting and analysing results (CR Appendix A).

2.84.18 Kelle, U. (1995) *Computer-aided Qualitative Data Analysis: Theory, Methods and Practice*. London: Sage. ISBN 0803977611 References

2.84.19 Kirby, K.N. (1993) *Advanced Data Analysis with SYSTAT*. New York: Van Nostrand Reinhold. ISBN 0442308604

Bridges the gap between statistics texts and SYSTAT manuals and provides step by step instructions for carrying out complete data analysis (CR 2.80).

2.84.20 Lewando-Hundt, G., Beckerieg, S., El Alem, A. & Abed, Y. (1997) Comparing manual with software analysis in qualitative research: undressing NUD*IST. *Health Policy and Planning*, 12 (4) 372–80 16 References

Authors review the differences and similarities between using manual and software analysis. The aim was to establish the relative ease of each method, examine to what extent the analysis was facilitated by either method and if both could be used as a means of testing the internal validity of qualitative analysis by two different people. The study from which the data was collected is described and their conclusions are reported. Software is best seen as an aid and support but it does not replace conceptual thinking (CR 2.25, Appendix A).

2.84.21 Lewins, A. (1996) The CAQDAS networking project: multi-level support for the qualitative research community. *Qualitative Health Research*, 6 (2) 298–303 2 References

Describes the background to this project which aimed to encourage debate and disseminate information concerning the use of computer assistance in qualitative data analysis in the social and behavioural sciences. Information on software development, online resources, seminars, training and support services is given (CR 2.86).
URL: http://www.soc.surrey.ac.uk/caqdas/

2.84.22 Morison, M. & Moir, J. (1998) The role of computer software in the analysis of qualitative data: efficient clerk, research assistant or Trojan horse? *Journal of Advanced Nursing*, 28 (9) 106–16   39 References

Paper aims to assist researchers considering the use of computer software to assess the consequences and be aware of how the analytical process may be changed. The role of CAQDAS (computer-assisted qualitative data analysis networking project) is discussed (CR 2.86).

2.84.23 Moseley, L. & Mead, D. (1992) The integration of a database and a statistical programme in the analysis of a large scale survey in nursing. *Nursing Practice*, 5 (3) 23–8 4 References

Reports the analysis of a large-scale survey of the use of primary nursing care models in hospitals in Wales. A statistical package and database were both used to utilize the advantages of both (CR 2.52, 2.66, 2.75).

2.84.24 Pateman, B. (1998) Computer-aided qualitative data analysis: the value of NUD*IST and other programs. *Nurse Researcher*, 5 (3) 77–89   19 References

Author examines the arguments for and against using computer programs for qualitative data analysis and reports his personal experience of using QSR NUD*IST in a small study (CR Appendix A).

2.84.25 Ryan, B.F., Joiner, B.L. & Ryan, T.A. Jr. (1992) *MINITAB Handbook* 3rd edition. Boston, MA: PWS-Kent Publishing Co. ISBN 0534933661   References

Book is designed to be used with MINITAB, a general-purpose statistical system. It emphasizes aspects of statistics particularly suitable for computer use, and includes many examples and exercises (CR Appendix A).

2.84.26 Saba, V.K. & McCormick, K.A. (1995) *Essentials of Computers for Nurses* 2nd edition. Maidenhead, Berks: McGraw-Hill. ISBN 0071054189 Chapter 14, Research applications, 330–61   References

Six major uses of computers in nursing research are discussed: information retrieval, data processing, statistical analysis, graphic displays, database management systems and text editing. Examples of computer usage in clinical nursing research are given. Issues which need to be considered are given and suggestions are made for hands-on experiences. Objectives and study questions are included. Book contains a glossary of computer terms (CR 2.94).

2.84.27 Scolari. (1997) *QSR NUD* IST 4.0* London: Sage Publications Software.
URL: http://www.scolari.co.uk (for information or to download a demonstration copy)

QSR NUD*IST provides software for the development, support and management of qualitative data analysis (QDA) projects. QDA projects involve the analysis of unstructured data such as text from interviews, historical or legal documents, or non-textual documentary material such as videotapes, in order to analyse and understand this material (CR 2.46, 2.68, 2.72, 2.76, Appendix A).

2.84.28 Stine, R. & Fox, J. (eds) (1996) *Statistical Computing Environments for Social Research*. Thousand Oaks, CA: Sage. ISBN 0761902708

Book describes seven statistical computing environments – APL2STAT, GAUSS, Lisp-Stat, Mathematica, S, SAS/IML and Stata – which can be used in graphical and exploratory modelling.

2.84.29 Walker, B.L. (1993) Computer analysis of qualitative data: a comparison of three packages. *Qualitative Health Research*, 3 (1) 91–111   13 References

Describes and compares three computer

programmes designed to assist in the analysis of narrative text. These are Ethnograph, GATOR and Martin. A particular study is used to describe the links between research purposes and programme capabilities, and the influence the latter may have on research methods or analysis (CR 2.86, Appendix A).

2.84.30 Weitzman, E. & Miles, M.B. (1995) *Computer Programs for Qualitative Data Analysis*. Thousand Oaks, CA: Sage. ISBN 0803955375

2.85 RESEARCH AND THE INTERNET

This section includes some of the literature relating to research and the Internet. It includes more general articles and specific ones will be found in individual sections. Further information may be found in section 1.8, electronic services.

Example

Miller, S., King, T., Lurie, P. & Choltz, P. (1997) Certified nurse-midwife and physician collaborative practice: piloting a survey on the Internet. Preliminary findings of this study were presented at the University of California, San Francisco Antepartum and Intrapartum Management Conference, 9 June 1995. *Journal of Nurse-Midwifery*, 42 (4) 308–15   36 References

A pilot study was designed to describe the clinical areas of collaboration, financial structures and sources of conflict for nurse-midwives involved in nurse-midwife/physician practice. A questionnaire was posted on an electronic bulletin board. Results are reported (CR 2.15, 2.23, 2.52, 2.75).

Annotations

2.85.1 Anthony, D. (1994) The nursing net: using the systems. *Nurse Researcher*, 2 (2) 84–91   8 References

Explores the value for nurses of using e-mail, news groups, file transfer, remote access,

Gopher, and the World Wide Web to obtain and share information.

2.85.2 Farmer, J. & Richardson, A. (1997) Information for trained nurses in remote areas: do electronically networked resources provide an answer? *Health Libraries Review*, 14 (2) 97–103   11 References

Paper reports a research project which examined the potential of the Internet, and other networked resources, to improve access for nurses in remote areas. A review of current literature in the field is also discussed. Authors believe that access to these resources is of considerable value but training in their use is also necessary (CR 2.12).

2.85.3 Fawcett, J. & Buhle, E.L. (1995) Using the Internet for data collection: an innovative electronic strategy. *Computers in Nursing*, 13 (6) 273–9   22 References

Article describes an innovative strategy for data collection using computer network forums on the Internet. The success of this strategy is illustrated by a report of the results of a survey of the needs and coping mechanisms of cancer survivors (CR 2.52, 2.64).

2.85.4 Fleiaas, J. (1998) Spinning tales from the WWW: qualitative research in an electronic environment. *Qualitative Health Research*, 8 (2) 283–92   4 References

Author describes the process of using qualitative research strategies to gather data from a web-based project which examined the stories of children with serious health problems. Barriers that were encountered are discussed, together with strategies employed to solve them (CR 2.36, 2.64).

2.85.5 Hardey, M. (1996) Research, innovation and practice: the role of the World Wide Web. *Nursing Standard Online*, 11 (11), 4 December URL: http://www.nursing-standard.co.uk/vol11-11/ol-art.htm   23 References

Author believes that the World Wide Web is not only a more economical way to disseminate information than the traditional text, but is particularly suitable for nursing as a discipline. The role of hypermedia, electronic journals and their future are all discussed.

2.85.6 Korn, K. (1996) Computer comments.

Nursing research on the information super-highway. *Journal of the American Academy of Nurse Practitioners*, 8 (12) 587–8   4 References

2.85.7   Lakeman, R. (1997) 'Using the Internet for data collection in nursing research.' Presented as a paper at a qualitative research conference for health researchers held at the Eastern Institute of Technology, Taradale, New Zealand, January 1997. *Computers in Nursing*, 15 (5) 269–75   14 References

Article describes how the Internet may be used as a tool for data collection in nursing research. An overview of the Internet population is outlined and discussed as a constraint on the type of research that can be undertaken. The use of e-mail and World Wide Web questionnaires are discussed, as is the possibility of virtual focus groups. Some of the advantages and disadvantages of using the Internet for these purposes are outlined (CR 2.64, 2.69, 2.75).

2.85.8   Murray, P.J. (1995a) Connecting points. Using the Internet for gathering data and conducting research: faster than mail, cheaper than the phone. *Computers in Nursing*, 13 (5) 206, 208–9   5 References

Reports that so far little has been published in the nursing literature about the issues involved in using computer-mediated communications for research. Three examples are given of ways in which researchers have actually used the medium (CR 2.64).

2.85.9   Murray, P.J. (1995b) Research data from cyberspace: interviewing nurses by e-mail. *Health Informatics*, 1 (2) 73–6   21 References

Paper discusses the use of e-mail as a means of interviewing research subjects. The author's experiences in using this method outlines the problems and advantages of this medium (CR 2.85).

2.85.10   Murray, P.J. (1996) Research and the Internet: some practical and ethical issues. *Nursing Standard Online*, 10 (28), 3 April
URL: http://www.nursing-standard.co.uk /week28/ol-art.htm   8 References

Paper briefly discusses some of the issues that nurses undertaking research via the Internet,

whether they are clinically-based nurse researchers, students or educators, may like to consider. Ethical issues are also discussed (CR 2.17).

2.85.11   Prohaska, J.L. & Chang, B.L. (1996) Computer use and nursing research. Using the Internet to enhance nursing knowledge and practice. *Western Journal of Nursing Research*, 18 (3) 365–70   4 References

Article provides a basic description of the Internet and its many uses for nurses who may be beginners in the language of electronic networks.

2.85.12   Pulzer, M. (1996) Research technology: the Internet. *Modern Midwife*, 6 (10) 30–1   No references

Article outlines the opportunities modern technology offers to the time-pressed midwife-researcher.

2.85.13   Royle, J.A., Blythe, J., DiCenso, A., Baumann, A. & Fitzgerald, D. (1997) Do nurses have the information resources and skills for research utilization? *Canadian Journal of Administration*, 10 (3) 9–30   36 References

Reports a study which aimed to assess existing information sources, the information management skills of nurses and what additional resources and training are required in hospitals in two regions of Ontario. Sixty-nine respondents, who were vice-presidents or directors of nursing, agreed that nurses need better information resources and skills to access and evaluate professional literature. The Internet provides the potential for sharing resources and expertise (CR 2.95, 3.17).

2.85.14   Soetikno, R.M., Mrad, R., Pao, V. & Lenert, L.A. (1997) Quality of life research on the Internet: feasibility and potential biases in patients with ulcerative colitis. *Journal of the American Informatics Association*, 4 (6) 426–35   18 References

Reports an online survey for patients with ulcerative colitis and those who had undergone surgery for the condition. Its aim was to establish the feasibility and validity of this approach by using self-administered questionnaires to study the effects of the disease on the quality of life. To understand how people on the World Wide Web might differ from those in practice, and the potential biases in conducting epidemiological research in volunteers recruited on the Internet, respondents were compared with those in a surgical practice. Results are reported (CR 2.25, 2.27, 2.41, 2.75).

2.85.15 Warburton, B. (1996) Research technology: electronic mail. *Modern Midwife*, 6 (11) 30–1 1 Reference

Author explains how researchers are increasingly turning to e-mail to track down information and communicate with others in their field.

2.86 ANALYSING QUALITATIVE DATA

Qualitative data are frequently expressed in words and the researcher must organize this material into groups and patterns in order to understand its meaning. Some qualitative data will also lend itself to description through the use of measures of central tendency, dispersion and correlation coefficients. Several computer programs are now available. Some are documented here, others in section 2.84 and Appendix A.

Definitions

Constant comparison – a procedure used in qualitative research wherein newly collected data are compared in an ongoing fashion with data collected earlier, to refine theoretically relevant categories

Qualitative analysis – the organization and interpretation of non-numerical information for the purpose of discovering important underlying dimensions and patterns of relationships

Qualitative metasynthesis – . . . the theories, grand narratives, generalizations, or interpretative translations produced from the integration or comparison of findings from qualitative studies

---

Annotations

2.86.1 Appleton, J.V. (1995) Analyzing qualitative interview data: addressing issues of validity and reliability. *Journal of Advanced Nursing*, 22 (5) 993–7 24 References

Describes the steps taken in one qualitative research study which explored the health visitor's role with vulnerable families to address the issues of validity and reliability (CR 2.24, 2.25, 2.36, 2.68).

2.86.2 Atkinson, S. & Abu El Haj, M. (1996) Domain analysis for qualitative public health data. *Health Policy and Planning*, 11 (4) 438–42 8 References

Authors describe an approach to analysing the content of qualitative data, based on the identification within the data content of key topics, referred to as domains, and the relationships between them. The method presented was used with open interviews but is applicable to any unstructured source of data (CR 2.36, 2.68).

2.86.3 Ball, M.S. & Smith, G.W.H. (1992) *Analyzing Visual Data*. Newbury Park, CA: Sage. ISBN 0803934351 References

The major form of visual presentation addressed by this book is the still photograph. Chapters cover the use of photographs in disciplines of words: anthropology, ethnography and sociology. Analysing the content of visual representations, symbolist and structuralist analyses and the social organization of visual experiences are all discussed (CR 2.42, 2.72, 2.88).

2.86.4 Bryman, A. & Burgess, R.G. (eds) (1995) *Analyzing Qualitative Data*. London: Routledge. ISBN 0415060621 References

A group of experienced researchers explore and explain the ways in which they have analysed qualitative data. Examples are given from ethnographers, case-study workers, lone researchers, team-based investigators and specialist approaches, including discourse analysis (CR 2.36, 2.39, 2.42, 2.89).

2.86.5 Burnard, P. (1991) A method of analysing interview data in qualitative research. *Nurse Education Today*, 11 (6) 461–6 9 References

Outlines the use of one method, thematic content analysis, for analysing qualitative interview data. Fourteen stages are described and questions of validity are addressed (CR 2.25, 2.68, 2.88).

2.86.6 Burnard, P. (1992) Some problems in understanding other people: analysing talk in research, counselling and psychotherapy. *Nurse Education Today*, 12 (2) 130–6 20 References

Discusses problems in analysing interview transcripts, including hidden agendas, subject's 'mood' during the interview, use of words, personal and public meanings, metaphors and categories (CR 2.68, 2.78).

2.86.7 Burnard, P. (1994) Searching for meaning: a method of analysing interview transcripts with a personal computer. *Nurse Education Today*, 14 (2) 111–17 13 References

Paper describes a method of focusing on meaning units as the basis of developing and categorizing systems for the analysis of interview transcripts. The use of Word Perfect is described (CR 2.68, 2.70, 2.88).

2.86.8 Burnard, P. (1995) Unspoken meanings: qualitative research and multi-media analysis. *Nurse Researcher*, 3 (1) 55–64 17 References

The shortcomings of interviews, transcription and textual analysis as qualitative research methods are examined (CR 2.68, 2.84, 2.89).

2.86.9 Coffey, A. & Atkinson, P. (1996) *Making Sense of Qualitative Data*. Thousand Oaks, CA: Sage. ISBN 0803970536 References

Describes and illustrates a number of approaches to analysing qualitative data.

2.86.10 Dey, I. (1993) *Qualitative Data Analysis: a User-friendly Guide for Social Scientists*. London: Routledge. ISBN 041505852X References

Book aims to fill the gap in texts on qualitative data analysis. It is written for undergraduates and postgraduates who need to handle data-using computers. A variety of ways in which computers can be used are discussed, providing background knowledge and learning experiences. Hypersoft is used as the medium through which methodological problems can be approached. Appendix 2 provides details of Hypersoft (CR 2.84).

2.86.11 Feldman, M.S. (1994) *Strategies for Interpreting Qualitative Data*. Thousand Oaks, CA: Sage. ISBN 0803959168 References

Book outlines four key strategies for interpreting qualitative data: ethnomethodology, semiotics, dramaturgy and deconstruction. The strengths and weaknesses of each are identified and author suggests when they may best be used. The techniques of each method are applied to a single data set by way of illustration and the differences are highlighted (CR 2.42, 2.89).

2.86.12 Fielding, N.G. & Fielding, J.L. (1986) *Linking Data*. Beverly Hills, CA: Sage. ISBN 0803925182 References

Book concentrates on techniques for linking and analysing data obtained from both qualitative and quantitative research methods (CR 2.29, 2.36, 2.87).

2.86.13 Hamill, C. & McAleer, J. (1996) Analysing qualitative data using a software package. *Nurse Researcher*, 4 (1) 70–8 14 References

Author describes the use of Ethnograph software which can assist in analysing large amounts of qualitative data. One disadvantage is that it operates in a DOS environment (CR 2.36, 2.84, Appendix A).

2.86.14 Hammersley, M. (1997) Qualitative data archiving: some reflections on its prospects and problems. *Sociology*, 31 (1) 131–42 41 References

Discusses two important functions that archiving can serve: facilitating the process of assessing research findings and providing a basis for secondary analysis, both as a supplement to primary data and as a basis for extensive historical or comparative studies (CR 2.36, 2.76, 2.90, 2.91).

2.86.15 Henderson, N.R. (1995) A practical approach to analysing and reporting focus group studies: lessons from qualitative market research. *Qualitative Health Research*, 5 (4) 463–77 5 References

Article gives some insight into how a small qualitative research company analyses focus group data and prepares reports. Approaches and techniques used by other groups can assist nurses when using this method of data collection (CR 2.36, 2.69).

2.86.16 Hickey, G. & Kipping, C. (1996) A multi-stage approach to the coding of data from open-ended questions. *Nurse Researcher*, 4 (1) 81–91 7 References

An approach is outlined which involves the use of content analysis in open-ended questions. It is useful for coding large amounts of diverse data and can be adapted for use in other projects (CR 2.88).

2.86.17 Jensen, L.A. & Allen, M.N. (1996) Meta synthesis of qualitative findings. *Qualitative Health Research*, 6 (4) 553–60 16 References

Describes a framework for synthesizing qualitative findings and discusses issues surrounding the use of this technique. The practical importance of interpretative meta-synthesis is discussed in relation to theory development (CR 2.7).

2.86.18 Miles, M.B. & Huberman, A.M. (1994) *Qualitative Data Analysis: an Expanded Sourcebook* 2nd edition. Thousand Oaks, CA: Sage. ISBN 0803955405 References

A practical sourcebook for all researchers who make use of qualitative data. Strong emphasis is put on new types of data displays and 49 methods are described and illustrated, with practical suggestions for their use. This new edition includes an appendix giving criteria for choosing from available software (CR 2.83, 2.94).

2.86.19 Minnick, A., Roberts, M.J., Young, W.B., Kleinpell, R.M. & Micek, W. (1995) An analysis of post-hospitalization telephone survey data. *Nursing Research*, 44 (6) 371–5 9 References

Article describes response-rate differences and reasons for non-participation among 4,600 adults taking part in a study of care outcomes by gender, age, ethnicity and race. Issues relating to obtaining data from telephone interviews are discussed (CR 2.52, 2.70).

2.86.20 Morrison, P. & Bauer, I. (1993) A clinical application of the multiple sorting technique. *International Journal of Nursing Studies*, 30 (6) 511–18 33 References

Paper gives an example of using the multiple sorting technique for structuring and analysing qualitative interviews (CR 2.68).

2.86.21 Northcott, N. (1996) Cognitive mapping: an approach to qualitative data analysis. *NT Research*, 1 (6) 456–64 26 References

Discusses the use of cognitive mapping as a way of handling a large quantity of qualitative data. Material obtained from a case study, generated from audio-recorded interviews, is used for illustration (CR 2.39, 2.68).

2.86.22 Pearson, P. (1997) Integrating qualitative and quantitative analysis. *Nurse Researcher*, 4 (3) 69–80 21 References

Using two examples where both quantitative and qualitative data have been examined, the author discusses the advantages and some of the problems of integrating these data (CR 2.29, 2.36, 2.87).

2.86.23 Richards, T.J. & Richard, L. (1994) Using computers in qualitative research, in Denzin, N.K. & Lincoln, Y.S. (eds), *Handbook of Qualitative Research*. Thousand Oaks, CA: Sage. ISBN 0803946791 Chapter 28, 445–62 39 References

Chapter examines the methodological features of qualitative data analysis to consider how, how much and how well it can be computerized. An overview is given of general-purpose and special packages, their value and how they may be used. Pointers to future software development are provided in order to stimulate methodological debate. Nine software packages are listed (CR 2.36.13, 2.84).

2.86.24 Riley, J. (1996) *Getting the Most from Your Data: a Handbook of Practical Ideas on How to Analyze Qualitative Data*. Bristol: Technical and Educational Services. ISBN 0947885315

A practical text covering many ideas for the analysis of qualitative data.

2.86.25 Ross, K. (1994) Making sense of qualitative data, in Buckeldee, J. & McMahon, R. (eds), *The Research Experience in Nursing*. London: Chapman & Hall. ISBN 0412441101 Chapter 9, 131–46 10 References

Describes the analysis 'maze' experienced when investigating reasons for clinical practitioners changing their professional orientation and becoming nurse educationalists. Author discusses how she found a way through this difficulty (CR 2.16.4).

2.86.26 Russell, C.K. & Gregory, D.M. (1993) Issues for consideration when choosing a qualitative management system. *Journal of Advanced Nursing*, 18 (11) 1806–16 20 References

Paper presents major issues to researchers who are considering using computer or manual qualitative management systems. These include availability, accessibility, comfort, appropriateness, efficiency, thoroughness and contextualization. Appendix contains selected lists of qualitative computer programs and addresses. These are grouped under the following headings: database manager, text-retriever, structural analysis and theory-building programmes (CR 2.84).

2.86.27 Sandelowski, M., Docherty, S. & Emden, C. (1997) Focus on qualitative methods. Qualitative meta-synthesis: issues and techniques. *Research in Nursing and Health*, 20 (4) 365–71 47 References

Article considers the appropriateness and feasibility of attempting qualitative meta-synthesis. Several efforts to create such synthesis are discussed together with methodological issues.

2.86.28 Silverman, D. (1993) *Interpreting Qualitative Data: Methods for Analyzing Talk, Text and Interaction*. London: Sage. ISBN 0803987587 References

This text, which is based on worked-through examples and student exercises, spans the range of different approaches in the qualitative tradition. It focuses on the strengths of particular methodologies, observation, analysis and validity in qualitative research, ethnography, symbolic interactionism and conversational analysis. Ways in which communication can be studied through the analysis of interviews, texts and transcripts are described (CR 2.9, 2.24, 2.25, 2.36, 2.42, 2.68, 2.72, 2.89).

2.86.29 Silverman, D. (ed.) (1997) *Qualitative Research: Theory, Method and Practice*. London: Sage. ISBN 0803976666 References

Contributors to this book reflect on the analysis of observations, texts, talk and interviews. Key themes include the centrality of the relationship between analytic perspectives and methodological issues; the need to broaden our conception of qualitative research beyond issues of subjective 'meaning' towards issues of language; representation and social organization; searching for ways to build links between social science traditions and having a dialogue between social science and the community (CR 2.68, 2.72, 2.76, 2.78).

2.86.30 Stern, P.N. (1991) Are counting and coding appropriate in qualitative research?, in Morse, J.M. (ed.), *Qualitative Nursing Research: a Contemporary Dialogue* Revised edition. Newbury Park, CA: Sage. ISBN 0803940793 Chapter 9, 147–62 19 References

Chapter explores two questions: whether measuring data by counting with percentages or ratios, i.e. quantitative tools, have any place in qualitative designs, and whether investigation of a given situation can be trusted to code, form categories and general constructs alone, or whether they must be examined by a panel of experts (CR 2.29, 2.36).

2.86.31 Taft, L.B. (1993) Computer-assisted qualitative research. *Research in Nursing and Health*, 16 (5) 379–83 11 References

Article differentiates between mechanical and conceptual activities in qualitative analysis and discusses the interplay between them. Advantages of computer technology in data management and concerns about their use are discussed. Guidelines are given for their judicious application in qualitative research (CR 2.36, 2.84).

2.86.32 Twinn, S. (1997) An exploratory study examining the influence of translation on the validity and reliability of qualitative data in nursing research. *Journal of Advanced Nursing*, 26 (2) 418–23 25 References

Six Cantonese speakers were interviewed about their attitudes towards having Pap smears. The three stages of data analysis are described, together with the difficulties of translation where subtleties of language occurred. The implications of this are discussed (CR 2.24, 2.25, 2.68).

2.86.33 University of Surrey. (no date) CAQDAS networking project.
URL: http://www.soc.surrey.ac.uk/caqdas/biblio.htm

The computer-assisted data analysis software project, funded by the Economic and Social Research Council, aims to disseminate an understanding of the practical skills needed to use software which has been designed to assist qualitative data analysis. It provides demonstration versions of various qualitative analysis packages, information on short courses, a bibliography on computer software and information about the qual-software mailing list (CR 2.84).

2.86.34 Wainwright, S.P. (1994) Analysing data using grounded theory. *Nurse Researcher*, 1 (3) 43–9   9 References

Describes how use of grounded theory methods of analysis can inform interpretations of data from semi- and unstructured interviews (CR 2.45, 2.68).

2.86.35 Wise, C., Plowfield, L.A., Kahn, D.L. & Steeves, R.H. (1992) Using a grid for interpretation and presenting qualitative data. *Western Journal of Nursing Research*, 14 (6) 796–800   6 References

Discusses the use of a simple tool, the data grid, for displaying categories of data and assisting in their analysis (CR 2.94).

2.86.36 Yamaguchi, K. (1991) *Event History Analysis*. Newbury Park, CA: Sage. ISBN 080393324X   References

Provides a systematic introduction to models, methods and applications of event history analysis.

2.87 ANALYSING QUANTITATIVE DATA

Statistical tests enable quantitative data to be made meaningful and intelligible. Having chosen the appropriate test and carried it out, the researcher is then in a position to reduce, organize, evaluate, interpret and communicate the results. Descriptive and/or inferential statistics will be utilized, depending on the problem and data obtained.

Definitions

Exploratory data analysis – a type of statistical analysis that uses a special collection of largely graphical descriptive statistics for summary research findings

Quantitative data analysis – the manipulation of numerical data through statistical procedures for the purpose of describing phenomena or assessing the magnitude and reliability of relationships among them

Annotations

2.87.1 Aiken, L.S. & West, S.G. (1996) *Multiple Regression: Testing and Interpreting Interactions*. Newbury Park, CA: Sage. ISBN 0761907122   References

Book provides a clear set of prescriptions for estimating, testing and probing interactions in regression models. The latest research is also included.

2.87.2 Anthony, D. (1997) Regression analysis. *Nurse Researcher*, 4 (4) 54–62   5 References

Author explains how to carry out regression analysis which explores the possible relationship between two variables. Suitable statistical packages are also mentioned.

2.87.3 Beard, M.T., Edwards, K., Marshall, D. & Johnson, M.N. (1995) Research methodology: Part II, essentials for factor analysis. *ABNF Journal*, 6 (4) 107–12   5 References

Using a case-method presentation, the basic elements of factor analysis are described.

2.87.4 Brieger, W.R. (1994) Pile sorts as a means of improving the quality of survey data: malaria illness symptoms. *Health Education Research*, 9 (2) 257–60   9 References

Reports a trial which used the pile sort technique to strengthen quantitative survey data. Computer analysis with ANTHROPAC software improved the quality and enhanced its use for culturally appropriate discussions with patients and for health education programmes (CR 2.52, 2.84, Appendix A).

2.87.5 Bryman, A. & Cramer, D. (1995)

Quantitative Analysis for Social Scientists Revised edition. London: Routledge. ISBN 0415113075   References

Provides social science students with a non-technical introduction to the use of statistical techniques. The most up-to-date version of SPSS (Statistical Package for the Social Sciences) is used and no previous knowledge is assumed (CR Appendix A).

2.87.6   Diggle, P.J., Liang, K.-Y., & Zeger, S.L. (1994) *The Analysis of Longitudinal Data.* Oxford: Clarendon Press. ISBN 0198522843   References

Describes statistical models and methods for the analysis of longitudinal data (CR 2.48).

2.87.7   Ferketich, S.L. & Mercer, R.T. (1992) Aggregating family data. *Research in Nursing and Health*, 15 (4) 313–17 10 References

Describes problems with aggregation of data when only a small number of family members are used as respondents.

2.87.8   Firebaugh, G. (1997) *Analyzing Repeated Surveys.* Thousand Oaks, CA: Sage. ISBN 0803973985   References

Author explicates different methods for studying social change through analysing data from repeated surveys. Four basic uses are identified – description, decomposition, explanation of aggregate trends and assessment of changing individual parameters (CR 2.52).

2.87.9   Fox, J. (1991) *Regression Diagnostics: an Introduction.* Newbury Park, CA: Sage. ISBN 080393971X   References

Explains the techniques for exploring problems that compromise a regression analysis, and for deciding whether certain assumptions seem reasonable.

2.87.10   Fox, J. (1997) *Applied Regression Analysis, Linear Models, and Related Methods.* Thousand Oaks, CA: Sage. ISBN 080394540X   References

Using graphs and numerous examples using real data from the social sciences, this book considers the role of statistical data analysis in social research. Many topics are covered which will enable an appropriate analysis of data.

2.87.11   Hagenaars, J.A. (1990) *Categorical Longitudinal Data: Log-linear Panel, Trend and Cohort Analysis.* Newbury Park, CA: Sage. ISBN 0803929579   References

The problems which may occur with statistical analysis of longitudinal data are covered, together with solutions shown by actual examples. The tools developed over the last decade are discussed (CR 2.48, 2.86).

2.87.12   Hagle, T.M. (1996) *Basic Math for Social Scientists: Problems and Solutions.* Thousand Oaks, CA: Sage. ISBN 0803972857 References

Provides an introduction to basic mathematical problems in the quantitative analysis of social science data.

2.87.13   Hollis, S. (1994) Statistical analysis: not just 'p < 0.05'. *Nurse Researcher*, 1 (4) 48–67   7 References

Author explores and explains the intricacies of statistical analysis (CR 2.20).

2.87.14   LeFort, S.M. (1993) The statistical versus clinical significance debate. *Image: Journal of Nursing Scholarship*, 25 (1) 57–62 36 References

Paper compares and contrasts statistical and clinical significance to provide an overview of the issues surrounding their use, as described in methodological literature from a variety of disciplines. Some implications for nursing research are discussed.

2.87.15   Leik, R.K. (1997) *Experimental Design and the Analysis of Variance.* Thousand Oaks, CA: Sage. ISBN 0803990065 References

Book provides comprehensive coverage of the concepts behind ANOVA as well as its implementation. It emphasizes the importance of assisting students to understand the principles before embarking on computation.

2.87.16   Lewis-Beck, M. (ed.) (1994) *Factor Analysis and Related Techniques.* London: Sage/Toppan Company. ISBN 080395431X References

Book covers all aspects of factor analysis together with principal components. Also covered are confirmatory analysis and covariance structure models.

2.87.17 Lunsford, T.R. & Lunsford, B.R. (1996) Methodology: parametric data analysis. *Journal of Prosthetics and Orthotics,* 8 (2) 65–76 12 References

Presents the concepts involved in analysing parametric data.

2.87.18 Martens, P.J. (1995) A mini lesson in statistics: what causes treatment groups to be deemed 'not statistically different'? *Journal of Human Lactation,* 11 (2) 117–21 13 References

The null effects in research, which resulted from studies of the effects of artificial baby milk gift packs is discussed. Type I and Type II errors are explained and reasons for 'not statistically different' results are detailed.

2.87.19 Maruyama, G.M. (1997) *Basis of Structural Equation Modelling.* Thousand Oaks, CA: Sage. ISBN 0803974094 References

Through the use of narrative explanation, the author describes the logic underlying structural equation modelling (SEM) approaches. Its relationship to techniques like regressions and factor analysis is described, together with its strengths and weaknesses. Carefully constructed exercises are included.

2.87.20 Ottenbacher, K.J. (1995) Why rehabilitation research does not work (as well as we think it should). *Archives of Physical Medicine and Rehabilitation,* 76 (2) 123–9 39 References

Identifies three problems in the analysis and interpretation of investigations based on statistical testing of hypotheses, which have a bearing on the quest to establish effective rehabilitation research. Specific recommendations are made to improve the usefulness of quantitative research methods.

2.87.21 Polit, D.F. (1996a) *Data Analysis and Statistics for Nursing Research.* Stamford, CT: Appleton & Lange. ISBN 0838563295

Book is intended for nursing students undertaking a course on statistics and data analysis. It is written in a non-technical manner, assumes no prior knowledge and its emphasis is on understanding how to use and interpret statistics, not how to calculate them. Computer printouts are included to help students understand them, with actual and fictitious

examples being given. Each chapter is summarized and exercises are included (CR 2.2, 2.80).

2.87.22 Polit, D.F. (1996b) *Application Manual to Accompany Data Analysis and Statistics for Nursing Research.* Stamford, CT: Appleton & Lange. ISBN 0838563341

2.87.23 Rose, D. & Sullivan, O. (1996) *Introducing Data Analysis for Social Scientists* 2nd edition. Buckingham: Open University Press. ISBN 0335196179 References

This revised and updated edition assumes no previous knowledge of statistics or computer use and aims to assist students taking a first course in quantitative analysis. The principles of analysing these data are explained and a floppy disc of SPSS (Statistical Package for the Social Sciences) is included (CR Appendix A).

2.87.24 Tacq, J. (1997) *Multivariate Analysis Techniques in Social Science Research: from Problem to Analysis.* London: Sage. ISBN 076195273X References

Book gives a range of actual research examples in the social sciences to show how to make the most appropriate choice of technique. All classical multivariate techniques are covered. The step-by-step explanation works through each analysis both by calculation and by reproducing the computer output from SPSS for Windows. A summary is also included of all the statistical concepts needed for dealing with more advanced techniques (CR 2.83).

2.87.25 Toothaker, L.E. (1993) *Multiple Comparison for Researchers.* Newbury Park, CA: Sage. ISBN 0803941773 References

Discusses all aspects of multiple comparison procedures. These are: when they may be of value; types of procedures; comparisons between them; violations of assumptions and robustness; multiple comparisons for the two-way ANOVA; and factorial or randomized blocks.

2.87.26 Vermunt, J.K. (1997) *Log-linear Models for Event Histories.* Thousand Oaks, CA: Sage. ISBN 0761909370

Book presents a general approach to missing data problems in event history analysis, where this is based upon the similarities between log-linear, hazard and event history models.

2.87.27   Walsh, M. (1988) Beyond statistical significance. *Applied Nursing Research*, 1 (2) 101–3   10 References

Article discusses the question of whether statistical significance is a necessary condition for clinical significance. When caring for people it is not so much the 'average' difference that is of interest, but rather the individual's difference.

2.87.28   Weisberg, H.F. (1991) *Central Tendency and Variability*. Newbury Park, CA: Sage. ISBN 0803940076   References

Book covers levels of measurement, measures of centre and spread, and shows how to generalize sample results to the population. The use of exploratory data analysis is also discussed (CR 2.28).

ANALYSIS OF DATA

2.88   CONTENT ANALYSIS

'Recorded words and sentences provide rich and varied sources of data about people and the contexts in which they live. In order to use these data, objective and systematic procedures need to be employed to render them valid and reliable' (Waltz, Strickland & Lenz, 1984: 285).

Definition

Content analysis – a procedure for analysing written or verbal communications in a systematic and objective fashion, typically with the goal of quantitatively measuring variables

---

Example

Elliott, B.J. (1994) A content analysis of the health information in women's weekly magazines. *Health Libraries Review*, 11 (2) 96–103 12 References

Provides a descriptive analysis of the content, relating to health, in eight popular women's magazines over a four-week period.

Annotations

2.88.1   Burnard, P. (1994) Analyzing data using a word processor. *Nurse Researcher*, 1 (3) 33–42   15 References

Describes one way of analysing the content of textual material obtained during interviews using a word processor (CR 2.68, 2.84, 2.86).

2.88.2   Burnard, P. (1996) Teaching the analysis of textual data: an experiential approach. *Nurse Education Today*, 16 (4) 278–81   26 References

Paper offers a group method for teaching the analysis of textual data. Terms are defined, an outline for a preliminary theory input is given and the group method is described. Problems and variants of the method are also discussed.

2.88.3   Cavanagh, S. (1997) Content analysis: concepts, methods and applications. *Nurse Researcher*, 4 (3) 5–16   29 References

Discusses content analysis as a qualitative methodology, considerations about its use, assessing reliability and validity, and ways in which these data can be analysed (CR 2.24, 2.25, 2.86).

2.88.4   A Concept Dictionary of English with Computer Programs for Content Analysis. (1990) Edited by Laffal, J. Essex, CT: Gallery. ISBN 0913622060

Book is a thesaurus-type dictionary of over 42,000 words, classified into 168 concept categories. The development of the system is described and a number of applications in textual analysis is discussed. Several computer programs on diskette are provided (CR 2.89).

2.88.5   Kelly, A.W. & Sime, A.M. (1990) Language as research data: application of computer content analysis in nursing research. *Advances in Nursing Science*, 12 (3) 32–40   27 References

Discusses use of the Minnesota Contextual Content Analysis Program in categorizing, reducing data and interpreting manifest and latent meaning in linguistic communications (CR 2.84, 2.89).

2.88.6 Krippendorf, K. (1980) *Content Analysis: an Introduction to its Methodology.* Beverly Hills, CA: Sage. ISBN 0803914970 References

Intended for a fairly wide audience, this book can serve as a text and practical guide to content analysis in research contexts. An overview of the technique is given, together with a comprehensive discussion of the key elements which need to be considered when it is used. Chapters on computer-based content analysis techniques, reliability and validity are included (CR 2.24, 2.25, 2.84).

2.88.7 Mackenzie, J. (1994) Analysing data: alternative methods. *Nurse Researcher*, 1 (3) 50–6 11 References

Two approaches to content analysis are described, one from a pragmatic point of view and the other a more complex discussion of the methodological and philosophical issues involved (CR 2.68).

2.88.8 Morgan, D.L. (1993) Qualitative content analysis: a guide to paths not taken. *Qualitative Health Research*, 3 (1) 112–21 8 References

Author argues that qualitative content analysis is distinctive in its approach to coding and interpretation of counts from codes. Researchers need to consider carefully whether counting codes is an appropriate method of analysis (CR 2.9, 2.86, 2.89).

2.88.9 Moseley, L.G., Mead, D.M. & Murphy, F. (1997) Applying lexical and semantic analysis to the exploration of free-text data. *Nurse Researcher*, 4 (3) 46–68 19 References

Discusses the categorization of a large number of free-text responses by using a computer. A study of primary nursing provided the data, part of which was to understand the leadership styles of ward sisters (CR 2.84).

2.89 CONTEXTUAL/NARRATIVE ANALYSIS

'Contextual analysis assumes that objects, and most obviously words, have more in common, the more the context they are in is alike. Context means the linguistic environment of words or within data surroundings of a recording unit' (Krippendorf, 1980: 117). Both qualitative and quantitative analytical techniques may be used for these data.

Definitions

Contextual analysis – analysis which focuses on the individual's behaviour or attitudes, with reference to a group context
Contextualization – the placement of data into a larger perspective
Discourse analysis – a general term covering a wide variety of approaches to the analysis of recorded talk (sometimes used interchangeably with conversation analysis)
Network analysis – an efficient way of contextualizing actors' behaviour, based on description and inductive modelling of a specific aspect of this context: the relational pattern or 'structure' of the social setting in which action is observed
Semiotics – the study of signs and their meanings

Example

Jackson, D. (1995) Nursing texts and lesbian contexts: lesbian imagery in the nursing literature, *Australian Journal of Advanced Nursing*, 13 (1) 25–31 84 References

Using textual analysis, the paper locates and explains the images of lesbians which have been presented in introductory nursing texts. Problems associated with 'labelling' people are discussed and implications for scholarly practice are highlighted.

Annotations

2.89.1 Atkinson, P. & Coffey, A. (1997) Analyzing documentary realities, in Silverman, D. (ed.), *Qualitative Research: Theory,*

Method and Practice. London: Sage. ISBN 0803976666 Part III, Chapter 4, 45–62 21 References

Chapter applies theories, from literary theory of narrative and genre, to the documents through which organizations represent themselves and the records and documentary data they accumulate (CR 2.36.59).

2.89.2   Carley, K. (1993) Coding choices for textual analysis: a comparison of content analysis and map analysis, in Marsden, P.V. (ed.), *Sociological Methodology.* Oxford: Blackwell. ISBN 1557864640 Volume 23 75–126

Describes and compares content and map analysis, two procedures for coding and understanding texts.

2.89.3   Cortazzi, M. (1993) *Narrative Analysis.* London: Falmer Press. ISBN 1850009635 References

Book discusses the gathering and analysis of narrative material drawing on models within the disciplines of sociology, psychology, literature analysis and anthropology. Illustrations are made by quotations and analysis of teachers' narratives (CR 2.86).

2.89.4   Coulthard, M. (ed.) (1994) *Advances in Written Text Analysis.* London: Routledge. ISBN 0415095204   References

Provides an overview of approaches to written text analysis. It includes classic and specially commissioned papers containing a variety of foci. Examples used come from pure science, social science, academic journals, weekly magazines, newspapers and literary narrations.

2.89.5   Coyle, A. (1995) Discourse analysis, in Breakwell, G.M., Hammond, S. & Fife-Schaw, C. (eds), *Research Methods in Psychology.* London: Sage. ISBN 0803977654 Part III, Chapter 16, 243–58   References

Chapter covers assumptions and applications of discourse analysis, sampling discourse, techniques, working with data and its evaluation. Problems with discourse analysis are also highlighted (CR 2.1.8).

2.89.6   Heartfield, M. (1996) Nursing documentation and nursing practice: a discourse

analysis. *Journal of Advanced Nursing,* 24 (1) 98–103   26 References

Paper reports on a study which examined nursing documentation as nursing practice. A research design, discourse analysis, developed by Foucault, enables examination of how written descriptions of patient events, taken from the notes, result from hegemonic influences that construct a knowledge and therefore a practice of nursing.

2.89.7   Heath, C. (1997) The analysis of activities in face-to-face interaction using video, in Silverman, D. (ed.), *Qualitative Research: Theory, Method and Practice.* London: Sage. ISBN 0803976666. Part V, Chapter 12, 183–200   42 References

Chapter discusses the analysis of face-to-face interaction through video. An extended example of a medical consultation is used to illustrate the relevance of this technique to studies in the workplace, including human–computer interaction (CR 2.36.59, 2.72).

2.89.8   Heath, C. & Luff, P. (1993) Explicating face-to-face interaction, in Gilbert, N. (ed.), *Researching Social Life.* London: Sage. ISBN 0803986823 Chapter 15, 306–26 References

Chapter discusses the methodological considerations underlying conversational analysis, and the analytic orientations of recent work studying face-to-face interactions (CR 2.1.25).

2.89.9   Heritage, J. (1997) Conversation analysis and institutional talk: analyzing data, in Silverman, D. (ed.), *Qualitative Research: Theory, Method and Practice.* London: Sage. ISBN 0803976666 Part V, Chapter 11, 161–82 64 References

Chapter presents an introduction on how conversation analytic methods can be used in the analysis of institutional talk. An example of a short telephone conversation between a school employee and mother of a child who may be a truant is used for illustration (CR 2.36.59, 2.70).

2.89.10   Iverson, G.R. (1991) *Contextual Analysis.* Newbury Park, CA: Sage. ISBN 0803942729   References

Discusses contextual analysis, which examines the role of group content on actions and attitudes of individuals. Guidance is given on selecting the most appropriate statistical model.

2.89.11 Kritzer, H.M. (1996) The data puzzle: the nature of interpretation in quantitative research. *American Journal of Political Science*, 40 (1) 1–32 References

Discusses interpretation in both qualitative textual analysis and quantitative statistical analysis (CR 2.86, 2.87).

2.89.12 Lazega, E. (1997) Network analysis and qualitative research: a method of contextualization, in Miller, G. & Dingwall, R. (eds), *Context and Method in Qualitative Research*. London: Sage. ISBN 0803976321 Part III, Chapter 9, 119–38 References

Discusses how network analysis may be combined with qualitative methods to analyse organizational and institutional settings. It is described as a method for contextualizing the knowledge and behaviour among members of a social setting, and the author also shows how the approach may be linked to themes in the symbolic interactionist theory (CR 2.36.40, 2.45).

2.89.13 Malrieu, J.P. (1994) Coloured semantic networks for content analysis. *Quality and Quantity*, 28 (1) 55–81 References

Proposes two methods of textual analysis which can benefit from semantic networks, path distributions and texts clustering (CR 2.88).

2.89.14 Manning, P.K. & Cullum-Swan, B. (1994) Narrative, content and semiotic analysis, in Denzin, N.K. & Lincoln, Y.S. (eds), *Handbook of Qualitative Research*. Thousand Oaks, CA: Sage. ISBN 0803946791 Chapter 29, 463–77 118 References

Chapter gives a brief history of documentary or textual analysis and outlines the changing paradigms within which these research approaches are used. Semiotics are used which permit systematic analysis of symbolic systems (CR 2.36.13, 2.97).

2.89.15 Miller, G. (1997) Contextualizing texts: studying organizational texts, in Miller, G. & Dingwall, R. (eds), *Context and Method in Qualitative Research*. London: Sage. ISBN

0803976321 Part II, Chapter 6, 77–91 References

Author argues for an ethnographic approach to the study of organizational texts. The ways in which texts are embedded in the mundane social relations and activities of organizations, and how the practical meanings assigned to them are inextricably linked to organizational contexts are discussed (CR 2.36.40, 2.42).

2.89.16 Potter, J. (1997) Discourse analysis as a way of analyzing naturally occurring talk, in Silverman, D. (ed.), *Qualitative Research: Theory, Method and Practice*. London: Sage. ISBN 0803976666 Part V, Chapter 10, 144–60 46 References

Chapter discusses discourse analysis as a way of analysing naturally occurring talk. Author shows the way in which it allows us to address how versions of reality are produced, to seem objective and separate from the speaker. Illustrations are drawn from television interviews with Diana, Princess of Wales and Salman Rushdie, and a newspaper report of a psychiatrist's comment (CR 2.36.59).

2.89.17 Prior, L. (1997) Following in Foucault's footsteps, in Silverman, D. (ed.), *Qualitative Research: Theory, Method and Practice*. London: Sage. ISBN 0803976666 Part III, Chapter 5, 63–79 38 References

Author suggests that texts can constitute a starting point for qualitative analysis in their own right and shows how it is possible to focus on how a text instructs us to see the world. Using diverse examples, he shows how Foucault's work can properly be used as a thought-provoking toolbox (CR 2.36.59).

2.89.18 Psathas, G. (1995) *Conversation Analysis: the Study of Talk-in-interaction*. Thousand Oaks, CA: Sage. ISBN 0803957475 References

Book provides an introduction to conversation analysis, outlines its procedures and major accomplishments. Also included are discussions on verbal sequence, institutional constraints on interaction and the deep structure of talk.

2.89.19 Schegloff, E.A. (1993) Reflections on quantification in the study of conversation. *Research on Language and Social Interaction*, 26 (1) 99–128 49 References

Explores the possibilities and disadvantages of using quantification approaches to conversational analysis (CR 2.87).

2.89.20 Watson,   R.   (1997)   Ethnomethodology and textual analysis, in Silverman, D. (ed.), *Qualitative Research: Theory, Method and Practice*. London: Sage. ISBN 0803976666 Chapter 6, 80–98   23 References

Author argues, using examples from many sources, that texts are so pervasive that we may not pay sufficient attention to them. Drawing on the ethnomethodological work of Garfinkel and Sacks, it is shown how texts depend upon the common-sense properties of everyday language and that readers are active in encouraging or producing particular interpretations (CR 2.36.59, 2.42).

2.89.21 Wooffitt, R. (1993) Analyzing accounts, in Gilbert, N. (ed.), *Researching Social Life*. London: Sage. ISBN 0803986823 Chapter 14 287–305   References

Examines language, data, methodological issues, linguistic repertoires, assembling descriptions and the organization of descriptive sequences (CR 2.1.25).

2.90   LEVELS OF DATA ANALYSIS – PRIMARY

There are three levels of data analysis: primary, secondary and meta-analysis. Primary analysis in the health field usually involves examining archives such as personal or public health records.

Definition

Primary data analysis – the initial analysis of data, whether those data were collated originally for research or other purposes

Example

Kirby, R.L. & Ackroyd-Stolarz, A. (1995) Wheelchair safety – adverse reports to the United States Food and Drugs Adminis-

tration. *American Journal of Physical Medicine and Rehabilitation*, 74 (4) 308–12 5 References

Describes an examination of the Food and Drugs Administration (FDA) databases to gain insight into the types, causes and extent of injuries sustained by wheelchair users. Six hundred and fifty one records received by the FDA between 1975 and 1993 were studied. Results are reported and the implications for clinicians, users, manufacturers and regulatory bodies are discussed.

Annotation

2.90.1   Black, C., Roos, L.L., Rosser, W. & Dunn, E.V. (1992) Analyzing large data sets, in Tudiver, F., Bass, M.J, Dunn, E.V., Norton, P.G. & Stewart, M. (eds), *Assessing Interventions: Traditional and Innovative Methods*. Newbury Park, CA: Sage. ISBN 0803947704 Chapter 17, 169–81   27 References

Chapter defines large data sets, identifies different types and describes their relevance for primary research. Some important issues in analysing them are discussed (CR 2.9.21).

2.91   LEVELS OF DATA ANALYSIS – SECONDARY

The next level of data analysis is called secondary analysis. The data used for this may be raw data, statistical databases or archival material.

Definition

Secondary data analysis – a form of research in which data collected by one researcher are re-analysed by another investigator, usually to test new research hypotheses

Example

Sandelowski M. & Black, B.P. (1994) The epistemology of expectant parenthood. *Western Journal of Nursing Research*, 16 (6) 601–22   75 References

Reports   on   the   secondary   analysis   of

information obtained from 288 interviews with childbearing couples in a longitudinal study. This showed that parents aimed to get to know the foetus above all else (CR 2.6, 2.48, 2.68).

Annotations

2.91.1 Abel, E. & Sherman, J.J. (1991) Use of national data sets to teach graduate students research skills. *Western Journal of Nursing Research*, 13 (6) 794–7 6 References

Discusses the use of national data sets as a method of teaching data analysis. Use of secondary data as an efficient, cost-effective method is rarely found in the literature (CR 3.17).

2.91.2 Bain, M.R.S., Chalmers, J.W.T. & Brewster, D.H. (1997) Routinely collected data in national and regional databases, an under-used resource. *Journal of Public Health Medicine*, 19 (4) 413–18 32 References

Authors believe that routinely collected data provide a valuable and often under-used source of information. With some imagination, and as long as adequate care is taken, the potential of these data goes far beyond the limited applications with which they have been associated, namely population health assessments and health service planning.

2.91.3 Barrett, R.E. (1994) *Using the 1990 US Census for Research*. Thousand Oaks, CA: Sage. ISBN 0803953909 References

Volume explains the 'ins and outs' of using American census data for research. It covers history of the census, its design, procedures and problems, and preparing data for analysis (CR 2.79).

2.91.4 Hilton, T.L. (1992) *Using National Data Bases in Educational Research*. Hillsdale, NJ: Laurence Erlbaum Associates. ISBN 080580840X References

Book is designed to enable educational researchers make better use of the many large, longitudinal and cross-sectional data files now readily available in the USA. It is not a 'how to' book, but should facilitate research at the planning and design stage. Studies show what can and cannot be done with large national databases (CR 2.14, 2.92).

2.91.5 Jacobson, A.F., Hamilton, P. & Galloway, J. (1993) Obtaining and evaluating data sets for secondary analysis in nursing research. *Western Journal of Nursing Research*, 15 (4) 483–94 23 References

Discusses the advantages and limitations of secondary analysis, locating sources of data, evaluating potential data sets, assistance with its analysis and some examples.

2.91.6 Nail, L.M. & Lange, L.L. (1996) Using computerized clinical nursing databases for nursing research. *Journal of Professional Nursing*, 12 (4) 197–206 28 References

Article suggests strategies for using computerized clinical nursing databases (CCNDBs). Three major steps are outlined: locating and accessing CCNDBs; assessing their content and quality; and extracting and analysing the data (CR 2.17, 2.64, 2.79, 2.84).

2.91.7 Procter, M. (1993) Analyzing other researchers' data, in Gilbert, N. (ed.), *Researching Social Life*. London: Sage. ISBN 0803986823 Chapter 13, 255–69 References

Examines the pros and cons of secondary analysis, descriptive and explanatory research, data sources, obtaining data and conceptualizing in secondary analysis (CR 2.1.25).

2.91.8 Reed, J. (1992) Secondary data in nursing research. *Journal of Advanced Nursing*, 17 (7) 877–83 13 References

Article discusses some of the problems inherent in using secondary data. It is illustrated by a study which examined the assessment of mobility in elderly care wards.

2.91.9 Stewart, D.W. (1993) *Secondary Research: Information Sources and Methods* 2nd edition. Beverly Hills, CA: Sage. ISBN 0803950373 References

Monograph is designed as an introduction to locating, using, evaluating and integrating information which is available from printed materials and computer-based data. Book includes issues in evaluating research, information sources, including computer-assisted information searches, and integrating data from multiple sources. Exercises are included and more relevant topic areas could easily be substituted for any particular discipline.

2.92   LEVELS OF DATA ANALYSIS – META-ANALYSIS

'The third level of data analysis is meta-analysis which enables the researcher to summarize and integrate findings from several studies. It can be performed using either raw data from original studies or summary measures to generate effect sizes' (Woods & Catanzaro, 1988: 335).

Definition

Meta-analysis – . . . a quantitative method of combining the results of independent studies (usually drawn from published literature) and synthesizing summaries and conclusions which may be used to evaluate therapeutic effectiveness, plan new studies

Example

Brown, S.A. & Grimes, D.E. (1995) A meta-analysis of nurse practitioners and nurse midwives in primary care. *Nursing Research*, 44 (6) 332–9   64 References

Reports a meta-analysis which evaluated patient outcomes of nurse practitioners and midwives compared to those of physicians in primary care. Trends in data were felt to be more important than individual statistical findings. The lack of rigour and logical formulation of several studies left many questions unanswered and gaps in the literature suggest a research agenda for the future.

Annotations

2.92.1   Egger, M. & Smith, G.D. (1998) Meta-analysis: bias in location and selection of studies. *British Medical Journal*, 3 January, 316 61–6   53 References

Discusses the different types of bias which may occur in meta-analyses. These are: publication, location, English language, database, citation, multiple publication, provision of data, poor methodology and quality of small studies (CR 2.27).

2.92.2 to 2.92.14   Evaluation and the Health Professions. (1995) Special issue 18 (3). The meta-analytic revolution in health research. Part I

The following entry differs in format as it documents two special issues of the journal *Evaluation and the Health Professions*. These articles have not been annotated.

2.92.2   Bangert-Drowns,   R.L. Misunderstanding meta-analysis. 304–14   12 References

2.92.3   Bausell, R.B. Introduction. 235–7 4 References

2.92.4   Bausell, R.B., Li, Y.-F., Gau, M.-L. & Soeken, K.L. The growth of meta-analytic literature from 1980–1993. 238–51   11 References

2.92.5   Preiss, R.W. & Allen, M. Understanding and using meta-analysis. 315–35 55 References

2.92.6   Soeken, K.L., Bausell, R.B. & Li, Y.-F. Realizing the meta-analytic potential. 336–44   3 References

2.92.7   Wieland, D., Stuck, A.E., Siu, A.L., Adams, J. & Rubenstein, L.Z. Meta-analytic methods for health services research: an example from geriatrics. 252–82   57 References

2.92.8   Yeaton, W.H., Langenbrunner, J.C., Smyth, J.M. & Wortman, P.M. Exploratory research synthesis: methodological considerations for addressing limitations in data quality. 283–303   40 References

Evaluation and Health Professions. (1995) Special issue 18 (4). The meta-analytic revolution in health research. Part II

2.92.9   Bausell, R.B. Introduction. 347–8 3 References

2.92.10   Hall, J.A. & Rosenthal, R. Interpreting and evaluating meta-analysis. 393–407   40 References

2.92.11   Kavale, K.A. Meta-analysis at 20: retrospect and prospect. 349–69   88 References

2.92.12   Miller, N. & Pollock, V.E. Use of meta-analysis for testing theory. 370–92 62 References

2.92.13 Sakala, C. & Hunter, J.E. The Cochrane pregnancy and childbirth database: implications for perinatal care policy and practice in the US. 428–66   91 References

2.92.14 Schmidt, F. & Hunter, J.E. The impact of data-analysis methods on cumulative research knowledge: statistical significance testing, confidence intervals and meta-analysis. 408–27   39 References

2.92.15 Eysenck, H.J. (1995) Problems with meta-analysis, in Chalmers, I. & Altman, D.G. (eds), *Systematic Reviews.* London: BMJ Publishing Group. ISBN 0727909045. Chapter 6, 64–74   20 References

Discusses some problems which occur in meta-analysis: regressions are often not linear, effects are often multivariate rather than univariate, coverage can be restricted, bad studies may be included, the data summarized may not be homogeneous, grouping different causal factors may lead to meaningless estimated effect sizes and the failure to relate data to theories may obscure discrepancies (CR 2.12.10).

2.92.16 Greener, J. & Grimshaw, J. (1996) Using meta-analysis to summarize evidence within systematic reviews. *Nurse Researcher,* 4 (1) 27–38   30 References

Authors discuss the relationship between meta-analysis and systematic review (CR 2.12).

2.92.17 Hunter, J.E., & Schmidt, F.L. (1989) *Methods of Meta-analysis: Correcting Error and Bias in Research Findings.* Newbury Park, CA: Sage. ISBN 0803932227   References

Book reviews all the methods proposed for cumulating knowledge across studies, including the narrative review, counting statistically significant findings, and the averaging of quantitative outcome measures (CR 2.27).

2.92.18 Jensen, L.A. & Allen, M.N. (1996) Meta-synthesis of qualitative findings. *Qualitative Health Research,* 6 (4) 553–60   18 References

Describes a framework for synthesizing qualitative findings and issues around the technique are discussed (CR 2.86).

2.92.19 Onyskiw, J.E. (1996) The meta-analytic approach to research integration. *Canadian Journal of Nursing Research,* 28 (3) 69–85   40 References

Article describes the meta-analytic approach to research integration, discusses the advantages it offers and highlights some methodological issues.

2.92.20 Oxman, A.D. & Guyatt, G.H. (1992) A consumers' guide to subgroup analysis. *Annals of Internal Medicine,* 116 (1) 78–84   43 References

Guidelines are given for making decisions about whether to believe or act upon the results of sub-group analyses of data from randomized trials or meta-analyses (CR 2.29).

2.92.21 Oxman, A.D. & Stachenko, S.J. (1992) Meta-analysis in primary care: theory and practice, in Tudiver, F, Bass, M.J., Dunn, E.V., Norton, P.G. & Stewart, M. (eds), *Assessing Interventions: Traditional and Innovative Methods.* Newbury Park, CA: Sage. ISBN 0803947704 Chapter 19, 191–207 60 References

Chapter highlights the major issues and decisions to be made when undertaking a meta-analysis. Examples are included from recently published literature.

2.92.22 Reynolds, N.R., Timmerman, G., Anderson, J. & Stevenson, J.S. (1992) Meta-analysis for descriptive research. *Research in Nursing and Health,* 15 (6) 467–75   52 References

A case is made for the value of meta-analysis as a technique for integrating descriptive research. An overview of different meta-analytic approaches to data analysis using the correlational index with descriptive research is described (CR 2.36, 2.86).

2.92.23 Rosenthal, R. (1991) *Meta-analytic Procedures for Social Research* Revised edition. Newbury Park, CA: Sage. ISBN 080394246X   References

Covers latest techniques in the field, as well as providing a comprehensive text on meta-analytic procedures.

2.92.24 Smith, G.D. & Egger, M. (1998) Meta-analysis: unresolved issues and future developments. *British Medical Journal,* 17 January, 316 221–5   40 References

Although this technique has been established as important in clinical epidemiology, several issues remain unresolved. These include: the inclusion of unpublished, non-peer-reviewed data, individual patient data which is needed to answer important questions; and the clinical application of results. The role of the Cochrane Collaboration in the field of systematic reviews is highlighted (CR 2.12).

2.92.25 Smith, M.C. & Stullenbargcr, E. (1991) A protoype for integrative review and meta-analysis of nursing research. *Journal of Advanced Nursing*, 16 (11) 1272–83 39 References

Describes a prototype which will enable systematic compilation of results from non-experimentally designed studies (CR 2.12).

2.92.26 Smith, M.C. & Stullenbarger, E. (1995) An integrative review and meta-analysis of oncology nursing research: 1981–1990. *Cancer Nursing*, 18 (3) 167–79 73 References

Study describes ten years of patient-related oncology nursing research in the USA. It assesses the effectiveness of interventions and tests a prototype for research synthesis projects. Recommendations are made for further work (CR 2.12).

2.92.27 Stock, W.A., Benito, J.G. & Lasa, N.B. (1996) Research synthesis: coding and conjectures. *Evaluation and the Health Professions*, 19 (1) 104–17 13 References

Authors offer guidelines that make it more likely for high-quality information to be extracted and coded from primary research reports. They address issues from the selection of items and construction of coding materials to sustaining reliability and vigilance across extended periods of coding. A few thoughts are offered on the future of meta-analysis (CR 2.24, 2.90).

2.92.28 Waddell, D.L. (1992) The effects of continuing education on nursing practice: a meta-analysis. *Journal of Continuing Education in Nursing*, 23 (4) 164–8 18 References

A meta-analysis of published and unpublished studies was conducted to reconcile the apparent conflicting results which examined the effects of continuing education on nursing practice. The overall mean effect size supplemented the hypothesis that continuing education positively affects practice. Findings related to mediating efforts were inconclusive.

2.93 INTERPRETING THE FINDINGS

The final steps in any research project are to interpret the data, so that it becomes meaningful within the context of a particular piece of research and it may then take its place in the literature.

Annotations

2.93.1 Anderson, A.J.B. (1989) *Interpreting Data: a First Course in Statistics*. London: Chapman Hall. ISBN 0412295709 References

Designed for students undertaking a statistics module, this book clarifies the basic requirements of data collection, examines the reliability of published data and the validation and analysis of data by computer. Examples are included from a wide range of disciplines and exercises conclude each chapter (CR 2.24, 2.25, 2.84).

2.93.2 Denzin, N.K. (1994) The art and politics of interpretation, in Denzin, N.K. & Lincoln, Y.S. (eds), *Handbook of Qualitative Research*. Thousand Oaks, CA: Sage. ISBN 0803946791 Chapter 31, 500–15 68 References

Chapter discusses how the complex art of interpretation and story-telling is practised. The constructivist, grounded theory, feminist, Marxist, cultural studies and poststructural perspectives are explored, and predictions are made for the future (CR 2.10, 2.36.13, 2.45, 2.97).

2.94 PRESENTING DATA

Once data has been carefully analysed, the next step is to present it in the most clear way so that other readers will have no difficulty in its interpretation. Depending on the type of research undertaken, data may be presented in the form of tables, graphs, charts, figures, verbatim accounts or other means.

Annotations

2.94.1 Her Majesty's Stationery Office. (1997) *Plain Figures*. London: HMSO. ISBN 0117020397 References

Demonstrates and discusses ways of presenting numbers effectively so that their value can be realized. It also aims to help the reader interpret data more competently and confidently. No statistical tests are discussed and the book concentrates on bringing together advice and research findings on statistical presentation.

2.94.2 Hicks, C. (1994) Using tables and graphs to present research findings. *Nurse Researcher*, 2 (1) 54–74 11 References

Discusses the different types of data which may be obtained and suggests how it may be presented graphically to bring the data to life.

2.94.3 Jacoby, W.G. (1997) *Statistical Graphics for Univariate and Bivariate Data*. Thousand Oaks, CA: Sage. ISBN 0761900837

Providing strategies for examining data more effectively, this volume focuses on displaying univariate and bivariate methods graphically (CR 2.87).

2.94.4 Kosslyn, S.M. (1993) *The Elements of Graph Design*. Oxford: W.H. Freeman. ISBN 071672362X References

A step-by-step approach showing how to create effective displays of quantitative data. Crucial communication between the design, data and the reader are made for those who prepare, use and interpret graphic data.

2.94.5 McKinney, V. & Burns, N. (1993)

The effective preparation of graphs. *Nursing Research*, 42 (4) 250–2 18 References

Discusses the use and effective preparation of graphs.

2.94.6 Office of Health Economics. (1997) *Compendium of Health Statistics* 10th edition. London: Office of Health Economics. No ISBN

Provides a comprehensive statistical description of the National Health Service in the UK. Various ways of presenting data are shown.

2.94.7 Pearson, L. (1997) Quantitative analysis: the principles of data presentation. *Nurse Researcher*, 4 (4) 41–53 9 References

Paper introduces some of the main principles of data presentation in relation to quantitative analysis. Ways of enhancing the clarity and integrity of the data are suggested (CR 2.87).

2.94.8 Sprent, P. (1988) *Understanding Data*. Harmondsworth, Middlesex: Penguin. ISBN 0140772065 References

A practical text which aims to develop skills in selection and presentation of numerical data. Data is discussed and presented in a number of different contexts. Exercises to consolidate learning are interspersed throughout the text.

2.94.9 Wallgren, A., Wallgren, B., Persson, R., Jorner, U. & Haaland, J.-A. (1996) Graphing statistics and data: creating better charts. Thousand Oaks, CA: Sage. ISBN 0761905995 References

Book covers all aspects of organizing and presenting data, using real examples. Readers are shown step by step how to work from the raw data to a finished chart.

COMMUNICATING NURSING RESEARCH

2.95   EVALUATING RESEARCH FINDINGS

'A research critique is an objective, systematic attempt to identify, appreciate and weigh the merits and demerits of a particular piece of scientific research' (Phillips, L.R.F., 1986: 364). Literature included in this section will help nurses to develop their skills in evaluating published works and then in making decisions about relevance to practice.

Definition ｜

Evaluating research findings – a creative, constructive and positive process conducted for the purpose of identifying the strategies and limitations of a research project

---

Major text

Phillips, L.R.F. (1986) *A Clinician's Guide to the Critique and Utilization of Nursing Research*. Norwalk, CT: Appleton-Century-Crofts. ISBN 0838511627   References

Annotations

2.95.1   Avis, M. (1994a) Reading research critically I. An introduction to appraisal: designs and objectives. *Journal of Clinical Nursing*, 3 (4) 227–34   32 References

An approach to appraising published research is suggested. Simple guidelines and evaluation are included for three types of research.

2.95.2   Avis, M. (1994b) Reading research critically II. An introduction to appraisal: assessing the evidence. *Journal of Clinical Nursing*, 3 (5) 271–7   18 References

Guidelines for evaluating the quality of evidence and the validity of conclusions are suggested, and a checklist of evaluation points is presented.

2.95.3   Black, T.R. (1994) *Evaluating Social Science Research: an Introduction*. London: Sage. ISBN 0803988524   References

Provides a basic introduction to assessing the meaning and validity of research in social science, education and other fields (CR 2.25).

2.95.4   Burns, N. & Grove, S.K. (1995) *Understanding Nursing Research*. Philadelphia: W.B. Saunders ISBN 0721644368 References

The major theme of this book is critiquing the steps of the research process with the goal of using findings in clinical practice. Quantitative and qualitative methods are both included and extensive use is made of published studies. Supporting materials include an instruction manual and student study guide (CR 2.29, 2.36, 2.102).

2.95.5   Gehlbach, S.H. (1993) *Interpreting the Medical Literature* 3rd edition. New York: McGraw-Hill.   ISBN   0071054510   References

Book aims to provide medical students and clinicians with an approach to reading and understanding research articles in medical journals.

2.95.6   Girden, E.R. (1996) *Evaluating Research Articles from Start to Finish*. Thousand Oaks, CA: Sage. ISBN 0761904468 References

Using examples of both good and flawed studies, author shows how to read both quantitative and qualitative articles critically from start to finish. Targeted questions are used to assist in the critiquing process of each major section in an article (CR 2.29, 2.36).

2.95.7 Greenhalgh, T. (1997) *How to Read a Paper: the Basis of Evidence-based Medicine.* London: British Medical Journal Publishing Group. ISBN 0727911392 References

Book is an introduction to the value and potential applications of evidence-based medicine in the clinical setting. Examining each stage of the research process, guidance is given on how to assess its content, accuracy and applicability for practice.

2.95.8 Harrell, J.A. (1995) Reading research reports: should I apply the findings to my practice? *Tar Heel Nurse*, 57 (2) 26–7 3 References

Article provides general guidelines for nurses to consider when evaluating a research report for applicability to clinical practice (CR 2.102).

2.95.9 Hek, G. (1996) Guidelines to conducting a critical research evaluation. *Nursing Standard*, 30 October, 11 (6) 40–3 3 References

Outlines reasons why nurses need to develop evaluation skills and gives a step-by-step approach to critiquing an article.

2.95.10 Jack, B. & Oldham, J. (1997) Taking steps towards evidence-based practice: a model for implementation. *Nurse Researcher*, 5 (1) 65–71 22 References

Identifies the components of evidence-based practice and presents a model for its implementation. A strategy developed by one trust is described (CR 2.101, 2.102).

2.95.11 Katz, R.T., Campagnolo, D.I., Goldberg, G., Parker, J.C., Pine, Z.M. & Whyte, J. (1995) Critical evaluation of clinical research. *Archives of Physical Medicine and Rehabilitation*, 76 (1) 82–93 16 References

Paper contains a suggested core of material that will enable doctors to review critically research published in the medical literature.

2.95.12 Light, R.J. & Pillemer, D.B. (1984)

Summing up the Science of Reviewing Research. Cambridge, MA: Harvard University Press. ISBN 0674854314 References

Discusses the art of combining information from several studies in a practical way. General guidelines and step-by-step procedures are included with examples given from several disciplines. A checklist for evaluating reviews is given. The book is written in non-technical language and is likely to become a methodological classic (CR 2.12, 2.92).

2.95.13 Locke, L.F., Spirduso, W.W. & Silverman, S.J. (1998) *Reading and Understanding Research.* Thousand Oaks, CA: Sage. ISBN 0761903062 References

Authors introduce and frame the notion of reading research within a wider context. Information is given on finding, selecting and evaluating reports for trustworthiness. A step-by-step guide is given to reading reports from both qualitative and quantitative studies (CR 2.29, 2.36).

2.95.14 Moorbath, P. (1993) Selection of sources on critiquing research and reviewing literature. *Nurse Researcher*, 1 (1) 74–8 References

Provides a selected list of reading material on critiquing and reviewing literature, including introductory books. Four entries are listed about publishing processes (CR 2.12, 2.99).

2.95.15 Morse, J.M., Dellasega, C. & Doberneck, B. (1993) Evaluating abstracts: preparing a research conference. *Nursing Research*, 42 (5) 308–10 1 Reference

Discusses the difficulties associated with evaluating abstracts of proposed conference papers and suggests alternative approaches to this task.

2.95.16 Ogier, M.E. (1998) *Reading Research: How to Make Research more Approachable* 2nd editition. London: Baillière Tindall. ISBN 0702023388 References

This booklet gives a brief, introductory step-by-step guide to reading research. The new edition reflects changes in locating research using the new technologies (CR 2.2).

2.95.17 Phillips, L.R.F. (1986) *A Clinician's*

Guide to the Critique and Utilization of Nursing Research. Norwalk, CT: Appleton-Century-Crofts. ISBN 0838511627 References

Book is designed to complement existing texts and aims to provide the information needed to conduct an objective research critique and to use this to make decisions about research utilization. Major units in the text focus on the current research–practice gap in nursing, development of critiquing skills and the utilization of clinical nursing research. Each chapter is summarized and includes additional learning activities and a bibliography. Two examples of published research are used to illustrate each aspect of the critiquing process (CR 2.102, 3.8).

2.95.18 Polit, D.F. (1996) *Essentials of Nursing Research: Methods, Appraisal and Utilization* 4th edition. Philadelphia: Lippincott-Raven. ISBN 0397553684 References

Text is written for consumers of nursing research to assist in evaluating the adequacy of research findings in terms of their scientific merit and utilization potential. Chapters contain information on what to expect in research reports and guidelines for conducting a critique, using one real and one fictitious example. Book contains methodological and substantive references (CR 2.95).

2.95.19 Rose, G. (1982) *Deciphering Sociological Research.* London: Macmillan. ISBN 0333285581 References

This book, which complements existing texts, provides an approach to analysing sociological research. Systematic methods are given for deciphering reports and 12 selected examples, which are edited versions of articles originally published in sociological journals, provide the data for analysis. These illustrate a range of approaches to research and are chosen from three major areas of sociology; deviance, education and stratification. The link between theory and empirical evidence is thoroughly explored in the analyses.

2.95.20 Sajiwandani, J. (1996) Ensuring the trustworthiness of quantitative research through critique. *NT Research*, 1 (2) 135–42 8 References

Paper explains what is meant by trustworthy research, how research critics work, the skills which are required, and the characteristics of a research critique. A model for evaluating a piece of research is given, together with a checklist for critiquing quantitative studies (CR 2.87).

2.95.21 Smith, H.W. (1991) *Strategies of Social Research: Methodological Imagination* 3rd revised edition. Austin, TX: Holt. ISBN 0030230772 References

This Open University reader comprises four major parts: sociology as a science; the production of data; improving data quality; and the analysis and presentation of data. The emphasis is on evaluating research rather than doing it. Each chapter ends with readings for advanced students and suggested research projects. Case histories are used to illustrate ethical and moral problems in social research (CR 2.17).

2.95.22 Tornquist, E.M., Funk, S.G., Champagne, M.T. & Wiese, R.A. (1993) Advice on reading research: overcoming the barriers. *Applied Nursing Research*, 6 (4) 177–83 19 References

Discusses some problems of research reports, how they may be structured to increase clarity, and suggests an approach to reading and evaluation.

2.95.23 Ventry, I.M. & Schiavetti, N. (1986) *Evaluating Research in Speech Pathology and Audiology* 2nd edition. London: Macmillan. ISBN 0024229407 References

Although written for advanced-level students in speech pathology and audiology this book may also be useful to nursing students. It is not a 'how to do it' book, but rather shows how to read, understand and evaluate research done by others. Parts describe the underlying framework used to generate guidelines for evaluation, the main sections of a research article and it contains two annotated articles to lead the reader through the process of evaluation.

2.96 RESEARCH PROPOSALS

'A research proposal is a written document specifying what the investigator proposes to study. Proposals serve to communicate the research problem, its significance, and

planned procedures for solving the problem'
(Polit & Hungler, 1991: 535)

Definition

Research proposal – the written plan and
justification for a research project prepared
before it begins. It is also used when applying
for financial support to do the research

Example

Morse, J.M. (1996) The qualitative proposal,
in Morse, J.M. & Field, P.A., *Nursing
Research: the Application of Qualitative
Approaches* 2nd edition. London: Chapman
& Hall. ISBN 0412605104 Appendix A,
161–93 [Appendix B, 194–6 Critique of the
proposal]

Reproduces a proposal which was submitted
to the National Center for Nursing Research,
National Institutes of Health (USA), funded
as a three-year foreign award in 1989, to
conduct a series of studies on comfort and its
application within nursing. A critique of the
proposal is also included (CR 2.36.47).

Annotations

2.96.1 Anonymous. (1995) Nurses' perception of involvement in Thunder Project.
Clinical Nurse Specialist, 9 (2) 88–91
4 References

The American Association of Critical Care
Nurses (AACN) Thunder Project was developed to provide critical-care nurses with a
research protocol ready for institutional
review and implementation. This included
providing a research package (protocol, educational and data collection materials) and a
topic of clinical significance. Site co-ordina-
tors and research associates were identified to
implement all study activities. An evaluation
was made of the process and deemed to be
successful. Barriers to implementation were
highlighted, including obtaining informed
consent and physician approval and/or co-
operation (CR 2.14, 2.17, 2.101, 2.102, 3.16).

2.96.2 Bond, S. (1994) Writing a grant application. *Nurse Researcher*, 2 (1) 34–42
1 Reference

Author gives advice on measures that can be
taken to increase the chances of success in
gaining research funding (CR 3.13).

**2.96.3 Brooker, C., Read, S., Morrell, C.J.,
Repper, J., Jones, R. & Akehurst, R.** (1997)
Coming in from the cold? An analysis of
research proposals submitted by the nursing
section at ScHARR, 1994–97. *NT Research*,
2 (6) 405–13　25 References

Examines the characteristics of 50 proposals
submitted by nurses over a three-year period.
Approximately 50 per cent were successful.
Results are discussed.

2.96.4 Carlisle, C. (1994) Writing a research
proposal. *Nurse Researcher*, 2 (1) 24–33
8 References

Article covers the purposes of writing a
research proposal, its content, structure and
how to avoid some common errors.

2.96.5 Chubin, D.E. (1994) Grants peer
review in theory and practice. *Evaluation
Review*, 18 (1) 20–30　References

Discusses grants peer reviews as an evaluation methodology for research impact
assessment. Suggestions are made to remedy
the shortcomings of peer reviews in decision-
making when selecting research proposals for
funding (CR 3.13).

**2.96.6 Cohen, M.Z., Knafl, K. & Dzurec,
L.C.** (1993) Grant writing for qualitative
research. *Image: Journal of Nursing Scholarship*, 25 (2) 151–6　13 References

Paper summarizes the analysis of 19 qualitative grant proposal summary statements to
illuminate their strengths and weaknesses, as
identified by grant reviewers (CR 2.36, 3.13).

2.96.7 Coley, S.M. & Scheinberg, C.A.
(1991) *Proposal Writing*. Newbury Park, CA:
Sage. ISBN 0803932324　References

Covers all aspects of proposal writing for
beginners and moderately experienced grant
writers. Appendices contain information on
estimating time, a sample proposal, critique
and funding resource information (CR 3.13).

2.96.8 Davitz, J.R. & Davitz, L.L. (1997)
*Evaluating Research Proposals: a Guide for
the Behavioural Sciences* 3rd edition. Englewood Cliffs, NJ: Prentice-Hall. ISBN
0133485668　References

Book designed for students who are planning or critically evaluating research studies. The points to be considered when evaluating research proposals are discussed and a series of questions accompanies each section.

2.96.9 Ezell-Kalish, S.E., McCullum, T., Henry, Y., Schoenthaler, A. & Grady, S. (1981) *The Proposal Writer's Swipe File: 15 Winning Fund-raising Proposals . . . Prototypes of Approaches, Styles and Structures.* Washington, DC: Taft Corporation. ISBN 0914756451

Provides a resource book of successful research proposals. Examples, covering a wide range of disciplines, were written by professional proposal writers and give insight into how fund-raising proposals should be constructed, organized, styled and presented.

2.96.10 Fessey, C. (1997) Preparing research proposals for contract research. *Nurse Education Today*, 17 (1) 3–6   4 References

Article provides feedback to nurses who sent in proposals for an English National Board research contract, but which were unsuccessful. The common characteristics are discussed which will help to guide those submitting proposals in future.

2.96.11 Fuller, E.O., Hasselmeyer, E.G., Hunter, J.C., Abdellah, F.G. & Hinshaw, A.S. (1991) Summary statements of the NIH Nursing Research Grant Applications. *Nursing Research*, 40 (6) 346–51   8 References

Reports a study which investigated summary statements between October 1968 and June 1988 to identify reasons for recommending approval or disapproval of grant applications.

2.96.12 Geever, J.C. (1997) *The Foundation Center's Guide to Proposal Writing* 2nd edition. New York: The Foundation Center. ISBN 0879547030

2.96.13 Gitlin, L.N. & Lyons, K.J. (1996) *Successful Grant Writing: Strategies for Health and Human Service Professionals.* New York: Springer. ISBN 0826192602   References

Book is specially written for those in academic and practice settings. A range of strategies and work models are presented. Parts cover the perspective of funding agencies and the grantee, writing the proposal, models for their development and life after its submission (CR 3.13).

2.96.14 Holmes, S.B., Becher, M., Karande, U. & Riley, K. (1989) Research on every rung of the clinical ladder. *American Journal of Nursing*, 89 (2) 246, 248, 250   5 References

Describes the setting up of a nursing research committee whose aims were to review and approve research proposals, recommend changes in practice based on research findings, serve as a resource and co-ordinate research activities (CR 2.101, 2.102, 3.7).

2.96.15 Jacox, A.K. (1980) Nursing's statement: testifying in Washington, in Davis, A.J. & Krueger, J.C. (eds), *Patients, Nurses, Ethics.* New York: American Journal of Nursing Company. ISBN 0937126845   References. A testimony presented on 3 May 1977 at a public hearing before the National Commission for the Protection of Human Subjects of Biomedical and Behavioural Research, National Institute of Health, Bethesda, Maryland.

Presenter reports on the difficulties encountered in getting research proposals accepted by research committees. Author contends that committees are composed largely of physicians and representatives of the biomedical sciences. This creates a powerful pressure to encourage research designs that are experimental rather than non-experimental. The place and value of nursing research is explored and examples where permission has been refused are used illustrate these points. Physicians in their role as gatekeepers are discussed and the case for nursing representation on committees is outlined (CR 2.17).

2.96.16 Johnson, J.E. (1994) How to write a winning proposal: strategies for nursing executives. *Journal of Nursing Administration*, 24 (4S) 10–11   No references

Outlines the essential features required in a research proposal.

2.96.17 Kirk-Smith, M. (1996) Winning ways with research proposals and reports. *Nursing Times*, 13–19 March, 92 (11) 36–8   2 References

Explains the steps involved in drawing up research proposals and reports, with emphasis on the importance of planning (CR 2.97).

2.96.18 Locke, L.F., Spirduso, W.W. & Silverman, S. (1993) *Proposals that Work: a Guide for Planning Dissertations and Grant Proposals* 3rd edition. Newbury Park, CA: Sage. ISBN 0803950675   References

Book gives practical advice on all aspects of writing research proposals This edition also includes chapters on ethics, literature searching, pilot testing, grant opportunities and an expanded section on qualitative proposal writing. Appendices contain general standards for judging the acceptability of a thesis or dissertation proposal, an annotated bibliography and a sample form for informed consent (CR 1.5, 2.13, 2.17, 2.23, 3.13).

2.96.19 Marshall, C.M. & Rossman, G.B. (1995) *Designing Qualitative Research* 2nd edition. Thousand Oaks, CA: Sage. ISBN 080395249X   References

This revised and updated edition offers guidance on all aspects of preparation for qualitative research proposals (CR 2.36, 2.73).

2.96.20 Medical Research Council. (1994) *Developing High Quality Proposals in Health Services Research* London: Medical Research Council. No ISBN

Booklet provides guidance on developing research proposals (CR 3.13).

2.96.21 Meerabeau, L. (1997) Why are our grant applications continually rejected? *Nurse Researcher*, 5 (1) 5–13   6 References

Based on experience as a research manager at the Department of Health, the author poses questions which any prospective researcher needs to consider when making a grant application. Access to funds is discussed and recent changes are highlighted (CR 3.13).

2.96.22 Miller, D.C. (1991) The art and science of grantsmanship, in Author, *Handbook of Research Design and Social Measurement* 5th edition. Newbury Park, CA: Sage. ISBN 0803942192   Part 7, B3, 596–641 References (extensive)

Covers all aspects of proposal writing, contract research, pre- and post-doctoral fellowships, funding institutions both government and private, together with information sources. Advice is also given on costing research projects (CR 2.54.14, 2.99, 3.13).

2.96.23 Morse, J.M. (1994) Designing funded qualitative research, in Denzin, N.K. & Lincoln, Y.S. (eds) *Handbook of Qualitative Research*. Thousand Oaks, CA: Sage. ISBN 0803946791   Chapter 13, 220–35 62 References

Identifies and describes the major design issues when planning a qualitative research project. Author suggests ways in which researchers may overcome the paradoxes inherent in qualitative inquiry (CR 2.36.13, 3.13).

2.96.24 Munhall, P.L. (1994) *Qualitative Research Proposals and Reports: a Guide.* New York: National League for Nursing. ISBN 0887376061 Publication no. 19–2609

This 'how to' book discusses formatting and reporting on qualitative research reports and abstracts.

2.96.25 Naylor, M.D. (1990) An example of a research grant application: comprehensive discharge planning for the elderly. *Research in Nursing and Health*, 13 (5) 327–47   45 References

Gives an example of a successful research proposal and includes evaluations by the nursing research section of the National Institute of Nursing Research.

2.96.26 Ogden, T.E. (1995) *Research Proposals: a Guide to Success* 2nd edition. New York: Raven Press. ISBN 0781703131 References

Book is a complete guide to the preparation of research proposals written from the perspective of a grant reviewer. Focusing on the National Institute of Health (NIH) system in the USA, the book covers basic grantsmanship for the novice and unsuccessful applicant, and advanced grantsmanship for scientists beginning academic and research careers. Appendices include information sources at NIH, categorical institute programmes and examples of pink sheets, preliminary data and informed consent.

2.96.27 Richards, D. (1990) Ten steps to successful grant writing. *Journal of Nursing Administration*, 20 (1) 20–3   6 References

A step-by-step approach to writing a research proposal is given.

2.96.28 Rix, G. & Cutting, K. (1996) Research interests: a study of proposals submitted for approval. *Nurse Researcher*, 3 (3) 71–9   8 References

Paper examines the research interests of nurses and midwives, based on proposals submitted for ethical approval in one health district in South Wales.

2.96.29   Schmelzer, M. (1995) Writing a grant proposal. *Gastroenterology Nursing*, 18 (3) 104–6   5 References

Author discusses basic rules for improving the quality of research grant proposals.

2.96.30   Stevenson, C. & Beech, I. (1998) Playing the power game for qualitative researchers: the possibility of a post-modern approach. *Journal of Advanced Nursing*, 27 (4) 790–7   31 References

Discusses the type of language and meaning which may be used by qualitative researchers when submitting research proposals, compared with that of ethical/research awarding committees, and the clashes which may ensue. Postmodernism, as advocated by Wittgenstein, is used to explore this problem and suggestions are made which may help to overcome the difficulties (CR 2.17, 2.36).

2.96.31   Stewart, R.D. & Stewart, A.L. (1992) *Proposal Preparation* 2nd edition. New York: Wiley. ISBN 0471552690   References

Although largely aimed at business enterprises, this book shows how to present the information required for successful research applications to funding bodies. It also describes how they are evaluated, which gives clues about the preparation of a winning proposal.

2.96.32   Tornquist, E.M. & Funk, S.G. (1990) How to write a research grant proposal. *Image: Journal of Nursing Scholarship*, 22 (1) 44–51   1 Reference

Provides guidelines for writing all parts of a research proposal.

2.96.33   Turner, S.O. (1996) Career guide: how to write a winning proposal. *American Journal of Nursing*, 96 (7) 64–5   No references

Gives step-by-step advice about writing research proposals.

2.96.34   Watzlaf, V.J.M., Addeo, L. &

Nous, A. (1995) Education review: a computer assisted instructional tool to assist students in developing an epidemiological research proposal. *Topics in Health Information Management*, 16 (2) 64–71   1 Reference

Article describes how a computer-assisted instructional (CAI) tool was created to assist students in the development of an epidemiological research proposal. Surveys showed which were the particular problem areas and these were incorporated into the new Research and Grant Writer tool. Positive feedback was received on its use (CR 2.41).

2.97   WRITING ABOUT RESEARCH

'To write is to convey to others the facts, and the relationships between facts, that have been discovered.' (Goodall 1994: 6)

Definitions

Plagiarism – the incorporation of the work of one person into the work of another without citing the source
Research report – a document that summarizes the main features of a study, including the research question . . . methods used to address it . . . findings . . . interpretation and implications

Annotations

2.97.1   Becker, H.S. (1986) *Writing for Social Scientists: How to Start and Finish Your Thesis, Book or Article*. Chicago: University of Chicago Press. ISBN 0226041085   References

An unusual book about how to improve writing skills. It focuses on the elusive work habits which contribute to good writing. Discussion on how to overcome others' criticisms, revise again and again, and develop the skills of writing clear prose are all discussed. A chapter is included on the personal and professional risks involved in scholarly writing.

2.97.2   Berry, R. (1994) *The Research*

Project: How to Write It 3rd edition. London: Routledge. ISBN 0415110904   References

Designed for students at school, college or university, this book covers all aspects needed to develop, carry out and write up a research project. An example of a well-researched, well-written paper with full bibliography and notes is also included.

2.97.3   Burnard, P. (1992) *Writing for Health Professionals: a Manual for Writers.* London: Chapman & Hall. ISBN 0412474409   References

Book contains practical advice on the processes involved in academic writing.

2.97.4   Closs, S.J. (1994) Writing a research thesis. *Nurse Researcher* 2 (1) 43–53 2 References

Provides a basic guide to writing a full research report. Careful initial consideration about style and content will assist in this complex task.

2.97.5   Cormack, D.F.S. (1994) *Writing for Health Care Professions.* Oxford: Blackwell Scientific. ISBN 0632034491   References

Gives advice to health care professionals on all aspects of writing papers. Publishing opportunities are also discussed (CR 2.99).

2.97.6   Cuba, L. (1997) *A Short Guide to Writing about Social Science* 3rd edition. New York: Longman. ISBN 0673524949   References

Covers many aspects of writing about social science.

2.97.7   Ely, M., Vinz, R., Downing, M. & Anzol, M. (1997) *On Writing Qualitative Research: Living by Words.* London: Falmer Press. ISBN 0750706031   References

Written for beginners and experienced researchers, this book is about creating research writing that is useful, believable and interesting. Blending rigorous scholarship and a clear academic style, authors examine the process, rhetorical devices and other tools that researchers use to evoke the complexity of their experience. Authors include accounts of their own research writing experiences to show how data can be presented in a meaningful way (CR 2.36).

2.97.8   Fairbairn, G.J. & Winch, C. (1996) *Reading, Writing and Reasoning: a Guide for Students* 2nd edition. Buckingham: Open University Press. ISBN 033519740X   References

Gives advice on all problematic aspects of reading for meaning, developing analytical and coherent thinking in writing and course work (CR 3.17).

2.97.9   French, S. & Sim, J. (1993) *Writing: a Guide for Therapists.* Oxford: Butterworth Heinemann. ISBN 0750605804   References

Provides information on all aspects of writing research reports, essays, clinical notes and papers for publication.

2.97.10   Gilbert, N. (1993) Writing about social research, in Author (ed.), *Researching Social Life.* London: Sage. ISBN 0803986823 Chapter 16, 328–44   References

Chapter gives advice on writing and publishing social research. An article from *American Sociological Review* is dissected to show how it is organized. Some difficulties in getting social research to influence policy are discussed (CR 2.1.25, 2.99, 3.11).

2.97.11   Giltrow, J. (1995) *Academic Writing: Writing and Reading across the Disciplines* 2nd edition. Peterborough, Ontario: Broadview Press. ISBN 1551110555   References

This text is designed to help students produce scholarly papers. Examples are included throughout which illustrate techniques for all stages of the process.

2.97.12   Glatthorn, A.A. (1998) *Writing the Winning Dissertation: a Step-by-step Guide.* Thousand Oaks, CA: Corwin Press Publications. ISBN 0803966784   References

Book covers in detail how to lay the foundations for a project, find a problem, develop a proposal, organize and write each chapter. Common problems are identified and advice is given (CR 2.96).

2.97.13   Golden-Biddle, K. & Locke, K.D. (1997) *Writing Matters: Crafting Theoretical Points from Qualitative Research.* Thousand Oaks, CA: Sage. ISBN 0803974310   References

Provides both theoretical and practical

guidance for students and researchers who need to transform data organized around the metaphor of 'story'. Each chapter covers a different aspect of creating stories: disclosing, telling and revising for publication. Writing issues are addressed as the manuscript is taken from inception to publication (CR 2.89).

2.97.14   Goodall, C.J. (1994) Writing and research: an introduction. *Nurse Researcher*, 2 (1) 4–12   8 References

Article addresses various issues including the art of communication, the motivation for, and fear of, undertaking research, together with the medium of the message (CR 2.2).

2.97.15   Goodman, N.W. & Edwards, M.B. (1991) *Medical Writing: a Prescription for Clarity*. Cambridge: Cambridge University Press. ISBN 052140701X   References

Provides practical help for authors when writing theses or material for publication.

2.97.16   Hall, G.M. (ed.) (1994) *How to Write a Paper*. London: British Medical Journal Publishing. ISBN 0727908227 References

Gives information on how to get a paper accepted for publication and explains what editors are looking for. Each aspect is discussed to help prospective authors (CR 2.99).

2.97.17   Hawksley, B. (1996) Ready referencing. *Practice Nurse*, 11 (4) 264–6, 268 10 References

Author outlines the main methods of citing sources and compiling a bibliography.

2.97.18   Kazdin, A.E. (1995) Preparing and evaluating research reports. *Psychological Assessment*, 7 (3) 228–37   References

Discusses the preparation and evaluation of research reports and how they contribute to the research process. Description, explanation and contextualization are studied by examining the manuscript and generating questions for evaluation (CR 2.89, 2.95).

2.97.19   Lester, J.D. (1996) *Writing Research Papers: a Complete Guide* 8th edition. New York: Addison-Wesley. ISBN 0673982211 References

This standard text covers all aspects of writing

research papers. Appendix contains an index to sources by discipline.

2.97.20   Morse, J.M. & Field, P.A. (1996) Reporting qualitative research, in Authors, *Nursing Research: the Application of Qualitative Approaches* 2nd edition. London: Chapman & Hall. ISBN 0412605104 Chapter 8, 141–60   References

Gives specific advice on writing in general and for publication. Particular reference is made to the reporting of qualitative research (CR 2.36.47).

2.97.21   Murrell, G., Huang, C. & Ellis, H. (1990) *Research in Medicine: a Guide to Writing a Thesis in the Medical Sciences*. Cambridge: Cambridge University Press. ISBN 0521399254   References

Provides advice for the beginner and covers all the steps involved from choosing a project to submitting a thesis. The practicalities of planning and financing a project are covered, and insights are given into the frustrations and satisfactions of doing research (CR 2.16, 3.13).

2.97.22   Orna, E. with Stevens, G. (1995) *Managing Information for Research*. Buckingham: Open University Press. ISBN 0335193978   References

A book for first-time researchers which discusses transferring knowledge gained during research into written form. Also included is information on managing time, organizing and transferring data and coping with feelings of isolation and loss of confidence.

2.97.23   Parry, A. (1993a) How to . . . construct an outline for a research report. *Physiotherapy*, 79 (4) 257–8   No references

Outlines the main topic headings for a research report to be submitted for publication.

2.97.24   Parry, A.W. (1993b) Writing for physiotherapy: guidelines for authors. *Physiotherapy*, 79 (3) 229–31   No references

Outlines role of the journal in promoting the principles and practice of physiotherapy, and the processes involved in accepting articles for publication. Types of manuscripts are discussed, together with other sorts of editorial material and its preparation (CR 2.99).

2.97.25 Richardson, L. (1990) *Writing Strategies: Reaching Diverse Audiences*. Newbury Park, CA: Sage. ISBN 0803935226 References

Book gives writers stylistic conventions about different media to assist when presenting work to diverse audiences (CR 2.99).

2.97.26 Sheridan, D.R. & Dowdney, D.L. (1997) *How to Write and Publish Articles in Nursing* 2nd edition. New York: Springer. ISBN 0826149812 References

Manual offers nurses a step-by-step approach to writing journal articles. Techniques, exercises, practical checklists and forms for each stage in the writing and marketing process are included. Guidance is given on using online databases, e-mail and the Internet. Appendices include lists of nursing journals, publications for writers and writing and literary associations (CR 2.99).

2.97.27 Smith, J.P. (1997) References, copyright and plagiarism. *Journal of Advanced Nursing*, 26 (1) 1 Editorial

Outlines the rules relating to referencing, copyright and plagiarism, and gives advice to prospective authors (CR 2.17).

2.97.28 Turabian, K.L. (1996) *A Manual for Writers of Term Papers, Theses and Dissertations* 6th edition. Chicago: University of Chicago Press. ISBN 0226816273 References

The British edition of an American 'vade mecum', intended to assist all those preparing academic work for advanced-level courses or presenting papers in scholarly journals. It gives comprehensive guidance on all aspects of style, presentation, examples of entries of reference styles, notes, bibliographical entries and annotated sample pages. Throughout, the needs of computer users are emphasized.

2.97.29 Watson, G. (1987) *Writing a Thesis: a Guide to Long Essays and Dissertations*. London: Longman. ISBN 0582494656 References

Gives practical guidance to students undertaking major written work for the first time. It covers the approach to scholarship, choosing and delineating a subject and techniques of writing and documentation.

2.97.30 Webb, C. (1992) The use of the first person in academic writing: objectivity, language and gatekeeping. *Journal of Advanced Nursing*, 17 (6) 747–52 19 References

Examines the 'problem' of writing in the first person, the role of language in thinking, qualitative, action and feminist research and gatekeeping in refereed journals (CR 2.10, 2.36, 2.37).

2.97.31 Wolcott, H.F. (1990) *Writing up Qualitative Research*. Newbury Park, CA: Sage. ISBN 0803937938 References

Purpose of book is to ensure that all data collected is included in the final account, and its quality is good. Information on getting started and keeping going is covered, together with tightening up, finishing and getting published (CR 2.36, 2.99).

2.98 DISSEMINATING RESEARCH FINDINGS

'. . . Dissemination [of research] is frequently neglected or fails to receive the time, planning and emphasis that it requires. Emphasis has been placed on carrying out the research, while strategic planning and funding for the dissemination of results have been neglected' (Dickson, 1996: 6).

Definitions

Diffusion – . . . is haphazard, lacks a target and is generally unplanned and uncontrolled
Dissemination – . . . it not only implies a more aggressive flow of information from the source, . . . but also targeting and tailoring the information for the intended audience

---

Example

Williams, K.S., Crichton, N.J. & Roe, B. (1997) Disseminating research evidence: a controlled trial in continence care. *Journal of Advanced Nursing*, 25 (4) 691–8 25 References

Study aimed at overcoming barriers to dissemination by providing a research-based handbook for continence care. Improvements in knowledge were found in the experimental group who received a copy of the handbook (CR 2.29).

Annotations

2.98.1 Akinsanya, J.A. (1994) Making research useful to the practising nurse. *Journal of Advanced Nursing*, 19 (1) 174–9 30 References

Paper examines the problems of developing research in nursing, and the challenge of establishing its relevance and usefulness to the practising nurse (CR 2.102, 3.8, 3.16).

2.98.2 Buffum, M.D. (1996) Staff action: the nurse researcher in the clinical setting. *Journal of Neuroscience Nursing*, 28 (6) 399–406   27 References

Article describes the nurse researchers' role in involving staff nurses in research evaluation and utilization (CR 3.16).

2.98.3 Cronenwett, L.R. (1995) Effective methods for disseminating research findings to nurses in practice, in Titler, M.G. & Goode, C.J. (eds), *The Nursing Clinics of North America: Research Utilization*. Philadelphia: W.B Saunders. ISSN 0029-6465   429–38 16 References

Discusses the challenges, goals and methods of disseminating research findings.

2.98.4 Dickson, R. (1996) Dissemination and implementation: the wider picture. *Nurse Researcher*, 4 (1) 5–14   27 References

Article discusses some components that are believed to be necessary in the process of disseminating research findings (CR 2.102).

2.98.5 Dunn, E.V., Norton, P.G., Stewart, M., Tudiver, F. & Bass, M.J. (eds) (1994) *Disseminating Research/Changing Practice.* Thousand Oaks, CA: Sage. ISBN 0803957068 References

Book covers general aspects of dissemination, issues of methodology and changing practitioner behaviour.

2.98.6 Dunn, V., Crichton, N., Roe, B., Seers, K. & Williams, K. (1997) Using research for practice: a UK experience of the BARRIERS Scale. *Journal of Advanced Nursing*, 26 (6) 1203–10   21 References

Reports use of the BARRIERS Scale in a British study which aimed to identify and measure barriers to utilization. Comparisons are made with other North American nurses from studies used during development of the scale (CR 2.101, 2.102).

2.98.7 Freemantle, N. & Watt, I. (1994) Dissemination: implementing the findings of research. *Health Libraries Review*, 11 (2) 133–7   8 References

Discusses dissemination techniques, the role of information professionals and challenges for the future (CR 2.102, 3.9).

2.98.8 French, B. (1996) Networking for research dissemination: collaboration between education and practice. *NT Research*, 1 (2) 113–19   29 References

In order to ensure that sources of information about effective practice are easily accessible and the skills to find, evaluate and utilize them are developed, author suggests a collaborative approach between education and practice, using a network of link personnel.

2.98.9 Hunt, J. (1996) Barriers to research utilization. *Journal of Advanced Nursing*, 23 (3) 423–5   4 References   Editorial

Editorial leads discussion on the barriers which still prevent nursing practice being based on research. The responsibilities of researchers are outlined and the political imperative is discussed (CR 3.9).

2.98.10 Kitson, A. & Currie, L. (1996) Clinical practice development and research activity in four district health authorities. *Journal of Clinical Nursing*, 5 (1) 41–51 9 References

Reports the findings of a postal survey which examined developments and research activity in four health authorities. These endeavours tended to be small-scale and unsupported, with nursing staff trying to implement findings or be innovative without the necessary expertise and support (CR 2.52).

2.98.11 Luker, K.A. & Kenrick, M. (1995) Towards knowledge-based practice: an evaluation of a method of dissemination. *International Journal of Nursing Studies*, 32 (1) 59–67   19 References

Paper describes a method for the dissemination of research-based information to nurses.

The approach involved the development and evaluation of a clinical information pack relating to the management of leg ulcers. Results of a study are reported, and other factors are uncovered, relating to the relationship between research and clinical practice and the way information is disseminated to practitioners.

2.98.12 Robinson, D. (1996) Developing the contribution of research in nursing practice. *Psychiatric Care*, 3 (2) 45–50   19 References

Describes the contribution of research in nursing within a forensic setting and with application to the wider National Health Service.

2.98.13 Robinson, J. (1994) Research for whom?: the politics of research dissemination and application, in Buckeldee, J. & McMahon, R. (eds), *The Research Experience in Nursing*. London: Chapman & Hall. ISBN 0412441101 Chapter 11, 165–88   31 References

Describes the results of a study which investigated perinatal deaths in a health authority. The responses made by members, and the apparent threats posed to them by hidden assumptions about patient care, are discussed. The researcher was able to attend subsequent health authority meetings where initially anger and hostility were shown. A chairman's report eventually enabled the group to build new policy proposals, with strategies for their implementation. Later evidence showed some changes but also entrenched attitudes. The competence of nurse researchers is discussed and lessons for the future are identified (CR 2.16.4, 2.102, 3.11).

2.98.14 Smith, P. & Masterson, A. (1996) Promoting the dissemination and implementation of research findings. *Nurse Researcher*, 4 (2) 15–29   26 References

A case study is used to demonstrate strategies for promoting the dissemination and implementation of research findings. Some of the difficulties involved in both major processes are discussed and ideas for their resolution are shared (CR 2.37, 2.39, 2.102, 3.16).

2.98.15 Tierney, A. (1995) Dissemination, in *Foundation of Nursing Studies. Annual Report 1995*. London: Foundation of Nursing studies. No ISBN

Outlines the role of the Foundation of Nursing Studies in the dissemination of nursing research findings.

2.98.16 White, J.M., Leske, J.S. & Pearcy, J.M. (1995) Models and processes of research utilization, in Titler, M.G. & Goode, C.J. (eds), *The Nursing Clinics of North America*: *Research Utilization*. Philadelphia: W.B. Saunders. ISSN 0029-6465 409–20   27 References

Reviews three models of research utilization spanning three decades of development: Conduct and Utilization of Research in Nursing (CURN), the Stetler Model, and Iowa Model of Research in Practice. Seven characteristics of models were identified and used to critique each one (CR 2.102).

2.99   PUBLICATION PROCESSES

An increasing number of nurses are now writing for publication and it is the responsibility of all researchers to communicate their findings to colleagues. Many journals include instructions to authors regularly or periodically, and editors are available to give advice. Papers submitted for publication are frequently refereed by experts to ensure the highest standards of scholarship.

The general principles of copyright law do not vary greatly between countries, however specific national legislation may differ. Please consult local librarians for guidance or the national copyright receipt office.

Definitions

Abstract – a brief description of a completed or proposed investigation in research journals, usually located at the beginning of an article
Refereed journal – a journal that makes decisions about the acceptance of manuscripts on the basis of recommendations from peer reviewers

Annotations

2.99.1 Aaronson, L.S. (1994) Milking data or meeting commitments: how many papers from one study? *Nursing Research*, 43 (1) 60–2   No references

Discusses the appropriateness or otherwise of publishing several papers from a single study. The norms of different research methods, science, scientific integrity and using old data are discussed.

2.99.2   Abraham, I.L., Chalifoux, Z.L., Evers, G.C.M. & De Geest, S. (1995) Conditions, interventions, and outcomes in nursing research: a comparative analysis of North American and European/International journals (1981–1990). *International Journal of Nursing Studies*, 32 (2) 173–87   18 References

Study compares the conceptual foci and methodological characteristics of research projects which tested the effects of nursing interventions, published in four general nursing research journals. Dimensions and variables of comparison included: nature of subjects; design issues; statistical methodology and power; and types of intervention and outcomes. Results showed that reported nursing intervention studies in European/International and North American journals were similar in the parameters examined, but in need of overall improvement. There is no empirical support for the common (explicit or implicit) ethnocentric American bias that leadership in nursing intervention research resides with and in the USA (CR 2.27).

2.99.3   American Psychological Association. (1994) *Publication Manual of the American Psychological Association* 4th edition. Washington, DC: APA Books   ISBN 1557982414   References

Gives detailed guidance to authors on the content and organization of a manuscript, expression of ideas, editorial style, typing instructions and a sample paper, submitting the paper, proof-reading and the journal programme of the association. The bibliography includes references to the history of the manual and suggested reading. Brief guidance is given on preparation of materials other than journal articles. This new edition contains many revisions and has features on current technological tools, contemporary language issues and publishing standards. A full section on the ethics of scientific publishing is included, covering reporting results, the peer reviewer, plagiarism, author's and peer

reviewer's responsibilities, duplicate publication of data and its verification and treatment of research participants (CR 2.17).

2.99.4   Ashworth, P. (1996) Writing and submitting abstracts for conference presentation. *Nurse Researcher*, 4 (1) 39–48   11 References

Discusses the place, process and content of abstracts to help nurses master the skills of presentation.

2.99.5   Barnum, B.S. (1995) *Writing and Getting Published: a Primer for Nurses*. New York: Springer. ISBN 0826186904   References

Book is mainly intended for new authors who wish to develop writing skills and navigate the publishing process. Established authors may also find some sections useful.

2.99.6   Beyea, S.C. & Nicoll, L.H. (1998) Writing and submitting an abstract. *AORN Journal*, 67 (1) 273–4   No references

Addresses strategies for writing a competitive research abstract for congress or any other conference.

2.99.7   Biddle, C. & Aker, J. (1996) How does the peer review process influence ANNA journal article readability? *ANNA Journal*, 64 (1) 65–8   9 References

Reports on a study which examined the readability of the *ANNA Journal*, quantifying the effect of peer review on case and research reports from 1992 to 1994. Two computer indices, Gunning and Flesch, as well as human comparative analysis, were used. Results are reported.

2.99.8   Birchenhall, P. (1997) Reasons for rejection. *Nurse Education Today*, 17 (2) 85–6   No references   Editorial

Discusses the main reasons for rejecting manuscripts, providing readers with pointers for submitting successful papers.

2.99.9   Blancett, S.S., Flanagin, A. & Young, R.K. (1995) Duplicate publication in the nursing literature. *Image: Journal of Nursing Scholarship*, 27 (1) 51–6   37 References

Study aimed to identify examples of duplicate publication in the nursing literature and determine what types of article are being published in this way. From a sample of 642 articles, published by 77 authors during a five-year period, 181 were classified as duplicate. Forty-one authors published at least one form of duplicate article. Fifty-nine did not reference the primary article. Authors point out that duplicate publication in itself is not unethical, but doing this without referencing is, and may violate copyright law (CR 2.17).

2.99.10 Bowbrick, P. (1995) Blowing the whistle on referees. *Times Higher Education Supplement*, 10 February, 1162 11

Discusses the value of refereeing systems, the types of paper published and biases among referees (CR 2.27).

2.99.11 British Medical Journal. (1995) *How To Do It* 3rd edition. London: British Medical Journal Publishing Group. ISBN 0727909061   References

A series of short articles from the *British Medical Journal*, several of which relate to publication processes, authorship, editing and writing.

2.99.12 Burnard, P. (1995) Writing for publication: a guide for those who must. *Nurse Education Today*, 15 (2) 117–20 5 References

Outlines the principles which need to be observed for getting work into print. Information is given on work to be done before preparing a manuscript, its actual preparation and what needs to be done after submission (CR 2.97).

2.99.13 Clark, A.J. (1993) Responsible dissemination of scholarly work. *Journal of Neuroscience Nursing*, 25 (2) 113–17 32 References

Article addresses potential abuses of research and reasons for their occurrence. Recommendations for prevention of authorship abuse and the maintenance of high standards in disseminating scholarly work are made (CR 2.17).

2.99.14 Cohen, L.J. (1989) Reframing manuscript rejection. *Nurse Educator*, 14 (2) 4–5 2 References   Guest editorial

Discusses how to rewrite an article which has been rejected for publication.

2.99.15 Crosby, L.J. (1990) The abstract: an important first impression. *Journal of Neuroscience Nursing*, 22 (3) 192–4   3 References

Discusses the critical items which need to be included in abstracts and two are given as examples.

2.99.16 Cummings, L.L. & Frost, P.J. (eds) (1995) *Publishing in the Organizational Sciences* 2nd edition. Thousand Oaks, CA: Sage. ISBN 0803971451   References

Book explains the entire context of scholarly publishing and how it should contribute towards advancing knowledge and successful management practice.

2.99.17 Curran, S. (1990) *How to Write a Book and Get it Published: a Complete Guide to the Publishing Maze*. London: Thorsons. ISBN 0722521464   References

A practical guide to the types of book that publishers want. Advice is given on most aspects of book publishing (CR 2.97).

2.99.18 Directory of European Nursing Journals. (1996) Edited by Anderson, Y. Copenhagen: Workshop of European Nurse Researchers. ISBN 8772661879

Booklet provides information for nurse researchers who wish to extend their knowledge of nursing journals that publish research (CR 1.3, Appendix B).

2.99.19 Dladla, A.B.W., Gumede, L., Lin, J. & Puckree, T. (1997) Publication trends in the *SA Journal of Physiotherapy* for the decade 1985–1994. *South African Journal of Physiotherapy*, 53 (1) 14–16   7 References

Purpose of this study was to determine trends in the types and first authorship of articles appearing over a decade. One hundred and forty articles were classified into research or non-research, type of research methods used and the status of authors. Results are discussed and trends showing the state of the profession are outlined.

2.99.20 Dowd, S.B. & Schulz, D.L. (1996) Responsible dissemination of scholarly work in radiology. *Radiologic Technology*, 67 (5) 407–14   22 References

Article describes the peer review process, discusses problems of authorship, examines questionable research practices and presents guidelines for the responsible dissemination of research (CR 2.98).

2.99.21 Easterbrook, P.J., Berlin, J.A., Gopalan, R. & Matthews, D.R. (1991) Publication bias in clinical research. *Lancet*, 13 April, 337 (8746) 867–72   28 References

Reports a study which analysed 487 research projects, approved by the Central Oxford Research Ethics Committee between 1984 and 1987, for evidence of publication bias. This was found to exist and authors urge that caution should be taken when basing conclusions only on reviews of published data (CR 2.17, 2.27, 2.29).

2.99.22 Ellis, H. (1995) Review a book, in *British Medical Journal, How To Do It* 4th edition. London: British Medical Journal Publishing Group. ISBN 0727909061

A personal account of the experience of reviewing medical books, usually textbooks and monographs of general surgery. Some of the problems and pleasures are described.

2.99.23 Farquar, M. & McAllister, G. (1993) Publishing literature reviews: why, who, where, when and how? *Nurse Researcher*, 1 (1) 64–73   8 References

The various forms of literature reviews are discussed, together with why, for whom, where, when and how they should be published (CR 2.12).

2.99.24 Flanagin, A. (1993) Writing and publishing: fraudulent publication. *Image: Journal of Nursing Scholarship*, 25 (4) 359   5 References

Statement presented at the annual meeting of the International Academy of Nursing Editors in Edmonton, Canada on 18 August 1993. It is intended as a guide to educate authors and editors about authorship and fraudulent publication (CR 2.17).

2.99.25 Flanagin, A. (1994) Fraudulent publication. *Journal of Nursing Administration*, 24 (4) 60–1   5 References

Briefly discusses scientific misconduct, fraud, the editor's role and retractions (CR 2.17).

2.99.26 Hamblet, J.L. (1996) Ethical issues in publication. *Seminars in Perioperative Nursing*, 5 (2) 102–7   19 References

Discusses the ethical issues of veracity, justice, beneficence and nonmaleficence which play a part in any phase of writing for publication (CR 2.17).

2.99.27 Hicks, C. (1995) The shortfall in published research: a study of nurses' research and publication activities. *Journal of Advanced Nursing*, 21 (3) 594–604   20 References

Reports a study which surveyed 230 nurses to determine the reasons for low publication rates. Results showed that although many nurses undertook research, few published their findings. The chief reason for this was lack of confidence and the author suggests possible ways forward (CR 2.52, 3.17).

2.99.28 Horrobin, D.F. (1990) The philosophical basis of peer review – and the suppression of innovation. *Journal of American Medical Association*, 9 March, 263 (10) 1438–41   24 References

Article discusses the suppression of innovation by the process of peer review. Many examples are given of scientific papers not being published in the 'usual' journals. Author believes that possible improvements in patient care may have been delayed or not implemented at all.

2.99.29 Jackson, D., Raftos, M. & Mannix, J. (1996) Through the looking glass: reflections on the authorship and content of current Australian nursing journals. *Nursing Inquiry*, 3 (2) 112–17   14 References

Examines the refereed content published in four Australian nursing journals over a recent 12-month period. Articles were categorized according to subject matter and authorship, by gender and discipline. Findings showed a marked change from earlier analyses where other disciplines were over-represented.

2.99.30 Janforum. (1997) On being published in the *Journal of Advanced Nursing*: personal, professional and international impact. *Journal of Advanced Nursing*, 26 (6) 1278–80

Six authors discuss experiences following publication of their work in this journal. International contacts and feedback, confidence, career path entered, participation in scientific discourse and the professional debate about nursing are highlighted.

2.99.31 Juhl, N. & Norman, V.L. (1989) Writing an effective abstract. *Applied Nursing Research*, 2 (4) 189–93 3 References

Describes how to write an abstract using two versions of one based on a particular study. Criteria for critiquing abstracts are given and the first version is revised according to these guidelines.

2.99.32 King, C.R., McGuire, D.B., Longman, A.J. & Carroll-Johnson, R.M. (1997) Peer review, authorship, ethics and conflicts of interest. *Image: Journal of Nursing Scholarship*, 29 (2) 163–7 48 References

Paper explores the problems in peer review, authorship, ethics and conflict of interest related to writing and publishing. The quality and integrity of nursing publications are affected by all these factors but an understanding of them will ensure fewer difficulties (CR 2.17, 2.97).

2.99.33 Kirkham, S.R. (1993) Processing papers for *Palliative Medicine*. *Palliative Medicine*, 7 (2) 89–91 Editorial

Explains the processes which take place once an article for publication is received by the editor.

2.99.34 Lee, Y.Y., Wang, C.J. & Liu, S.Y. (1995) Trend analysis of nursing research published in the *Journal of Nursing*: 1982–1992 [Chinese]. *Nursing Research (China)*, 3 (2) 161–70 18 References

Article analysed 178 research papers by nurses published over a ten-year period. Frequency, percentage and chi-square were used for data analysis. Results are reported and discussed together with suggestions for the future.

2.99.35 Legat, M. (1991) *An Author's Guide to Publishing*. London: Robert Hale. ISBN 0709046642 References

This standard work has been extensively revised and updated and includes information on submitting work, contracts, author/publisher relationships, legal matters and the rewards of writing. It also contains a list of organizations for authors in the UK.

2.99.36 Lindquist, R.A. (1993) Strategies for writing a competitive research abstract.

Dimensions of Critical Care Nursing, 12 (1) 46–53 6 References

Article discusses the preparation of research abstracts for submission to scientific meetings of professional organizations. Key components of abstracts are discussed, together with choosing an appropriate meeting and type of presentation, developing and writing an abstract. An example of a draft and final abstract is given.

2.99.37 Lock, S. (1991a) *A Difficult Balance: Editorial Peer Review in Medicine*. London: British Medical Journal Publishing Group. ISBN 0727903101 References

Discusses the processes of peer review of scientific research when applications are made for a grant, an abstract is submitted to a scientific journal or a paper is submitted for publication.

2.99.38 Lock, S. (1991b) *The Future of Medical Journals: in Commemoration of 150 Years of the British Medical Journal*. London: British Medical Journal Publishing Group. ISBN 0727903128 References

A collection of papers given at a conference at Leeds Castle, Kent, by editors of major general medical journals throughout the world, together with experts in science, sociology and epidemiology. They discuss the foundations and effectiveness of modern journals and debate possibilities for the future.

2.99.39 Luey, B. (1990) *Handbook for Academic Authors* 2nd edition. Cambridge: Cambridge University Press. ISBN 0521396468 References

Book provides information on publishing journal articles, revising dissertations, finding and working with publishers. The mechanics of authorship, electronic publishing, costs and prices are also discussed. Bibliography makes reference to many other sources (CR 2.97).

2.99.40 McConnell, E.A. (1995) Journal publishing characteristics for 42 nursing publications outside the United States. *Image: Journal of Nursing Scholarship*, 27 (3) 225–9 5 References

Forty-two out of 102 journal editors from 14 countries responded to a request for information about their journals: their characteristics, leadership, review process and journal staff. Such information will enable nurses to send papers to the most appropriate place for potential publication.

2.99.41 Miller, D.C. (1991) How to take rejection, in Author, *Handbook of Research Design and Social Measurement* 5th edition. Newbury Park, CA: Sage. ISBN 0803942192 Chapter 7D6, 658–62 6 References and Notes

Discusses reasons for the rejection of manuscripts, a typology of reviewers, 'how to take it' and the adaptive response (CR 2.54.14).

2.99.42 Morse, J.M. (1996) 'Revise and resubmit': responding to reviewers' reports. *Qualitative Health Research*, 6 (2) 149–51 Editorial

The editor of *Qualitative Health Research* gives advice to authors about the process of revising articles to be resubmitted for publication.

2.99.43 Mulhall, A. (1996) Publishing original research: principles and practice. *Nurse Researcher*, 4 (1) 49–61 26 References

Paper aims to raise awareness of issues surrounding the publication of research.

2.99.44 Nativio, D.G. (1994) Writing and publishing guidelines. *ANNA Journal*, 21 (6) 359, 367 8 References

Statement is intended as a guide to educate authors and editors about authorship.

2.99.45 Nativio, D.G. (1995) Authorship. *Journal of Cultural Diversity*, 2 (3) 93–4 8 References

Reports a position paper presented at the 1993 International Academy of Nursing Editors conference in Edmonton, Alberta, Canada, on the questions: who is an author, and in collaborative works how should the order of authorship be decided?

2.99.46 Nicholson, R.H. (1993) Old world news: truth lies somewhere, if we knew but where: American authors not citing work published outside the US. *Hastings Center Report*, 23 (5) 5 4 References

Concern is expressed about misconceptions relating to treatment methods for patients over the age of 65 with end-stage renal disease. Evidence is available in both British and European journals and author questions if American scientists and academics read material published elsewhere. Literature from other fields is cited where references were also primarily from American journals. There is a possibility that readers could be misinformed about work done by scientists elsewhere in the world. Where tenure and promotion depend on success in the citation stakes, this could be an unethical practice (CR 2.17).

2.99.47 Orr, J.A. (1993) A brief review of papers published in the *Journal of Advanced Nursing*, 1983–1992. *Journal of Advanced Nursing*, 18 (8) 1337–9 Janforum

Paper classifies articles into 22 categories and gives numbers on research methods between 1983 and 1987 (16) and 1988 and 1992 (40). These covered debates about research methodologies, report writing and the interpretation of results.

2.99.48 Parry, A. (1993) How to write an abstract or summary. *Physiotherapy*, 79 (7) 472–3 1 Reference

Discusses different types of abstract for journal articles, theses, reports of clinical trials, applications for funds and conferences. Some general points are also included.

2.99.49 Roberts, K. (1995) Early Australian nursing scholarship: the first decade of the *Australian Journal of Advanced Nursing*. The *Australian Electronic Journal of Nursing Education.* References

Part 1: Scholars.
URL: http://www.scu.edu.au/schools/nhcp/aejne/vol1-1/ajn1.htm
and
Part 2: Scholarship.
URL: http://www.scu.edu.au/schools/nhcp/aejne/vol1-1/ajan2.htm
and
Part 3: Relationships between scholars and scholarship.
URL: http://www.scu.edu.au/schools.nhcp/aejne/vol1-1/ajan3.htm

This three-part article reports a study which examined papers in the first decade of the *Australian Journal of Advanced Nursing* (*AJAN*), the primary vehicle for disseminating Australian nursing scholarship. It describes the personal and professional characteristics of the authors and compares this with scholars from the USA. The types of article were examined with over half being research reports, one-third were theoretical scholarship with a few clinical articles. The relationships between scholars and scholarship were also explored.

2.99.50 Robinson, D., Collins, M. & Monkman, J. (1997) A practical guide to writing for publication. *Nurse Researcher*, 5 (1) 53–64 No references

Article developed from writers' workshops held in two hospitals. A wide range of issues is included which would guide both novices and the more experienced writer (CR 2.97).

2.99.51 Rushforth, D. (1994) Guidance for first-time contributors. *Mental Health Nursing*, 14 (2) 10–12 8 References

Article offers some suggestions to writers embarking for the first time on the preparation of a paper for publication.

2.99.52 Schmitt, M.H. (1993) Knowledge or nursing knowledge? *Research in Nursing and Health*, 16 (5) 321–2 4 References Editorial

Reports reasons for concern about papers submitted for publication and why they may be rejected by this journal.

2.99.53 Segesten, K. (1995) Creating a Swedish top-ten list of scientific nursing journals. *Scandinavian Journal of Caring Sciences*, 9 (2) 123–6 7 References

Reports a study of preferences for, and utilization of, scientific nursing journals by leading Swedish nurse researchers and American deans of top-ranked university schools of nursing. All articles with a nurse as primary author and published in the *Scandinavian Journal of Caring Sciences*, 1989–1993, were analysed for references to nursing journals. Lists were compiled reflecting the various preferences.

2.99.54 Smith, R. (1997) Misconduct in research: editors respond. *British Medical Journal*, 26 July, 315 (7102) 201–2 8 References

Reports the setting up of the Committee on Publication Ethics (COPE) following several high-profile cases of professional misconduct by senior clinicians. The committee will serve

editors, rather than authors or readers, and will give advice, consider all aspects of potential or actual misconduct, publish an annual report, draft guidelines, promote research into publication ethics and consider offering training (CR 2.17).

2.99.55 Soriano, M.G., Otaolaurruchi, C.R. & Pascual, M.J.F. (1997) The 10-year evolution of public health care publications and community nursing in six Spanish journals [Spanish]. *Enfermería Clínica*, 7 (2) 63–71 18 References

The study examined 241 articles from six Spanish journals from 1984 to 1993 to ascertain the number of research articles, subjects investigated, the most frequent study designs and references used. The number had increased significantly during the period under examination and the most frequent study designs were descriptive.

2.99.56 Waldron, T. (1992) Is duplicate publishing on the increase? *British Medical Journal*, 18 April, 304 (6833) 1029 4 References

Author examined the *British Journal of Industrial Medicine* from 1988 to 1990 to see whether, and how many, articles had been published elsewhere. An increased number over time was observed. The problems, consequences and preventative measures are discussed (CR 2.17).

2.99.57 Yarbro, C.H. (1995) Duplicate publication: guidelines for nurse authors and editors. *Image: Journal of Nursing Scholarship*, 27 (1) 57 9 References

Reports a statement given at the 13th annual meeting of the International Academy of Nursing Editors in 1994 which is intended to guide authors and editors on the appropriateness or otherwise of duplicate publication.

2.100 TALKING ABOUT RESEARCH

In addition to writing about research, opportunities arise for students or experienced researchers to present their work to colleagues verbally. This may be in the classroom, to a small group of interested people or a formal presentation at a conference.

Annotations

2.100.1 Fowles, E.R. (1992) Poster presentations as a strategy for evaluating nursing students on a research course. *Journal of Nursing Education*, 31 (6) 287   3 References

Outlines the value of poster presentations for learning and as an assessment tool. A list of criteria is given to guide the presentation.

2.100.2 Gray, M. (1995) Giving a poster presentation: a personal view. *Nurse Researcher*, 3 (1) 74–81   3 References

Guides readers through the process of preparing and presenting poster material at conferences.

2.100.3 Hayes, P. (1994) Researchers: blow your own horn! *Clinical Nursing Research*, 3 (2) 83–5   Editorial

Editor urges nurses to talk and write about their work so that knowledge about nursing is spread among other health care professionals (CR 2.97).

2.100.4 Kaplan, B.J. (1997) *A Nurse's Guide to Public Speaking*. New York: Springer. ISBN 0826192505   References

Tailored specifically for nurses, this guide will assist in the development of public speaking skills. Advice is given on preparing and delivering a speech, how to organize it, how to assess the room and audience, and how to perform relaxation exercises. Quotes from experienced speakers are included in the text.

2.100.5 Kirkpatrick, H. & Martin, M.-L. (1991) Communicating nursing research through poster presentations. *Western Journal of Nursing Research*, 13 (1) 145–8   4 References

Gives specific information on the presentation of poster sessions.

2.100.6 Martin, P.A. (1994) Poster sessions: tips for the novice viewer. *Applied Nursing Research*, 7 (4) 208–10   5 References

Paper gives some guiding principles and explanations for and about poster sessions which will enable novices to gain more from these encounters.

2.100.7 Mathieson, A. (1996) The principles and practice of oral presentation. *Nurse Researcher*, 4 (2) 41–54   5 References

Provides advice on making good conference presentations.

2.100.8 McDaniel, R.W., Bach, C.A. & Poole, M.J. (1993) Poster update: getting their attention. *Nursing Research*, 42 (5) 302–4   5 References

Discusses essential information needed on a poster, the resources necessary and its presentation.

2.100.9 Miracle, V.A. & King, K.C. (1994) Presenting research: effective paper presentations and impressive poster presentations. *Applied Nursing Research*, 7 (3) 147–51   13 References

Article gives guidelines on preparing for an oral presentation, together with poster presentations. Authors believe these are both valuable ways of disseminating research findings (CR 2.98).

2.100.10 Russell, C.K., Gregory, D.M. & Gates, M.F. (1996) Aesthetics and substance in qualitative research posters. *Qualitative Health Research*, 6 (4) 542–52   17 References

Guidelines are presented for qualitative posters based upon the evaluation of such posters at research conferences and a review of the literature. Areas included are content, text, materials, component arrangement and visual appearance.

2.100.11 Todoroff, C. (1997) *Presenting Science with Impact*. Toronto, Canada: Trifolium Books. ISBN 1895579872   References

Book gives practical advice on making presentations, from initial organization to the final meeting. Each stage is broken down and described in detail.

2.101 CREATING A RESEARCH UTILIZATION ENVIRONMENT

'Creation of a research utilization environment is a pre-condition to implementing appropriate research findings. Nurse managers, educators, researchers and clinicians all have responsibilities in relation to this.

Creating support networks, providing opportunities for learning, communicating in a clear way and the willingness to participate in research are all required' (Phillips, L.R.F., 1986: 462).

Definition

Research utilization – a process directed towards transferring specific research-based knowledge into actual clinical practice

Example

Ashcroft, T & Kristjanson, L.J. (1994) Utilization in maternal–child nursing: application of the CURN model. *Canadian Journal of Nursing Administration*, 7 (3) 90–102 16 References

Article describes how the CURN (Conduct and Utilization of Research in Nursing) approach was used in a maternal–child area of a Canadian tertiary care hospital. One patient care problem was identified that required the application of recent findings and the results are reported.

Annotations

2.101.1 Brown, D.S. (1997) Nursing education and nursing research utilization: is there a connection in clinical settings? *Journal of Continuing Education in Nursing*, 28 (6) 258–62   12 References

Reports a survey of 753 nurses in North Carolina which showed that nurses with higher levels of education are more involved in research activities and research utilization. Recommendations to improve research utilization in clinical and academic settings are provided (CR 3.17).

2.101.2 Butler, L. (1995) Valuing research in clinical practice: a basis for developing a strategic plan for nursing research. *Canadian Journal of Nursing Research*, 27 (4) 33–49 18 References

Reports a survey conducted to examine staff and leadership nurses' attitudes towards research as part of their work, with a view to developing a strategic plan for nursing research in clinical practice. Factors which explain research use and participation in designing and conducting research differed for the two groups.

2.101.3 Butler, L. (1996) Deciding on research in times of fiscal restraint: can nursing risk the cost? *Canadian Oncology Nursing Journal*, 6 (4) 178–80   9 References

Describes how a nursing division responded to a hospital's mission by developing a program of nursing research. The research component was aligned with oncology and the various staff roles are discussed (CR 3.11, 3.16).

2.101.4 Camiah, S. (1997) Utilization of nursing research in practice and application strategies to raise research awareness amongst practitioners: a model for success. *Journal of Advanced Nursing*, 26 (6) 1193–202 34 References

Describes a study where the views of nurse practitioners regarding the utilization of nursing research in practice and their awareness of research relevant to their practice were elicited. Four major strategies are suggested to raise awareness.

2.101.5 Caroselli, C. (1995) Research utilization: reducing the pain. *Orthopaedic Nursing*, 14 (2) 32–7   19 References

Describes ways of initiating the process of research utilization. Suggestions are given for finding resources as well as practical tips for what can be a very satisfying way to implement cost-effective high-quality care.

2.101.6 Clark, K.H., Cronenwett, L.R., Thompson, P.A. & Reeves, S.A. (1991) Turning the organization upside down: creating a culture for innovation and creativity. *Nursing Administration Quarterly*, 16 (1) 7–14 2 References

Authors describe the concepts, processes and outcomes which developed as a conscious effort was made to turn their organization upside down. This enabled a culture of innovation and creativity to emerge.

2.101.7 Edwards-Beckett, J. (1990) Nursing research utilization techniques. *Journal of Nursing Administration*, 20 (11) 25–30 44 References

Describes a literature review which aimed to

identify methods to promote research utilization in practice settings. Nine general themes were used and suggestions are made for appropriate input by individuals, groups, organizations and professions (CR 2.12).

2.101.8 Funk, S.G., Champagne, M.T., Tornquist, E.M. & Wiese, R.A. (1995) Administrators views on barriers to research utilization. *Applied Nursing Research*, 8 (1) 44–54   22 References

Reports a study which aimed to identify the barriers to research utilization as seen from the administrators' point of view. Twenty-eight items were singled out, the results discussed and possible solutions identified.

2.101.9   Green, S. & Houston, S. (1993) Promoting research activities: institutional strategies. *Applied Nursing Research*, 6 (2) 97–102 4 References

Paper describes many innovative ideas developed and adopted in one hospital to promote research activities.

2.101.10   Hefferin, E.A., Horsley, J.A. & Ventura, M.R. (1991) Promoting research-based nursing: the nurse administrators' role, in Ward, M.J., & Price, S.A. (eds), *Issues in Nursing Administration: Selected Readings*. St Louis: Mosby Year Book. ISBN 0801660637 Chapter 25, 215–24   39 References

Reports a survey among hospital-based nurse administrators and researchers to determine research-related issues. The roles of all nurses are outlined (CR 3.16).

2.101.11   Hicks, C. (1994) The role of the middle manager in health care research: some problems and perspectives. *Health Services Management Research*, 7 (4) 282–6 16 References

Reports a pilot study which examined the impact of developing research competencies in a group of middle managers, on the assumption that they might influence other staff. The difficulties that were encountered are highlighted and suggestions are made for overcoming them (CR 2.23).

2.101.12   Kitson, A. & Currie, L. (1996) Clinical practice development and research activities in four district health authorities. *Journal of Clinical Nursing*, 5 (1) 41–51 9 References

Reports a postal survey in 1992 which elicited information from four health authorities regarding the development and research activity in which they were involved. The aim was to provide staff with a mechanism for networking good practice and identify any areas of replication. Results are reported and findings confirm other work showing small-scale work and unsupported nurses who were trying to implement findings and be innovative in practice (CR 2.13).

2.101.13   Knight, S., Bowman, G. & Thompson, D.R. (1997) A strategy for developing research in practice. *NT Research*, 2 (2) 119–25   13 References

Describes how one National Health Service trust, in partnership with a university, has formulated and created a strategy for developing research in nursing practice. This aims to support nurses and midwives in understanding research and applying it where appropriate.

2.101.14   Lacey, E.A. (1994) Research utilization in nursing practice: a pilot study. *Journal of Advanced Nursing*, 19 (5) 987–95 15 References

Paper reviews recent empirical studies about research utilization. A small pilot study which attempted to measure research utilization among general nurses is described. Some preliminary results showed a positive attitude in the group of British nurses studied, but the biggest deterrent to use of research findings seemed to be a perceived lack of autonomy (CR 2.23).

2.101.15   Macguire, J.M. (1990) Putting research findings into practice: research utilization as an aspect of the management of change. *Journal of Advanced Nursing*, 15 (5) 614–20   22 References

Identifies ten areas of potential difficulty which need to be examined before research findings may be implemented in practice. These need to be addressed at all organizational levels, rather than putting blame on individuals for non-implementation of research findings.

2.101.16   Mackay, R., Cruickshank, J. & Matsund, K. (1991) Developing a hospital nursing research programme. *Australian Journal of Advanced Nursing*, 8 (2) 10–14 11 References

Describes the development of a programme of research activities organized by a nursing research department in one hospital (CR 2.102).

2.101.17 Martin, M.-L. & Forchuk, C. (1994) Linking research and practice. *International Nursing Review*, 41 (6) 184–7 12 References

Reports how a service agency facilitated the links between nursing research and practice at a Canadian hospital (CR 2.102).

2.101.18 Martin, P.A. (1993) Clinical settings need organizational support for research. *Applied Nursing Research*, 6 (2) 103–4 3 References

Discusses the importance of an organizational research culture and climate for the promotion of nursing research activities. The elements necessary are outlined from the literature.

2.101.19 Mitchell, A., Janzen, K., Pask, E. & Southwell, D. (1995) Assessment of nursing research utilization needs in Ontario health agencies. *Canadian Journal of Administration*, 8 (1) 77–91 17 References

Reports a survey, conducted by the Nursing Research Interest Group of the Registered Nurses' Association of Ontario, to determine whether health agencies have implemented programmes to assist staff nurses in utilizing research findings, and if they would accept resources to assist in the development of these skills. A need was identified for assistance in encouraging research-based nursing practice.

2.101.20 Nolan, M. & Behi, R. (1996) From methodology to method: the building blocks of research literacy. *British Journal of Nursing*, 5 (1) 54–7 18 References

Discusses some of the barriers to research utilization and argues that in order to overcome these both decision- and knowledge-driven approaches are required (CR 2.14).

2.101.21 Nolan, M.T., Larson, E., McGuire, D., Hill, M.N. & Haller, K. (1994) A review of approaches to integrating research and practice. *Applied Nursing Research*, 7 (4) 199–207 32 References

Report presents a review and comparison of several approaches to research utilization: the

Western Interstate Commission for Higher Education in Nursing (WICHEN); Regional Program for Nursing Research Development; the Conduct and Utilization of Research in Nursing (CURN); the Stetler Model; the American Association of Critical Care Nurses (AACN) Approach; and the University of North Carolina Approach.

2.101.22 Parker, M.E., Gordon, S.C. & Brannon, P.T. (1992) Involving nursing staff in research: a non-traditional approach. *Journal of Nursing Administration*, 22 (4) 58–63 18 References

Describes a study which aimed to create a positive environment, expressing nursing values. Nurse administrators, researchers and practitioners all worked together to examine the climate in which research could both be conducted and utilized (CR 2.15, 3.16).

2.101.23 Pearcey, P. & Draper, P. (1996) Using the diffusion of innovation model to influence practice: a case study. *Journal of Advanced Nursing*, 23 (4) 714–21 33 References

Authors suggest that a 'bottom up' approach to encourage research utilization may be appropriate, using the techniques of action research (CR 2.37, 2.39).

2.101.24 Rizzuto, C. & Mitchell, M. (1990) Outcomes of a research consortium project. *Journal of Nursing Administration*, 20 (4) 13–17 3 References

Gives a final report on the work of a unique collaborative model for facilitating the conduct of nursing research in service settings (CR 2.15).

2.101.25 Rodgers, S. (1994) An exploratory study of research utilization by nurses in general medical and surgical wards. *Journal of Advanced Nursing*, 20 (5) 904–11 27 References

This exploratory study examined potential factors that may affect research utilization through a review of the literature and field work carried out in two hospitals in Scotland. Findings indicate the complexity of the issue and the author believes that the multiple factors must be addressed simultaneously.

2.101.26 Rosswurm, M.A. (1992) A research-based practice model in a hospital setting. *Journal of Nursing Administration*, 22 (3) 57–60   10 References

Discusses the critical factors required to develop and support a nursing research department in a community medical centre. A research-based practice model is proposed.

2.101.27   Royle, J.A., Blythe, J., Ingram, C., DiCenso, A., Bhatnager, N. & Potvin, C. (1996) The research utilization process: the use of guided imagery to reduce anxiety. *Canadian Oncology Nursing Journal*, 6 (1) 20–5   38 References

This study aimed to introduce a framework for research-based care, enhance research utilization in a selected setting and evaluate the outcomes of this work. The facilitators and barriers to research utilization are discussed (CR 2.61).

2.101.28   Rutledge, D.N. (1995) Building organizational capacity to engage in research utilization. *Journal of Nursing Administration*, 25 (10) 12–16   11 References

Reports the work of the Orange County Research Unit in Nursing Project (OCRUN) which aimed to educate nurses on their role-specific research utilization competency development. Paper reports positive changes and gives a series of recommendations for the future.

2.101.29   Selby, M.L., Riportella-Muller, R. & Farel, A. (1992) Building administrative support for your research: a neglected key for turning a research plan into a funded project. *Nursing Outlook*, 40 (2) 73–7   9 References

Article addresses administrative issues that nurse researchers must consider when submitting a grant proposal to health care institutions or universities. An adequate budget and clear agreements with all agencies are crucial for the successful implementation of a research plan (CR 2.96, 3.13).

2.101.30   Sperhac, A.M., Haas, S.A. & O'Malley, J. (1994) Supporting nursing research: a representation program. *Journal of Nursing Administration*, 24 (5) 28–31   3 References

Describes the design and conception of two funded programmes which support clinical nursing research in a paediatric hospital.

2.101.31   Tiffany, C.R. & Lutjens, L.R.J.
(1998) *Planned Change Theories for Nursing: Review, Analysis and Implications*. Thousand Oaks, CA: Sage. ISBN 076190235X

Book provides an overview of three widely accepted change theories, as well as a new systems-orientated theory. The implications for nursing practice and research are discussed.

2.101.32   Titler, M.G. (1997) Utilization: necessity or luxury?, in McCloskey, J.C. & Grace. H.K. (eds), *Current Issues in Nursing* 5th edition.   St Louis: Mosby.   ISBN 0815185944 Chapter 15, 104–17   54 References

Chapter presents an overview of the history and process of research utilization. The potential barriers, strategies used to overcome them, and future ways in which they may be streamlined are discussed.

2.101.33   Tranmer, J.E., Kisilevsky, B.S. & Muir, D.W. (1995) A nursing research utilization strategy for staff nurses in the acute care setting. *Journal of Nursing Administration*, 25 (4) 21–9   24 References

Reports a project which aimed to serve as a model for the incorporation of research findings into practice settings, other than a neonatal intensive care unit where the original work was done. Its implications are discussed.

2.101.34   Varcoe, C. & Hilton, A. (1995) Factors affecting acute-care nurses' use of research findings. *Canadian Journal of Nursing Research*, 27 (4) 51–71   24 References

Study describes staff nurses' perceptions of hospital support for research and their expectations. Relationships between organizational and individual factors and their use of research is discussed. Results suggest that the organizational context is important but nurses' value of, interest in and expectations to use research may mediate this influence.

2.101.35   Wright, S.G. (1997) *Changing Nursing Practice* 2nd edition. San Diego, CA: Singular Publishing Group Inc. ISBN 1565937589   References

Book explores the concept of change and discusses the complex skills which nurses need in order to become change agents. Many examples are included which illustrate 'how to' change nursing practice.

2.101.36 Wright, S.G. & Dolan, M. (1991) Coming down from the ivory tower: putting research into practice. *Professional Nurse*, 7 (1) 38, 40–1   9 References

Discusses ways used to encourage staff in a nursing development unit to become research aware, and how this is beginning to be achieved.

2.102   APPLYING RESEARCH TO PRACTICE

'The ultimate goal is not the use of research, it is to deliver high-quality, cost-effective care to achieve desirable patient outcomes and to deliver care from a professional practice model.' (Crane, 1995: 575)

Definition

Implementing research findings – to use in practice

Example

Dufalt, M. A., Bielecki, C.X., Collins, E. & Willey, C. (1995) Changing nurses' pain assessment practice: a collaborative research utilization approach. *Journal of Advanced Nursing*, 21 (4) 634–45   55 References

This quasi-experimental study showed the effectiveness of a collaborative research model, directed towards transferring specific knowledge of pain assessment into practice. Nurses who participated significantly improved their competence in research utilization and in their attitudes towards research (CR 2.15, 2.35).

Annotations

2.102.1 Allen, A. (1993) Changing theory in nursing practice. *Senior Nurse*, 13 (10) 43–5, 49   27 References

Describes how change theory can be used to overcome some of the difficulties associated with the implementation of research findings.

2.102.2 Anonymous (1996) How nursing research makes a difference. *International Nursing Review*, 43 (2) 49–52, 58   41 References

Article gives examples of evidence to show that nursing care has significant effects on health outcomes and costs of care. Also acknowledged is the need to do further work in linking research to practice and policy-making.

2.102.3 Baessler, C.A., Blumberg, M., Cunningham, J.S., Curran, J.A., Fennessey, A.G., Jacobs, J.M., McGrath, P., Perrong, M.T. & Wolf, Z.R. (1994) Medical-surgical nurses' utilization of research methods and products. *MEDSURG Nursing*, 3 (2) 113–17, 120–1   31 References

Reports a study, using the Research Utilization Questionnaire, in which 212 registered nurses were asked to describe the use of the methods and products of research in their disciplines, and to identify their attitudes towards the use of research-based knowledge in clinical practice.

2.102.4 Balcombe, K.P. (1996) Management. Effects of the purchaser/provider split on research implementation. *British Journal of Nursing*, 5 (19) 1206–9   7 References

The challenges and relationships of this new phase in health services organization are explored using Nolan and Grant's (1993) framework. The implementation of nursing research findings should be part of the contracting process and all those involved need knowledge about research and professional values to maximize benefits to the patient.

2.102.5 Barnsteiner, J.H., Ford, N. & Howe, C. (1995) Research utilization in a metropolitan children's hospital. *Nursing Clinics of North America*, 30 (3) 447–55   3 References

Describes a model of research utilization for directing clinical practice. Staff organization, together with formal and informal mechanisms for knowledge dissemination and utilization, are discussed (CR 2.98).

2.102.6 Beaudry, M., Van den Bosch, T. & Anderson, J. (1996) Research utilization: once-a-day temperatures for afebrile patients. *Clinical Nurse Specialist*, 10 (1) 21–4   24 References

The need for clinical research utilization is

discussed, and ideas for implementation, using an adaptation of the Conduct and Utilization of Research in Nursing model, are described. The taking of temperatures is used as an example and relevant studies are listed which were used as the basis for change. The research base of the topic is summarized and an example is given of practice guidelines.

2.102.7   Berggren, A.C. (1996) Swedish midwives' awareness of attitudes to the use of selected research findings. *Journal of Advanced Nursing*, 23 (3) 462–70   59 References

Describes a small study of Swedish midwives which examined awareness of research findings, opinions of their value and whether they were used in practice. Results showed that findings were used when the midwives believed the care of mother and baby would be improved. Author suggests that the innovation-diffusion process is examined from an organizational perspective to improve further the quality of care.

2.102.8   Blegen, M.A. & Goode, C. (1994) Interactive process of conducting and utilizing research in nursing service administration. *Journal of Nursing Administration*, 24 (9) 24–8   17 References

Reports how three research studies were conducted and the knowledge systematically applied to the practice of nursing service administration. Authors believe that findings can be more widely used in organizing and managing the care of hospital patients.

2.102.9   Bradish, G., Goddard, P., Hatcher, S., Myslick, B., Vlasic, W., Wilson, B. & Laschinger, H.K.S. (1996) Applying the Stetler-Marram model to a nursing administration problem: a graduate student learning experience. *Canadian Journal of Nursing Administration*, 9 (1) 57–70   21 References

Describes a graduate learning experience in which the Stetler-Marram Research Utilization Model was applied to a fictitious case in nursing administration.

2.102.10   Carter, D. (1996) Barriers to the implementation of research findings in practice. *Nurse Researcher*, 4 (2) 30–40   38 References

Reviews the literature from 1972 to 1995 to examine reasons for the failure to implement

research findings. Areas covered include theory, research and practice, knowledge of research, the theory–practice gap and the process of change (CR 2.12, 2.101, 3.8).

2.102.11   Cavanagh, S.J. & Tross, G. (1996) Utilizing research findings in nursing: policy and practice considerations. *Journal of Advanced Nursing*, 24 (5) 1083–8   48 References

Paper reviews some issues relating to implementing research findings in practice, examines research studies in this area and discusses a strategy for the future.

2.102.12   Chapman, H. (1996) Why do nurses not make use of a solid research base? *Nursing Times*, 17 January, 92 (3) 38–9   8 References

Paper explores some reasons why nursing has failed to become a research-based profession.

2.102.13   Clarke, H.F. (1996) Utilizing research findings in practice: issues and strategies, in Kerr, J.S. & MacPhail, J. (eds), *Canadian Nursing: Issues and Perspectives* 3rd edition. St Louis: Mosby. ISBN 0815152256 Chapter 13, 162–80   56 References

Discusses health care system issues relating to the utilization of research findings, professional practice of nursing, innovative adaptive behaviour and future challenges.

2.102.14   Closs, S.J. & Cheater, F.M. (1994) Utilization of nursing research: culture, interest and support. *Journal of Advanced Nursing*, 19 (4) 762–73   61 References

Utilization of nursing research is acknowledged to be a highly complex task and this article explores aspects of research culture, together with the interest and support needed within organizations. Also considered are the research–practice gap, the role of researchers and educational issues. Comparisons are also made with the more positive research culture in the USA (CR 3.8).

2.102.15   Crane, J. (1995) The future of research utilization, in Titler, M.G. & Goode, C.J. (eds), *The Nursing Clinics of North America: Research Utilization*. Philadelphia: W.B. Saunders. ISSN 0029-6465   565–77 37 References

Author charts the progress of research utilization, the agencies and organizations involved, education of nurses and use of the Internet, which have laid the foundations for and will assist in the development of research utilization (CR 2.85).

2.102.16 Donaldson, N.E. (1992) If not now, then when? Nursing's research utilization imperative, in *Communicating Nursing Research. Silver Threads – 25 Years of Nursing Excellence* Volume 25. Boulder, CO: Western Institute of Nursing. No ISBN 29–44 68 References

Discusses the discipline of knowledge utilization, the evolution of nursing inquiry and variables which influence dissemination and utilization. Recommendations are made for practice and education (CR 2.101).

2.102.17 Fitzpatrick, J., Stevenson, J.S. & Polis, N.S. (eds) (1994) *Nursing Research and its Utilization: International State of the Science.* New York: Springer. ISBN 0826180906 References

Book includes sections on how research has been used in various specialist areas; perspectives on the delivery of care; research training and guidance for those wishing to have a career in research. International perspectives include nursing research in the Western Pacific Region, in Holland and challenges which exist in conducting cross-national nursing research (CR 3.3, 3.16, 3.17, 3.22).

2.102.18 Foundation of Nursing Studies. (1996) *Reflection for Action.* London: Foundation of Nursing Studies. No ISBN References

Paper reports on four conferences held in the UK (1994–96) which provided opportunities to debate the issues surrounding the dissemination and implementation of research. An evaluation is made of a series of workshops on the effective implementation of research and a phenomenological study which investigated the research culture of nurses, health visitors, midwives and managers is reported (CR 2.29, 2.98).

2.102.19 Freemantle, N. & Watt, I. (1994) Dissemination: implementing the findings of research. *Health Libraries Review*, 11 (2) 133–7 8 References

Research evidence suggests that effective dissemination will depend upon multiple means to communicate key messages rather than a single measure. Information professionals have a role in ensuring that the key evidence is promoted and is reliable (CR 2.98).

2.102.20 Funk, S.G., Tornquist, E.M. & Champagne, M.T. (1995) Barriers and facilitators of research utilization, in Titler, M.G. & Goode, C.J. (eds), *The Nursing Clinics of North America: Research Utilization.* Philadelphia: W.B. Saunders. ISSN 0029-6465 395–407 79 References

Authors identify the barriers to research utilization, how institutions can facilitate and suggest an integrated approach for the future.

2.102.21 Horsley, J.A. (1983) *Using Research to Improve Nursing Practice: a Guide. CURN project.** Orlando: Grune & Stratton. ISBN 080891510X References

[*Conduct and Utilization of Research in Nursing project, Michigan Nurses Association.] Book attempts to move research and practice closer together by describing the processes involved in incorporating research-based knowledge into practice. Emphasis is put on the activities undertaken by the organization involved in change, rather than by individuals. These are creating a climate for practice change, planning, implementing and then evaluating the processes.

2.102.22 Kajermo, K.N., Nordström, G., Krusebrant, Å. & Björvell, H. (1998) Barriers to and facilitators of research utilization as perceived by a group of registered nurses in Sweden. *Journal of Advanced Nursing*, 27 (4) 798–807 35 References

Describes a survey which described 237 nurses' perceptions of research utilization at two hospitals in Sweden. Twenty-nine barriers were identified, with the three most problematic being: insufficient time on the job to implement new ideas; research reports/ articles are not readily available; and the facilities were inadequate for implementation. Results are discussed.

2.102.23 Kenrick, M. & Luker, K.A. (1996) An exploration of the influence of managerial factors on research utilization in district nursing practice. *Journal of Advanced Nursing*, 23 (4) 697–704 33 References

Reports a small study which explored managerial arrangements in five health care districts. The influence these had on the way in which research findings were used in practice is discussed.

2.102.24 Kitson, A., Ahmed, L.B., Harvey, G., Seera, K. & Thompson, D.R. (1996) From research to practice: one organizational model for promoting research-based practice. *Journal of Advanced Nursing*, 23 (3) 430–40 53 References

Paper describes a framework used to integrate research, development and practice. Its strengths and weaknesses are discussed.

2.102.25 Mateo, M.A. & Kirchhoff, K.T. (eds) (1999) *Using and Conducting Nursing Research in Clinical Settings* 2nd edition. Philadelphia, PA: W.B. Saunders. ISBN 0721671659 References

Book aims to assist clinical nurses to integrate and use research in practice and complements existing methodological texts. It covers research in clinical settings, using it in practice, conducting and disseminating findings. An annotated bibliography includes research texts, instrumentation, design, statistics and publications. Journals publishing research articles are listed and book includes two directories which give researchers' names and interests (CR 1.5, 2.1, 2.54, 3.22, Appendix B). [Annotation refers to 1991 (1st) edition]

2.102.26 McIntosh, J. (1995) Barriers to research implementation. *Nurse Researcher*, 2 (4) 83–91   13 References

Article identifies barriers to utilizing research and indicates some strategies used to eradicate them.

2.102.27 Meah, S., Luker, K.A. & Cullum, N.A. (1996) An exploration of midwives' attitudes to research and perceived barriers to research utilization. *Midwifery*, 12 (2) 73–84 24 References

A study of 32 midwives in North-West England showed that they aspired to deliver research-based care, but a number of barriers were identified to prevent this occurring. Research was felt to be physically inaccessible, complex and they lacked the knowledge and confidence to appraise findings and assess their appropriateness for implementation.

2.102.28 Mhlongo, T.P. & Brink, H. (1996) Research utilization. *Curationis: South African Journal of Nursing*, 19 (1) 6–10 23 References

Authors state that in South Africa the research–practice gap is maximized by the lack of facilities and research utilization projects in nursing education programmes. Various conceptual, empirical and pragmatic issues are discussed to explore the complex influences which may prevent integration of research into practice (CR 3.8).

2.102.29 Mottola, C.A. (1996) Research utilization and the continuing staff development educator. *Journal of Continuing Education in Nursing*, 27 (4) 168–75, 192, 195 34 References

The current turbulent health care environment necessitates utilization of current research findings to maintain efficient and effective functioning of nursing staff. Familiarity with recent research utilization projects and barriers which may impede this can assist educators to bridge the gap between knowledge and practice (CR 3.8).

2.102.30 Nelson, D. (1995) Research into nursing practice. *Accident and Emergency Nursing*, 3 (4) 184–9   32 References

Paper aimed to establish whether research by practitioners is being used in practice. A small-scale study showed that many action research projects were not being formally utilized. A lack of research culture, and managerial and peer support contributed to this problem. Further integration between college, management and students is required (CR 2.37).

2.102.31 NHS Executive Anglia & Oxford R&D Directorate. (1997) *Methods to Improve the Implementation of Research Findings*. London: NHS Executive North Thames RO.
URL: http://libsun1.jr2.ox.ac.uk/nhserdd/ aordd/overview/impintro.htm

Reports on a programme to identify an agenda for the promotion and implementation of research and development findings in the National Health Service.

2.102.32 Pearcey, P.A. (1995) Achieving research-based nursing practice. *Journal of Advanced Nursing*, 22 (1) 33–9   20 References

Reports a study which aimed to identify the self-perceived research skill needs of qualified nurses with a view to developing training workshops. Results showed 93 per cent of participants were dissatisfied with their research skills. Ways forward are suggested.

2.102.33 Robinson, D., Gajos, M. & Whyte, L. (1997) Evidence-based nursing through clinical practice. *Nursing Standard*, 16 April, 11 (30) 32–3   9 References

Describes how a working group examined ways to overcome difficulties with applying research findings in practice. A distance-learning package was created to assist in developing staff skills and was felt to be relevant to registered nurses in all contexts.

2.102.34 Stocking, B. (1995) Why research findings are not used by commissions – and what can be done about it. *Journal of Public Health Medicine*, 17 (4) 380–2   No references

Examines issues which the author believes to be reasons why research findings are not used: these are that the research is not there, many managers are not knowledgeable, public health (and others) does not act as a product champion of knowledge, change is more difficult than expected, and purchasing is the only lever (CR 3.11).

2.102.35 Titler, M.G. & Goode, C.J. (eds) (1995) *The Nursing Clinics of North America: Research Utilization.* Philadelphia: W.B. Saunders. ISSN 0029-6465 30 (3)

This issue gives an overview of the theoretical aspects of research utilization describing what is known about the barriers and facilitators. The differences are also described between evaluating the impact of using research findings in practice and conducting the research itself. Different research utilization models are reviewed, compared and critiqued, and methods for effective dissemination are outlined. A selection of examples are given which represent the complexities of research utilization activities.

2.102.36 Titler, M.G., Kleiber, C., Steelman, V., Goode, C., Rakel, B., Barry-Walker, J., Small, S. & Buckwalter, K. (1995) Infusing research into practice to promote quality care. *Nursing Research*, 43 (5) 307–13   27 References

Describes the Iowa Model of Research in Practice, a heuristic model used for infusing research into practice to improve the quality of care. Its components are given, with examples. The potential impact on patients, staff and fiscal outcomes is discussed.

2.102.37 Vaughan, B. & Edwards, M. (1996) *Interface Between Research and Practice.* London: King's Fund Centre. ISBN 1857170849   References

Paper gives examples of how research can be utilized in practice and how projects may be developed from practice. Material is based on work carried out in Nursing Development Units.

2.102.38 Walsh, M. (1997) How nurses perceive barriers to research implementation. *Nursing Standard*, 11 (29) 34–9   12 References

Paper examines the perceived barriers to research in a sample of 63 hospital and 78 community nurses. The major problems identified related to the clinical setting and understanding research reports.

2.102.39 Wuest, J. (1995) Breaking the barriers to nursing research. *Canadian Nurse*, 91 (4) 29–33   14 References

Author believes that the two major barriers to integrating nursing research and practice are the prevailing perception of research as a remote nursing science and the absence of a supportive infrastructure.

2.102.40 Zacharia, R. & Lundeen, S.P. (1997) Research and practice in an academic community nursing center. *Image: Journal of Nursing Scholarship*, 29 (3) 255–60   29 References

Paper identifies issues and describes strategies used in developing a successful programme of clinical research focused on vulnerable populations served by one centre. Factors affecting the integration of research are outlined and steps taken to overcome them are highlighted (CR 3.16).

PART 3: THE BACKGROUND TO RESEARCH IN NURSING

DEVELOPMENT OF NURSING RESEARCH

HISTORICAL PERSPECTIVES

3.1 AFRICA, AMERICA (SOUTH & CENTRAL), AND ASIA

The history of nursing research development in many parts of the world shows varying levels of progress and sophistication. Positive and rapid growth is reported in some countries, whereas in others the process may be just beginning.

Annotations

3.1.1 Boontong, T. (1990) The status of nursing research in Thailand, in National Center for Nursing Research/International Council of Nurses. *Nursing Research Worldwide: Current Dimensions and Future Directions*. Bethesda, MD: National Center for Nursing Research/Geneva, Switzerland: International Council of Nurses. No ISBN 27–138   11 References

Reports on the health care system in Thailand, the distribution of health personnel, historical background to nursing research, number of researchers and their education, types of research conducted and its funding, current trends, priorities and the role of the National Nurses' Association in promoting research (CR 3.22.9).

3.1.2 Cianciarullo, T.I. & Salzano, S.D. (1990) Nursing and nursing research in Brazil, in National Center for Nursing Research/International Council of Nurses, *Nursing Research Worldwide: Current Dimensions and Future Directions*. Bethesda, MD: National Center for Nursing Research/Geneva, Switzerland: International Council of Nurses. No ISBN 139–49 24 References

Reports on the status of nursing in Brazil, the history of nursing research and its generation. Profiles of researchers, types of research and its application in practice, graduate programmes, funding agencies, research priorities, limitations and the role of the Brazilian Nurses' Association are all discussed (CR 3.22.9).

3.1.3 Golander, H. & Krulik, T. (1996) Nursing research in Israel. *Annual Review of Nursing Research*, 14 207–24

3.1.4 Higuchi, Y. (1990) Nursing research in Japan, in National Center for Nursing Research/International Council of Nurses, *Nursing Research Worldwide: Current Dimensions and Future Directions*. Bethesda, MD: National Center for Nursing Research/Geneva, Switzerland: International Council of Nurses. No ISBN 113–20 12 References

Outlines the educational programmes prepared for nurse researchers, the agencies involved, setting the research agenda, types and areas of research. Four case studies are included (CR 3.22.9).

3.1.5 Hunt, N. (1995) Nursing research in South Africa. *Curationis: South African Journal of Nursing*, 18 (2) 1

3.1.6 Kim, E. (1990) Nursing research in Korea, in National Center for Nursing Research/International Council of Nurses, *Nursing Research Worldwide: Current Dimensions and Future Directions*. Bethesda, MD: National Center for Nursing Research/ Geneva, Switzerland: International Council of Nurses. No ISBN 160–9   15 References

Describes the country of Korea, its health care delivery system, historical background of nursing research, status and preparation of researchers. Also discussed are trends, funding, the need for improvement, priorities for nursing research and the role of the Korean Nurses' Association (CR 3.22.9).

3.1.7 Kim, M.-I. (1994) Nursing research in the Western Pacific region and future directions, in Fitzpatrick, J.J., Stevenson, J.S. & Polis, N.S. (eds) *Nursing Research and its Utilization*. New York: Springer. ISBN 0826180906   Chapter 20, 203–10   1 Reference

Reports on a study which examined the status of nursing resources in the Western Pacific region in 1991, the International Council of Nurses' Directory of Nursing Research Units and future directions (CR 2.102.17, 3.14.6).

3.1.8 Kim, M.-I. (1998) Nursing research in Asia. *International Nursing Review*, 45 (1) 21–2

Summarizes the nursing research status in eight Asian countries: Australia, China, India, Japan, Korea, Mongolia, the Philippines and Thailand (CR 3.2).

3.1.9 Lange, I. & Campos, C. (1998) Nursing research in Chile. *International Nursing Review*, 45 (1) 23–5   10 References

Reports on recent developments, future outlook and makes proposals for research priorities (CR 3.20).

3.1.10 Mangay-Maglacas, A. (1992) Nursing research in developing countries: needs and prospects. *Journal of Advanced Nursing*, 17 (3) 267–70   Guest editorial

Describes the growth of, and interest in, nursing research in developing compared with developed countries. Resources for research, the need for training facilities, personnel and funding are outlined, together with priorities which need to be established (CR 3.20).

3.1.11 Mendes, I.A.C. & Trevizan, M.A. (1996) The evolution of nursing research in Brazil. *Annual Review of Nursing Research*, 14 225–42

3.1.12 Oguisso, T. (1996) Professional nursing in Brazil. *International Nursing Review*, 43 (3) 81–4

Reports on the development of the Brazilian Nurses' Association which has been instrumental in achieving much for the nursing profession.

3.1.13 Olade, R.A. (1990) A survey of nursing research in Nigeria. *International Nursing Review*, 37 (4) 299–302   11 References

Reports a survey which examined the status of nursing research in Nigeria. The background is discussed, as are the infrastructure for research, funding, climate, nursing practice, education, services and the future.

3.1.14 Tlou, S.D. (1998) Nursing research in Africa. *International Nursing Review*, 45 (1) 20

Reports the research priorities in Africa based on input from colleges of nursing and national associations (CR 3.20).

3.2 AUSTRALIA AND NEW ZEALAND

Development of nursing research in Australia and New Zealand is beginning to gain momentum and literature here reports some of the achievements and hopes for the future.

Annotations

3.2.1 Chick, N.P. (1987) Nursing research in New Zealand. *Western Journal of Nursing Research*, 9 (3) 317–34   65 References

Provides an overview of the development of nursing research in New Zealand. This includes its history, progress in educating nurses for research, research as a career pathway, avenues for publication, information retrieval systems, consumership, funding, policy and research priorities (CR 3.13, 3.16, 3.17, 3.20).

3.2.2 Fry, A. (1993) A visit to the National Center for Nursing Research, USA. *Australian Journal of Advanced Nursing*, 11 (1) 5–13 32 References

Reports on a visit to the National Center for Nursing Research at the National Institutes of Health, Bethesda, Maryland. Its structure, functions and some funded programmes are outlined. Issues regarding the future of nursing research in Australia are discussed, including the formulation of the Nursing Research Targets (CR 3.10).

3.2.3 Gray, G. & Pratt, R. (eds) (1992) *Issues in Australian Nursing* Volume 3. Melbourne: Churchill Livingstone. ISBN 0443044376 References

Book covers a wide range of topics under the headings of health care, nursing practice, education and the profession. Although related to nursing in Australia, it provides useful comparative material for nurses elsewhere.

3.2.4 Pittman, E. (1989) Making the most of new opportunities: clinical nursing research in the 1990s, in Gray, G. & Pratt, R. (eds), *Issues in Australian Nursing* Volume 2. Melbourne: Churchill Livingstone. ISBN 0443040338 Chapter 26, 393–407 References

Examines three major research issues in Australia: wider recognition of the value of clinical nursing research; collaboration between academic and clinical nurses; and building institutional bases for nursing research.

3.2.5 Saarinen, J. (1995) Ideological and logistical barriers to the development of nursing research: real or imagined? *Contemporary Nurse: a Journal for the Australian Nursing Profession*, 4 (2) 69–75 22 References

Explores the real or perceived barriers to the development of nursing research in Australia which include ideological concerns, economic constraints and factors within the infrastructure. Suggestions are made as to how these problems may be overcome.

3.2.6 Sellick, K., McKinley, S., Botti, M., Kingsland, S. & Behan, J. (1993) How many hospitals have a nursing research policy? A Victorian survey. *Australian Journal of Advanced Nursing*, 10 (4) 20–5 11 References

Article reports results of a questionnaire which sought information on 29 hospitals' nursing research policies, structures, education and the level of organizational support (CR 2.75).

3.2.7 Sellick, K., McKinley, S., Botti, M., Kingsland, S. & Behan, J. (1996) Victorian hospital nurses' research attitudes and activity. *Australian Journal of Advanced Nursing*, 13 (4) 5–14 18 References

Four hundred and fifty eight registered nurses from seven Victorian hospitals were surveyed to establish their attitudes to nursing research and levels of research activity, and whether working in a hospital with research policies had any influence. Results are reported and the main hindrances to conducting research were seen to be workloads and lack of time.

3.2.8 Sigsby, L.M. & Bullock, L. (1996) Nursing education and research in New Zealand. *Image: Journal of Nursing Scholarship*, 28 (3) 269–72 21 References

Discusses the status of New Zealand nursing education and research based on knowledge, experience and an informal survey of a small sample of nurse researchers. Current research and its dissemination are discussed. Reasons for limited publication of research to date are given (CR 2.102).

3.2.9 Smith, M.G. & Shadbolt, Y.T. (eds) (1984) *Objects and Outcomes: New Zealand Nurses' Association 1909–1983*. Wellington: New Zealand Nurses' Association. ISBN 0908669097

Documents the development of the Association, its structure and functions, professionalism and unionism, nursing services, basic and post-basic education, politics and power, the international idea and the *New Zealand Nursing Journal*. Mention is also made of the Nursing Education Research Foundation.

3.3 EUROPE

The development of nursing research in Europe is at several different stages, with some countries having much experience and expertise, while others are beginning to create an appropriate structure within which it may start to flourish.

Annotations

3.3.1 Abraham, I.L. (1986) Chronological analysis of nursing research content in an international context, in Stinson, S.M. & Kerr, J.C. (eds), *International Issues in Nursing Research*. London: Croom Helm. ISBN 0709944373 Part 4, Chapter 15, 259–88 References

Chapter discusses the development of the European nursing research movement and the major issues which surround it. Results of a study which examined the content of 5,035 articles published between 1976 and 1980 in four European countries are reported. Its aim was to define the current state of nursing and future directions as seen in the literature. Evidence showed that nursing research investigation was being promoted, facilitated and attention given to the dissemination and utilization of research findings (CR 2.98, 2.102, 3.22.12).

3.3.2 Biomedical and Health Research Programme (BIOMED). (1993) *Royal College of Nursing Euroforum*, 4 (Winter) 4

Programme follows on from, and builds upon, the 4th Medical and Health Research Programme 1987–1991. Its objectives are given and current areas of research are listed.

3.3.3 Bjorn, A. (1993) A cross-cultural perspective in Europe, in Kitson, A. (ed.), *Nursing: Art and Science*. London: Chapman & Hall. ISBN 0412470705 Chapter 5, 61–71 9 References

Chapter focuses on universalities and similarities of nursing in Europe, developments in the last decade and differences. Development of key collaborative projects is described (CR 2.15, 2.53).

3.3.4 Clift, J., Domajnko, N., Pretnar-Kunstek, V. & Sustersic, O. (1996) Nursing in Slovenia. *International Nursing Review*, 43 (5) 151–3 4 References

Following its recent independence, nursing is establishing university degree programmes, active participation in international conferences and contributing to international publications. Nursing research is being carried out by individuals and also through the World Health Organization Collaborating Centre.

3.3.5 Council of Europe (1996) *Nursing Research/Council of Europe*. Strasbourg: Council of Europe. ISBN 9287131120 URL: http://europa.eu.int/eclas (European Community Libraries Catalogue)

3.3.6 Hamrin, E.K.F. (1990) Nursing research in Sweden. *International Journal of Nursing Studies*, 27 (2) 149–57 41 References

Discusses the development of, and interest in, nursing research. New opportunities, the relationship of nursing education to research, research training, significant accomplishments, funding, interest groups and prospects for the future are discussed (CR 3.13, 3.17).

3.3.7 Hohmann, U. (1996) The concern with nursing research in the future work of nurse graduates. Expectations from the viewpoint of the nurse researcher [German]. *Pflege*, 9 (3) 180–8 18 References

Nurse graduates from programmes being established in the Federal Republic of Germany will be seen as 'change agents' in their future employment. Their involvement will be conducting research, receiving, putting into practice and disseminating findings, together with initiating and commissioning research projects.

3.3.8 Lanara, V.A. & Raya, A.A.C. (eds) (1981) *Collaborative Research and its Implementation in Nursing*. Third Conference of European Nurse Researchers. Athens: Hellenic National Graduate Nurses' Association. No ISBN

Reports the development of nursing research in 16 European countries. It also contains a keynote speech by Baroness McFarlane of Llandaff entitled 'Standards of nursing care, can research help the nurse manager?' (CR 2.15).

3.3.9 Lauri, S. (1990) The history of nursing research in Finland. *International Journal of Nursing Studies*, 27 (2) 169–73 15 References

Outlines the history of nursing research in Finland. Aims and activities of the Research Institute of Nursing, university-level nurse education and research, nurse researchers and publication of studies and prospects for the future are discussed (CR 3.17).

3.3.10 Lerheim, K. (1990a) Nursing research developments in Norway. *International Journal of Nursing Studies*, 27 (2) 139–47 28 References

Discusses the origins of nursing research in Norway, research in the 1970s and 1980s, the influence of nursing organizations on nursing research, funding and the future.

3.3.11 Lerheim, K. (1990b) Workshop of European Nurse Researchers, a historical review: WENR 1978–1988, in Christensen, E.H. & Lerheim, K. (eds), *Proceedings of the 10th and 11th Workshop of European Nurse Researchers*. Copenhagen: Danish Nurses' Organization. ISBN 8772660635 4–11

Provides an overview of the development of the Workshop of European Nurse Researchers, how and where it links with other associations and institutions, the venues and broad subject areas of its 11 conferences, what has been accomplished over this period and a glimpse of the future.

3.3.12 Lorenson, M. (1990) Research resource development in Denmark. *International Journal of Nursing Studies*, 27 (2) 159–68 72 References

Discusses the development of nursing research in Denmark, the work of the Danish Nurses' Organization and the Danish Medical Research Council, educational opportunities for nursing research and future prospects.

3.3.13 Shortridge, L.M. (1994) Nursing research from a Dutch perspective, in Fitzpatrick, J.J., Stevenson, J.S. & Polis, N.S. (eds) *Nursing Research and its Utilization*. New York: Springer. ISBN 0836180906 Chapter 22, 217–21 18 References

Chapter discusses several differences between the development of nursing science in the Netherlands and the USA. These are: funding for education and research; the distinction between the scientific (university) and professional (vocational) approach to doctoral study; department structure; and research funding. Developments at the University of Utrecht are described (CR 2.102.17, 3.17).

3.3.14 Steka-Feffer, H. (1996) A short outline of the history of nurse training in Poland. *International History of Nursing Journal*, 1 (4) 72–6

Author traces the history of the Polish nursing associations from the start of the century to the present day.

3.3.15 Suominen, T. & Leino-Kilpi, H. (1998) Review of Finnish nursing research from 1958 to 1995. *Scandinavian Journal of Caring Sciences*, 12 (1) 57–62 25 References

Provides an overview of Finnish research, describes its content, sources of information and level of analysis.

3.3.16 Tierney, A. (1993) The Workgroup of European Nurse Researchers. *Royal College of Nursing Euroforum*, 4 (Winter) 4

Outlines the purpose of the Workgroup of European Nurse Researchers and gives an update on its activities.

3.3.17 Tierney, A.J. (1998) Nursing research in Europe. *International Nursing Review*, 45 (1) 15–18 12 References

Author reports on participation in the Workgroup of European Nurse Researchers and gives an overall view of nursing research in Europe. Because research is a relatively new activity and so variable in such a diverse region, a comprehensive view is limited. Strategic development, research activity, priorities and the challenges ahead are all discussed (CR 3.20).

3.3.18 Workshop of European Nurse Researchers. (1984) Developments in nursing research, in *Nursing Research: Does it Make a Difference?* Proceedings of the 7th Workgroup Meeting 2nd Open Conference of the Workgroup of European Nurse Researchers, 10–13 April. London: Royal College of Nursing. ISBN 0902606891 Section 1

Reports on research developments in many European countries are given under the following headings: introduction; education for/in nursing research; completed and ongoing research in nursing, dissemination of research findings; funds available for nursing research; and perspectives for the future. Some include references.

3.4 UNITED KINGDOM

In the UK nursing research began in the 1960s, about 80 years after Florence Nightingale had laid the foundations. Since that time, after a fairly slow beginning, the number of nurses who have had research training is rising and there is a marked increase in the volume of literature being published.

Annotations

3.4.1 Alexander, M. & Hunt, J. (1996) Nursing figures for the patient. *Times Higher Education Supplement*, 19 January, 1211 Synthesis iv

Outlines the history of nursing research in the UK and its relationship to medical research. Ways forward are suggested in the context of a new Department of Health Strategy.

3.4.2 Gardener, M.G. (1977) The history, philosophy and evaluation on the work of the Joint Board of Clinical Nursing Studies. *Journal of Advanced Nursing*, 2 (6) 621–32 12 References

Describes the establishment, philosophy, organization and evaluation of the work of the Joint Board of Clinical Nursing Studies. Mention is made of the small research department whose programme was to assist with the aims of establishing and maintaining a national standard.

3.4.3 Hancock, C. (1993) Promoting nursing research: the RCN's role. *Nurse Researcher*, 1 (2) 72–80 7 References

Discusses impediments to nursing research, current problems, the role of the Royal College of Nursing, current initiatives and the future.

3.4.4 Hayward, J.C. (1982) Nursing research, in Allan, P. & Jolley, M. (eds), *Nursing, Midwifery and Health Visiting since 1900*. London: Faber & Faber. ISBN 0571118399 Chapter 15, 196–214 References

Describes the development of nursing research in the UK and the educational facilities available for nurses. The setting up of

nursing research units and the ways in which research findings may be disseminated are outlined. Some studies into aspects of clinical nursing and nursing education, and future directions for research are mentioned (CR 2.101).

3.4.5 Hockey, L. (1979) Expanding the nursing horizon. *Nursing Mirror*, 25 October 149 (17) 32–5

Author believes that the misunderstanding of what research is, i.e. the rules of the game, its objectives and outcome, can be the greatest barrier to its development. The commitment to and roles of teachers, administrators and practitioners are explored. Her hopes for the future are outlined (CR 3.16).

3.4.6 Hockey, L. (1986) Frontiers of nursing research: real or imagined?, in *New Frontiers in Nursing Research*. Proceedings of the International Nursing Research Conference, Edmonton, Canada, 7–9 May 1986. University of Alberta: Faculty of Nursing. 20–4

Discusses the conventional territory of nursing research and the origins of its frontiers. The properties of these are identified and author asks if they are real or imagined. Nurses are urged to build bridges between disciplines so that nursing research can move forward.

3.4.7 Hockey, L. & Clark, M.O. (1984) Nursing research in Scotland, in Werley, H.H. & Fitzpatrick, J.J. (eds), *Annual Review of Nursing Research* Volume 2 New York: Springer. ISBN 0826143512 Chapter 13, 307–24 References

Chapter discusses Scotland's policy on nursing research, the structure and early development of the Nursing Studies Research Unit, Department of Nursing Studies, University of Edinburgh. The application of Donabedian's evaluative framework to the Women in Nursing study is outlined together with the unit's core programme of research.

3.4.8 Hopps, L.C. (1994) The development of research in nursing in the UK. *Journal of Clinical Nursing*, 3 (4) 199–204 39 References

Paper describes some of the early developments of research in nursing. The creation of policies for nursing research are discussed, together with implementing research in practice, changes in nurse education and the Department of Health Research Strategy launched in 1993 (CR 3.9).

3.4.9 Hunt, J. (1982) Nursing research in the United Kingdom, in Lerheim, K. (ed.), *Collaborative Research and its Implementation in Nursing.* 4th Conference of Nurse Researchers. Oslo: Norwegian Nurses' Association. 73–7   6 References

An overview of progress being made in the UK, including courses available, development of nursing research units, current projects, lectures, publications and funding. Mention is made of the involvement of the Royal College of Nursing in nursing research (CR 2.15, 3.13, 3.14, 3.23).

3.4.10 Joint Board of Clinical Nursing Studies. (1977) *The Research Objective in Joint Board Courses: an Introductory Guide.* London: Joint Board of Clinical Nursing Studies. Occasional Paper 1

First UK publication designed to assist nurse teachers in introducing research into post-basic curricula. Suggestions are made as to how this may be achieved. Appendices contain an outline of the research process, a glossary and reference materials.

3.4.11 Joint Board of Clinical Nursing Studies. (1980) *Review of the Work of the Joint Board of Clinical Nursing Studies, 1970–1980.* London: Joint Board of Clinical Nursing Studies. No ISBN

Describes the background, structure, finances, philosophy and work of the Joint Board in connection with post-basic clinical courses. The future of these courses is also discussed. Part 4 outlines the projects undertaken by the research staff, which included assessment in relation to clinical nursing skills, the planning and execution of Joint Board courses and a follow-up study on nurses holding the Board's certificates. A course evaluation package, and one designed to assist teachers in introducing research into courses were developed by professional and research staff (CR 3.17).

3.4.12 Keith, J.M. (1988) Florence Nightingale: statistician and consultant epidemiologist. *International Nursing Review*, 35 (5) Issue 281 147–50   16 References

Article explores a lesser-known aspect of the work of Florence Nightingale, her expertise and use of statistics and epidemiology. A major health problem in New Zealand in 1860 is used for illustration.

3.4.13 King's Fund Centre. (1986) *Scholarship and the Growth of Nursing Knowledge.* Report from a symposium held at the King's Fund Centre, 18 February 1986. London: King's Fund Centre. No ISBN   References

Symposium was held to celebrate the first ten years of the *Journal of Advanced Nursing.* Papers cover the contribution of the journal to the body of nursing knowledge:

Chapman, C.M.	The contribution of the *Journal of Advanced Nursing* to the body of nursing knowledge, 1–5.
Clarke, M.	Scholarship and nursing education, 7–22.
Cox, A.M.	Scholarship and nursing management, 23–37.
Pembrey, S.	Scholarship and nursing practice, 39–52.
Wilson Barnett, J.	Research: its relationship to practice and representation in the *Journal of Advanced Nursing*, 53–66.

3.4.14 LeLean, S.R. (1980a) Research in Nursing: an overview of DHSS initiatives in developing research in nursing 1. *Nursing Times*, 17 January, 76 (2) 5–8 Occasional Paper

The need for, and the history of, the development of nursing research is described, with particular reference to the work of the Department of Health and Social Security. Among the items discussed are introducing research in basic nurse education, the Nursing Research Liaison Group scheme, research courses and fellowships. The evolution of the Index of Nursing Research and the role of librarians in relation to it is outlined (CR 3.9).

3.4.15 LeLean, S.R. (1980b) Research in nursing: an overview of DHSS initiatives in developing research in nursing 2. *Nursing Times*, 24 January, 76 (3) 9–12 Occasional Paper   35 References

An overview is given of some research commissioned by the Nursing Research Liaison Group. The problems in undertaking research in nursing are identified and suggestions are made for future development (CR 3.9).

3.4.16 LeLean, S.R. & Clarke, M. (1990) Research resource development in the UK. *International Journal of Nursing Studies,* 27 (2) 128–32   72 References

Traces the development of nursing research in the UK over the last 30 years. Its origins are outlined and the following areas are covered: the role of government departments; the National Health Service; professional organizations; the higher education sector; research funding; training for research; the present position; and future prospects (CR 3.9, 3.13, 3.17).

3.4.17 Mead, D. (1996) Using nursing initiatives to encourage the use of research. *Nursing Standard,* 31 January, 10 (19) 33–6   26 References

Outlines the history of nursing research in the UK and discusses the progress made. Some of the problems of taking research forward are discussed and details are given of new initiatives within the Department of Health Research and Development Strategy. Information synthesis and dissemination are discussed, and the role of the Royal College of Nursing in promoting research is outlined (CR 2.98, 2.102, 3.9, 3.14).

3.4.18 Payne, S. (1993) Constraints for nursing in developing a framework for cancer care. *European Journal of Cancer Care,* 2 (3) 117–20   7 References

Paper highlights some key constraints inhibiting the development of cancer nursing research. The need for research training and a co-ordinated programme of basic and applied research is identified. The difficulties of obtaining funding and adequate supervision for higher degrees are discussed (CR 3.13, 3.18).

3.4.19 Simpson, M. (1981) Issues in nursing research, in Hockey, L. (ed.), *Current Issues in Nursing.* Recent Advances in Nursing 1. Edinburgh: Churchill Livingstone. ISBN 0443021864 Chapter 2, 29–32   References

The growth and development of nursing research, training and funding of nurse researchers, and the foundation of nursing research units are all discussed. The importance of research to the profession and for policy-making is described, and the roles of both the Department of Health and Social Security and the Joint Board of Clinical Nursing Studies are discussed (CR 3.9, 3.11).

3.4.20 Smith, J.P. (1986) The end of the beginning. *Senior Nurse,* 5 (1) 14–15   9 References

Discusses the developments in nursing research in the UK, including the growth of the Royal College of Nursing Research Society, nursing research departments and research fellowships. It is suggested that much nursing research needs to be replicated, nurses should document innovations, and develop the ability to analyse their work and roles (CR 2.13).

3.4.21 Stacey, M. (1984) Future directions in health care research, in *Nursing Research: Does it Make a Difference?* Proceedings from the 7th Workgroup Meeting, 2nd Open Conference of the Workgroup of European Nurse Researchers, 10–13 April 1984. London: Royal College of Nursing. ISBN 0902606891 126–48   References

The growth of nursing research over the last 30 years is described. The problems encountered by nurses when trying to implement research findings, although they were not involved in the research, is demonstrated by reference to the report of the Platt Committee in 1959. Difficulties experienced by nurses trying to combine their jobs with day-release studies are described. The future of health care research in the UK is discussed, particularly with regard to funding and complex social relationships and roles (CR 2.102, 3.12, 3.13, 3.16).

3.4.22 Tierney, A. (1996) Nursing research at the University of Edinburgh. *Nursing Standard,* 10 (48) 32

Report highlights the continuing commitment to innovative research for nurses at the University of Edinburgh.

3.4.23 Tierney, A.J. (1990) Nursing research in Scotland: a review and analysis from a personal perspective, in National Center for Nursing Research/International Council for Nurses, *Nursing Research Worldwide: Current Dimensions and Future Directions.* Bethesda, MD: National Center for Nursing Research/Geneva, Switzerland: International

Council of Nurses. No ISBN 85–95 No references

Reports on the health care system in the UK, gives an historical outline of the development of nursing research in Scotland, the current position and future prospects (CR 3.22.9).

3.5 UNITED STATES OF AMERICA AND CANADA

The development of nursing research is at its most advanced in the USA and nurses all over the world can continue to learn from their prolific literature. Although nursing practice and research operate within varying 'political' systems, we all have much to share for the benefit of patients and clients.

Annotations

3.5.1 Allen, J.C. (1990) *Consumers' Guide to Doctoral Degree Programmes in Nursing.* New York: National League for Nursing. ISBN 0887374557 Publication no. 15–2293

Book provides an historical overview of doctoral education in nursing and discusses approval and review processes for these programmes. Degree options, assessing quality and financing education are also discussed. Individual programme descriptions are included for the USA (CR 3.13).

3.5.2 Baer, E.D. (1987) 'A co-operative venture' in pursuit of professional status: a research journal for nursing. *Nursing Research*, 36 (1) 18–25 64 Notes and References

Describes the origins and purpose of the journal, *Nursing Research*. Themes explored are educational issues, establishing the editorial process, defining and developing nursing research, centralizing research in nursing, the search for a theory base and financing the journal.

3.5.3 Brimmer, P. (1986) The American Nurses' Association: its role in nursing research, in Stinson, S.M. & Kerr, J.C.A. (eds), *International Issues in Nursing Research.* Beckenham: Croom Helm. ISBN 0709944373 Chapter 16, 289–312 References

Documents the role of the American Nurses'

Association (ANA) and the development of nursing research since 1978. Its structure, policies, financing and programmes are discussed. Because of legislative difficulties preventing the ANA from undertaking some types of research, the American Nurses' Foundation was established. Its aims are to fund research projects, analyse health policy and identify issues of concern to nursing, and assist the educational and research aims of the ANA. The work of the American Academy of Nursing, whose aims are to advance new concepts in nursing and health care, identify and explore issues in health, examine the dynamics within nursing and identify and propose solutions, is also described (CR 3.22.12).

3.5.4 Brown, B.J. (1985) Past and current status of nursing's role in influencing governmental policy for research training in nursing, in McCloskey, J.C. & Grace, H.K. (eds), *Current Issues in Nursing* 2nd edition. Boston, MA: Blackwell Scientific. ISBN 086542019X Part 7, Chapter 51, 697–712 References

The history of nurses' involvement in legislation in the USA is reviewed, together with their current influence. The benefits of involvement, ways in which this may be increased, and goals for influencing legislation are discussed (CR 3.11).

3.5.5 Brown, J.S., Tanner, C.A. & Padrick, K.S. (1984) Nursing's search for scientific knowledge. *Nursing Research*, 33 (1) 26–32 19 References

The characteristics of nursing research today, trends and changes over the past 30 years are outlined. A sample of 137 studies published between 1952 and 1980 were analysed. The conclusions drawn were that nursing research had increased substantially in amount, become more clinically focused, demonstrated a higher theoretical orientation and was more sophisticated and sound in the methods employed. Limitations noted were insufficient conceptualization and the failure to build a cumulative science (CR 2.6, 2.7).

3.5.6 Canadian Nurses' Association. (1984) *The Research Imperative for Nursing in Canada: a 5-year Plan Towards Year 2000.* Ottawa: Canadian Nurses' Association. ISBN 0920381030

Documents a plan for the development of nursing research under three major headings:

development of nurse researchers; nursing research; and nursing research reality (establishment of a general expectation among nurses, governments and the public of nursing research as the basis for care within the discipline). The plan includes goals, objectives, detailed strategies and recommended actions.

3.5.7 Canadian Nurses' Association. (1990) *Research Imperative for Nursing in Canada: the Next 5 Years 1990–1995.* Ottawa: Canadian Nurses' Association. ISBN 092038160X

The Canadian Nurses' Association (CNA) is committed to continue with the strategic plan which began in 1984, and this new five-year plan recognizes the importance of collaborative effort in the development of nursing research. Sub-goals have been established and actions for CNA have been delineated.

3.5.8 D'Antonio, P. (1997) Towards a history of research in nursing. *Nursing Research*, 46 (2) 105–10   49 References

Article suggests ways in which the history of research in nursing might be positioned as a case study of the interplay between the social and scientific in the generation of new data, knowledge and considerations. Interconnected examples of social context and gender are used to show how recasting nurses as critical actors in, and interpreters of, the world of science and research may prove to be historians' contribution to the profession's drive for sustained legitimacy and authority.

3.5.9 Degner, L.F. (1990) The status of nursing research in Canada, in National Center for Nursing Research/International Council of Nurses, *Nursing Research Worldwide: Current Dimensions and Future Directions.* Bethesda, MD: National Center for Nursing Research/Geneva, Switzerland: International Council of Nurses. No ISBN 96–104   14 References

Reports the status of nursing research in Canada and discusses the context for research, historical background, numbers of nurse researchers, programmes to prepare them, funding, types of research, current trends and the role of the Canadian Nurses' Association and other organizations (CR 3.22.9).

3.5.10 Department of Health and Human Services, Public Health Service, National Institutes of Health. (1989) *Report of 1989 NIH Task Force on Nursing Research.* Bethesda, MD: NIH. Publication no. 89–487

Report outlines the creation and functioning of the National Center for Nursing Research, the characteristics of nursing research and the development of a national nursing research agenda. The main part of the report includes extra-mural grant applications, awards and intra-mural project data, the implementation plan and update of the 1984 Task Force recommendations, statements of nurse consultants together with conclusions and recommendations of the NIH Task Force.

3.5.11 Field, P.A. (1990) *Advancing Doctoral Preparation for Nurses: Charting a Course for the Future.* Proceedings of a conference on doctoral education, 27–28 September 1990. Edmonton, Alberta, Canada: University of Alberta

Papers cover the history of doctoral education for nurses, and nursing in the USA, together with developments in Europe and Canada. Social, political and economic influences, a university perspective, advancing doctoral preparation for nurses, and the philosophical underpinnings of, pathways to and the substance and content of doctoral programmes are all discussed (CR 3.3, 3.17).

3.5.12 Fitzpatrick, M.L. (1986) A historical study of nursing organization: doing historical research, in Munhall, P.L. & Oiler, C.J. (eds), *Nursing Research: a Qualitative Perspective.* Norwalk, CT: Appleton-Century-Crofts. ISBN 0838570488   Chapter 11, 195–225

Describes the history of American nursing during the 20th century through the development of its organizations. The development of the American Nurses' Association, among others, is described (CR 2.46).

3.5.13 Fondiller, S.H. (1986) The American Nurses' Association and National League for Nursing: political relationships and realities, in White, R. (ed.), *Political Issues in Nursing: Past, Present and Future* Volume 2. Chichester: Wiley. ISBN 0471909130 Chapter 7, 119–43   References

Chapter documents the history of the ANA and NLN, examines collaboration and conflicts, new structural arrangements, the question of entry to the profession, political activities and the future.

3.5.14 Gortner, S.R. (1983) The history and philosophy of nursing science and research. *Advances in Nursing Science*, 5 (2) 1–8 21 References

A general discussion on the development of nursing research in the USA over the last 150 years. Particular reference is made to the choice of research ideas, education of nurses and the philosophical and scientific basis of nursing research (CR 2.8).

3.5.15 Gortner, S.R. (1986) Impact of the Division of Nursing Research, in Stinson, S.M. & Kerr, J.C. (eds), *International Issues in Nursing Research*. Beckenham: Croom Helm. ISBN 0709944373 Part 2, Chapter 7, 113–30 References

Chapter describes the development of the Division of Nursing Research, support for research, research training, institutional resources, the development of a scientific base for practice and scientific communication through conferences (CR 3.22.12).

3.5.16 Guyer, R.L. (1998) People doing science.
URL: http://science-education.nih.gov/nihHTML/ose/snapshots/multimedia/pds/nursing

Outlines the career of the present Director of the National Institute of Nursing Research, Dr Patricia Grady, and the development of nursing research in the UK and USA. It reiterates her belief in the value of collaborative research (CR 2.15, 3.4, 3.5).

3.5.17 Hamilton, D.B. (1996) The seventh star: Dorothy Ford Buschmann and the founding of Sigma Theta Tau. *Image: Journal of Nursing Scholarship*, 28 (2) 177–80 20 References

This historical study examined the role of Dorothy Buschmann in helping to design the philosophy and constitution of Sigma Theta Tau. She believed that the foundations of professional nursing were love, honour and courage, and that the enduring value of nursing was its contribution to the social good.

3.5.18 Himot, L.B. (1993) Nursing today, in Chitty, K.K. (ed.), *Professional Nursing: Concept and Challenges*. Philadelphia: W.B. Saunders. ISBN 0721640613 Chapter 5, 94–112 8 References

Describes nursing today, settings in which registered nurses practise, examples of roles and how these may be expanded, and discusses the impact of salary compression (CR 3.16).

3.5.19 Hinshaw, A.S. (1990) Facilitating nursing research: a national perspective, in National Center for Nursing Research/International Council of Nurses, *Nursing Research Worldwide: Current Dimensions and Future Directions*. Bethesda, MD: National Center for Nursing Research/Geneva, Switzerland: International Council of Nurses. No ISBN 73–84 28 References

Outlines the evolution of nursing research in the USA, challenges, future directions and national facilitation of nursing research (CR 3.22.9).

3.5.20 Hinshaw, A.S. (1992) Nursing research: weaving the past and the future, in Aiken, L.H. & Fagin, C.M. (eds), *Charting Nursing's Future: Agenda for the 1990s*. Philadelphia, PA: J.B. Lippincott. ISBN 0397548001 Chapter 30, 485–503 97 References

Chapter documents the history of nursing research in the USA and the progress made. Suggested areas for future research include those identified by the National Nursing Research Center and the National Nursing Research agenda. These include low birth weight, mother and infant, HIV prevention and care, long-term care for the elderly, symptom management, health promotion for adolescents and technology dependency across the life-span. Other discipline-based priorities are also identified (CR 2.23, 3.20).

3.5.21 Hinshaw, A.S. & Merritt, J. (1988) Moving nursing research to the National Institutes of Health, in *Perspectives in Nursing 1987–1989*. New York: National League for Nursing. ISBN 0887373844 93–103 References

Discusses the history of the National Center for Nursing Research, its mission in relation to that of the National Institute of Health, the current structure, research programmes and future initiatives.

3.5.22 International Nursing Review. (1993) National Centre for Nursing Research redesignated as the 17th Institute of the National Institute of Health. *International*

Nursing Review, 40 (5) Issue 311 129 News feature

The re-designation of this unit will assist in its purpose of providing a strong science base for nursing practice. There is no change in its budget, but an important signal will be sent to the public and nursing community. Nursing research will be strengthened at the national level, its visibility raised within the health research community and this indicates a permanence and stability for this type of research (CR 3.13).

3.5.23   MacPhail, J. (1996) Scope of research in nursing practice, in Kerr, J.C. & MacPhail, J. (eds), *Canadian Nursing: Issues and Perspectives* 3rd edition. St Louis: Mosby. ISBN 0815152256 Chapter 12, 146–61   37 References

Outlines the development of nursing research in Canada, and the organization and funding of national research conferences. Chapter also analyses the content of conferences held, their organization and the influence of a foundation on research in nursing practice (CR 3.13).

3.5.24   Martinson, I.M. (1997) Nursing research: obstacles and challenges. *Image: Journal of Nursing Scholarship*, 29 (4) 322–3 9 References [Original article condensed – *Image* (1976) 8 (1) 3–5]

Records the 'state of the art' and future as seen by an Associate Professor of Nursing in 1976 (CR 3.5.25).

3.5.25   Nagelkerk, J., Henry, S.B. & Brooten, D. (1997) Commentary about Martinson's 'Nursing research: obstacles and challenges'. *Image: Journal of Nursing Scholarship*, 29 (4) 324–5   11 References

Examines the changes in nursing research which have taken place in the USA since Martinson's article was written and charts some of the successes (CR 3.5.24).

3.5.26   Norbeck, J.S. (1990) Nursing research in the United States of America, in National Center for Nursing Research/International Council of Nurses, *Nursing Research Worldwide: Current Dimensions and Future Directions.* Bethesda, MD: National Center for Nursing Research/Geneva, Switzerland: International Council of Nurses. No ISBN 121–6   15 References

Outlines the history of nursing research in the USA, the number and programmes available for preparation of nurse researchers, types of research, funded positions, number of employed researchers and the greatest needs, trends and priorities for the future. The role of the National Nurses' Association is also explained (CR 3.22.9).

3.5.27   Rodger, G.L. (1991) Canadian nurses succeed again! The launch of Canada's first doctoral degree in nursing. *Journal of Advanced Nursing*, 16 (12) 1395–6 Guest editorial

Describes the strategy and political action which led to Canada's first doctoral degree in nursing (CR 3.17).

3.5.28   Stevenson, J.S. (1987) Forging a research discipline. *Nursing Research*, 36 (1) 60–4   30 Notes and References

Article reports the history of nursing research over the last 35 years in the USA. Aspects discussed are its development in the military and Veterans' Administration, funding, the centralization of resources, national and regional associations, conferences and networking through journals. Suggestions for the future are also made.

3.5.29   Stinson, S.M., Lamb, M. & Thibaudeau, M.-F. (1990) Nursing research: the Canadian scene. *International Journal of Nursing Studies*, 27(2) 105–22 51 References

Provides an overview of the development of nursing research in Canada. Sections cover factors governing science policy, key national, provincial/territorial nursing organizations and how this affects research. Research literature, libraries, nursing research manpower, networking, funding and the future are also discussed.

3.5.30   White, D.L. & Hamel, P.K. (1990) National Center for Nursing Research: how it came to be, in Lindeman, C.A. & McAthie, M. (eds), *Nursing Trends and Issues.* Springhouse, PA: Springhouse Corporation. ISBN 0874342325 Chapter 14, 396–400   7 References

Describes how the National Centre for Nursing Research achieved formal agenda status and nursing accomplished its goal in the legislative arena.

3.5.31 Wilmot, V. (1986) Health science policy and health research funding in Canada, in Stinson, S.M. & Kerr, J.C. (eds), *International Issues in Nursing Research*. Beckenham: Croom Helm. ISBN 0709944373 Part 2, Chapter 5, 76–96 References

Discusses the evolution of science policy in Canada and the problems experienced in health science research. As in the UK, biomedical research commands popular support and the major share of funds. This position is being hotly contested and the passing in 1984 of the Canada Health Act may have important implications for change. Federal expenditure management systems are discussed, as it is change within these which would enable financial support for nursing research to take place (CR 3.10, 3.12, 3.22.12).

3.6 STATE OF THE ART

The development of nursing research has taken place over varying periods of time in different countries, but reported progress is ongoing and exciting in some parts of the world, and frustrating in others. To take stock of 'where we are' from time to time can help to consolidate the efforts being made to improve practice.

Annotations

3.6.1 Abdellah, F.G. & Levine, E. (1994) *Preparing Nursing Research for the 21st Century: Evolution, Methodologies, Challenges*. New York: Springer. ISBN 0862184405 References

Purpose of this book is to present a commentary, in jargon-free and understandable language, on the state of the art of nursing research. Many questions are asked and the authors attempt to provide answers. The three sections trace the evolution of nursing research from its beginnings as observational studies, to the controlled studies of today, identify methodologies that have emerged as the tools of nursing research, and discuss the impact of research on health policy formulation and what needs to be done if nursing is to influence the national health agenda. Also discussed are some potential funding strategies for research. Nursing research in the next

century is examined, including the current gaps and breakthroughs needed (CR 2.29, 2.36, 2.43, 2.61, 2.92, 3.5, 3.11, 3.13, 3.17).

3.6.2 Hockey, L. (1986) Nursing research in the United Kingdom: the state of the art, in Stinson, S.M. & Kerr, J.C. (eds), *International Issues in Nursing Research*. Beckenham: Croom Helm. ISBN 0709944373 Part 4, Chapter 13, 216–35 References

A wide-ranging chapter covering a personal view on the position of nursing research in Britain in relation to seven requirements: individual academic curiosity, research education, activity, appropriate climate, finance, dissemination of information and research utilization. Focus is also on research activities in nursing education, practice and management. The chapter concludes with an appraisal of past performance and a glimpse of the future (CR 3.22.12).

3.6.3 Hockey, L. (1994) *Conference Summation*. First International Conference on Community Health Nursing Research, Edmonton, Alberta, Canada, 26–29 September 1993. References

Plenary address gives a developmental overview of community health nursing research, the contemporary scene and some glimpses into the future. A few notes of caution are expressed and ways forward are discussed (CR 3.4, 3.5).

3.6.4 Larson, E. (1984) The current state of nursing research. *Nursing Forum*, 21 (3) 131–4 11 References

Discusses the state of research in the USA and outlines some studies undertaken by nurses. The late entry of nursing into politics and the paucity of funds currently available are discussed. The Institute of Medicine report on nursing and nursing education advocates the development of a federally sponsored centre for nursing research (CR 3.13).

3.6.5 Merwin, E. & Mauck, A. (1995) Psychiatric nursing outcome research: the state of the science. *Archives of Psychiatric Nursing*, 9 (6) 311–31 110 References

A review of the nursing literature from 1989 to 1994 shows that few psychiatric studies are published in major research journals. Only a small number of studies build on prior research, resulting in a weak scientific base for evaluating the outcomes of psychiatric nursing care. Strategies for increasing the quantity and quality of research are presented (CR 2.12, 2.43).

3.6.6   Mulhall, A. (1995) Nursing research: what difference does it make? *Journal of Advanced Nursing*, 21 (3) 576–83   37 References

Discusses the history, current status and organization of nursing research in the UK. The differing agendas of policy-makers, practitioners and researchers are explored, together with the constraints which may hinder its development and utilization (CR 2.102, 3.4, 3.11).

3.6.7   Rafferty, A.M. & Traynor, M. (1997) On the state of play in nursing research. *Journal of Interprofessional Care*, 11 (1) 43–8 22 References

Paper presents some snapshot views of the problems of, and prospects for, developing a research culture in nursing. Authors argue that nursing research is enmeshed in political, social and gendered forces. Any achievement has to be set within the framework of nursing's relative youth and its own intellectual history within academe, along with the impact that different research traditions have exerted upon it. The American experience is briefly outlined and markers of development in the UK are discussed.

3.6.8   Stodulski, A. (ed.) (1995/6) *RCN Study of UK Nursing Journals*. London: Royal College of Nursing Library. ISBN 1873852428

Provides an assessment of research content in UK nursing journals, gives an account of refereeing and peer reviewing policies. A directory gives full publication details for each journal (CR 2.99).

A PROFESSION'S RESPONSIBILITY

3.7 RESEARCH, PRACTICE AND PROFESSIONAL RESPONSIBILITY

In many countries today there is an increasing emphasis on cost-effectiveness when there seems to be an unlimited demand for health care. All nurses want to give their patients and clients the best possible research-based care, but 'political' pressures from within and outside the organization can sometimes make this very difficult. Literature in this section highlights some of the problems.

Definition

Journal club – a group that meets regularly (usually in clinical settings) to discuss and critique research reports appearing in research journals, often with the goal of assessing the utilization potential of the findings

---

Annotations

3.7.1 Abbott, P. (1993) Why do we need review literature? *Nurse Researcher*, 1 (1) 14–22 7 References

Article discusses the professional responsibilities of all nurses, with research providing the basis for practice (CR 2.12).

3.7.2 Ágústsdóttir, A., Holcombe, J., Wright, P., Daffin, P. & Ogletree, G. (1995) Publication of patient-related oncology nursing research. *Oncology Nursing Forum*, 22 (5) 827–30 14 References

Survey aimed to identify publication rates of patient-related studies in oncology nursing research. Findings showed that the majority of papers submitted for presentation at the Oncology Nursing Society Congresses from 1981 to 1990 were not published and therefore unavailable for use in clinical practice. This is a serious threat to knowledge development (CR 2.52, 2.92).

3.7.3 Akinsanya, J.A. (1991) The usefulness of research to the surgical nurse: a critique. *Surgical Nurse*, 4 (1) 4, 6–8 14 References

Article discusses the relevance of nursing research, areas of study reported in the literature, its value, implementation of findings and the contribution of clinical nurse researchers (CR 2.102, 3.17).

3.7.4 Aspery, C. (1993) How to set up a journal club. *British Journal of Midwifery*, 1 (1) 17 20 7 References

Discusses the value of journal clubs and their role in professional development. Some practical advice is given.

3.7.5 Baessler, C.A., Blumberg, M., Cunningham, J.S., Curran, J.A., Fennessey, A.G., Jacobs, J.M., McGrath, P., Perrong, M.T. & Wolf, Z.R. (1994) Medical-surgical nurses' utilization of research methods and products. *MEDSURG Nursing*, 3 (2) 113–17, 120–1, 141 31 References

Using the Research Utilization Questionnaire, paper describes the methods and products of research by 212 registered nurses, and their attitudes towards research-based knowledge in clinical practice. Results showed that it was difficult for respondents to change their practice, but they were willing to do so if findings were relevant. Articles from nursing research journals were ranked low as sources of knowledge, while that from patients was high (CR 2.101, 2.102).

3.7.6 Baumgart, A.J. (1996) Promoting nursing practice through nursing research.

International Nursing Review, 43 (2) 45–8, 57
7 References

Article discusses fostering research-based practice, documenting the work and worth of nursing and enhancing public understanding of nursing work.

3.7.7   Blair, C.E. (1997) Nursing research: advancing practice and the profession. *Psychiatric Care*, 4 (2) 56–8, 60–1   12 References

Author argues that incorporating research findings into clinical practice promotes the standardization of nursing interventions, helps nurses meet the needs of clients effectively and increases nurses' autonomy and credibility.

3.7.8   Challen, V., Kaminski, S. & Harris, P. (1996) Research-mindedness in the radiography profession. *Radiography*, 2 (2) 139–51 29 References

Project aimed to identify the level of research-mindedness among practising clinical radiographers. Results showed that most work was done to fulfil course requirements and little had been published. Subjects believed they should be involved for self-development and enhancing the profession. Authors suggest the setting up of interest groups and providing short courses on research methods.

3.7.9   Clark, E. & Renfrew, M. (1992) *Research Awareness and the Midwife.* London: Distance Learning Centre, South Bank University. ISBN 0948250631   References

This module forms part of a series entitled *Midwifery Update* and provides an introduction to the use of research in midwifery. Chapters cover the place of research in midwifery, sources of knowledge, the midwife's role in research, applying research in everyday practice and what further steps might be taken to learn more about the subject (CR 2.6, 2.10, 3.16, 3.17).

3.7.10   Cleverly, D. (1998) Nursing research: taking an active interest. *Nurse Education Today*, 18 (4) 267–72   26 References

Paper discusses the issues raised by the still unfolding transformation of nurse education attitudes to research, from the traditional stance that it was something which other people did, to the realization that quality research is central to the development of the profession. The problems and challenges of the Research Assessment Exercise are also examined (CR 2.99, 3.9, 3.13, 3.17).

3.7.11   Griffiths, P. (1993) To believe or not to believe. *Nursing Times*, 6 January, 89 (1) 39 No references

Outlines the pitfalls of relying on hearsay or second-hand interpretation of original research.

3.7.12   Hammick, M. (1995) A research and journal club: a medium for teaching, professional development and networking. *European Journal of Cancer Care*, 4 (1) 33–7 7 References

Reports the establishment of a monthly research and journal club to meet the needs of students and qualified staff. A varied, practitioner-led programme provided a flexible approach which ensured maximum participation. Topics included current practices and research methods (CR 3.17).

3.7.13   Hicks, C. (1993) A survey of midwives' attitudes to and involvement in research: the first stage in identifying needs for a staff development programme. *Midwifery*, 9 (2) 51–62   19 References

Study investigated reasons for limited research output in midwifery. Findings suggested that a major reason for low publication rates was not failure to do research, but a reluctance to submit findings for publication. Results are interpreted within the context of developing future staff training programmes (CR 2.75).

3.7.14   Hicks, C. (1996) The potential impact of gender stereotypes for nursing research. *Journal of Advanced Nursing*, 24 (5) 1006–13 27 References

Discusses reasons for the perceived shortfall of published research in nursing. Author believes there may be reasons other than structural or organizational. A small study showed that gender stereotypes could play a significant part.

3.7.15   Hicks, C., Hennessy, D., Cooper, J. & Barwell, F. (1996) Investigating attitudes to research in primary health care teams. *Journal*

of Advanced Nursing, 24(5) 1033–41 19 References

Reports a study which aimed to develop a diagnostic instrument for identifying the research training needs of health care professionals. Results showed that the majority perceived research as being unimportant and peripheral to their jobs, and the responsibility of others. Their understanding of research and its methodologies was discordant within and across professional groups. The implications of these findings are discussed (CR 3.17).

3.7.16 Holzemer, W. & Tierney, A. (1996) How nursing research makes a difference. *International Nursing Review*, 43 (2) 49–52, 58 38 References

Authors report on selected studies demonstrating how nursing research has provided information to assist in care planning and programme development.

3.7.17 Hunsley, S.L. (1995) Orientation and preceptorship: the new research clinicians lifeline. *Journal of Neuroscience Nursing*, 27 (3) 194–9 8 References

Article suggest a practical programme to help new research clinicians efficiently and effectively integrate into the work environment. It establishes an orientation pattern, develops a preceptor programme and incorporates tools to enhance both roles (CR 3.16, 3.17).

3.7.18 Kirchhoff, K.T. (1993) Issues and challenges in clinical nursing research, in Maas, M.L., Titler, M.G. & Buckwalter, K.C. (eds), *The Nursing Clinics of North America: Advances in Clinical Research*. Philadelphia: W.B. Saunders. 28 (2) June 271–8 ISSN 0029-6465 8 References

Several major issues are explored including subject accrual, compatibility of the research protocol with the clinical site, and gaining co-operation from groups of health professionals. Approvals required, protocol maintenance when others are involved, and compromises which may be necessary are also discussed (CR 2.14, 2.15, 2.17, 2.22).

3.7.19 Kyei, M.B. (1993) Nurses' knowledge and options about the research process in the Netherlands. *Journal of Advanced Nursing*, 18 (10) 1640–4 29 References

Study aimed to discover to what extent Dutch nurses in clinical areas had acquired research-based knowledge. Many nurses claimed knowledge of the process and agreed with the relevance of nursing research to practice. They identified the need for more research education and suggested some priorities (CR 2.102, 3.20).

3.7.20 Lancet. (1993) Does research make for better doctors? *Lancet*, 30 October, 342 (8879) 1063–4 10 References Editorial

Discusses doctors' roles and responsibilities relating to research (CR 3.16).

3.7.21 Leighton-Beck, L. (1997) Networking: putting research at the heart of professional practice. *British Journal of Nursing*, 6 (2) 120–2 3 References

Discusses the origins, value and developing role of networks in Scotland which provide advice to clinical nurses on potential and existing research which may help to improve patient care (CR 2.101, 2.102).

3.7.22 Logan, J. & Davies, B. (1995) The staff nurse as research facilitator. *Canadian Journal of Administration*, 8 (1) 92–110 24 References

Describes the Nursing Research Facilitator (NRF) Project which aims to enhance professional practice through research activities. A one-day workshop was held and staff nurse volunteers undertook to scan research journals and discuss findings with colleagues. Positive feedback was received from facilitators and managers, and awareness of research was raised. There was evidence that staff needed ongoing support from their managers (CR 3.16, 3.17).

3.7.23 Logue, R. (1996) Is nursing research detrimental to nursing education and practice? *Nurse Researcher*, 4 (1) 63–9 No references

Paper expresses some personal concerns about the relationship between nursing education, practice and research.

3.7.24 MacPhail, J. (1996) Research mindedness in the profession, in Kerr, J.C. & MacPhail, J. (eds), *Canadian Nursing: Issues and Perspectives* 3rd edition. St Louis: Mosby. ISBN 0815152256 Chapter 10, 118–34 43 References

Examines research-based nursing practice, deterrents to conducting research, disseminating findings and its application. Strategies are suggested to promote research and research-based practice.

3.7.25 Mander, R. (1995) Midwife researchers need to get their work published. *British Journal of Midwifery*, 3 (2) 107–10 11 References

Author states that midwives show a marked reluctance to publish. Recommendations are made to encourage this important aspect of professional responsibility.

3.7.26 Martin, C.R., Bowman, G.S., Knight, S. & Thompson, D.R. (1998) Progress with a strategy for developing research in practice. *NT Research*, 3 (1) 29–34 5 References

Reports progress on a strategy for developing research in practice. It is planned to be evolutionary, to focus on research related to practice, taking into account organizational and external factors.

3.7.27 Martin, P.A. (1995) Finding time for research. *Applied Nursing Research*, 8 (3) 151 No references

Author suggests five tools which may help clinicians or faculty members to find time for research. These are: make research a priority; collaborate in the research endeavour; break projects into manageable parts; structure work so that one activity yields multiple outcomes of which one is research; and garner resources for research work. She believes that these tools work whether the research activity is reading, applying or conducting research.

3.7.28 Milne, J. & Hurdley, V. (1998) A strategy for research awareness among midwives. *British Journal of Midwifery*, 6 (6) 374–8 35 References

This strategy, designed to overcome some obstacles associated with doing and using research, focuses on four main areas: education and training; access to facilities; changing the climate, culture and practice; policy and documentation.

3.7.29 Nagy, S., Crisp, J. & Brodie, L. (1992) Journal reading practices of RNs in New South Wales public hospitals. *Australian Journal of Advanced Nursing*, 9 (2) 29–33 12 References

Reports a study which examined use of professional journals by registered nurses. Ten per cent reported frequently incorporating research findings into practice and 44 per cent never did so. Implications for nursing are discussed (CR 2.102).

3.7.30 O'Connor, T. (1996) Nursing needs research . . . Jill White . . . Chair of department of nursing and midwifery at Victoria University. *Kai Tiaki: Nursing New Zealand*, 2 (3) 20–1

On the theme 'better health through nursing research', discussed on International Nurses' Day, Professor White talks about how New Zealand nurses can help to achieve this goal (CR 3.2).

3.7.31 Pranulis, M.F. (1991) Research programmes in a clinical setting. *Western Journal of Nursing Research*, 13 (2) 274–7 13 References

Discusses the problems of defining, setting up and evaluating clinical research programmes because of the different viewpoints of academics and clinicians.

3.7.32 Reed, J. & Robbins, I. (1991) Research rituals. *Nursing Times*, 5 June, 87(23) 50–1 2 References

Relates the findings of Menzies' classic study on defence mechanisms to nurse researchers.

3.7.33 Sheehy, C.M. & Wuebbles, B.H. (1996) Nursing research in the hospital and beyond. *Seminars for Nurse Managers*, 4 (2) 122–9 4 References

Authors highlight the fact that nursing care takes place in many places in addition to the hospital, and nurses transcend the conventional expectation of being implementers rather than originators, and inter-disciplinary team members rather than team leaders. A framework, and scenarios illustrating strategies, are given so that nursing research can integrate and maximize the use of resources.

3.7.34 Smith, P. (ed.) (1997) *Research-mindedness for Practice: an Interactive Approach for Nursing and Health Care*. New York: Churchill Livingstone. ISBN 044305293X References

Book aims to help nurses become research-minded, decode research jargon, explore and explode myths, to increase confidence in asking questions and in thinking analytically and critically. It also encourages them to apply research-mindedness to practice.

3.7.35 Smith, P. (ed.) (1998) *Nursing Research: Setting New Agendas*. London: Edward Arnold. ISBN 0340661941 References

Book explores the relationship between nursing research and practice. It is written from the combined perspectives of educators, researchers and practitioners and discusses ways in which research can be taken forward.

3.7.36 Tierney, A. (1993) Research literacy: an essential pre-requisite for knowledge-led practice. *Nurse Researcher*, 1 (1) 79–83 2 References

Article examines the 'Strategy for research in nursing, midwifery and health visiting' recently produced by the Department of Health. In particular it looks at suggestions about raising the level of research appreciation in nursing and improving skills in accessing and reading research reports (CR 2.102, 3.9).

3.7.37 Vail, S. & Hicks, S.E. (1996) Issues and trends: the growing importance of health research. *Canadian Nurse*, 92 (3) 59–60 6 References

Authors state that client care should be based on solid research, but implementing an 'evidence-based' approach is difficult to achieve without adequate funding (CR 3.13).

3.7.38 Webb, C. & Mackenzie, J. (1993) Where are we now? Research-mindedness in the 1990s. *Journal of Clinical Nursing*, 2 (3) 129–33 16 References

Reports a study which aimed to identify the level of knowledge about, and colleagues' attitudes towards, research. Findings showed that few nurses read journals regularly, that negative attitudes were expressed towards research articles, and that observation showed a limited application of research in practice.

3.7.39 Wells, N. & Baggs, J.G. (1994) A survey of practising nurses' research interests and activities. *Clinical Nurse Specialist*, 8 (3) 145–51   24 References

Reports a survey of 279 nurses which examined their research attitudes, past and current

research activities and available resources. Results are discussed and suggestions are made for encouraging nurses to develop and practise research skills (CR 2.52).

3.7.40 Wright, A., Brown, P. & Sloman, R. (1996) Nurses' perceptions of the value of nursing research for practice. *Australian Journal of Advanced Nursing*, 13(4) 15–18 11 References

Reports the results of a study which questioned 410 nurses' perceptions of whether nursing research is a valuable guide for clinical practice. Most believed that research is important for advancing care, but few applied findings to practice, participated in research or read research journals (CR 2.52, 2.75).

3.7.41 Wright, S.G. (1990) *Building and Using a Model of Nursing* 2nd edition. London: Edward Arnold. ISBN 0340526270 Chapter 6, 117–23   References

It is suggested that nursing research is an important component of a nursing model. There is brief discussion of the importance of research awareness in clinical nursing. Five items are identified as necessary for this change to occur: research awareness to be included in all objectives; skilled research nurse support to be available; ease of access to nursing literature; resources to be available at clinical level; and peer support groups to be fostered by managers.

3.8   RESEARCH/PRACTICE GAP

'Nurses who incorporate research evidence into their clinical decisions are being professionally accountable to their clients and are also helping nursing to achieve its own professional identity' (Polit & Hungler 1999: 3).

Definition

Research/practice gap – the lag between the rate at which research results are produced and utilized

---

Example

Mallett, J. & Bailey, C. (eds) (1996) *Royal Marsden NHS Trust Manual of Clinical Nursing Procedures* 4th edition. Oxford: Blackwell. ISBN 0632040688   References

Aim of this book is to link available research findings with practical policies and procedures. Each policy/procedure includes reference material (where available), the procedure itself and a nursing care plan. Book has been extended and updated for this new edition.

Annotations

3.8.1   Bostrom, J. & Wise, L. (1994) Closing the gap between research and practice. *Journal of Nursing Administration*, 24 (5) 22–7   23 References

Reports use of the Retrieval and Application of Research in Nursing Project (RARIN). This aims to improve the quality of nursing care by facilitating the transfer of new and clinically relevant information to current practice.

3.8.2   Burrows, D.E. & McLeish, K. (1995) A model for research-based practice. *Journal of Clinical Nursing*, 4 (4) 243–7   17 References

Paper provides a model identifying possible strategies to help nurses develop research-based practice.

3.8.3   Collins, M. & Robinson, D. (1996) Bridging the research–practice gap: the role of the link nurse. *Nursing Standard*, 10 (25) 44–6   12 References

Article describes the gap between research and practice, and highlights the rationale behind an initiative at a psychiatric hospital where ward-based link people were put in place to reduce this problem (CR 3.16).

3.8.4   Fallis, W.M. & Gupton, A. (1995) What bugs you about nursing practice?: closing the gap between research and practice. *Clinical Nursing Research*, 4 (2) 123–6   1 Reference Editorial

Reports ways in which a group of nurses in Manitoba undertook a multi-phase project to bring research closer to practice and acclimatize nurses to the research process.

3.8.5   Haynes, R.B., Hayward, R.S.A. & Lomas, J. (1995) Bridges between health care research evidence and clinical practice. *Journal of the American Medical Informatics Association*, 29(6) 342–50   96 References

Authors believe the reason for the research/practice gap is the extensive processing that evidence requires before application. This article discusses a three-step model for creating a bridge between research evidence and management of clinical problems.

3.8.6   Hicks, C. & Hennessey, D. (1997) Mixed messages in nursing research: their contribution to the persisting hiatus between evidence and practice. *Journal of Advanced Nursing*, 25 (3) 595–601   20 References

Authors discuss reasons for the limited amount of research evidence on which to base care. They advocate use of a more eclectic approach to research, using both quantitative and qualitative approaches (CR 2.29, 2.36).

3.8.7   Jaretz, N.J. & Rosenbloom, S.K. (1994) Bridging the clinical–research gap through nursing collaboration. *Archives of Psychiatric Nursing*, 8 (5) 298–302   10 References

Article describes an attempt to bridge the gap between clinical and research needs through nursing collaboration, focusing on the specific issue of managing treatment-resistant psychotic patients (CR 2.15).

3.8.8   Mason, C. (1992) Research in practice: rhetoric or reality? *Nursing Standard*, 25 March,   6 (27) 36–9   11 References

Examines some of the rhetoric associated with research-based practice. What research can and cannot do, the amount now being done, and some possible topics for the future are all discussed. Suggestions are made as to how nurses can become more research literate (CR 3.17).

3.8.9   McCloughlin, A., Aitcheson, S. & Irvine, H. (1993) The appliance of science. *Nursing Times*, 29 September, 89 (39) 52–3   2 References

Describes the formation of a research interest group which aimed to bridge the gap between research theory and practice and so improve patient care.

3.8.10 Rafferty, A.M., Allcock, N. & Lathlean, J. (1996) The theory/practice gap: taking issue with the issue. *Journal of Advanced Nursing*, 23 (4) 685–91   44 References

Authors argue that the tension between theory, practice and research can be usefully exploited in teaching and research. The myths, metaphors, reconstructing resources, reconstituting roles, theory and practice, and synthetic solutions are all discussed. The gap will always be present and it can help students make sense of their experience when confronting the ambiguities, uncertainties and contradictions within nursing.

3.8.11 Sleep, J. (1992) Research and the practice of midwifery. *Journal of Advanced Nursing*, 17 (12) 1465–71   39 References

Paper considers conceptual and pragmatic issues in order to explore the complexity of influences which may affect integration of research into midwifery practice.

3.8.12 Thomson, M.A. (1998) Closing the gap between nursing research and practice. *Evidence-based Nursing*, 1(1) 7–8   33 References   Editorial

Editorial summarizes what is known about the effectiveness of continuing professional education/behaviour change strategies and makes suggestions for choosing appropriate activities.

THE ROLE OF GOVERNMENT

GOVERNMENT AND NURSING RESEARCH

3.9 UNITED KINGDOM

Papers in this section document some aspects of the part the UK government has played in the development of nursing research and the wider context within which it operates.

Annotations

3.9.1 Anthony, D. (1997) Funding research in nursing: results of the RAE [Research Assessment Exercise]. *Nursing Standard*, 11 (20) 32–3   2 References

Reports that only one academic nursing department was rated highly enough in the Research Assessment Exercise to get meaningful research funding. The implications for nursing research are discussed (CR 3.13).

3.9.2   Baroness Jay of Paddington (1998) A strategy to create a research-friendly environment. *NT Research*, 3(3) 91–2   2 References

The Minister of State for Health outlines the current activities of nursing research and steps taken by government to encourage its development.

3.9.3 Centre for Policy in Nursing Research. (1997) *The NHS R&D Context for Nursing Research: a Working Paper.* London: Centre for Policy in Nursing Research. No ISBN References

Paper describes the progress to date on setting nursing research into a policy context, gives a summary of recent policy initiatives, and discusses their assumptions and implications. Ways in which government have attempted to control professional activity, the background to their research and development strategy, and a summary of key issues for nursing are all discussed.

3.9.4   Chambers, M. & Coates, V. (1992) Research in nursing. Part 2. *Senior Nurse*, 12 (6) 32–5   51 References

Examines some political issues relating to nursing research. These include the position of women in society, the status of nursing, the influence of the medical profession upon research development and how projects are funded (CR 3.13).

3.9.5   Department of Health (1992) *Review of the Role of DH-funded Research Units: Strategies for Long-term Funding of Research and Development.* London: Department of Health. No ISBN

Reports on the units established under the Rothschild guidelines, their finance, staffing, research projects, problems relating to the career structure of staff and recommendations for the future.

3.9.6   Department of Health. (1993a) *Report of the Task Force on the Strategy for Research in Nursing, Midwifery and Health Visiting.* London: Department of Health. No ISBN References

This report contributes to the National Health Service Research and Development Strategy. The issues examined were the importance of nursing, midwifery, health visiting and research to health and patient care, the scope and contribution of research, the wider context, and objectives of the strategy. Recommendations are made on the structure and organization of research, research education and training, funding, and the integration of research, development and practice (CR 2.98, 2.102, 3.7, 3.8, 3.11, 3.12, 3.13, 3.17).

3.9.7 Department of Health. (1993b) *Research for Health*. London: Department of Health. No ISBN   References

Summarizes progress and charts the direction of the Department of Health's Research and Development (R&D) Strategy. It reports the creation of a new national register of research based upon regional collections, which will interface, in due course, with the databases of the Medical Research Council, major charities and other health departments. The Cochrane Centre, the first element of the information systems strategy was opened in 1992 and prepares, maintains and disseminates systematic, up-to-date reviews of randomized controlled trials of health care. International collaboration is taking place and similar units are opening in other countries (CR 2.12, 2.29).

3.9.8 Department of Health. (1994) *Supporting Research and Development in the NHS*. A report to the Minister of Health by a research and development task force chaired by Professor Anthony Culyer. London: HMSO. ISBN 0113218311

Reports on the deliberations and recommendations of the Culyer Committee on the future of research and development in the National Health Service.

3.9.9 Department of Health. (1995) *Research and Development: Towards an Evidence-based Service*. London: Department of Health. Reference No. G60/001 2835 1R 500 June

An information pack containing details of the National Health Service programme, the Department's policy research programme and wider research issues (CR 3.11).

3.9.10 Department of Health. (1996) *Research Capacity Strategy for the Department of Health and the NHS*. London: HMSO. No ISBN

3.9.11 Department of Health: England. (1997) *Research and Development in the Department of Health and National Health Service*. London: Department of Health. URL: http://www.open.gov.uk/doh/rdd1.htm

This website outlines the work of the Research and Development Directorate and gives instructions on downloading and obtaining details of the NHS programme. Contents of the Research and Development Information Pack are listed.

3.9.12 Field, J. (1997) Judging research quality in post-compulsory education and training: lessons of the 1996 Assessment Exercise. *Studies in the Education of Adults*, 29 (1) 101–8   10 References

Paper provides a description and analysis of the fate of research in the 1996 Research Assessment Exercise. A brief description of the procedures followed is given, aspects of the results are analysed and key issues are identified.

3.9.13 Higher Education Funding Councils. (1996) *1996 Research Assessment Exercise*, Index to papers. URL: http://www.niss.ac.uk/education/hefc/rac/rae96/

Lists papers relating to the Research Assessment Exercise from 1994 to 1997 (CR 3.17).

3.9.14 Hurst, K. & Thompson, D. (1992) Make or break. *Health Service Journal*, 12 March, 102 (5293) 27   2 References

Explores the strengths, weaknesses, opportunities and threats which face nurse researchers in the new contracting environment.

3.9.15 Kiger, A. (1994) Nursing education and the research assessment exercises. *Nurse Researcher*, 1 (3) 85–95   8 References

Article explains how the 1992 Research Assessment Exercise was carried out and gives key questions and pointers which need to be considered if nursing research is to develop further.

3.9.16 Kitson, A. (1997) Lessons from the 1996 Research Assessment Exercise. *Nurse Researcher*, 4 (3) 81–93   23 References

Examines the results of the 1996 Research Assessment Exercise and suggests a positive national strategy is needed to improve the profile of nursing research.

3.9.17 Lorentzon, M. (1993) Research for health: managing the nursing input. *Journal of*

Nursing Management, 1 (1) 39–46   37 References

Paper focuses on nursing research and its management in Britain, and examines the roles of nurse managers, researchers, clinicians and educationalists. The history of research development is described and a systematic examination of four British, and two American journals is made to explore the various aspects of research management. The challenges facing nurses are outlined and various groups of nurses are encouraged to collaborate (CR 2.15, 3.6, 3.10).

3.9.18   Medical Research Council. (1994) *The Council's Role in Health Services and Public Health Research.* London: Medical Research Council. No ISBN

Booklet discusses the Medical Research Council's role in health-related research, strategic issues, relationships with government departments, collaborative activities, training and grant applications.

3.9.19   National Health Service Management Executive of the Department of Health. (1992) *Assessing the Effect of Health Technologies.* London: Department of Health. No ISBN

Discusses outcomes for evaluating the effects of new technology, research designs, using the evidence obtained and developing appropriate assessment strategies.

3.9.20   Nolan, M. & Behi, R. (1995) Research in nursing: a conceptual approach. *British Journal of Nursing*, 4 (1) 47–50   16 References

Discusses the Department of Health Strategy for Research and Development which aims to unite research and practice and develop a conceptual approach. Authors believe that nurses should be knowledgeable doers in order to apply research findings (CR 3.11).

3.9.21   Nursing Research Initiative for Scotland (NRIS).
URL: http://fhis.gcal.ac.uk/nris/opening.html#heading4

This initiative, funded by the Scottish Office, was set up in 1994 to provide a focus for direct patient care research. This Internet home page gives an introduction to the unit, current staff, aims, the research and development programme and other useful information.

3.9.22   Nyatanga, L. (1995) The Research Assessment Exercise (RAE): criteria and issues. *Nurse Education Today*, 15 (6) 395–6   3 References   Editorial

Outlines the background, context, funding, panels, assessment criteria and method of working which contribute to this exercise. Other issues are also highlighted.

3.9.23   Peckham, M. & Smith, R. (eds) (1996) *Scientific Basis of Health Services.* London: British Medical Journal Publishing. ISBN 0727910299   References

Book examines the links between scientific advances and medicine. Subjects include setting priorities, evidence-based clinical practice, the impact of management on outcomes, clinical guidelines and implementation of research findings (CR 2.102, 3.20).

3.9.24   Read, S. (1994) The strategy for research in nursing in England: initial impact. *Nurse Researcher*, 1 (3) 72–84   13 References

Reports the progress made by the task force appointed to consider the scope and objectives of research in England and its interface with other areas of health service research (CR 3.6, 3.11).

3.9.25   Robinson, J. (1993) Nursing and the research assessment exercise: what counts? *Nurse Researcher*, 1 (1) 84–93   11 References

Discusses the recent research assessment exercise (RAE) carried out by the Higher Education Funding Council (HEFC) in British universities. Author believes that the RAE has serious implications for nursing as an academic discipline and some of the issues arising are discussed (CR 3.17).

3.9.26   Royal College of Nursing Research Advisory Group. (1993) Strategic thinking. *Nursing Standard*, 9 June, 7 (38) 22–4 No references

Members of the Royal College of Nursing Advisory Group discuss the objectives and recommendations of the Department of Health Strategy for Research. The research infrastructure and the place of nursing within it are examined. Opportunities that are available for nurses to undertake research, and the support needed, are outlined (CR 3.16).

3.9.27   Royal College of Nursing/Royal College of Midwives. (1993) *Strategy for*

Research in Nursing, Midwifery and Health Visiting. Annexes 1–4. London: Royal College of Nursing/Royal College of Midwives. No ISBN   References

These annexes complement the report of the Task Force for Research in Nursing, Midwifery and Health Visiting and their purpose is to elaborate on and explore four of the key issues. These are: identifying research and development priorities; research education and training; dissemination and implementation of research findings; and careers in research (CR 3.16, 3.17).

3.9.28 Salvage, J. (1998) Evidence-based practice: a mixture of motives? *Nursing Times,* 10 June, 94 (23) 61–4   19 References

Paper suggests that the government's R&D initiative mixes altruism with pragmatism. Its aims include cost containment and the control of the professions, alongside its more overt commitment to improving the quality of care. Efforts are being made to tackle the shortcomings of nursing research but nurses attempting to influence the R&D agenda need to be aware of its political nuances.

3.9.29 Scott, E. (1997) Research and development in nursing. *Nursing Times,* 3 September, 93 (36) 32–3   7 References

Paper introduces the National Health Service research and development programme and reviews the opportunities and obstacles which have emerged as health service R&D has expanded, and nurses aim to raise the level of their research capability.

3.9.30 Watson, R. (1997) UK universities' Research Assessment Exercise 1996: critique, comment and concern. *Journal of Advanced Nursing,* 26 (4) 641–2   4 References Editorial

Discusses the results of the most recent 1996 Research Assessment Exercise and expresses concerns about the poor overall rating by university nursing departments, with one major exception. Possible reasons are suggested and the role played by journals in publishing research material is discussed. Author urges the panel next time round to judge nursing in a more realistic way.

3.9.31 Wojtas, O. (1996) A healthy body of evidence. *Times Higher Education Supplement,* 19 January, 1211 Synthesis I

Outlines the new medical research strategy of the Department of Health. The fundamental need is for more scientific data so that care is based on the best available evidence.

3.10   UNITED STATES OF AMERICA AND CANADA

The National Institute of Nursing Research in the USA is funded by the government and works to promote research activity in advancing nursing practice, to establish priorities and to make grants available.

Annotations

3.10.1 American Association of Colleges of Nursing. (1997) *Appropriations for the National Institute of Nursing Research (at National Institutes of Health).* Washington, DC: American Association of Colleges of Nursing.
[Government Affairs Issues Summary: 105th Congress, First Session].
URL: http://www.aacn.nche.edu/GovtAff/Ninrapp.html

Outlines the position taken for the fiscal year 1998, the reasoning behind it and action taken. The Institute was awarded $63.597 for the financial year 1998 (CR 3.13).

3.10.2 Davitt, D.C. (1993) The Center for Nursing Research: a case study in agenda setting. PhD thesis (unpublished). St Louis University, St Louis, MO

A non-experimental, retrospective case study is reported, which determined the process utilized to attain formal agenda status of the National Center for Nursing Research at the National Institutes of Health.

3.10.3 de Chesnay, M. (1996) National Institute of Nursing Research update: interview with Dr. Patricia Grady. *Advanced Practice Nursing Quarterly* 2 (3) 20–2

An update is given on research funded by the National Institute for Nursing Research (NINR) and the Director shares her thoughts on the future, NINR priorities and the importance of advanced practice nurses in the research arena (CR 3.20).

3.10.4 Grady, P.A. (1996) Landmark anniversary for nursing research at the National Institute of Health. *Image: Journal of Nursing Scholarship*, 28 (1) 4–5 Guest editorial

Reports on the growth, achievements and future activities of the National Institute of Nursing Research (CR 3.5).

3.10.5 National Institutes of Health
URL: http://www.nih.gov/

The home page of the NIH includes news and events, health information, grants and contracts, scientific resources, institutes and offices, and information for employees (CR 3.13).

3.10.6 National Institute of Nursing Research
URL: http://www.nih.gov/ninr/

The home page of the NINR includes details about the Institute, its staff, mission and history, news and information, legislative activities, research programmes – grants and funding, training, scientific advances and other resources (CR 3.13).

3.11 RESEARCH AND POLICY-MAKING

Research is essential to policy-makers for planning appropriate facilities to improve the health care of all patients and clients. The nature of research into nursing, with all its complexities and potential cost implications, has meant that both personnel and funds have not always been available. Decisions have sometimes been made without sufficient background information resulting in wasted resources and less than satisfactory care.

Annotations

3.11.1 Beasley, C. (1997) Taking research and development forward: why the profession must be involved. *NT Research*, 2 (2) 147–9 1 Reference

Discusses the achievements of the NHS Executive North Thames in research and development and discusses ways in which nurses can play a part in regional and national agendas.

3.11.2 Bloor, M. (1997) Addressing social problems through qualitative research, in Silverman, D. (ed.), *Qualitative Research: Theory, Method and Practice*. London: Sage. ISBN 0803976666 Part VII, Chapter 14, 221–38 33 References

Using two case studies of male prostitutes in Glasgow and eight therapeutic communities, author states his belief that rigorous qualitative research can have relevance for service provision even though it may not have much impact at government level (CR 2.36.59).

3.11.3 Centre for Policy in Nursing Research. (1997a) *Annual Report 1997*. London: Centre for Policy in Nursing Research, London School of Hygiene and Tropical Medicine. No ISBN References

Report outlines the initial work undertaken by the staff of this centre, financed initially by the Nuffield Provincial Hospitals Trust. This has comprised ground-clearing exercises, designed to establish the context and data required for setting priorities for research in nursing and research policy. Two working papers have been published. Future projects are outlined (CR 3.9.3, 3.17.14, 3.20).

3.11.4 Centre for Policy in Nursing Research. (1997b) *The National Health Service R&D Context for Nursing Research: a Working Paper*. London: Centre for Policy in Nursing Research, London School of Hygiene and Tropical Medicine. No ISBN References

Provides a progress report on the newly established Centre for Policy in Nursing Research. Its three main sections cover the context of the NHS research and development strategy, the strategy itself and the modernization of nursing. The main issues identified are discussed: developing methods to access the complexities of nursing; identifying appropriate outcome measures; the theoretical basis of nursing; identification of priorities; and the linking of research outcomes to policy. A possible new career structure for nurse researchers is mentioned (CR 2.7, 2.43, 2.54, 2.61, 3.16, 3.20).

3.11.5 Conn, V.S. & Armer, J.M. (1996) Meta-analysis and public policy: opportunity for nursing impact. *Nursing Outlook*, 44 (6) 267–71   29 References

Describes ways in which meta-analysis can be used to influence public policy. Its strengths are outlined and examples are given which have the potential to inform policy (CR 2.92).

3.11.6   Craig, G. (1996) Qualitative research in an NHS setting: uses and dilemmas. *Changes*, 14 (3) 180–6   20 References

Paper argues that evidence-based medicine gives precedence to quantitative research. Qualitative research tends to be marginalized and less well understood. Recent initiatives in the NHS Research and Development Programme may compound this problem and has led to a blurring of boundaries between both methods and personnel (CR 2.29, 2.36).

3.11.7   Department of Health Management Executive. (1993) *A Vision for the Future: the Nursing, Midwifery and Health Visiting Contribution to Health and Health Care.* London: Department of Health, National Health Service Management Executive. Circular EL/93/32, 27 April 1993. Targets 8 and 9

Paper examines the implications for nurses, midwives and health visitors of recent National Health Service key policy initiatives. Targets 8 and 9 require leaders to demonstrate the existence of local networks to disseminate good practice based on research, and to show at least three areas where clinical practice has changed as a result of research findings (CR 2.102, 3.9).

3.11.8   Gipps, C.V. (1993) The profession of educational research. *British Educational Research Journal*, 19 (1) 3–16   25 References

Reports the crisis in education research policy-making caused by central intervention and restriction on reporting. Research findings are mis-reported in the press and policy-making processes have become truncated, ignoring discussion, debate and research evidence. Author believes that current reforms in education will not lead to resourceful, active learners. Researchers are urged to work together with teachers and the British Educational Research Association to publish findings.

3.11.9   Green, J. & Thorogood, N. (1998) Researching health policy, in Authors, *Analysing Health Policy: a Sociological Approach.* London: Longman. ISBN 0582298016 Chapter 6, 156–93   References

Chapter looks at issues raised, both theoretical and methodological, when undertaking health policy research.

3.11.10   Hantrais, L. & Mansen, S. (eds) (1996) *Cross-national Research Methodology in the Social Sciences.* London: Pinter. ISBN 1855673452   References

Critically examines the methodological and managerial issues which arise in cross-national research, with particular emphasis on economic and social policy in the European Union (CR 3.3, 3.22).

3.11.11   Hinshaw, A.S. (1992) The impact of nursing science on health policy, in *Communicating Nursing Research. Silver Threads – 25 Years of Nursing Excellence* (Volume 25). Boulder, CO: Western Institute of Nursing. 15–26   No ISBN   17 References

Discusses definitions and characteristics of health policy research, framing research to influence policy, methodological approaches and opportunities for influence.

3.11.12   John, M. (1993) Educating the policy maker. European comparative research: case studies and appraisal. *Research Papers in Education*, 8 (1) 3–17   23 References

Article examines the value of comparative research studies relating to disability, and focuses on them as contributions to policy, knowledge, practice, theory and as part of the process in educating European policy-makers about relevant issues. The roles and responsibilities of researchers come under scrutiny and selected case studies are used to explore relationships between such research, the policies it sets out to inform, and the nature of policy itself (CR 2.39, 3.16).

3.11.13   Keighley, T. (1994) The new politics of nursing research. *Nurse Researcher*, 2 (1) 76–84   12 References

Author revisits the new nursing research agenda based on the Research and Development Strategy for the National Health Service. A knowledge of the political climate is essential to see how this may be achieved.

3.11.14   Lewis, S. (1995) Quality, context and distributive justice: the role of utilization research and management. *International Journal for Quality in Health Care*, 7 (4) 325–31   7 References

Author states that utilization research and management are essential tools to pursue quality objectives. Use of these tools will lead to a new era of accountability in giving improved quality of care (CR 2.102).

3.11.15   Lilford, R.J. & Harrison, S. (1994) Health services research: what it is, how to do it and why it matters. *Health Services Management Research*, 7 (4) 214–19   25 References

Article explains how health service research differs from clinical research, even when using similar methods. Author believes it will become of increasing importance to health policy-makers and managers.

3.11.16   McIntyre, L. (1996) The role of the researcher cum health policy advocate. *Journal of the Canadian Dietetic Association*, 57 (1) 35–8   26 References

Paper discusses the proper role of the researcher-cum-policy advocate and suggests strategies which will enhance that role. The choice of research question and use of multiple strategies for disseminating research results are both important to the health advocacy process (CR 2.18, 2.98, 3.16).

3.11.17   Meerabeau, L. (1996) Managing policy research in nursing. *Journal of Advanced Nursing*, 23 (4) 692–6   18 References

Paper explores the use of research in policy-making. Relationships between the worlds of researchers and policy-makers are discussed and an example, 'The research initiative on human resources and effectiveness', is given to show how research topics are formulated (CR 2.20).

3.11.18   Nichols-Casebolt, A. & Spakes, P. (1995) Policy research and the voices of women. *Social Work Research*, 19 (1) 49–55   23 References

In many instances the outcomes of studies reflect male researchers' biases and assumptions, and the reliance on quantitative methods obscures multiple perspectives and diversity among research subjects. Using an example of a town hall research project, this article discusses how the diverse 'voices' of women can be amalgamated into an analysis of policy issues (CR 2.10, 2.27, 2.29).

3.11.19   O'Neill, M. & Pederson, A.P. (1992) Building a methods bridge between public policy analysis and health public policy. *Canadian Journal of Public Health/Revue Canadienne de Santé Publique*, 83 (Suppl. 1) S25–30   35 References

Explores the idea that the explicit values of healthy public policy suggest the need to pay more attention to epistemological and theoretical principles when making methodological choices, rather than simply using multiple methods (CR 2.6, 2.7, 3.10).

3.11.20   Peckham, M. (1991) Research and development for the National Health Service. *Lancet*, 10 August, 338 (8763) 367–71   13 References

Discusses the National Health Service and research, and its research and development programme. The content and scope is outlined, including priorities which will be set. Creating space for new developments, clinical research, evaluative clinical science, disseminating findings, manpower and training, and the role of industry are all discussed (CR 2.98, 3.9, 3.20).

3.11.21   Rafferty, A.M. & Traynor, M. (1997) Quality and quantity in research policy for nursing. *NT Research*, 2 (1) 16–27   21 References

Paper considers two mapping exercises designed to survey research activity within nursing, midwifery and health visiting, to ascertain current strengths and weaknesses in the research capacity. Interviews with key opinion leaders and stakeholders of research have been and are being conducted. One theme to emerge is the dominance of medicine as a reference point for analysis, and the extent to which nurses share problems and prospects with other groups. The future for research in nursing may have more in common with these groups and could provide a useful point of reference (CR 2.68).

3.11.22   Rappert, B. (1997) Users and social science research: policy, problems and possibilities. *Sociological Research Online*, 2 (3) URL: <http://www.socresonline.org.uk/socresonline/2/3/10.html>   References

Paper examines some of the consequences of greater user involvement in the UK Economic and Social Research Council, by drawing on both empirical evidence and more speculative argumentation. In doing so it poses some of the dilemmas for conceptualizing proper user involvement.

3.11.23 Strong, P.M. (1997) One branch of moral science: an early approach to public policy, in Miller, G. & Dingwall, R. (eds), *Context and Method in Qualitative Research.* London: Sage. ISBN 0803976321 Part IV, Chapter 13, 185–97 References

Author describes how qualitative research may contribute to a new public ethic and liberal metaphysics, both of which focus on improving society, while recognizing that utopian dreams for a fully just world are unlikely to be realized (CR 2.36.40).

3.11.24 Terenzini, P.T. (1993) On the nature of institutional research and the knowledge and skill it requires. *Research in Higher Education,* 34 (1) 1–10   17 References

Examines three forms of organizational intelligence: technical/analytical, issues and contextual intelligence. The nature of preparation that is required, which will allow appropriate and competent research to be undertaken, is discussed.

3.11.25 Thomas, A., Chataway, J. & Wuyts, M. (eds) (1998) *Finding Out Fast: Investigative Skills for Policy and Development.* London: Sage, in association with the Open University. ISBN 0761958371   References

Book is a guide to research which informs policy and public action, particularly on issues of development. Guidance and ideas on how to research, evaluate and use information fast is given. It also discusses the dangers of misusing methods which interpret the need for speed as an excuse for not allocating proper resources to analysis and investigation.

3.11.26 World Health Organization. (1996) World needs a research network for health. Geneva: World Health Organization. Press release WHO/71, 18 October
URL: http: //www.who.ch/press/1996/pr96-71. html

This press release outlines the deliberations of the WHO Global Advisory Committee on Health Research following their meeting on 15–18 October 1996 in Geneva. The group will be preparing an agenda entitled 'Science and technology for global health development' for submission to the World Health Assembly in May 1998, which will enable member states to be better prepared to meet future public health challenges.

3.12 RESEARCH IN HEALTH CARE

Health services research is an area where governments spend a considerable amount of money, albeit far less than that spent on defence. All health care professionals have the responsibility to read and use research findings where appropriate to ensure the highest standards of care.

Annotations

3.12.1 Ahrens, E.H. Jr. (1992) *The Crisis in Clinical Research: Overcoming Institutional Obstacles.* New York: Oxford University Press. ISBN 0195051564   References

Examines the broad picture of American medicine, doctors, medical schools and the institutional settings where research takes place. The current status of clinical research and its future outlook are examined. Author questions whether it is possible for academic physicians to continue the three roles of teaching, service and research because each is so time-consuming and imbalances are created. Recommendations are made for correcting these (CR 3.10, 3.11, 3.13).

3.12.2 Colquhoon, D. & Kellehear, A. (eds) (1993) *Health Research in Practice: Political, Ethical and Methodological Issues.* London: Chapman & Hall. ISBN 0412474700   References

Explores some of the major issues and problems in health care research. All chapters are based on the experience of authors from a wide range of disciplines. The theoretical and practical problems in conducting research are discussed (CR 2.10, 2.15, 2.16, 2.17, 2.46, 2.49, 2.52, 2.53, 3.11).

3.12.3 Daly, J., Willis, E. & McDonald, I. (eds) (1992) *Researching Health Care: Designs, Dilemmas, Discipline.* London: Routledge. ISBN 0415070783 References

Discusses issues of policy relating to the

effectiveness of appropriate research methods in health care, the randomized controlled trial, non-experimental quantitative study designs and qualitative research methods (CR 2.29, 2.36).

3.12.4 Ingram, N. (1996) The research basis of health care decision making. *Journal of Advanced Nursing*, 23 (4) 692–6 18 References

The research basis of decision-making in health care services is discussed and appropriate types of data are suggested. Some philosophical assumptions are explored.

3.12.5 Ong, B.N. (1993) *The Practice of Health Services Research*. London: Chapman & Hall. ISBN 0412543400   References

Examines the development of social science research and its contribution to health services planning and management. Ethnography, action research, surveys, evaluation, multi-method research and some broader issues in using research findings are discussed (CR 2.37, 2.42, 2.43, 2.52, 2.102).

3.12.6 Styles, M.M. (1990) A common sense approach to research. *International Nursing Review*, 37 (1) 203–6, 218   9 References

Article aims to start a debate about the political significance of knowledge, appropriate paradigms, the presentation of knowledge, power brokers, professional priorities and evaluation (CR 2.6, 2.43, 3.20).

FUNDING FOR RESEARCH

3.13   FUNDING FOR RESEARCH

Probably the most crucial issue relating to research is that of the amount of funding available. Governments, private institutions, industry and individual donors all have many calls on the funds which they are able and willing to allocate to any particular form of research. Nursing has frequently been fairly low on the list of priorities.

Annotations

3.13.1   Abdellah, F.G. & Levine E. (1994) The funding of nursing research, in Authors, *Preparing Nursing Research for the 21st Century: Evolution, Methodologies, Challenges.* New York: Springer. ISBN 0826184405 Part III, Chapter 12, 211–27

Chapter addresses the funding crisis affecting the new investigator, setting priorities for research funding and discusses selected federal funding sources that give priority to health policy research (CR 3.5).

3.13.2   American Nurses Foundation (annual) *Nursing Research Grants Program.* Washington, DC: American Nurses Foundation
URL: http://www.nursingworld.org/anf/98grant.htm

Outlines information on these annual awards, provides dates for application and guidance on obtaining an application package.

3.13.3   Annual Registers of Grant Support 1998: a Directory of Funding Sources. Edited by Bowker staff (1997) New Providence, NJ: Bowker & Ingram. ISBN 0835239306 Nursing 998–1006 Entry numbers 2797–821

Book is the standard reference source on non-repayable financial support in the USA which will be of value to hospitals, community service groups, medical research facilities and other institutional applicants. Information given includes name, address, telephone, fax, name of programmes, type, purpose, legal basis, eligibility, financial data, awards and application information.

3.13.4   AORN research grant program. (1998)
URL. http.//www.aorn.org/research/grants/rschover.htm

Website gives an overview of this grant program for members of the AORN. Funding opportunities, levels, guidelines for grants, funding sources and application deadlines are included.

3.13.5   Crombie, I.K. & Du V. Florey, C. (1998) *The Pocket Guide to Grant Applications.* London: BMJ Books. ISBN 0727912194

Book gives advice on how to approach organizations and includes a floppy disk with guidelines on drawing up grant applications.

3.13.6   Department of Health. (1997) *R&D in the NHS: Implementing the Culyer Report.* London: Department of Health
URL: http://www.open.gov.uk/doh/culyer2.htm

Outlines the new strategy for funding R&D in the National Health Service and lists documents which are available on the Internet.

3.13.7   Directory of Biomedical and Health Care Grants 1998. (1997) 12th edition. Phoenix, AZ: Oryx Press. ISBN 1573560367

This is one of four specialized directories that serve portions of the research and community development sectors. These are the *Directory of Research Grants, Directory of Grants in the Humanities, Directory of Biomedical and Health Care Grants* and *Funding Sources for Community and Economic Development.* GRANTS database is available online through Knight-Ridder Information Inc. (File 85) and Knowledge Expert Data System. This directory includes over 3,400 funding programmes concerned with human health and biomedicine. Most originate in the USA and Canada, but other countries are also represented. A brief guide to proposal planning is given, and a list of World Wide Web sites for those organizations with a presence on the Internet, together with e-mail addresses where available (CR 2.96).

3.13.8   Duffy, M.E. (1999) *Websites for Nurse Researchers: Public and Private Grant-related WWW Resources*
URL: http://www.nursing.uc.edu/nrm/duffy 81598.htm

Author lists several grant-related Websites. These include: ASKNIH; Community of Science; CRISP; Computer Retrieval of Information on Scientific Projects; Foundation Center; Grants and Related Resources: Michigan State University Collection Guides; Grantsmanship Center; GrantsWeb; The Research Administrators Resource Network; National Institutes of Health Guide Table of Contents via E-Mail; Proposal Tool Kit, and the Texas Research and Administrators Group (CR 2.99).

3.13.9   Economic   and   Social   Research Council (ESRC) (no date)
URL: http://www.esrc.ac.uk/

The ESRC is the UK's largest independent funding agency for research and postgraduate training into social and economic issues. They ensure that researchers have the training, resources and infrastructure to continue to make advances which will broaden public knowledge and contribute to the decision-making of policy-makers and businesses (CR 3.17).

3.13.10   The Foundation Center (1997) *The Foundation Directory 1997.* New York: Foundation Centre. ISBN 0614300401

Standard reference work for information about 8,729 private and community grant-making foundations in the USA. Sources for nursing are included. Information is given on

donors, type, financial data, fields of interest, limitations, publications and application information.

3.13.11   Grady,   P.A. (1997) News from NINR. *Nursing Outlook*, 45 (4) 154

The differences between a programme announcement and a request for application are described, areas of scientific opportunity for 1998 are indicated and research project grants and FIRST awards are discussed.

3.13.12   The Grants Register, 1998 (1997) 16th edition. Edited by Austin, R. New York: St Martin's Press Inc. ISBN 031217585X London: Macmillan   Reference.   ISBN 0333646142
URL: http://www.macmillan-reference.co.uk

Contains a subject and eligibility guide to awards, the grants register, index of awards and those discontinued, and an index of awarding organizations.

3.13.13   Kerr, J.C. (1996) The financing of nursing in Canada, in Kerr, J.C. & MacPhail, J. (eds), *Canadian Nursing: Issues and Perspectives* 3rd edition. St Louis: Mosby. ISBN 0815152256 Chapter 11, 135–45   20 References

Discusses Federal support for nursing research, research supported by university schools of nursing and in health care agencies.

3.13.14   Lauffer, A. (1997) *Grants, etc.* 2nd edition. Beverly Hills, CA: Sage. ISBN 0803954689   References

Book includes a step-by-step checklist of project design essentials, a section on Internet access filled with key website links and information on creating web pages. A wide range of examples will assist fund-seekers of all kinds (CR 2.96).

3.13.15   Miner, L.E. (ed.) (1997) *Directory of Research Grants 1997 with a Guide to Proposal Planning and Writing* 22nd edition. Phoenix, AZ: Oryx Press. ISBN 0897749480

This directory offers factual and concise descriptions of nearly 6,000 research funding programmes. Listings are non-repayable research funding for projects in medicine, the physical and social sciences, the arts, humanities and education. Information includes programme focus and goals, restrictions, eligibility, funding amounts, deadlines and sponsor name and address. Also included is a list of website addresses for those organizations which have established a presence on the Internet (CR 1.3, 2.96).

3.13.16 National Institute of Nursing Research. (1997) *National Institute of Nursing Research – Grants*
URL: http: //cos.gdb.org/best/fedfund/nih-select/nr.html

This website enables nurses to search for grants awarded by the National Institute of Nursing Research.

3.13.17 Read, S. & Roberts-Davis, M. (1995) An informative strategy to support nursing and midwifery research. *Health Informatics*, 1 (3) 108–12   16 References

Paper gives an overview of research funding for nurses in the UK and the criteria normally applied by those funding research (CR 2.96).

3.13.18 Ries, J.B. & Leukefeld, C.G. (1995) *Applying for Research Funding: Getting Started and Getting Funded.* Thousand Oaks, CA: Sage. ISBN 0803953658   References

Book covers the components needed when applying for research funding: key connections, research in the real world, what and when to write, checking for infractions and dealing with the reviewer's decision (CR 2.96).

3.13.19 Ries, J.B. & Leukefeld, C.G. (1997)

The Research Funding Guidebook: Getting It, Managing It, and Renewing It. Thousand Oaks, CA: Sage. ISBN 0761902317   References

Book begins with rejection and makes suggestions on how to re-submit applications to make them more competitive. The practical issues after funding is obtained are discussed. Also includes a checklist for progress and guidance on time management.

3.13.20 Robinson, K. (1996) Funding resources for nurse researchers. *Nurse Researcher*, 4 (2) 57–64   6 References

Author believes that nurses have new access to funds following National Health Service restructuring of education and research in the UK.

3.13.21 Selby-Harrington, M.L., Donat, P.L. & Hibbard, H.D. (1993) Guidance for managing a research grant. *Nursing Research*, 42 (1) 54–8   5 References

Article gives practical advice to help newly funded principal investigators manage federal research grants. The administrative issues that are covered are equally applicable to privately funded research.

3.13.22 Worldwide Nurse. (no date) *Nursing Research – Funding Information.*
URL: http: //www.wwnurse.com/nursing/research-funding.shtml

Website lists sources of funding.

NURSING RESEARCH CENTRES

3.14 NURSING RESEARCH CENTRES

Probably one of the major ways in which a consistent research programme can be carried out is for units, centres or departments in colleges or universities to establish their priorities, and obtain private funding or be financed by government sources. Staff members will usually be engaged in research, as well as having teaching commitments, although this can cause conflicts in terms of time.

Annotations

3.14.1 Centre for Policy in Nursing Research. (1998)
URL: http://www.lshtm.ac.uk/php/hsru/cpnr.htm

Website presents the aims of this new centre, established jointly by the Department of Public Health and Policy at the London School of Hygiene and Tropical Medicine and the Royal College of Nursing. These are: to help develop a co-ordinated strategy for nursing research in the UK; disseminate models of good research practice; identify current needs for research and training; and to help set a national agenda for nursing research (CR 3.17, 3.20).

3.14.2 Christ, G.H. & Weinstein, L. (1995) Developing a research unit within a hospital social work department. *Health and Social Work*, 20 (1) 60–9   23 References

Article describes the establishment of a research unit as an integral part of a hospital social work department. Methods are discussed for building support within the institution, the process of initiation, deciding on study topics and bridging the gap between clinical and research staff. The evolution of the relationship between clinical and research staff was characterized by four different phases: curiosity, competitiveness, co-operation and collaboration. The benefits and costs of the unit are also discussed.

3.14.3 Crow, S. (1996) A guide to the ENB's research and development programme [English National Board]. *Nursing Standard*, 10 (52) 39–43   4 References

Article presents the historical progress of research and development at the English National Board in relation to its statutory function. The commissioning process is explained in general terms to assist prospective applicants to understand how the Board assesses research proposals and awards contracts (CR 2.96, 3.13).

3.14.4 Feldman, H.R., Bidwell-Cerone, S., Haber, J.E., Hott, J.R. & Penney, N.E. (1994) Survey of nursing research in New York State: XVI. *Journal of the New York State Nurses' Association*, 25 (3) 30–1

Reports the results of the 16th survey undertaken by the Council on Nursing Research Clearing House. Its purposes are to: list current research done by nurses and their colleagues in New York State; facilitate networking of nurse researchers; stimulate and encourage novice researchers in nursing. Nurses are encouraged to add their completed research to this annual survey.

3.14.5 Foundation of Nursing Studies. (1996) *Part of Tomorrow's Nursing Practice, Today. Annual Report 1996.* London: Foundation of Nursing Studies. No ISBN

Report outlines the work undertaken by the Foundation which includes conferences, workshops and projects, and discusses their dissemination strategy for research findings.

A position paper entitled 'Reflection for action', which explores the barriers to research implementation and how they may be overcome, was published (CR 2.102).

3.14.6 International Council of Nurses.
(1990) *Directory of Nursing Research Units* 2nd edition. Geneva: International Council of Nurses. No ISBN ICN/89/202

Directory cites 115 nursing research units worldwide which were identified by national nurses' associations in membership with the International Council of Nurses. Information includes unit name and address, contact person, type of setting, number of professional staff, disciplines included, research activities and support, and conducted research. The latter are reported under the following categories: recipients of care; nursing practice; theory; education; research on nurses; organizations; management and administration; and research methodology. Also includes methodological approaches used, additional research activities, and whether consultancy is provided to outside professionals with or without fees (CR 1.3).

3.14.7 International Nursing Review.
(1994) Germany's first and only research unit. *International Nursing Review*, 41 (1) Issue 313 6 News

Reports the setting up of the Agnes Karll Institute for nursing research in 1991. Its focal points of research are based on the World Health Organization's 'Health for all' objectives (CR 3.3).

3.14.8 McMillan, I. (1992) Research development. *Nursing Times*, 9 December, 88 (50) 19 No references

Reports the creation of a new mental health nursing research unit in London. Links have been made with two universities and a medical school, and two topics have been identified as priorities.

3.14.9 Network for Psychiatric Nursing Research.
URL: http://www.man.ac.uk/rcn/ukwide/npnr.html

Based in the UK, this network offers a comprehensive search and information service for health professionals working in mental health nursing research. Its aim is to disseminate and develop research and practice initially within the UK.

3.14.10 Oguisso, T. (1990) How ICN is promoting research. *International Nursing Review*, 37 (4) Issue 292 295–8   9 References

Article examines the role of the International Council of Nurses in promoting nursing research. Study seminars and international congresses were organized, and a Task Force created whose members collected information about the development of research in their respective countries. Guidelines to promote research activity for National Nurses' Associations were also developed.

3.14.11 Queensland University of Technology. (1997) *The Centre for Mental Health Nursing Research.*
URL: http://qut.edu.au/qut/centres/tcmhnr.html

Website outlines the aims and objectives of this Centre.

3.14.12 Royal College of Nursing. (1998) *Research and Development Co-ordinating Centre.*
URL: http://www.man.ac.uk/rcn/

Reports on the development of a website launched in the UK early in 1998. Its purpose is to provide a means of sharing information on research and practice development in nursing, and it is designed to be fully interactive. The website will be permanently 'under construction' so that the latest information will be available on research networks, policy issues, funding, training, forthcoming conferences, research in progress, dissemination and utilization. Information will be gathered at local, regional, national and international levels.

3.14.13 Royal College of Nursing Research Society. (1998)
URL: http://www.man.uk/rcn/index.html

This website lists the relationship between nursing and research, states the aims of the society and invites nurses to join forces and move forward the research base for nursing.

3.14.14 Russell Sage Foundation.
URL: http://www.epn.org/sage.html

This American Foundation is devoted exclusively to research in the social sciences. Past and future work is outlined and its major goal now is to strengthen the methods, data and theoretical core of the social sciences as a means of improving social policies.

3.14.15　Sampselle, C.M. & Reame, N. (1992) The clinical research centre: important resource for the nurse investigator. *Nursing Research*, 41 (3) 184–5　4 References

Discusses the aims of clinical research centres (CRCs) and the value to nursing of this resource. A CRC model at the University of Michigan hospitals, and how resources from the current 75 centres may be accessed, are described.

3.14.16　Traynor, M. (1993) Daphne Heald Research Unit: 10 years on. *Nursing Standard*, 10–16 March, 7 (25) 26–7　9 References

Briefly outlines the work of this unit in four specialist areas: stoma care, diabetes care, sickle cell project and early discharge after surgery. Current work includes two linked studies examining the impact of recent legislation, focusing on four community trusts and the nursing care and treatment of people with AIDS.

3.14.17　University of Newcastle. (1998) *Centre for Nursing Research and Practice Development.*
http://www.newcastle.edu.au/department/ns/Centre.html

This Australian centre aims to assist staff and research students undertake and publish nursing research and win research grants. Currently funded projects are listed and pointers to interesting links are given.

3.14.18　University of Sheffield, School of Health and Related Research (ScHARR).
URL: http://www.sosig.ac.uk/roads/cgi/search

Acts as a focus for health services research/health technology assessment within the University of Sheffield and conducts research into a broad variety of clinical settings, including ageing, general practice, nursing, rehabilitation, mental and public health. Website includes lists of research and teaching, and publications, some of which, including 'Guide to evidence-based practice' (1997), are available online.

3.14.19　University of Sheffield, Centre for Research and Development in Nursing and Midwifery Practice.
URL: http: //www.shef.ac.uk/uni/academic/N-Q/nm/research/centre.htm

This website is at present under construction (checked on 4 September 1998).

3.14.20　University of York. (1996) *Centre for Evidence-based Nursing.* York: Department of Health Studies.
URL: http: //www.york.ac.uk/depts/hstd/centres/evidence/ev-intro.htm

This website gives the background and objectives of the Centre for Evidence-based Nursing, current projects, recent publications, the Cochrane Wounds Group, and links to external information sources.

3.14.21　University of York, Social Policy Research Unit.
URL: http: //york.ac.uk/inst/spru/welcome.htm

This unit carries out policy-related research using methodological skills, academic knowledge and an understanding of policy-making. It focuses on two major areas – health and social care and social security. Basic details of objectives, approach, research programmes and staff are given (CR 3.11).

3.14.22　Wojtas, O. (1995) Nursing research centre set for launch. *Times Higher Education Supplement*, 24 February, 1164　2

Reports on the establishment of a new policy centre for nursing research by the London School of Hygiene and Tropical Medicine and the Royal College of Nursing. It aims to establish a co-ordinated strategy for nursing research and build up a group of high-profile researchers (CR 3.11.4).

PROFESSIONAL GROUPS

3.15 PROFESSIONAL GROUPS

Professional groups have played many important roles in the development of nursing research, and continue to do so both locally, nationally and internationally.

Annotations

3.15.1 Henderson, S. & Perrier, P. (1995) A national survey of SNA research commissions: implications for Maine's nurses. *Maine Nurse*, July 27–28

Reports the results of a survey of American State Nurses' Associations which aimed to ascertain their research roles and activities. A considerable variety of projects, actions, policies and debates emerged which the Maine State Nurses' Association will use to develop their own activities (CR 2.96, 3.11).

3.15.2 Kikuchi, J. (1994) Institute for Philosophical Nursing Research. *Canadian Journal of Nursing Research*, 26 (2) 91–3 No references
URL: nursing.ualberta.ca/HomePage.nsf/Nursing/PNR-CFA

Reports on the aims, objectives, activities, administration and future directions of the Institute for Philosophical Nursing Research (CR 2.5).

3.15.3 Martin, P.A. (1994) Building a local research consortium. *Applied Nursing Research*, 7 (2) 107–9 11 References

Discusses the formation of a local group of nurses with similar research aspirations which could provide support and encourage development of research skills. It could also assist in balancing the research and clinical aspects of nurses' roles. Membership, meetings, agendas and programmes are all discussed (CR 3.16).

3.15.4 Rempusheski, V.F., Wolfe, B.E., Dow, K.H. & Fish, L.C. (1996) Peer review by nursing research committees in hospitals. *Image: Journal of Nursing Scholarship*, 28 (1) 51–3 32 References

Article discusses the role of nursing research committees and believes that they are leading a shift towards activities that strengthen nursing science and scientists. Eight strategies to support this role are suggested.

3.15.5 Thede, L. (1995a) *NurseRes – a listserv Discussion Group for Nurse Researchers.* Kent, Ohio: School of Nursing, Kent State University
URL: http://tilenet/listserv/nurseres.html

Outlines the development of this electronic discussion group for nurse researchers. Information is given on access and services.

3.15.6 Thede, L. (1995b) *NurseRes-DB-Database of Nurse Researchers and their Interests.* Kent, Ohio: School of Nursing, Kent State University
URL: http://ds.internic.net/cgi-bin/enthtml/health/nurseres-db.b

This database of nurse researchers contains names, e-mail addresses, institution, interests and level of availability. [For more information contact Lthede@KentVM.Kent.Edu]

3.15.7 UNESCO. (1993) *World Directory of Academic Research Groups in Science Ethics.* Paris: UNESCO. Science Policy Studies and Documents No. 73.
URL: http://www.unesco.org

Provides information on sources and research institutes throughout the world (CR 1.3).

RESEARCH ROLES AND CAREERS

3.16 RESEARCH ROLES AND CAREERS

There is a variety of roles which nurses may fulfil in relation to research and all are important to ensure that professional practice is based on firm foundations. Some nurses will conduct research themselves, others will facilitate this process and most nurses will be informed consumers.

Definition

Research assistant – the individual who assists the principal investigator with such activities as subject recruitment, data collection and data analysis

---

Annotations

3.16.1 Anderson, C.A. (1994) The role of the academic setting in research career development, in Fitzpatrick, J.J., Stevenson, J.S. & Polis, N.S. (eds), *Nursing Research and its Utilization.* New York: Springer. ISBN 0826180906 Chapter 18, 183–9 3 References

Chapter discusses the importance of research, successful research careers and gives a brief history of research facilitation in nursing (CR 2.102.17, 3.17).

3.16.2 Andre, R. & Frost, P.J. (eds) (1996) *Researchers Hooked on Teaching: Noted Scholars Discuss the Synergies of Teaching and Research.* London: Sage. ISBN 0761906223 References

International contributors describe their experiences of balancing the tension between teaching and research. The themes which emerge are: teachers as models for each other

and their students; individualism versus collectivism in the institution and classroom; integrating individual research interests into the classroom; and finding one's voice.

3.16.3 Anonymous (1998) Are you cut out for a career in research? *Nursing Times Learning Curve,* 4 March, 2 (1) 14–15

Reports some of the routes taken by nurses into the field of nursing research and the difficulties they experienced. Questions are posed which may guide other nurses who are interested in pursuing their careers in research.

3.16.4 Baron, S., Gilloran, A. & Schad, D. (1995) Researching with nurses and patients: from subjects to collaborators? *Social Sciences in Health: International Journal of Research and Practice,* 1 (3) 175–88 47 References

Reports on methodological aspects of research into new ways of assessing quality of care for those with special needs, conducted with a team of community mental handicap nurses in Scotland. Existing models of clinical audit and of the concomitant researcher–researched relationship are examined: the positivist and action research models of the subject, the ethnographic model of the informant and the feminist model of the friend. An alternative is sought to enable clients with special needs to specify themselves what quality of care means so that different forms of researcher–researched relations can develop (CR 2.10, 2.37, 2.42).

3.16.5 Baumgart, A.J. (1996) Promoting nursing practice through nursing research. *International Nursing Review,* 43 (2) 45–8, 57 7 References

Reports that the International Council of Nurses is investing in programmes and projects that will strengthen the capabilities of the organization and its members to exercise research leadership. Three dimensions of such leadership are: fostering research-based practice; documenting the work and worth of nursing; and enhancing public understanding of nursing work.

3.16.6 Benton, D. (1995) Senior nursing research posts: formation, location and future. *Nurse Researcher*, 2 (3) 80–91   17 References

Reports a study which examined the characteristics of district nurse researchers. Author believes that this type of innovative post could be a way forward for those interested in research careers.

3.16.7 Buffum, M.D. (1996) Staff action: the nurse researcher in the clinical setting. *Journal of Neuroscience Nursing*, 28 (6) 399–406   27 References

Utilizing the author's experiences, the article describes the role of the nurse researcher in relation to staff nurse involvement at the San Francisco Veterans' Affairs Medical Center. An historical perspective is given and a programme which aimed to involve all nurses in utilizing research findings is described (CR 2.102).

3.16.8 Cartwright, J. & Limandri, B. (1997) The challenge of multiple roles in the qualitative clinician researcher–participant client relationship. *Qualitative Health Research*, 7 (2) 223–35   20 References

Article discusses the multi-dimensional relationships that developed between researcher and participants during an exploratory study of enrichment processes in family care-giving to frail elders. During the data collection phase the following unintended relationships were revealed: stranger–stranger, friend–friend, nurse–client and guest–host. Additional topics for discussion regarding the experience of undertaking research in people's homes are suggested (CR 2.36).

3.16.9 Cohen, F.L., Holm, K. & Cloninger, L. (1995) Equal team partners? The roles of principal investigators, co-principal investigators and co-investigators on federally supported research grants. *Image: Journal of Nursing Scholarship*, 27 (1) 76–9   12 References

A survey of 188 National League of Nursing-accredited graduate nursing programmes was completed to determine how the research roles of the various investigators were supported and to examine the difference in benefits. Results showed various differences in remuneration, cost recovery, use of research assistants and reduction of teaching time. Authors believe that everyone involved should be treated equally (CR 2.52).

3.16.10 Cohen, M.Z. (1995) The experience of surgery: phenomenological clinical nursing research, in Omery, A., Kasper, C.E. & Page, G.G. (eds) *In Search of Nursing Science.* Thousand Oaks, CA: Sage. ISBN 0803950942 Chapter 12, 159–74   47 References

Reports a phenomenological study which aimed to provide an understanding of the essential structure of the experience of having surgery. Author also reports on the extensive preparation given to staff nurse interviewers for one year prior to commencing the study to gain requisite experiences. These included discussing readings about phenomenological research, interviewing techniques and data analysis. The principal investigator discussed strengths, weaknesses and alternative approaches which could be used in interviews (CR 2.8.11, 2.49, 2.68).

3.16.11 Cormack, D.F.S. (ed.) (1990) *Developing Your Career in Nursing.* London: Chapman & Hall. ISBN 0412321300   References

A practical text giving advice on how to plan one's career. Several sections in the book cover aspects of nursing research and nurse researchers.

3.16.12 Csokasy, J.A. (1997) Building perioperative nursing research teams – Part I. *AORN Journal*, 65 (2) 396, 398, 400–1 10 References

and

3.16.13 Csokasy, J.A. (1997) Building perioperative nursing research teams – Part II. *AORN Journal*, 65 (4) 787, 789–90   10 References

This two-part article describes the use of the experiential learning model, developed by David Kolb, to facilitate a team approach to perioperative nursing research. Constraints and enablers to conducting and using research in perioperative care settings are discussed and suggestions are made for nurse managers which will help to facilitate clinical research.

3.16.14   Di Giulio, P., Arrigo, C., Gall, H., Molin, C., Nieweg, R. & Strohbucker, B. (1996) Expanding the role of the nurse in clinical trials. *Cancer Nursing*, 19 (5) 343–7 9 References

Authors believe that in order for the overall quality of clinical trials to be improved the role of the nurse should be expanded. They suggest that a nursing summary of the medical protocol, developed by those responsible for it, would provide a short and easy-to-read selection of protocol-relevant information and enable nurses to enhance their role. The advantages of doing this are discussed (CR 2.29).

3.16.15   Gift, A.G., Creasia, J. & Parker, B. (1991) Utilising research assistants and maintaining research integrity. *Research in Nursing and Health*, 14 (3) 229–33   10 References

Gives guidelines on hiring, contracting, orientating, monitoring, mentoring and evaluating the performance of research assistants.

3.16.16   Gregory, D., Russell, C.K. & Phillips, L.R. (1997) Beyond textual perfection: transcribers as vulnerable persons. *Qualitative Health Research*, 7 (2) 294–300 6 References

Discusses the role transcribers play and the protection they may need from ethical and institutional review committees to prevent emotional injury when dealing with sensitive information. They need to be fully informed about the nature of the research being undertaken and the type of data to be collected before being hired. Difficulties which may arise from interviews should be discussed and regular debriefing sessions should be arranged (CR 2.17).

3.16.17   Grofsik, J.S. & Sauers, J.A. (1997) Alternative career options. A cutting-edge job? Consider research. *RN* [Registered Nurse], 60 (9) 55–8   4 References

Discusses the possibilities of a career in clinical research.

3.16.18   Hicks, C. (1995a) A study of nurse managers' constructs of nurse researchers.

Journal of Nursing Management, 3 (5) 237–45 31 References

Two groups of nurse managers were asked to consider how many of 15 bipolar dimensions were possessed by a nurse described as either a 'good clinician' or a 'good researcher'. Results appeared to show that the two roles are not compatible and this is discussed in the context of the development of nursing research.

3.16.19   Hicks, C. (1995b) Good researcher, poor midwife: an investigation into the impact of central trait descriptions on assumptions of professional competence. *Midwifery*, 11 (2) 81–7   25 References

Author reports a serious shortfall in published midwifery research. A study was conducted to assess the way in which midwives construed their professional role and whether this acted as a deterrent to undertaking research. Results are reported and suggestions for change are identified.

3.16.20   Hicks, C. (1996) Nurse researcher: a study of contradiction in terms? *Journal of Advanced Nursing*, 24 (2) 357–63   26 References

Study tested the idea that the roles of nurse practitioners and researchers may not be compatible because of different expectations from colleagues. Findings showed that qualities attributed to each group were different which may prove to be an obstacle to research development in nursing (CR 3.7).

3.16.21   Hill, M.N., Bone, L.R. & Butz, A.M. (1996) Enhancing the role of community health workers in research. *Image: Journal of Nursing Scholarship*, 28 (3) 221–6   37 References

Article describes the rationale for inclusion of community health workers in research, their roles and responsibilities, and issues in their selection, training and supervision. Examples are given from the authors' experiences with interventions by nurse and community teams.

3.16.22   Hinshaw, A.S. (1994) Developing a research career: a trajectory for career development, in Fitzpatrick, J.J., Stevenson, J.S. & Polis, N.S. (eds) *Nursing Research and its Utilization*. New York: Springer. ISBN 0826180906 Chapter 16, 167–77 17 References

Chapter considers becoming a scientist, a trajectory for the career development of investigators and the opportunities for advancing scientific careers and issues involved in a career trajectory (CR 2.102.17).

3.16.23 Hoffart, N. (1995) Characteristics of nephrology nurse researchers and their research. *ANNA Journal*, 22 (1) 33–41 22 References

Describes findings from a survey undertaken to identify characteristics of nephrology nurse researchers together with descriptions of studies they had conducted. Recommendations to foster continued maturation of their research are offered. *The Directory of Nephrology Nurse Researchers* will be updated from data obtained in this survey.

3.16.24 Institute of Health Services Research. (1995) *Career Profiles of Researchers in Health and Social Care*. Luton: University of Luton. No ISBN

3.16.25 Jordan, S. (1990) Look before you leap: becoming a nurse researcher. *Nursing Times*, 14–20 March, 86 (11) 42 No references

Discusses some aspects of the role of a clinical nurse researcher.

3.16.26 Kirchhoff, K.T. (1993) The role of nurse researchers employed in clinical settings, in Fitzpatrick, J.J. & Stevenson, J.S. (eds), *Annual Review of Nursing Research* Volume 11. New York: Springer. ISBN 0826182305 Part II, Chapter 7, 169–81 55 References

Reviews literature on the role of nurse researchers employed in clinical settings from 1980 to 1992. Headings are enactment of a new role, strategies for success, research activities, productivity, programme reports, organizational attributes and directions for future research (CR 2.12).

3.16.27 Kirk, K. (1996) From practitioners to practitioner/researcher – Part 2. *Health Visitor*, 69 (10) 427 3 References

Author believes that health visitors already possess the level of skills required to undertake research (CR 2.4).

3.16.28 Knight-Bohnhoff, K., Horne-Lucero, L., Kory, L. & Fry, R. (1995) The challenge of trauma clinical trials: facilitation through understanding. *Journal of Trauma Nursing*, 2 (2) 43–9

Authors examine the roles and responsibilities of the clinical research nurse co-ordinator within the surgical intensive care unit when research trials are being conducted. Historical evolution of this role is reviewed and specific responsibilities are discussed. Ethical considerations are also presented (CR 2.17, 2.29).

3.16.29 Lewis, J. & Ritchie, J. (1995) *Advancing Research: Research Workforce Capacity in Health and Social Care*. London: Social and Community Planning Research. No ISBN

3.16.30 Logan, J. & Davies, B. (1995) The staff nurse as research facilitator. *Canadian Journal of Nursing Administration*, 8 (1) 92–110 24 References

Reports the outcomes of a one-day workshop which aimed to enhance professional practice through becoming more knowledgeable about research findings. Nurses attending felt more positive about research and developed a network to share tactics. There was an expressed need for ongoing support from managers.

3.16.31 Martin, P.A. (1996) Member responsibilities on a nursing research committee. *Applied Nursing Research*, 9 (3) 154–7 15 References

Article discusses the factors necessary for being a competent nursing research committee member. These are: knowing the research process; the subject's rights; the role of the committee; developing sensitivity to timelines; knowing exclusions or exclusion criteria; and identifying topics or populations needing more review time (CR 2.17).

3.16.32 Mateo, M.A. & Kirchhoff, K.T. (1995) Productivity of nurse researchers employed in clinical settings. *Journal of Nursing Administration*, 25 (10) 37–42 5 References

Authors describe the activities of nurses working in clinical practice that pertain to research, presentations, publications, and procurement of funds for studies. Major obstacles that prevent them carrying out their roles are presented.

3.16.33 McMahon, K., McEnhill, M. &

Youngquist, R. (1996) Utilizing volunteer research assistants in epidemiologic studies. *Journal of Aging and Social Policy*, 8 (1) 39–58 11 References

Discusses the use of volunteers, who were healthy older adults or retired workers, in a two-year cross-sectional study of factors which predict health ageing. Eighty-two volunteers were recruited and trained to fill roles usually undertaken by paid research assistants. They performed the key activities of telephone screening, interviewing, coding and data entry, following standards and within a time-frame comparable to similar studies. This resulted in cost savings of over $100,000 (CR 2.41).

3.16.34   O'Brien, S. (1996) The role of the nurse in medically oriented research. *Nursing Standard*, 10 (24) 32   No references

A clinical research nurse explains his role and emphasizes the benefits for nurses, and the influence they can have on medically orientated research (CR 3.23).

3.16.35   Ochert, A. (1996) Life on the bottom rung. *Times Higher Education Supplement*, 23 February, 1216 Research opportunities, xxxvi

Examines the effort being made to relieve the plight of contract research staff who earn a pittance and have slim hopes of promotion.

3.16.36   Oguisso, T. (1994) Nursing research training and career development around the world, in Fitzpatrick, J.J., Stevenson, J.S. & Polis, N.S. (eds), *Nursing Research and its Utilization*. New York: Springer. ISBN 0826180906 Chapter 19, 191–9 12 References

Chapter briefly reports on the state of nursing research worldwide (except in North America), research training and career structure (CR 2.102.17, 3.1, 3.3, 3.4, 3.6).

3.16.37   Ohman, K.A. (1996) Expanding collaborative efforts for research utilization. *Clinical Nurse Specialist*, 10 (2) 58–62 38 References

The role of the clinical nurse specialist in research and strategies for the promotion of research utilization are discussed. The collaborative role of the clinical nurse is highlighted as a key factor in promoting research utilization (CR 2.15, 2.101).

3.16.38   Patel, K. (1996) Contract staff win better conditions. *Times Higher Education Supplement*, 8 March, 1218   2

Reports that details of a framework for researchers' career management are to be published shortly. The draft 'concordat' is expected to place responsibility for their management on employing institutions. In return Research Councils and the Royal Society will expect there to be effective policies on training supervision and appraisal.

3.16.39   Pelke, S. & Easa, D. (1997) The role of the clinical research co-ordinator in multi-center clinical trials. *JOGNN – Journal of Obstetric, Gynecologic and Neonatal Nursing*, 26 (3) 279–85   14 References

Article clarifies the role of the clinical research co-ordinator for those about to assume these responsibilities and outlines planning procedures leading to successful implementation. Emphasis is placed upon establishing an interdependent relationship with the principal investigator, careful protocol assessment, team-building and staff feedback (CR 2.29).

3.16.40   Porter, S. (1996) Men researching women working. *Nursing Outlook*, 44 (1) 22–6 31 References

Author asks the question: can research by male nurses into the work of female practitioners be justified?

3.16.41   Pranulis, M.F. (1991) Research progress in a clinical setting. *Western Journal of Nursing Research*, 13 (2) 274–7   13 References

Article suggests that research projects are largely generated by academics which enhances their careers, but which may neglect clinically based research. A plea is made for both groups of nurses to come together, recognizing each other's contributions and developing programmes of clinically relevant research (CR 3.7).

3.16.42   Rempusheski, V.F. (1992) A researcher as resource, mentor, and preceptor. *Applied Nursing Research*, 5 (2) 105–7 5 References

Author suggests ways in which clinical nurses may contact a nurse researcher and other sources which may be consulted. Advice is given on how to determine a 'fit' between yourself and the researcher, defining one's interests and expressing commitment of time, energy and talents (CR 3.7).

3.16.43 Sapers, R. & Sweich, K. (1992) Experiences of acute care nurses who seek out a nurse researcher as preceptor. *Applied Nursing Research*, 5 (3) 154–6   1 Reference

Two nurses write about their experiences of working with an experienced researcher, how this was initiated, the objectives that were set and met, and what was gained.

3.16.44 Saunders, M.J. (1993) Director of quality improvement research. *Journal of Nursing Care Quality,* 7 (4) 39–43   13 References

Discusses ways in which quality care can be assisted by the appointment of a researcher whose role is to teach, encourage and develop all aspects of research. The use of action research is recommended (CR 2.37, 3.17).

3.16.45 Sawyer, L., Regev, H., Procter, S., Nelson, M., Messias, D., Barnes, D. & Meleis, A.I. (1995) Matching versus cultural competence in research: methodological considerations. *Research in Nursing and Health*, 18 (6) 557–67   51 References

Paper considers the complexities in using matching in research with diverse populations and challenges the idea that matching of researchers and participants is the only strategy for generating culturally valid knowledge. It also argues that cultural competence, as a synthesis of cultural knowledge, sensitivity and collaboration, could be used in facilitating the development of culturally-competent nursing knowledge.

3.16.46 Selby-Harrington, M.L., Donat, P.L.N. & Hibbard, H.D. (1994) Research grant implementation: staff development as a tool to accomplish research activities. *Applied Nursing Research*, 7 (1) 38–46   25 References

Article provides principal investigators (PIs)

with practical guidance for determining staffing needs and selecting staff for a research project. It also provides guidance for using staff development programmes to enhance research skills so they can assist in completing grant activities and grow into more seasoned researchers themselves.

3.16.47 Stotts, N.A. (1997) Nurse researchers: who are they, what do they do and what challenges do they face?, in McCloskey, J.C. & Grace, H.K. (eds), *Current Issues in Nursing* 5th edition. St Louis: Mosby. ISBN 0815185944 Chapter 6, 41–4   5 References

Chapter introduces nurses to the world of the researcher and asks who they are, what do they do and what are the challenges which they face?

3.16.48 Trilla, A. (1995) Components of a clinical trial: historical development, study personnel, and nursing roles. *ANNA Journal*, 22 (4) 375–9   7 References

Article discusses some of the many roles which nurses play within research, elements of a clinical trial and their historical influences (CR 2.29).

3.16.49 Willis, J. (1998) Are you cut out for a career in research? *Nursing Times Learning Curve*, 2 (1) 14–15

Article outlines some of the factors which need to be considered before embarking on a career in research. Some of the opportunities that are available are outlined.

3.16.50 Wilson-Barnett, J., Corner, J. & DeCarle, B. (1990) Integrating research and practice: the role of the researcher as teacher. *Journal of Advanced Nursing*, 15 (5) 621–5   20 References

Two recent studies are examined to show how researchers can assist practitioners in developing some research skills by working in close co-operation. This model is suggested as the way forward for increasing research-based practice.

RESEARCH EDUCATION

3.17 RESEARCH EDUCATION

Introducing nursing research early in learning programmes will enable students to see it in the context of patient/client care. The knowledge that is gained can later provide the foundation for expert practice.

Annotations

3.17.1 Adams, T. (1994) Teaching research methods to nursing students. *British Journal of Nursing* (Educational careers supplement), 13–26 October, 3 (18) 947–8, 950–1   9 References

Author suggests an eclectic approach using traditional, experiential and action-orientated methods. An example is given and ways in which research can be integrated into courses are described.

3.17.2 Ailinger, R.L., Lasus, H. & Choi, E. (1997) Using national data sets on CD ROM to teach nursing research. *Image: Journal of Nursing Scholarship*, 29 (1) 17–20   8 References

Reports use of national data sets to teach graduate nursing research. Such use of secondary data is cost-effective and a rich source of material. The findings of a pilot programme are discussed and ten steps to ensure better attainment of objectives were formulated (CR 2.91).

3.17.3 Axford, R.L. & Carter, B.E. (1995) Nursing research education practices in Australia. *Collegian: Journal of the Royal College of Nursing, Australia*, 2 (4) 23–8   11 References

Reports the wide variety of work and expectations regarding the research education of nurses in Australia. Respondents to a country-wide survey believe that a clear policy formulation is necessary across university, state and national levels so that education is appropriate, resources are used carefully and nurses are taught how to use research findings.

3.17.4 Baker, C.M. (1995) When to begin a doctoral programme in nursing. *International Nursing Review*, 42 (2) 61–4   16 References

Discusses the various processes which need to be considered before a doctoral programme is developed. Aspects include socio-cultural environment, academic context, programme resources, availability of students, career opportunities and a time-orientated planning model.

3.17.5 Barhyte, D.Y. & Redman, B.K. (1993) Factors related to graduate nursing faculty scholarship productivity. *Nursing Research*, 42 (3) 179–83   22 References

Reports a study which focused on the scholarly endeavours of the faculty teaching in graduate programmes in schools of nursing. Factors are identified in these academic environments that influence their productivity.

3.17.6 Beck, C.T. (1993) Integrating research into an RN to BSN clinical course. *Western Journal of Nursing Research*, 15 (1) 118–21   7 References

Reports on the use of a teaching strategy where students used a phenomenological approach to a patient/client experience from the client's perspective. Students reported the value of this exercise for learning about elements of the research process (CR 2.49).

3.17.7 Beck, C.T. (1997) Use of meta-analysis as a teaching strategy in nursing research courses. *Journal of Nursing Education*, 36 (2) 87–90   15 References

Article describes two teaching strategies using meta-analysis for sharpening both graduate and undergraduate nurses' critiquing skills. At graduate level, students can use an appraisal checklist of criteria for evaluating the actual meta-analysis, and undergraduates can assess the quality of studies included in a particular meta-analysis (CR 2.92).

3.17.8   Berry, J. & Kenny, C. (1994) Using a game to teach research and statistics. *Nurse Researcher*, 1 (4) 69–77   11 References

Discusses the development and initial evaluation of a board game which aims to teach students undertaking research modules on a degree course about very complex subjects.

3.17.9   Blackburn, R.T. & Bentley, R.J. (1993) Faculty research productivity: some moderators of associated stressors. *Research in Higher Education*, 34 (6) 725–45   28 References

Reports a study which aimed to generate knowledge on the relationship between stress, moderators and research productivity.

3.17.10   Burrows, D.E. (1997) A strategy for teaching research to adult branch diploma students. *Nurse Education Today*, 17 (1) 39–45   31 References

Describes a strategy based on the use of journal clubs and presentations of individuals' work to promote interest in, and the knowledge and skills required to understand and use, research in practice.

3.17.11   Butterworth, T. (1991) Continuity in research and teaching: the role of departments of nursing in higher education. *Nursing Standard*, 22 May, 5 (35) 31–6   References

Paper examines the role of nursing departments in universities in relation to research education, the problems of attracting and keeping experienced researchers, government controls on programmes and funding. Also discussed are the position of research units and developing multi-disciplinary programmes. The results are given of a survey of nursing research units in the UK which identified the broad areas of work being undertaken. Author urges further discussion on how research can find expression in clinical excellence (CR 3.9, 3.13, 3.14).

3.17.12   Byrne, M.M., Kangas, S.K. & Warren, N. (1996) Advice for beginning researchers. *Image: Journal of Nursing Scholarship*, 28 (2) 165–7   10 References

Advice given to beginning researchers included identifying a planned programme of research with a topic that we 'love' and doing work which is meaningful. Other suggestions were keeping an idea log, networking, mentoring and developing collegial relationships.

3.17.13   Cavanagh, S. & Coffin, D. (1993) Teaching nursing research. *Senior Nurse*, 13 (4) 51–4   21 References

Discusses the knowledge of educators' planning and delivery of research-based materials in the nursing curriculum. Strategies are examined and ways of communicating findings are discussed. An early introduction of research into courses aids understanding of its importance to patients and nurses.

3.17.14   Centre for Policy in Nursing Research. (1998) *Nursing Research and the Higher Education Context: a Second Working Paper* London: Centre for Policy in Nursing Research. No ISBN   References

Paper provides various contexts for understanding the dilemmas faced by nurses involved in higher education. The political context of higher education policy and issues facing medical education in the UK are discussed, together with a brief history of nurse education, UK events in an international context and the performance of nursing in the last two Research Assessment Exercises. The findings of a study examining the foundations of nursing knowledge, the level of supervision in a study of PhD students and current academic activity of the UK's university nursing departments, together with their views and experiences, are all reported. Points for consideration by heads of university departments, National Health Service (NHS) research commissioners, managers, education commissioners and the NHS Executive of the Department of Health are given (CR 2.6, 3.9, 3.11, 3.18).

3.17.15   Conn, V.S. (1995) Involving students in advanced practice nurses' and nurse educators' collaborative research. *Western Journal of Nursing Research*, 17 (5) 574–8   9 References

Describes   teaching   nursing   research   to

graduate students by involving them in collaborative research. Authors believe that this gives a context which is congruent with the realities of practice, and it may contribute to reducing the separation between service and education (CR 2.15).

3.17.16   Cowan, M.J., Heinrich, J., Lucas, M., Sigmon, H. & Hinshaw, A.S. (1993) Integration of biological and nursing sciences: a 10 year plan to enhance research and training. *Research in Nursing and Health*, 16 (1) 3–9 No references

Reports a proposed multi-year plan of funding mechanisms by the National Center for Nursing Research which aims to increase the use of biological theory and measurements in nursing research. Plans have been made for both research training and research programmes (CR 3.16).

3.17.17   Davis, B.D. & Burnard, P. (1992) Academic levels in nursing. *Journal of Advanced Nursing*, 17 (12) 1395–400 10 References

As new academic courses in nursing develop, some issues involved in the debate about educational levels are explored. Data were obtained from professors of nursing in the UK, masters students in a Dutch college and American literature. The characteristics of diploma, baccalaureate, masters and doctoral courses are outlined.

3.17.18   Dunn, B. (1991) Who should be doing research in nursing? *Professional Nurse*, 6 (4) 190, 192–4, 196   23 References

Discusses who should be undertaking research, how they should be educated, funding research and possible careers. Author advocates the establishment of a single government body to provide direction and guidance (CR 3.9, 3.13, 3.16).

3.17.19   Evans, J.H. (1992) *An Exploration of Graduate Nursing Research Education: Factors and Attitudes Influencing Choice of Paradigms, Models and Methodologies.* ED.D., Peabody College for Teachers of Vanderbilt University

Study investigated the framework of selected masters degree nursing programmes by describing and analysing the education and socialization of graduate students into the various research paradigms and

methodologies used by nurses. Findings highlighted various issues of importance to nursing administrators, faculty members, researchers and nursing organizations.

3.17.20   Farrington, A. (1996) Developing a research culture for nursing in higher education. *British Journal of Nursing*, 5 (1) 57–81 Reference

Discusses ways in which a research culture may be developed. A seamless mesh of research activity and information dissemination are believed to be essential. The long-term nature of these processes is acknowledged but they are essential if nursing is to play a full part in improving patient care.

3.17.21   Field, J. (1997) Judging research quality in post-compulsory education and training: lessons of the 1996 assessment exercise. *Studies in the Education of Adults*, 29 (1) 101–8   10 References

Paper provides a description and analysis of the fate of research into post-compulsory education and training in the 1996 Research Assessment Exercise. A brief description of the procedures that were followed is given, aspects of the results are analysed and key issues are identified (CR 3.9).

3.17.22   Fitch, M., Bolster, A., Alderson, D., Kennedy, G. & Woermke, D.H. (1995) Moving toward research-based cancer nursing practice. *Canadian Oncology Nursing Journal*, 5 (1) 5–8   3 References

Article describes an approach for introducing research to cancer nurses. Four projects are highlighted to show how questions were identified in clinical practice and systematic data collection used to help in decision-making.

3.17.23   Fogarty, T.J. & Saftner, D.V. (1993) Academic department prestige: a new measure based on the doctoral student labour market. *Research in Higher Education*, 34 (4) 427–49   64 References

Paper argues that since prestige is a multi-dimensional attribute that requires continuous re-affirmation between participants, the construct merits a new approach as applied to academic faculty. A short literature review sets the scene, a new measure and field test are described. Its implications and limitations are discussed (CR 2.12).

3.17.24 Goldrick, B.A., Larson, E. & Lyons, D. (1995) Conflict of interest in academia. *Image: Journal of Nursing Scholarship*, 27 (1) 65–9   30 References

Authors discuss conflicts of interest as they apply to nursing research and how these may affect practice and education. Resources for the development of guidelines to prevent these conflicts are given (CR 2.16).

3.17.25 Holloway, D.G. & Race, A.J. (1993) Developing a rationale for research-based practice: some considerations for nurse teachers. *Nurse Education Today*, 13 (4) 259–63   22 References

Discusses the implications of advocating a research focus on the problems arising in practitioner and action-based methodologies (CR 2.37).

3.17.26 Howard, E.P., Beauchesne, M.A., Shea, C.A. & Meservey, P.M. (1996) Research practicum: linking education to practice. *Nurse Educator*, 21 (6) 33–7   6 References

Describes the development and implementation of an innovative sequence of research courses at one graduate school of nursing. Students are involved in real-life aspects of conducting research in a practice discipline.

3.17.27 Hutchinson, S.A. & Webb, R.B. (1991) Teaching qualitative research: perennial problems and possible solutions, in Morse, J.M. (ed.), *Qualitative Nursing Research: a Contemporary Dialogue* (Revised edition). Newbury Park, CA: Sage. ISBN 0803940793 Chapter 17, 301–21   19 References

Chapter discusses the difficulties encountered and some possible solutions when teaching qualitative research courses to graduate students.

3.17.28 Kapp, S. & Wentz, G. (1997) Research forum. Baccalaureate student research. *JPO: Journal of Prosthetics and Orthotics*, 9 (1) 42–7

Describes ways in which research education has been built into the curriculum at the University of Texas Southwestern Medical Center at Dallas Prosthetics-Orthotics Program.

3.17.29 Ketefian, S. & Lenz, E.R. (1995)

Promoting scientific integrity in nursing research, Part II: Strategies. *Journal of Professional Nursing*, 11 (5) 263–9   16 References

Reports a survey of doctorate-granting schools on scientific integrity. Authors discuss publication and authorship practices, promotion and tenure policies and strategies to promote scientific integrity. Recommendations are made in a proactive manner rather than focusing on procedures for dealing with misconduct (CR 2.17, 3.7, 3.17.31).

3.17.30 Lacey, E.A. (1996) Facilitating research-based practice by educational intervention. *Nurse Education Today*, 16 (4) 296–301   20 References

The teaching of research in all nursing courses has enabled increased student awareness of its value to practice to develop. This article discusses the extent to which educational intervention can actually influence this practice.

3.17.31 Lenz, E.R. & Ketefian, S. (1995) Promoting scientific integrity in nursing research: Part 1. Current approaches in doctoral programs. *Journal of Professional Nursing*, 11 (4) 213–19   8 References

A survey of schools of nursing with doctoral programmes examined current approaches and elicited suggestions for strategies to promote scientific integrity (CR 3.17.29).

3.17.32 Macrina, F.L. & Munro, C.L. (1995) The case study approach to teaching scientific integrity in nursing and the biomedical sciences. *Journal of Professional Nursing*, 11 (1) 40–4   8 References

Discusses the experiences in teaching scientific integrity using a case-study approach. Issues covered include the underlying philosophy of this approach, preparation and use of cases, desired in-class teaching skills and the involvement of faculty in case preparation and teaching (CR 2.39).

3.17.33 Manley, K. (1996) Developing practice: the contribution of the masters prepared nurse. *Journal of Clinical Nursing*, 5 (6) 339–40   8 References   Editorial

Discusses some of the problems of assessing clinical practice at masters level. The role of universities, which may not recognize the differences within a practice-based discipline when evaluating research, are explored.

3.17.34   Martin, M. (1997) Critical education for participatory research. *Sociological Research Online*, 2 (2)
URL: http://www.socresonline.org.uk/socres online/2/2/8.html   21 References

Author believes that conventional training of health care professionals does not encourage critical reflection on practice. This case study of a masters course for health professionals working in primary care shows how an educational programme can help to develop the necessary skills (CR 2.39).

3.17.35   McSherry, R., Bond, M., Bassett, C. & Mudge, K. (1997) Unity is strength in joint research project. *Nursing Times*, 93 (16) 50–1
4 References

Authors outline ways in which they are helping staff to develop research skills so that they can analyse, evaluate and use research in their daily practice.

3.17.36   Millar, M.A. (1993) The place of research and development in nurse education. *Journal of Advanced Nursing*, 18 (7) 1039–42   27 References

Article discusses the relevance of research for nursing, education research and co-ordination of activity in light of the Department of Health document 'Strategy for health' (CR 3.9).

3.17.37   Moch, S.D., Robie, D.E., Bauer, K.C., Pederson, A., Bowe, S. & Shadick, K. (1997) Linking research and practice through discussion. *Image: Journal of Nursing Scholarship*, 29 (2) 189–91   12 References

Paper describes a case study which examined the process and outcomes of a researcher-initiated discussion group with nurses in clinical practice. Results showed that this could be a valuable way of enabling practitioners to learn more about research and it may assist in reducing the research–practice gap (CR 2.39, 3.7, 3.8).

3.17.38   Newman, M.A. (1997) The professional doctorate in nursing. *Image: Journal of Nursing Scholarship*, 29 (4) 361–2   2 References [Original article condensed, *Nursing Outlook* (1975), 23 (11) 704–6]

Reports a position paper written in 1975 about the development of professional doctorates in nursing. It is contrasted with the conventional PhD and the potential value to nursing practice is discussed (CR 3.5).

3.17.39   Noll, M.L. & Murphy, M.A. (1993) Integrating nursing information into a graduate course. *Journal of Nursing Education*, 32 (7) 332–4   5 References

Discusses ways of introducing computers, retrieval systems, data processing, database management, statistical packages and graphic displays into graduate courses.

3.17.40   O'Halloran, V.E., Pollock, S.E., Gottleib, T. & Schwartz, F. (1996) Improving self-efficacy in nursing research. *Clinical Nurse Specialist*, 10 (2) 83–7   14 References

Reports a project which aimed to increase research skills of practising nurses at one large health care facility. A participatory learning experience was developed and results showed increased confidence and the implementation of a number of research projects. The Delphi technique was used to identify priorities which were used to stimulate nurses to initiate and conduct clinical research (CR 2.66).

3.17.41   Parry, O., Atkinson, P. & Delamont, S. (1997) The structure of PhD research. *Sociology*, 31 (1) 121–9   21 References

Paper presents some findings from two national projects which focused on PhD research in Britain. It explored the characteristic structures which index natural science and social science doctoral study in both single and multi/inter-disciplinary fields. The research highlights ways in which PhD study can be organized to minimize some of the problems routinely experienced by students.

3.17.42   Parsons, C. (1995) The impact of postmodernism on research methodology: implications for nursing. *Nursing Inquiry*, 2 (1) 22–8   20 References

Article discusses the two major crises in research methodology: legitimization and representation. Educating nurses in research requires them to learn many skills but postmodern debates are also necessary so that contemporary issues can be woven into their practices (CR 2.3).

3.17.43 Pearcey, P.A. (1995) Achieving research-based nursing practice. *Journal of Advanced Nursing*, 22 (1) 33–9 21 References

Study examined the self-perceived research skills of 600 trained nurses with the aim of organizing workshops to meet their needs. Results showed that many were not happy with their skills, some of which were of an elementary nature. The implications of these findings are explored.

3.17.44 Pearson, A., Borbasi, S. & Gott, M. (1997) Doctoral education in nursing for practitioner knowledge and for academic knowledge: the University of Adelaide, Australia. *Image: Journal of Nursing Scholarship* 29 (4) 365–8 15 References

Paper argues the need for, and appropriateness of developing a doctoral programme in nursing, equivalent to, but different from, the PhD. Comparisons are made and the approach taken by the University of Adelaide is described.

3.17.45 Ranson, S. (1993) The management and organisation of education research. *Research Papers in Education*, 8 (2) 177–98 No references

An Economic and Social Research Council (ESRC)-commissioned study which examined how departments of education are developing their research profiles during a period of increasing competition for sponsorship. Strategic planning, organizing to develop a culture of research and the role of the ESRC are discussed. Suggestions are made for future development (CR 3.11).

3.17.46 Reed, J. (1995) Using a group project to teach research methods. *Nurse Education Today*, 15 (1) 56–60 5 References

Teaching research methods is problematic in nurse education, primarily because of the range of methodologies used and the ambiguity about the purpose of teaching – does it enable students to read or to do research? A strategy is described which may help to overcome some of these difficulties.

3.17.47 Royal College of Nursing of the United Kingdom. (1982) *Research-mindedness and Nurse Education*. London: Royal College of Nursing. No ISBN

Booklet, prepared by the RCN Research Society, which outlines ways in which research-mindedness can be encouraged. This is discussed in relation to pre- and post-registration education, nurse teachers, and library and information services.

3.17.48 Smith, P. (1994) Fulbright Scholarship: an opportunity for UK nurses. *Nurse Researcher*, 1 (4) 87–92 8 References

Provides details of the processes required to apply for Fulbright Scholarships, funded by the US government.

3.17.49 Sorrell, J. & Williams, S. (1993) Strategies for teaching nursing research. *Western Journal of Nursing Research*, 15 (3) 373–6 No references

Describes a collaborative model which enabled students to see the value of research and its clinical applications (CR 2.15).

3.17.50 Spiby, H. & Molloy, C. (1992) Encouraging research. *Nursing Times*, 1 January, 88 (1) 30–1 3 References

Reports a secondment scheme developed by a school of midwifery to enable midwives to learn about research. Its aims are listed and one midwife outlines her experiences (CR 3.6).

3.17.51 Tilley, S., Runciman, P. & Hockey, L. (1997) Research-based nurse education: understandings and personal accounts. *International Journal of Nursing Studies*, 34 (2) 111–18 18 References

Four nurse educators explored their understanding of the term 'research-based nursing education' (RBNE) and gave accounts of practice in different types of educational institution. Themes from the data are discussed, including the central role of questioning in teaching and learning. The study highlights contradictions and dilemmas arising when the constraints of nursing practice are 'married' to knowledge generation and freedom to learn. The implications of these tensions for higher education of nurses are discussed.

3.17.52 Trojan, L., Marck, P., Gray, C. & Rodger, G.L. (1996) A framework for planned change: achieving a funded PhD program in nursing. *Canadian Journal of Nursing Administration*, 9 (1) 71–86 16 References

Paper describes a process of planned change undertaken by a group of graduate nursing students at the University of Alberta. Their goal was to obtain funding for a PhD programme in nursing. Academic approval had already been received but funding was not readily available. Using a framework of planned change, based on concepts found in the literature on power, politics and political action, the nurses achieved their goal within 14 months.

3.17.53 University of Rochester, School of Nursing. (1997) *School of Nursing Cybercourse.*
URL: http://www.urmc.rochester.edu/son/courses/301/NUR301.htm

Outlines a course on research methods in nursing. Students will acquire a familiarity with the process of scientific inquiry and the application of quantitative and qualitative research to the development of nursing knowledge (CR 2.6, 2.29, 2.36).

3.17.54 Waters, C.M. (1996) Professional development in nursing research – a culturally diverse post-doctoral experience. *Image: Journal of Nursing Scholarship*, 28 (1) 47–50 35 References

Describes the key issues to be considered for culturally integrated professional development experiences between ethnic minority post-doctoral research fellows and white non-Hispanic nurse scientists. Factors critical to ensuring the survival and success of ethnic minority researchers are discussed.

3.17.55 Watson, D. (1998) Developing the capacity of nursing and midwifery research: the view from higher education. *NT Research*, 3 (2) 93–9 7 References

Author explores the problems and prospects for institutional support of nursing and midwifery research.

3.18   RESEARCH SUPERVISION AND MENTORSHIP

Providing students with appropriate and constructive supervision demands different skills from those of doing research. Teachers themselves may therefore need guidance, and institutions often set up short courses or arrange for staff to learn from each other by working together.

Definition

Research supervisor – ... an experienced researcher or academic trainer who advises students or employees in independent research

---

Annotations

3.18.1 Davies, J. (1996) Degrees of no liaison. *Times Higher Education Supplement*, 23 February, 1216 Research opportunities, xxxiv

Discusses the role of a PhD supervisor and reports the considerable variation which exists in British universities, with some students receiving ample help while others are abandoned.

3.18.2 Davis, L.L. & Grant, J.S. (1993) Guidelines for using psychometric consultants in nursing studies. *Research in Nursing and Health*, 16 (20) 151–5 16 References

The role of the psychometrician as research consultant is discussed and the questions that are commonly asked are identified. The consultation process when selecting, revising and developing data collection instruments is explored.

3.18.3 Delamont, S., Atkinson, P. & Parry, O. (1997) *Supervising the PhD: a Guide to Success.* Buckingham: Open University Press. ISBN 0335195164 References

Provides 'everything you wanted to know about PhD supervision but were afraid to ask'. Book is written to assist both the novice and experienced supervisors.

3.18.4 Gordon, F. & Wimpenny, P. (1997) Sex, gender and research supervision in nursing. *Nurse Researcher*, 4 (4) 63–77 43 References

Authors assert that patriarchal influences continue to pervade all aspects of life, including that of research supervision. Supervision relationships, research methods and nursing knowledge and supervision from a gender perspective are all discussed.

3.18.5 Holloway, I.M. (1995) Supervising nursing research projects: the case of qualitative research. *Nurse Education Today*, 15 (4) 257–62 26 References

Discusses the practical aspects of being a supervisor and student when undertaking qualitative research.

3.18.6 Jackson, N.E. (1982) Choosing and using a statistical consultant. *Nursing Research*, 31 (4) 248–50

Article gives advice about the preparation needed prior to consulting a statistician, and how to choose and communicate with one. The role of consultants is given, as is their contribution to the production of the final study.

3.18.7 Jacobi, M.C. (1991) Mentoring and undergraduate academic success: a literature review. *Review of Education Research*, 61 (4) 505–32 102 References

Provides a critical review of the mainly North American literature on mentoring from 1963 to 1991. Some definitions are given, together with sections on mentoring and undergraduate success and theoretical models of mentoring in higher education. Author lists specific questions for further investigation (CR 2.12).

3.18.8 Lurie, W. (1991) The impertinent question: the scientists' guide to the statistical mind, in Miller, D.C. (ed.), *Handbook of Research Design and Social Measurement* 5th edition. Newbury Park, CA: Sage. ISBN 0803942192 Part 5.1, 234–8 1 Reference

Section aims to sharpen the researchers' awareness of the dimensions of their hypotheses. Questions are posed which will enable statisticians to assist in this procedure (CR 2.20, 2.54.14).

3.18.9 Maggs, C. (1994) Mentorship in nursing and midwifery education: issues for research. *Nurse Education Today*, 14 (1) 22–9 81 references

Paper aims to begin to construct a research agenda for mentorship, free of statutory and regulatory constraints, about meaning and practice, as there has been no real critical appraisal of the literature to provide a research base.

3.18.10 Parsloe, P. (1993) Supervising students for higher degrees by research in a social work department. *Journal of Further and Higher Education*, 17 (3) 49–60 4 References

Examines the process of supervision from the supervisor's point of view. Areas discussed are the aims of supervision, the differences between research degrees, motives for doing a higher degree, choice of topic, getting started, processes of work and supervision, moods and stages and why be a supervisor.

3.18.11 Sheehan J. (1993) Issues in the supervision of post-graduate research students in nursing. *Journal of Advanced Nursing*, 18 (6) 880–5 26 References

Author makes some general points about post-graduate research degrees and then sets them within the nursing and social science contexts. The expectations of doctoral students, how they can be appropriately matched with supervisors, and the processes of mentoring are all discussed (CR 3.17).

3.18.12 Snowball, J., Ross, K. & Murphy, K. (1994) Illuminating dissertation supervision through reflection. *Journal of Advanced Nursing*, 19 (6) 1234–40 17 References

Describes a small study which explored the role of the dissertation supervisor, and examined the potential of using reflection as a tool for learning and enhancing professional practice.

3.19 STUDENT GUIDES TO RESEARCH

Books in this section will guide students through the various stages of doing and writing about research.

Annotations

3.19.1 Allan, G. & Skinner, C. (eds) (1991) *Handbook for Research Students in the Social Sciences*. London: Falmer Press. ISBN 1850009368 References

Discusses the nature of research degrees, study skills, management of research and research strategies in the social sciences (CR 3.17).

3.19.2 Allison, B. (1997) *The Students' Guide to Preparing Dissertations and Theses.* London: Kogan Page. ISBN 0749421932 References

Book is a detailed guide to all aspects of preparing dissertations and theses, and covers contents, presentation and style.

3.19.3 Barnes, R. (1996) *Successful Study for Degrees* 2nd edition. London: Routledge. ISBN 0415127416 References

Book gives advice on many elements required for undergraduate and post-graduate study. Sections cover study skills, developing higher-order questioning, reading academic texts, essays, seminars, dissertations, reliability, validity and meaning (CR 2.24, 2.25).

3.19.4 Bell, J. (1993) *Doing Your Research Project: a Guide for First-time Researchers in Education and Social Science* 2nd edition. Buckingham: Open University Press ISBN 0335190944 References

Book is a source of reference and guide to good practice for all novice researchers. In this new edition material has been substantially adapted and new chapters have been included.

3.19.5 Berry, R. (1994) *The Research Project: How To Write It* 3rd edition. London: Routledge. ISBN 0415110904 References

A guide for students just starting project work and those who are more experienced. Topics include choosing a subject, using the library, taking notes, and shaping and composing the project (CR 1.1).

3.19.6 Cryer, P. (1996) *The Research Student's Guide to Success.* Buckingham: Open University Press. ISBN 033519611X References

Book for post-graduate students working for research degrees in institutes of higher education. It identifies skills and strategies, gives practical advice and support, and discusses the pleasures and difficulties of doing research (CR 3.17).

3.19.7 Fairbairn, G.J. & Winch, C. (1991) *Reading, Writing and Reasoning: a Guide for Students.* Buckingham: Society for Research into Higher Education and Open University Press. ISBN 0335095968 References

Book is in three parts and covers reading, writing and talking, writing as a student and developing coherent trains of thought (CR 2.97, 2.100).

3.19.8 Higgins, R. (1996) *Approaches to Research: a Handbook for Those Writing Dissertations.* London: Jessica Kingsley Publisher. ISBN 1853023078 References

Takes a step-by-step approach to what is involved in choosing, organizing and presenting a research project.

3.19.9 Madsen, D. (1992) *Successful Dissertations and Theses: a Guide to Graduate Student Research from Proposal to Completion* 2nd edition. San Francisco: Jossey-Bass. ISBN 0783725507 References

Book gives practical advice on all aspects of writing dissertations and theses. This includes starting and completing the work, working with one's advisers, selecting the topic, preparing the proposal, following research procedures, organizing and writing the work, defending it, adapting it for publication and using the library. Two sample proposals are included, one using an historical approach and the other an experimental approach (CR 2.96, 3.18).

3.19.10 Mason, C. & McKenna, H. (1995) How to survive a PhD. *Nurse Researcher,* 2 (3) 73–9 18 References

Gives advice to those wishing to undertake PhD studies.

3.19.11 Phillips, E.M. & Pugh, D.S. (1994) *How To Get a PhD: a Handbook for Students and their Supervisors* 2nd edition. Buckingham: Open University Press. ISBN 0335192149 References

This practical text provides a realistic understanding of the process of doing research for a doctoral degree. Its main aim is to help students to understand and achieve the necessary skills, and to assist supervisors in planning and executing appropriate research programmes (CR 3.18).

3.19.12 Rudestam, K.E. & Newton, R.R. (1992) *Surviving Your Dissertation: a Comprehensive Guide to Content and Process.* Newbury Park, CA: Sage. ISBN 0803945620 References

Book is intended as a 'how to' guide for graduate students at all stages of their research. Described as a handbook, most elements relating to planning, completing and writing up projects are included.

3.19.13 Sharp, J.A. & Howard, K. (1996) *The Management of a Student Research Project* 2nd edition. Aldershot: Gower. ISBN 055607706X   References

Intended for students writing up and presenting the results of a research project. A step-by-step guide is given to all stages, with research methods and tools also being discussed.

3.19.14 Smith, R.V. (1990) *Graduate Research: a Guide for Students in the Sciences* 2nd edition. New York: Plenum Press. ISBN 0306434652   References

This workbook is designed for self-instruction by students in a wide variety of disciplines. Chapters cover the whole process of undertaking research and include: getting started, commitment, making choices, time management, ethics, developing library and writing skills, presenting papers, obtaining funds and getting a job.

RESEARCH PRIORITIES

3.20 RESEARCH PRIORITIES

There have been many studies which aimed to establish priorities for nursing research in clinical practice and nurse education. Some of those reported here have been undertaken comparatively recently, so there may be a considerable time lag before they are described in the literature.

Annotations

3.20.1 Adams, T. (1996) Informal family caregiving to older people with dementia: research priorities for community psychiatric nursing. *Journal of Advanced Nursing*, 24 (4) 703–10   97 References

Paper reviews the literature on the provision of community psychiatric nursing to demented elderly people and their informal family care-givers. Priorities for nursing care and research are also identified. The article places in context the present policy of refocusing psychiatric nursing on to people with serious and enduring mental disorders, but the author believes it should also include elderly, demented people and not just younger people with functional mental disorders (CR 2.12, 3.11).

3.20.2 Anonymous. (1997) *Child Health Services: Building a Research Agenda.* Report to the Committee on Appropriations US House of Representatives. Washington, DC: US Department of Health and Human Services Publications. Public Health Service AHCPR 97–RO55 April

The US House of Representatives Appropriation Committee gave guidance to the Agency for Health Care Policy and Research (AHCPR) on developing a research agenda for children on health care effectiveness, quality and outcome measures. This report describes the activities which ensued.

3.20.3 Bell, P.F., Daly, J. & Chang, E.M.L. (1997) A study of the educational and research priorities of registered nurses in rural Australia. *Journal of Advanced Nursing*, 25 (4) 794–800   21 References

The Delphi technique was used to identify the educational and research priorities of nurses working in rural Australia. Thirteen were given a high priority and study provided useful information about the needs for education and research (CR 2.66).

3.20.4 Broome, M.E., Woodring, B. & O'Connor-Von, S. (1996) Research priorities for the nursing of children and their families: a Delphi study. *Journal of Pediatric Nursing: Nursing Care of Children and Families*, 11(5) 281–7   25 References

Authors state that there has been no systematic identification of critical areas of inquiry needed to provide quality paediatric care in the next decade. A three-round Delphi study was set up to establish from paediatric nurse experts where priorities lay and these are reported (CR 2.66).

3.20.5 Butterworth, T. (1991) Generating research in mental nursing. *International Journal of Nursing Studies*, 28 (3) 237–46   40 References

Paper explores research priorities for mental health nursing in the UK. Areas identified include historical research, policy-related research, and the role of the mental health nurse as a provider of a therapeutic milieu, as therapist and teacher. Ways of promoting mental health research are outlined. The author stresses that valuable archival data must not be lost with the closure of psychiatric hospitals (CR 2.76).

3.20.6   Cronin, S.N. & Owsley, V.B. (1993) Identifying nursing research priorities in an acute care hospital. *Journal of Nursing Administration*, 23 (11) 58–62   16 References

Using the Delphi technique, data were obtained from a panel of nurses and a prioritized list was obtained after three rounds. The study motivated and guided research efforts, stimulated formation of research interest groups and attracted local researchers (CR 2.66).

3.20.7   Daly, J., Chang, E.M.L. & Bell, P.F. (1996) Clinical nursing research priorities in Australian critical care: a pilot study. *Journal of Advanced Nursing*, 23 (1) 145–51   19 References

Project aimed to identify areas for improving patient care and to inform nursing research policy to develop priorities with relevance to patients' needs. The Delphi technique was used to obtain information from clinical nurse specialists. Nine high-priority areas were identified (CR 2.23, 2.66, 3.11).

3.20.8   Fitch, M.I. (1996) Creating a research agenda with relevance to cancer nursing practice. *Cancer Nursing*, 19 (5) 335–42   23 References

Article describes the process used by one nursing department to identify significant clinical questions to create a research agenda. These were ascertained from the literature and interviewing all nursing staff, and results are reported (CR 2.68, 2.88).

3.20.9   Forrest, J.L., Lyons, K.J., Bross, T.M., Gitlin, L.N.& Kraemer, L.G. (1995) Reaching consensus on the national dental hygiene research agenda: a Delphi study. *Journal of Dental Hygiene*, 69 (6) 261–9   46 References

Using the Delphi technique, this study aimed to achieve consensus about research priorities for dental hygiene research consistent with the national agenda. Thirty-seven out of 66 topics that were identified were consistent with this agenda and showed just the first stage in long-term development plans to guide research efforts and promote the body of knowledge (CR 2.66).

3.20.10   Forte, P.S., Ritz, L.J. & Balestracci, D. Jr. (1997) Identifying nursing research priorities in a newly merged health care system. *Journal of Nursing Administration*, 27 (6) 51–5   11 References

Reports a Delphi study which identified two final topics centred on nursing administration research. The data served many purposes, including increased organizational awareness of nursing research and development of a nursing research council to facilitate future activities (CR 2.66).

3.20.11   Grady, P.A., Harden, J.T., Moritz, P. & Amende, L.M. (1997) Incorporating environmental sciences and nursing research: an NINR initiative. *Nursing Outlook*, 45 (2) 73–5   3 References

Reports the deliberations of a working group set up by the National Institute of Nursing Research to identify environmental health science research gaps, opportunities and challenges. Areas discussed were target populations, target areas for clinical studies, research infrastructure needs and promising areas for nursing research (CR 3.10, 3.13).

3.20.12   Hirschfeld, M.J. (1998) WHO priorities for a common research agenda. *International Nursing Review*, 45 (1) 13–14   2 References

Reports on the World Health Organization Nursing Unit's analysis of research at nursing/midwifery collaborating centres and suggests future foci for nursing projects (CR 2.15).

3.20.13   Jennings, B.M. (1995) Nursing research: a time for redirection. *Journal of Nursing Administration*, 25 (4) 9–11   29 References

Briefly outlines the history of nursing research in the USA and suggests that its focus has been too narrow. Author urges researchers to integrate clinical and administrative frameworks as one cannot do without the other (CR 3.5).

3.20.14   Kitson, A., McMahon, A., Rafferty, A.M. & Scott, E. (1997) High priority . . . setting priorities to raise the profile of nursing research. *Nursing Times*, 15–21 October, 93 (42) 26, 28–30   14 References

Authors examine a national research and

development priority-setting exercise to influence nursing practice.

3.20.15 Leibenluft, E. (1994) A research agenda for women's health. *Journal of Women's Health,* 3 (5) 377–82   26 References

Article gives areas where research on women's psychiatric problems have been adequately represented. It also identifies some which have received little attention, for example, substance abuse disorders, alcoholism and the psychiatric effects of the menopause in depressed women.

3.20.16 Lynn, M.R. & Cobb, B.K. (1994) Changes in nursing administration research priorities: a sign of the times. *Journal of Nursing Administration,* 24 (4S) 12–18   17 References

Describes the development of research priorities for nursing administrators based on the Healthy People 2000 Report. For comparative purposes, an overview of previous priorities is also included.

3.20.17 Lynn, M.R. & Layman, E. (1996) Research priorities: the nature of nursing administration research: knowledge building or fire stomping? *Journal of Nursing Administration,* 26 (5) 9–14   11 References

Reports on previous literature reviews on the state of nursing administration research. The themes, frameworks and methods used are discussed and the impact of research priorities on published research, targeted and cumulative research programmes are highlighted.

3.20.18 National Institute of Nursing Research, National Institutes of Health. (1993) *National Nursing Research Agenda: Setting Nursing Research Priorities.* Bethesda, MD: National Institute of Nursing Research. URL: http: //www.nih.gov/ninr/

Outlines the research priorities set out by the National Institute of Nursing Research for phases one and two.

3.20.19 Schmidt, K., Montgomery, L.A., Bruene, D. & Kenney, M. (1997) Determining research priorities in pediatric nursing: a Delphi study. *Journal of Pediatric Nursing: Nursing Care of Children and Families,* 12 (4) 201–7   12 References

Describes the results of a Delphi study which

identified 45 separate topics/themes of interest. In the second round, participants were asked to choose their top five and these are discussed (CR 2.66).

3.20.20 Sleep, J., Bullock, I. & Grayson, K. (1995) Establishing priorities for research in education within one college of nursing and midwifery. *Nurse Education Today,* 15 (6) 439–45   26 References

Many recent major changes in nurse education remain largely unevaluated. This article reports a four-round Delphi survey designed to set an agenda for research priorities within one college of nursing and midwifery. Twenty-eight items were prioritized, the top ten primarily focused on the pre-registration provision, encompassing preparation of students for professional practice and the changing role of the nurse/midwife teacher. Paper explores the implications of these findings for setting a research agenda within the organization (CR 2.66).

3.20.21 Sleep, J., Renfrew, M.J., Bowler, U., Dunn, A. & Garcia, J. (1995) Establishing priorities for research in midwifery within the UK: report of a Delphi survey of midwives' and students' views. *British Journal of Midwifery,* 3 (6) 323–31   46 References

Reports a three-round Delphi survey designed to inform a research agenda reflecting the issues of current concern within maternity services (CR 2.66).

3.20.22 Wilson-Barnett, J. (1996) Research directions in palliative care nursing. *International Journal of Palliative Nursing,* 2 (1) 5–6   7 References   Editorial

Outlines some of the areas which have been examined in palliative care, the personnel involved and the methods which have and could be used. Some areas for future research are identified.

3.20.23 Woledge, R. (1995) Physiotherapy research: finding out how it works. *British Journal of Therapy and Rehabilitation,* 2 (9) 461–2   No references   Editorial

Discusses the types of research which would be appropriate in physiotherapy.

3.20.24 Woods, N.F. (1994) The United States women's health research agenda analysis and critique. *Western Journal of Nursing Research*, 16 (5) 467–79   14 References

Describes the process used to develop a US women's health research agenda and its published critiques. Questions about the process and products of feminist research methods are discussed (CR 2.10).

3.20.25 Woods, N.F. (1995) Cancer research: future agendas for women's health. *Seminars in Oncology Nursing*, 11 (2) 143–7   9 References

Reviews the national research priorities for women's health and focuses on future work needed.

3.20.26 Yeaworth, R.C. (1997) Ethics and research priorities in academic administration. *Journal of Professional Nursing*, 13 (2) 69–75   8 References

Article discusses the micro and macro levels involved in the restructuring of health care, the downsizing of educational programmes, the strategic plans of particular institutions and granting agencies, and the effects these can have on research. The ethical aspects of these changes are considered (CR 2.17).

RESEARCH REVIEWS

3.21 RESEARCH REVIEWS

Books in this section give examples of research in practice which aim to help nurses understand its value when caring for patients and clients.

Annotations

3.21.1 Alexander, J., Levy, V. & Roch, S. (eds) (1993) *Midwifery Practice: a Research-based Approach*. Basingstoke: Macmillan. ISBN 0333576179 References

Provides a broad-ranging survey and analysis of key research literature placed in the context of clinical practice.

3.21.2 Ford, P. & Walsh, M. (1994) *New Rituals for Old: Nursing through the Looking Glass*. Oxford: Butterworth-Heinemann. ISBN 0750615818 References

Some accepted concepts in nursing are subjected to rigorous scrutiny, and selected research findings are analysed to open them up to debate. Authors believe that critical questioning will enable a sound knowledge base to be developed. Areas covered are concepts of empowerment and delivery of care.

3.21.3 Macleod Clark, J. & Hockey, L. (1979) *Research for Nursing: a Guide for the Enquiring Nurse*. Aylesbury, Buckinghamshire: HM+M Publishers. ISBN 085602077X References

Book is divided into four major sections. The first two parts comprise understanding research in which the basic research approach is outlined and an overview of design and methods given. Subsequent parts analyse studies relating to patient care and those relating to nurses, nursing management and education. Each study is examined under the following headings: main research question(s); research design and method; findings and implications. The final section briefly examines training for research, career possibilities, resources, and research as a change agent.

3.21.4 Macleod Clark, J. & Hockey, L. (eds) (1989) *Further Research for Nursing*. London: Scutari. ISBN 1871364140 References

A companion volume to *Research for Nursing: a Guide for the Enquiring Nurse*, which aims to help nurses understand the value of research in their practice. A general introduction to research is given, together with its relevance to nursing and an overview of research processes. The remainder of the book contains overviews of research in 12 topic areas. Each is illustrated by a précis of one or two specific studies. Several chapters are devoted to studies about specific patient groups and others to more general nursing issues.

3.21.5 Walsh, M. & Ford, P. (1990) *Nursing Rituals, Research and Rational Actions*. Oxford: Butterworth-Heinemann. ISBN 0750600977 References

Book highlights key areas of nursing practice where research evidence is available, but in many instances is not being used. Rituals of clinical practice and organization are explored, and recommendations for good practice are given.

3.21.6 Wilson-Barnett, J. & Batehup, L. (1988) *Patient Problems: a Research Base for Nursing Care*. London: Scutari Press. ISBN 1871364108 References

Book reviews research relating to some of the major challenges in patient care: problems with adjustment to illness and recovery, depression, communication problems, pain and sleep disturbance. Authors' aim has been to describe research which assists in providing assessment tools, to explore patients' responses to health problems and evaluate interventions aimed to solve them. Authors hope that similar books will be developed as the body of research knowledge increases (CR 2.12, 2.20, 2.55, 3.20).

INTERNATIONAL NURSING RESEARCH

3.22 INTERNATIONAL NURSING RESEARCH

'Individual research projects that are disconnected and scattered around the world may not have the necessary impact. The collaboration of a community of researchers, organized to explore and answer a set of related questions and considered from different socio-political and cultural perspectives, could empower nurses to make a difference in the health and health care of those who need it most.' (Meleis, 1989: 138) [adapted]

Example

Brooten, D., Thompson, J., Makoza, J., Kaponda, C., Mede, E., Kachapila, L. & Phoya, A. (1997) Collaborating for international research development in Malawi, Africa. *Image: Journal of Nursing Scholarship*, 29 (4) 369–73   11 References

Paper describes a collaborative research project by nurses from American and African schools of nursing, together with the Malawian Ministry of Health. Its aim was to give assistance to women leaders in Malawi for developing and conducting research to improve the health of mothers and babies in villages. The organization of this five-year project is described, together with its results and conclusions (CR 2.15).

Annotations

3.22.1 Bergman, R. (ed.) (1990) *Nursing Research for Nursing Practice: an International Perspective.* London: Chapman & Hall. ISBN 041233500X   References

Book includes contributions from researchers around the world. Each chapter gives a brief description of their major health care system, problems which have been encountered, the scope and development of nursing research and research on a selected topic. Chapter 1 discusses the role of international organizations in nursing research (CR 3.1, 3.3, 3.5, 3.20).

3.22.2 Degner, L.F. & McWilliams, M.E. (1994) Challenges in cross-national nursing research, in Fitzpatrick, J.J., Stevenson, J.S. & Polis, N.S. (eds), *Nursing Research and its Utilization.* New York: Springer. ISBN 0826180906 Chapter 21, 211–15 6 References

Chapter describes the practical issues involved in mounting a cross-national project in three countries – Canada, the UK and Sweden (CR 2.102.17).

3.22.3 Dier, K.A. (1988) International nursing: the global approach. *Recent Advances in Nursing*, 20 39–60 55 References

Examines the development of international nursing research from the Second World War up to the present, with particular attention being given to Third World countries. The evolution, global and country perspectives, social structure, cultural and health care values and a taxonomy of health care systems are all discussed. The functions of health personnel and the scope of international nursing are explored.

3.22.4 Henry, B.M. & Nagelkerk, J.M. (1992) International nursing research, in Fitzpatrick, J.J., Taunton, R.L. & Jacox, A.K. (eds), *Annual Review of Nursing Research* Volume 10. New York: Springer. ISBN 0826143598 Part 3, Chapter 11, 207–30 135 References

Chapter discusses the significance of international nursing research. Research published in journals from 1985 to 1989 was examined and 461 reports were identified under the headings of clinical, nurse education and nursing administrative research (CR 2.12).

3.22.5 International Council of Nurses, Council of National Representatives. (1993) Resolutions approved. *International Nursing Review*, 40 (5) 152   2 References

This resolution, one of 14 approved at a meeting held in Madrid, outlines the need for developments in training for nursing research and the dissemination of findings. National Nursing Associations are urged to collaborate, communicate and exchange findings, discuss experiences of utilization and initiate the development of joint activities (CR 2.98, 3.17).

3.22.6 Manfredi, M., Ailinger, R.L. & Collado, C. (1990) The process, benefits and costs of conducting multi-national nursing research. *International Journal of Nursing Studies*, 27 (4) 325–32   6 References

Discusses the process, benefits and costs of conducting a six-country research study on nursing practice in Latin America. The political, economic and professional outcomes are examined and suggestions are offered for further multi-national studies (CR 3.1).

3.22.7 Meleis, A.I. (1989) International research: a need or a luxury? *Nursing Outlook*, 37 (3) 138–42   13 References

Author urges the development of cross-national, collaborative studies in order to further nursing science. The policies that are required and personal considerations are discussed, global priorities and strategies for achieving these goals are given (CR 2.15).

3.22.8 Modly, D., Fitzpatrick, J.J., Poletti, P. & Zanotti, R. (1995) *Advancing Nursing Education Worldwide*. New York: Springer. ISBN 0826186505   References

Nurse leaders from 12 countries examine issues of significance to nurse educators around the world. The purpose of the book is to describe global trends in nurse education, share innovative approaches to it, report and develop cross-cultural and collaborative research and provide a model for future international collaborations (CR 2.15, 2.53).

3.22.9 National Center for Nursing Research and International Council of Nurses.

(1990) *Nursing Research Worldwide: Current Dimensions and Future Directions*. Bethesda, MD: National Center for Nursing Research/Geneva, Switzerland: International Council of Nurses. No ISBN   References

Book includes reports from the meeting in Geneva which aimed to review the current status of nursing research, identify research priorities, plan the development of an international agenda and make recommendations on how the National Center for Nursing Research (NCNR) and the International Council of Nurses (ICN) could each foster further development. Background papers from nine countries are included which document the current position and identify future directions. Several papers from ICN are included together with a NCNR brochure (CR 3.1, 3.4, 3.5).

3.22.10 Oyen, E. (ed.) (1990) *Comparative Methodology: Theory and Practice in International Social Research*. Newbury Park, CA: Sage. ISBN 0803983263   References

An international team of researchers explore the problems associated with the design and conduct of cross-national studies. Serious theoretical and methodological difficulties are still encountered and authors give examples of how these were overcome.

3.22.11 Skeet, M. (1987) Internationalisation of nursing, in Hockey, L. (ed.), *Current Issues (Recent Advances in Nursing 18, 109–28)* Edinburgh: Churchill Livingstone. ISBN 0443032807   13 References

Discusses internationalism, why nursing has become internationally minded and its activities in clinical practice, management and education. The work of the International Council of Nurses, the Red Cross and other groups of nurses are explored, together with the role of the individual nurse.

3.22.12 Stinson, S.M. & Kerr, J.C. (eds) (1986) *International Issues in Nursing Research*. Beckenham: Croom Helm. ISBN 0709944373   References

Book presents a review of specific international themes in nursing research. It includes methodological issues, policy and funding, preparation for nursing research, publication issues and the role of professional associations. Contributors are leading authorities in the UK, the USA and Canada (CR 2.99, 3.11, 3.13, 3.14).

INTER-DISCIPLINARY RESEARCH

3.23   INTER-DISCIPLINARY RESEARCH

Inter-disciplinary research can provide all health care professionals with opportunities to examine some of the complex issues involved in practice. Different perspectives on problems can give valuable insights which it may then be possible to translate into patient care.

Definitions

Cross-disciplinary research – task requires a combination of disciplines for its achievement
Multi- and inter-disciplinary research – organizational form used to carry out cross-disciplinary research

---

Annotations

3.23.1 Barratt, E. (1990) Doctors' response to nursing studies. *Nursing*, 12 April, 4(8) 23–4
8 References

Explores reasons why doctors may not always be supportive of nursing research and the author suggests that the professions often approach methodologies from different ends of the spectrum. The research/practice gap also exists in medicine and there are failures of communication where the roles of each group differ in approach and in their outlook towards care (CR 2.9, 3.8).

3.23.2   Bartunek, J.M. & Louis, M.R. (1996) *Insider/Outsider Team Research*. Thousand Oaks, CA: Sage. ISBN 0803971591 References

Discusses the recent growth of research partnerships and identifies problems that occur at various stages of team research (CR 2.14).

3.23.3 Epton, S.R., Payne, R.L. & Pearson, A.W. (eds) (1983) *Managing Inter-disciplinary Research*. Chichester: Wiley. ISBN 0471903175 References [2nd International Conference on the Management of Interdisciplinary Research held at Manchester Business School, UK, July 1981]

Book contains chapters on nomenclature, where this type of research may provide the best approach to solving problems, consideration of institutional and personal barriers and extracting lessons for management. Editors suggest that it should not be read as a formal record of proceedings, but rather capture the main themes and illustrate the variety of activity taking place. Also reported are the deliberations of the 1st Inter-disciplinary Research Management Conference held in Schloss Reisenburg in the Federal Republic of Germany, 22–28 April 1979.

3.23.4   Gueldner, S.H. & Stroud, S.D. (1996) Sharing the quest for knowledge through interdisciplinary research. *Holistic Nursing Practice*, 10 (3) 54–62   33 References

Article traces nurses' 20-year struggle to become a credible partner in interdisciplinary research and highlights the advantages and challenges characteristic in such collaboration. The authors describe their respective experiences as members of such teams, one in private practice and the other in an academic setting. Recommendations that nurture successful collaborations are proposed (CR 2.15).

3.23.5   Lorentzon, M. (1995) Multidisciplinary collaboration: life line or drowning pool for nurse researchers? *Journal of*

Advanced Nursing, 22 (5) 825–6 5 References Guest Editorial

Discusses the place of multi-disciplinary research in health care and the role of nursing within this. A balance between quantitative and qualitative methods is suggested and nurses are urged to take their place within this context (CR 2.15, 3.7).

3.23.6 Merwin, E. (1995) Building interdisciplinary mental health services research teams: a case example. *Issues in Mental Health Nursing*, 16 (6) 547–54 8 References

Reports a paper presented at the October 1994 Pre-Conference Mental Health Methods Workshop, sponsored by the National Institute of Mental Health at the American Public Health Association Annual Convention. The experience of building a team, creating roles, developing working relationships and the evolution of projects are all discussed. Suggestions are made within the context of proposal development, successful funding and implementation of a research study.

3.23.7 Rolley, F., Humphreys, J.S., Grogan, H., Hegney, D., Knight, S., Nichols, A. & Veitch, C. (1996) Fostering multi-disciplinary research and approaches to rural health issues: the concept of an international summer institute. *Australian Journal of Rural Health*, 4 (2) 80–8 8 References

Article outlines an Australian perspective on the rationale for, background to, and structure of an International Summer Institute, sponsored by the Social Science and Humanities Research Council of Canada for practitioners and researchers. Evaluation showed it to be one option for promoting multi-disciplinary approaches to rural health research.

REFERENCES

References recorded here relate to books and articles consulted during the development of this book. Page numbers of quotations are included in the main text. Numbers noted here refer to pages in the source texts listed in Appendix D – Sources of Definitions (pages 353 to 361).

Abdellah, F.G. & Levine, E. (1994) *Preparing Nursing Research for the 21st Century: Evolution, Methodologies, Challenges.* New York: Springer pp. 25, 67, 76, 157, 392

Apps, J. & Yeomans, M. (1995) Ethical issues in nursing research in Henry, K. & Pashley, G. (eds) *Community Ethics and Health Care Research.* Dinton, Nr Salisbury: Mark Allen

Bernard, J. (1973) My four revolutions: an autobiographical history of the American Sociological Association. *American Journal of Sociology* 78: p. 782

Breakwell, G.M., Hammond, S. & Fife-Schaw, C. (1995) *Research Methods in Psychology.* London: Sage

Brink, P.J. (1976) *Transcultural Nursing: a Book of Readings.* Englewood Cliffs, NJ: Prentice Hall pp. 1–5

Brown, S.R. (1996) Q methodology and qualitative research. *Qualitative Health Research* 6 (4)

Bryman, A. (1988) *Quantity and Quality in Social Research.* London: Unwin Hyman p. 94

Burns, N. & Grove, S.K. (1997) *The Practice of Nursing Research: Conduct, Critique and Utilization.* Philadelphia: W.B. Saunders pp. 569–611

Centre for Advanced Research in Phenomenology (1997)

URL: http://www.connect.net/ron/phenom.html

Commission on Research Integrity (1995) *Integrity and Misconduct in Research.* Washington, DC: US Department of Health and Human Services

Crane, J. (1995) The future of research utilization in Titler, M.G. & Goode, C.J. (eds) *The Nursing Clinics of North America: Research Utilization.* 30 (3) Philadelphia: W.B. Saunders

Cresswell, J.W. (1998) *Qualitative Inquiry and Research Design: Choosing Among Five Traditions.* Thousand Oaks, CA: Sage

Denzin, N.K. (1989) *The Research Act: a Theoretical Introduction to Sociological Methods.* 3rd edition Englewood Cliffs, NJ: Prentice Hall p. 269

Denzin, N.K. & Lincoln, Y.S. (eds) (1994) *Handbook of Qualitative Research.* Thousand Oaks, CA: Sage

Dickson, R. (1996) Dissemination and implementation: the wider picture. *Nurse Researcher* 4 (1)

Dictionary of Nursing Theory and Research 2nd edition (1995) Edited by Powers, B.A. & Knapp, T.R. Thousand Oaks, CA: Sage pp. 4, 12, 17, 20, 41, 49, 50, 51, 61, 64, 65, 69, 79–80, 89, 94, 102, 114, 130, 131, 157, 158, 164, 170

Dictionary of Social Science Methods (1983) Edited by Miller, P.McC. & Wilson, M.J. Chichester: John Wiley pp. 1–4, 21, 23, 30, 34, 62, 72, 88, 91, 92, 94, 96, 97, 102, 105, 112, 119

Dictionary of Statistics and Methodology: a Non-technical Guide for the Social Sciences (1993) Edited by Vogt, W.P. Newbury Park, CA: Sage ISBN 0803952775 pp. 59, 61, 89

Field, P.A. & Morse, J. M. (1985) *Nursing Research: the Application of Qualitative Approaches.* Rockville, MD: Aspen p. 85

Flanagan, J.C. (1947) *The Aviation Psychology Program in the Army Air Forces.* AAF Psychology Program Research Report No. 1 Washington, DC: Government Printing Office

Flanagan, J.C. (1954) The Critical Incident Technique. *Psychological Bulletin* 51 (4) pp. 327–58

Fox, D. (1982) *Fundamentals of Research in Nursing* 4th edition. Norwalk, CT: Appleton-Century-Crofts

Goodall, C.J. (1994) Writing and research: an introduction. *Nurse Researcher* 2 (1)

Hck, G., Judd, M. & Moule, P. (1996) *Making Sense of Research: an Introduction for Nurses.* London: Cassell

Holm, K. & Llewellyn, J.G. (1986) *Nursing Research for Nursing Practice.* Philadelphia: W.B. Saunders pp. 262, 270, 271, 274

Krippendorf, K. (1980) *Content Analysis: an Introduction to its Methodology.* Thousand Oaks, CA: Sage

Leininger, M.M. (1985) *Qualitative Research Methods in Nursing.* Orlando, FL: Grune & Stratton pp. 35, 38, 68, 69, 237

Leininger, M.M. (1987) Importance and uses of ethnomethods: ethnography and ethnonursing research. *Recent Advances in Nursing* p. 17

Lexicon of Psychology, Psychiatry and Psychoanalysis (1988) Edited by Kuper, L. London: Routledge p. 298

Lindlof, T.R. (1995) *Qualitative Communication Research Methods.* Thousand Oaks, CA: Sage p. 40

Linstone H.A. & Turoff, M. (eds) (1975) *The Delphi Method: Techniques and Applications.* Reading, MA: Addison-Wesley

Lomas, J. (1994) Diffusion, dissemination and implementation: who should do what? *Annals of the New York Academy of Sciences* New York: New York Academy of Sciences pp. 226–37

Mackenzie, J., Husband, C. & Gerrish, K. (1995) Researching in collaboration: a guide to successful partnerships. *Nurse Researcher* 3 (1)

Medical Research Council of Canada (1987) *Guidelines on Research Involving Human Subjects.* Ottawa: Supplies and Services, Canada p. 26

Meleis, A.I. (1989) International research: a need or a luxury? *Nursing Outlook* 37 (3)

New International Webster's Comprehensive Dictionary of the English Language (1996) Naples, FL: Trident Press International pp. 257, 591, 599, 844, 1968, 2122

Nolan, M. & Grant, C. (1993) Action research and quality of care: a mechanism for agreeing basic values as a precursor to change. *Journal of Advanced Nursing* 18 (2) pp. 305–11

Omery, A., Kasper, C.E. & Page, G.G. (eds) (1995) *In Search of Nursing Science.* Thousand Oaks, CA: Sage

Patton, M.Q. (1990) *Qualitative Evaluation and Research Methods* 2nd edition. Thousand Oaks, CA: Sage

Penguin Dictionary of Psychology (1985) Edited by Reber, A.S. Harmondsworth: Penguin p. 532

Phillips, D.C. (1987) *Philosophy, Science and Social Inquiry: Contemporary Methodological Controversies in Social Science and Related Applied Fields of Research.* Oxford: Pergamon

Phillips, L.R.F. (1986) *A Clinician's Guide to the Critique and Utilization of Nursing Research.* Norwalk, CT: Appleton-Century-Crofts pp. 149, 453, 454, 455, 456, 457, 458, 459, 462, 463, 464

Polgar, S. & Thomas, S.A. (1991) *Introduction to Research in the Health Sciences* 2nd edition. Melbourne: Churchill Livingstone p. 84

Polit, D.F. & Hungler, B.P. (1991) *Nursing Research: Principles and Methods* 4th edition. Hagerstown, MD: Lippincott p. 535

Polit, D.F. & Hungler, B.P. (1995) *Nursing Research: Principles and Methods* 5th edition. Philadelphia, PA: Lippincott pp. 635, 636, 638–9, 641, 642, 643, 644, 645, 648, 649, 650, 651, 652, 653, 656

Polit, D.F. & Hungler B.P. (1999) *Nursing Research: Principles and Methods* 6th Edition. Philadelphia PA: Lippincott p. 705

Rafferty, A.M. (1997/98) Writing, researching and reflexivity in nursing history. *Nurse Researcher* 5 (2)

Reader's Digest Universal Dictionary (1987) London: Reader's Digest Association Ltd pp. 347, 1083, 1161, 1212, 1543, 1551

Reason, P. & Rowan, J. (eds) (1981) *Human Inquiry: a Sourcebook of New Paradigm Research.* Chichester: John Wiley

Sandelowski, M. (1995) Triangles and crystals: the geometry of qualitative research. *Research in Nursing and Health* 18 (6)

Sandelowski, M., Docherty, S. & Emden, C. (1997) Qualitative metasynthesis: issues and techniques. *Research in Nursing and Health* 20 (4) pp. 365–6

Seaman, C.H. (1987) *Research Methods: Principles, Practice and Theory for Nursing* 3rd edition. Norwalk, CT: Appleton & Lange p. 433, 434

Treece, E.W. & Treece, J.W. Jr. (1986) *Elements of Research in Nursing* 4th edition. St Louis: Mosby pp 178–181, 318, 510

Wakefield, J.C. (1995) When an irresistible epistemology meets an immovable ontology. *Social Work Research* 19 (1)

Waltz, C.F., Strickland, O.L. & Lenz, E.R. (1984) *Measurement in Nursing Research.* Philadelphia, PA: Davis

Williamson, Y.M. (ed.) (1981) *Research Methodology and its Application to Nursing Research.* New York: John Wiley pp. 171, 172, 416, 417, 418, 419, 423, 424

Wilson, S.L. (1995) Single-case experimental designs, in Breakwell, G. M., Hammond, S. & Fife-Schaw, C. (1995) *Research Methods in Psychology.* London: Sage pp. 69–70

Woods, N.F. & Catanzaro, M. (1988) *Nursing Research: Theory and Practice.* St Louis: Mosby pp. 555, 558, 560, 562, 563, 564

Yin, R.K. (1984) *Case Study Research: Design and Methods.* Thousand Oaks, CA: Sage

APPENDIX A: COMPUTER-BASED RESEARCH METHODOLOGY DATABASES AND PROGRAMS

ANTHROPAC 4.92

Purpose: A menu-driven DOS program for collecting and analysing data on cultural domains. Program helps collect and analyse structured qualitative and quantitative data and its tools include techniques that are unique to anthropology.

Publisher: Analytic Technologies, 104 Pond Street, Natick MA 01760, USA
URL: http://www.analytictech.com/APAC.htm

ATLAS ti

Purpose: A software package for the visual qualitative analysis of large bodies of textual, graphical and audio data. It allows coding and annotation of text, images and audio material online; ability to build theory visually; browse and edit associated codes; express and browse the narrative structure of data using hypertext links; export data using the SPSS job generator for quantitative analysis; exchange text with OLE-2 applications by dragging and dropping; create Web pages for publishing research reports via the Internet using the html generator.

Publisher: Scolari, Sage Publications Ltd, 6 Bonhill Street, London EC2A 4PU, UK
URL: http://www.sagepub.co.uk/scolari/scolari.html
[to download a free demonstration copy or obtain more information]

CODE-A-TEXT

Purpose: A flexible tool for the analysis of recorded dialogues, interview transcripts and protocols with individuals or groups. In addition to text-based data, the system also accepts sound and video output. It will also enable storage and coding of any kind of data for both qualitative and quantitative methods of analysis.

Publisher: Scolari, Sage Publications Ltd, 6 Bonhill Street, London EC2A 4PU, UK
URL: http://www.scolari.co.uk
[a free demonstration copy is available on CD-ROM]

DECISION EXPLORER

Purpose: A set of tools for managing 'soft' issues – the qualitative information that surrounds complex or uncertain situations. [Available for use on Windows PCs or Apple Macintosh.]

Publisher: Scolari, Sage Publications Ltd, 6 Bonhill Street, London EC2A 4PU, UK
URL: http://www.sagepub.co.uk

DICTION 4.0

Purpose: A scientific method for determining the tone of a verbal message using a Windows-based program that searches for a passage for five general features as well as 35 sub-features. It can process an unlimited number of texts using a 10,000-word corpus, produce reports about the texts it processes and writes the results to numeric files for later statistical analysis. [Available for use on Windows PCs only.]

Publisher: Scolari, Sage Publications Ltd, 6 Bonhill Street, London EC2A 4PU, UK
URL: http://www.sagepub.co.uk

EPI INFO

Purpose: A series of microcomputer programs for word processing, data management, and epidemiological analysis, designed for health care professionals.

Publisher: Division of Surveillance, Epidemiology and Prevention Centers for Disease Control (CDC) Atlanta, GA 30333
URL: http://www.cdc.gov/epo/epi/epiinfo.htm

ETHNOGRAPH v5.0

Purpose: Facilitates the control and analysis of text-based data such as transcripts of interviews, focus groups, field notes, diaries, meeting minutes and other documents.

Publisher: Qualis Research Associates, PO Box 2070, Amherst MA 01004 USA
URL: http://www.qualisresearch.com/
[Distributed by Sage Publications Ltd, 6 Bonhill Street, London
EC2A 4PU
URL http://www.sagepub.co.uk]

GENSTAT 5 (General Statistical Programs)

Purpose: A high-level language for data manipulation and statistical analysis. Used mainly for analysis of experimental data.

Publisher: Numerical Algorithms Group Ltd, Wilkinson House, Jordan Hill Road, Oxford OX2 8DR, UK
NAG Inc., 1400 Opus Place, Suite 200, Downess Grove, Illinois IL 60515 5702, USA

NAG GmbH, Schleissheimerstrasse 5, W–8046 Garching bei München, Germany
URL: http://www.nag.co.uk/stats/TT.html

GLIM 4 (Generalized Linear Interactive Modelling)

Purpose: Used for generalized linear modelling techniques.

Publisher: Numerical Algorithms Group Ltd, Wilkinson House, Jordan Hill Road, Oxford OX2 8DR, UK
NAG Inc., 1400 Opus Place, Suitc 200, Downess Grove, Illinois IL 60515 5702, USA
NAG GmbH, Schleissheimerstrasse 5, W–8046 Garching bei München, Germany
URL: http://www.nag.co.uk/stats/GDGE/MKT65.html

METHODOLOGISTS TOOLCHEST 2.0

Purpose: An expert system consisting of nine modules, each addressing a specific aspect of the research process. It also includes Peer Review Emulator with FirstDraft*, Statistical Navigator*, Ex-Sample*, WhichGraph, Designer Research, Data Collection Selection, Measurement and Scaling Strategist, ETHX and Hyper-Stat, and definitions of 1000 research, statistics and data graphic terms. [Available on CD-ROM for use on Windows PCs only.]
* also sold separately

Publisher: Scolari, Sage Publications Ltd, 6 Bonhill Street, London EC2A 4PU, UK
URL: http://www.sagepub.co.uk/scolari/decision.html

MINITAB 12

Purpose: A general-purpose software package for statistical analysis covering the basic range of statistical analyses and high-resolution graphics.

Publisher: MINITAB Inc., 3081 Enterprise Drive, State College, PA 16801–3008, USA
URL: http://www.minitab.com/products/minitab/index.htm

QMethod

Purpose: A statistical program tailored to the requirements of Q studies.

Publisher: Kent State University, Kent OH 44240, USA
URL: http://listserv.kent.edu/archives/q-method.html
URL: http://www.rz.unibw-muenchen.de/~p41bsmk/qmethod/ (Q method page)

QSR NUD*IST 4 (Non-numerical Unstructured Data Indexing, Searching and Theory Building)

Purpose: Provides software for the development, support and management of qualitative data analysis (QDA) projects. QDA projects involving the analysis

of unstructured data such as text from interviews, historical or legal documents, or non-textual documentary material such as videotapes. This will enable documentary material to be analysed and understood.
[Available in versions for Windows PCs or Apple Macintosh.]

Publisher: Scolari, Sage Publications Ltd, 6 Bonhill Street, London EC2A 4PU, UK
URL: http: // www.scolari.co.uk
[for information or to download a demonstration copy]

Sage Publications/SRM database of social research methodology on CD-ROM

Purpose: Database containing over 40,000 key literature references in social science methodology from books and journals.

Publisher: Scolari, Sage Publications Ltd, 6 Bonhill Street, London EC2A 4PU, UK
(available on subscription)
URL: http://www.scolari.co.uk

SAS 6.12

Purpose: Research application offers a comprehensive range of ready-to-use tools for data entry, access and analysis specifically designed to meet the needs of research specialists.

Publisher: SAS Institute Inc., Box 8000, SAS Circle, Cary NC 27511, USA
URL: http://www.sas.com

SIR 3.0 (Scientific Information Retrieval)

Purpose: Integrated, research-orientated database management system which supports hierarchical and network relationships and interfaces directly with SPSS.

Publisher: SIR (Australia) Pty Ltd., 1/10-18 Cliff Street, Point Milsons, New South Wales 2061, Australia

SIR Inc., PO Box 1404, Evanston IL 60204, USA
URL: http://www.sir.com.au/index.html

SphinxSurvey Lexica & Plus2

Purpose: This software program facilitates straightforward questionnaire design, data entry, statistical processing and analysis, content and lexical analysis and the power to analyse qualitative data collected from open-ended responses.

Publisher: Scolari, Sage Publications Ltd, 6 Bonhill Street, London EC2A 4PU, UK
URL: http://www.scolari.co.uk

SPSS/Diamond (Statistical Package for the Social Sciences)

Purpose: An interactive graphical visualization tool for exploring relationships in multivariate data.

Publisher: SPSS Inc., 444 N Michigan Avenue, Chicago IL 60611, USA

SPSS UK, SPSS House, 5 London Street, Chertsey, Surrey KT16 8AP, UK
URL: http://spss.com

WinMAX

Purpose: This software for qualitative data analysis enables importation of texts, definition of, and building flexible code systems and keeping visual control. It also supports creativity and teamwork, provides easy retrieval, lexical searches and automatic coding, the ability to explore conceptual relationships and merge qualitative and quantitative data.

Publisher: Scolari, Sage Publications, 6 Bonhill Street, London EC2A 4PU, UK
URL: http://www.scolari.co.uk

References

Software products 1998 (1997) *The Software Users Yearbook* (13th edition). Oxford: Learned Information Europe Ltd. ISBN 1900871106
URL: http://www.learned.co.uk/databases

Information included for each item is its purpose, industry, configuration, languages, publisher, sales, version, availability and media.

Health care: 441 to 453
Human resources: 455 to 462

Note: As new software is constantly being created, readers are advised to consult the most up-to-date manuals and yearbooks or databases where available.

APPENDIX B: JOURNALS

A number of journals regularly report on or present research findings or discuss methodology. This list is not comprehensive; rather it should be seen as an indicator of the breadth of specialist journals.

AAOHN Journal (American Association of Occupational Health Nurses) (USA)

Academic Medicine (USA)

Accident and Emergency Nursing (USA)

Administrative Science Quarterly (USA)

Advanced Practice Nursing Quarterly (USA)

Advances in Nursing Science (USA)

Aging Today (USA)

American Journal of Critical Care

American Journal of Maternal Child Nursing

American Journal of Nursing

American Journal of Otolaryngology

American Journal of Physical Medicine and Rehabilitation

American Journal of Political Science

American Journal of Public Health

ANNA (American Nephrology Nurses Association) Journal

Annals of Allergy, Asthma & Immunology (USA)

Annals of Internal Medicine (USA)

Annual Review of Nursing Research (USA)

Annual Review of Psychology (USA)

Annual Review of Public Health (USA)

Anthropology and Education Quarterly (USA)

AORN Journal – Association of Operating Room Nurses (USA)

Applied Nursing Research (USA)

Applied Statistics (UK)

Archives of Physical Medicine and Rehabilitation (USA)

Archives of Psychiatric Nursing (USA)

Asian Journal of Nursing Studies (Hong Kong)

Assistive Technology (USA)

Australia New Zealand Journal of Mental Health Nursing

Australian Critical Care

Australian Electronic Journal of Nursing Education

Australian Health Review

Australian Journal of Advanced Nursing

Australian Journal of Rural Health

Australian Occupational Therapy Journal

Behaviour Research Methods, Instruments and Computers (USA)

Behaviour Therapy (USA)

Biological Psychiatry (USA)

British Educational Research Journal

British Journal of Addiction

British Journal of General Practice

British Journal of Learning Disabilities

British Journal of Midwifery

British Journal of Nursing

British Journal of Theatre Nursing

British Journal of Therapy and Rehabilitation

British Medical Journal
British Reports, Translations and Theses
  (Grey literature)
Bulletin de Méthodologie Sociologique
  (France)
Bulletin of Medical Ethics (UK)
Bulletin of the Medical Library
  Association (USA)
Cambridge Journal of Education (UK)
Cambridge Quarterly of Health Care
  Ethics (UK)
Canadian Journal of Community Mental
  Health
Canadian Journal of Medical Laboratory
  Science
Canadian Journal of Nursing
  Administration
Canadian Journal of Nursing Research
Canadian Journal of Public Health
Canadian Journal of Rehabilitation
Canadian Medical Association Journal
Canadian Nurse
Canadian Oncology Nursing Journal
Cancer Nursing (USA)
Cancer Practice: a Multidisciplinary
  Journal of Cancer Care (USA)
Cd Rom Professional (USA)
Changes: an International Journal of
  Psychology and Psychotherapy (UK)
Character and Personality (USA)
Chart (USA)
Child Welfare (USA)
Clinical Care Specialist – the Journal for
  Advanced Nursing Practice (USA)
Clinical Kinesiology: Journal of the
  American Kinesiotherapy Association
  (USA)
Clinical Nursing Research (USA)
Collegian: Journal of the Royal College
  of Nursing, Australia
Communicating Nursing Research
  (USA)
Community Medicine (Pakistan)
Complementary Therapies in Medicine
  (UK)
Complementary Therapies in Nursing
  and Midwifery (UK)

Computers in Nursing (USA)
Connecticut Nursing News (USA)
Connections (UK)
Contemporary Nurse: a Journal for the
  Australian Nursing Profession
Counseling Psychologist (USA)
Critical Care Nurse (USA)
Curationis: South African Journal of
  Nursing
Current Psychology: Research &
  Reviews – developmental, learning,
  personality, social (USA)
Cyberskeptic's Guide to Internet
  Research (USA)
Database (USA)
Dimensions of Critical Care Nursing
  (USA)
Dynamic Chiropractic (USA)
Educational Researcher (USA)
Emergency Care Nursing Quarterly
  (USA)
Enfermería Clínica (Spain)
European Journal of Cancer Care (UK)
European Journal of Education (UK)
European Journal of Public Health
  (Sweden)
Evaluation and Program Planning: an
  International Journal (UK)
Evaluation and the Health Professions
  (USA)
Evaluation Review: a Journal of Applied
  Social Research (UK)
Evaluation: the International Journal of
  Theory, Research and Practice (UK)
Evidence-based Nursing (UK)
Gastroenterology Nursing (USA)
Hastings Center Report (USA)
Health and Social Care in the
  Community (UK)
Health and Social Work (USA)
Health Care on the Internet (USA)
Health Education Journal (UK)
Health Education Research (UK)
Health Informatics (UK)
Health Law in Canada
Health Libraries Review (UK)
Health Policy and Planning (UK)

Health Service Journal (UK)

Health Services Management Research (UK)

Health Services Research (USA)

Health Visitor (UK)

Heart and Lung (USA)

Higher Education Quarterly (UK)

Historical Methods (USA)

Historical Research (UK)

Historical Social Research (Germany)

Holistic Nursing Practice (USA)

Hong Kong Nursing Journal

Hospice Journal – physical, psychological and pastoral care of the dying (USA)

Hospital Topics (USA)

Human Studies: a Journal for Philosophy and the Social Sciences (Netherlands)

Image: Journal of Nursing Scholarship (USA)

Information Technology in Nursing (UK)

Information World Review (UK)

Insight (USA)

Intensive Care Nursing (UK)

International History of Nursing Journal (UK)

International Journal for Quality in Health Care (UK)

International Journal of Nursing Practice (Australia)

International Journal of Nursing Studies (UK)

International Journal of Palliative Nursing (UK)

International Nursing Review (Switzerland)

Internet Reference Services Quarterly (USA)

Issues in Comprehensive Pediatric Nursing (USA)

Issues in Mental Health Nursing (USA)

JEMS – Journal of Emergency Medical Services (USA)

JMPT – Journal of Manipulative and Physiological Therapeutics (USA)

Journal of Advanced Nursing (UK)

Journal of Aging and Social Policy (USA)

Journal of Allied Health (USA)

Journal of Applied Behavioural Science (USA)

Journal of Child and Adolescent Psychiatric Nursing (USA)

Journal of Chiropractic Education (USA)

Journal of Clinical Epidemiology (USA)

Journal of Clinical Nursing (UK)

Journal of Clinical Oncology (USA)

Journal of Community Nursing (UK)

Journal of Community Practice (USA)

Journal of Continuing Education in Nursing (USA)

Journal of Counseling Psychology (USA)

Journal of Cultural Diversity (USA)

Journal of Dental Hygiene (USA)

Journal of Emergency Nursing (USA)

Journal of Family Therapy (UK)

Journal of Further and Higher Education (UK)

Journal of Gerontological Nursing (USA)

Journal of Health Services Research and Policy (UK)

Journal of Human Lactation (USA)

Journal of Interprofessional Care (UK)

Journal of Law, Medicine and Ethics (USA)

Journal of Learning Disabilities (UK)

Journal of Medical Education (USA)

Journal of Medical Ethics (UK)

Journal of Multi-cultural Nursing and Health (USA)

Journal of Neuroscience Nursing (USA)

Journal of Nurse Midwifery (USA)

Journal of Nursing Administration (USA)

Journal of Nursing Care Quality (USA)

Journal of Nursing Education (USA)

Journal of Nursing Management (UK)

Journal of Nursing Measurement (USA)

Journal of Nursing Science (USA)

Journal of Nursing Staff Development (USA)

Journal of Obstetric, Gynecological and Neonatal Nursing (USA)

Journal of Official Statistics (Sweden)

Journal of Pediatric Nursing – nursing care of children and families (USA)

Journal of Pediatric Oncology Nursing (USA)

Journal of Perianesthetic Nursing (USA)

Journal of Personality Assessment (USA)

Journal of PeriAnasthesia Nursing (USA)

Journal of Professional Nursing (USA)

Journal of Prosthetics and Orthotics (USA)

Journal of Psychiatric and Mental Health Nursing (UK)

Journal of Psychosocial Nursing and Mental Health Services (USA)

Journal of Public Health Medicine (UK)

Journal of Quality in Clinical Practice (Australia)

Journal of Social Behavior and Personality (USA)

Journal of Social Issues (USA)

Journal of the American Academy of Nurse Practitioners

Journal of the American Medical Association

Journal of the American Medical Informatics Association

Journal of the New York State Nurses Association (USA)

Journal of the Royal College of Physicians (UK)

Journal of Transcultural Nursing (USA)

Journal of Trauma Nursing (USA)

Journal of WOCN (Wound, Ostomy and Continence Nursing) (USA)

Journal of Women's Health (USA)

Journal of Wound Care (UK)

Kai Tiaki: Nursing New Zealand

Lancet (UK)

Legal Eagle Eye Newsletter for the Nursing Profession (USA)

Mail on Sunday (UK)

Marketing and Research Today (Netherlands)

Maternal Child Nursing Journal (USA)

Medical Care (USA)

Medical Education (UK)

Medical Reference Services Quarterly (USA)

Medical Research Council News (UK)

Medical Teacher (UK)

MEDSURG Nursing (USA)

Mental Handicap (UK)

Mental Health Nursing Journal (UK)

Michigan Nurse (USA)

Microworld (USA)

Midwifery (UK)

Midwives Chronicle (UK)

Military Medicine (USA)

Modern Midwife (UK)

N and H (Perspectives on Community) (USA)

Nature (UK)

Nature Medicine (UK)

Nordic Journal of Psychiatry (Norway)

NT Research (UK)

Nurse Author and Editor (USA)

Nurse Education Today (UK)

Nurse Educator (USA)

Nurse Educators' Microworld (USA)

Nurse Manager (USA)

Nurse Researcher (UK)

Nursing (USA)

Nursing Administration Quarterly (USA)

Nursing Clinics of North America

Nursing Connections (USA)

Nursing Economics (USA)

Nursing Ethics (UK)

Nursing Ethics: an International Journal for Health Care Professionals (UK)

Nursing Focus (UK)

Nursing Forum (USA)

Nursing History Review (USA)

Nursing Inquiry (Australia)

Nursing Journal of India

Nursing Management (USA)

Nursing New Zealand

Nursing Outlook (USA)
Nursing Practice (UK)
Nursing Practitioner (USA)
Nursing Research (China)
Nursing Research (USA)
Nursing Review (Australia)
Nursing Science Quarterly (USA)
Nursing Standard (UK)
Nursing Standard Online (UK)
Nursing Times (UK)
Nursing Times Learning Curve (UK)
Occupational Health (UK)
Occupational Therapy International
(USA)
Oncology Nursing Forum (USA)
Online (USA)
Online and CD ROM Review (UK)
Online Journal of Knowledge Synthesis
for Nursing (USA)
Oral History (UK)
Oral History Review (USA)
ORL–Head and Neck Nursing (USA)
Orthopaedic Nursing Journal (USA)
Paediatric Nursing (UK)
Palliative Medicine (UK)
Patient Education and Counseling
(USA)
Patient Education Management (USA)
Pediatric Nursing (USA)
Pediatrics (USA)
Pflege (Germany)
Philosophy of the Social Sciences (USA)
Physical and Occupational Therapy in
Geriatrics (USA)
Physical Therapy (USA)
Physiotherapy (UK)
Plastic Surgical Nursing (USA)
Practice Nurse (UK)
Prairie Rose (USA)
Professional Care of Mother and Child
(UK)
Professional Nurse (UK)
Program in Cardiovascular Nursing
(USA)
Psychiatric Care (UK)
Psychiatric Services (USA)
Psychological Assessment (USA)

Psychological Bulletin (USA)
Public Opinion Quarterly (USA)
Qualitative Health Research (USA)
Qualitative Inquiry (USA)
Qualitative Sociology (USA)
Quality & Quantity (Netherlands)
Quality in Health Care (UK)
Radiologic Technology (USA)
Radiology (UK)
RCN Euro Forum (UK)
Recent Advances in Nursing (UK)
ceased publication
Reflections (USA)
Rehabilitation (USA)
Rehabilitation Nursing Research (USA)
Research Communications and Review
Articles in Women's Studies (UK)
Research in Education (UK)
Research in Higher Education (USA)
Research in Nursing and Health (USA)
Research on Language and Social
Interaction (Canada)
Research Papers in Education: Policy &
Practice (UK)
Research, Policy & Planning (UK)
Respiratory Care (USA)
Review in Educational Research (USA)
Review Journal of Philosophy and Social
Science (USA)
RN (Registered Nurse) (USA)
Scandinavian Journal of Caring Sciences
(Norway)
Scholarly Inquiry for Nursing Practice
(USA)
Searcher: the Magazine for Database
Professionals (UK)
Seminars for Nurse Managers (USA)
Seminars in Oncology Nursing (USA)
Seminars in Peri-operative Nursing
(USA)
Senior Nurse (UK)
Small Group Research: an International
Journal of Theory, Investigation and
Application (USA)
Social History of Medicine (UK)
Social Science and Medicine (UK)
Social Science Computer Review (USA)

Social Science Research (USA)
Social Sciences in Health – International
  Journal of Research & Practice (UK)
Social Work Research (USA)
Sociological Methodology (USA)
Sociological Methods and Research
  (USA)
Sociological Research Online (UK)
Sociological Review (UK)
Sociology (UK)
Sociology of Health and Illness (UK)
South African Journal of Physiotherapy
Studies in the Education of Adults (UK)
Substance Abuse (USA)
Surgical Nurse (UK)
Survey Methodology (CN)
Tar Heel Nurse (USA)

Times Higher Education Supplement
  (UK)
Topics in Clinical Nursing (USA)
Topics in Health Information
  Management (USA)
Urologic Nursing (USA)
Western Journal of Nursing Research
  (USA)
Western Journal of Speech
  Communication (USA)
Woman & Health (USA)
Women's Studies International Forum: a
  multi-disciplinary journal for the rapid
  publication of research
  communications and review articles in
  women's studies (UK)

APPENDIX C: SAGE PUBLICATIONS

This appendix gives details of three series of books relating to research methodology, some of which have been included in this text. The information has been provided by Sage Publications Ltd and indicates books in print and forthcoming as at 7 July 1998. For up-to-date information, please visit:

In North, Central and South America
URL: http://www.sagepub.com

Rest of the world
URL: http://www.sagepub.co.uk

APPLIED SOCIAL RESEARCH METHODS SERIES

Methods for Policy Research. Ann Majchrzak, 1984
Cloth (0–8039–2059–8)
Paper (0–8039–2060–1)

Need Analysis: Tools for the Human Services and Education. Jack McKillip, 1987
Paper (0–8039–2648–0)

Linking Auditing and Meta-Evaluation: Enhancing Quality in Applied Research. Thomas A. Schwandt and Edward S. Halpern, 1988
Cloth (0–8039–2967–6)
Paper (0–8039–2968–4)

Ethics and Values in Applied Social Research. Allan Kimmel, 1988
Paper (0–8039–2632–4)

On Time and Method. Janice R. Kelly and Joseph E. McGrath, 1988
Cloth (0–8039–3046–1)
Paper (0–8039–3047-X)

Synthesizing Research: a Guide for Literature Reviews (3rd edition). Harris

M. Cooper, 1998
Cloth (0–7619–1347–5)
Paper (0–7619–1348–3)

Research in Health Care Settings. Kathleen E. Grady and Barbara Strudler Wallston, 1988
Cloth (0–8039–2874–2)
Paper (0–8039–2875–0)

Ethnography: Step by Step (2nd edition). David M. Fetterman, 1998
Cloth (0–7619–1384-X)
Paper (0–7619–1385–8)

Participant Observation: a Methodology for Human Studies.
Danny L. Jorgensen, 1989
Cloth (0–8039–2876–9)
Paper (0–8039–2877–7)

Interpretive Interactionism. Norman K. Denzin, 1989
Cloth (0–8039–3002-X)
Paper (0–8039–3003–8)

Ethnography: Step by Step. David M. Fetterman, 1989

Cloth (0–8039–2890–4)
Paper (0–8039–2891–2)

Integrating Research: a Guide for Literature Reviews (2nd edition). Harris M. Cooper, 1989
Cloth (0–8039–3430–0)
Paper (0–8039–3431–9)

Standardized Survey Interviewing Minimizing Interviewer-related Error. Floyd J. Fowler Jr. and Thomas W. Mangione, 1990
Paper (0–8039–3093–3)

Productivity Measurement: a Guide for Managers and Evaluators. Robert O. Brinkerhoff and Dennis E. Dressler, 1990
Paper (0–8039–3152–2)

Focus Groups: Theory and Practice. David W. Stewart and Prem N. Shamdasani, 1990
Cloth (0–8039–3389–4)
Paper (0–8039–3390–8)

Practical Sampling. Gary T. Henry, 1990
Cloth (0–8039–2958–7)
Paper (0–8039–2959–5)

Decision Research: a Field Guide. John S. Carroll and Eric J. Johnson, 1990
Cloth (0–8039–3268–5)
Paper (0–8039–3269–3)

Research with Hispanic Populations. Gerardo Marin and Barbara Vanoss, 1991
Cloth (0–8039–3720–2)
Paper (0–8039–3721–0)

Internal Evaluation: Building Organizations from Within. Arnold J. Love, 1991
Cloth (0–8039–3200–6)
Paper (0–8039–3201–4)

Computer Simulation Applications: an Introduction. Marcia Lynn Whicker and Lee Sigelman, 1991
Cloth (0–8039–3245–6)
Paper (0–8039–3246–4)

Scale Development: Theory and Applications. Robert F. DeVellis, 1991

Cloth (0–8039–3775-X)
Paper (0–8039–3776–8)

Studying Families. Anne P. Copeland and Kathleen M. White, 1991
Paper (0–8039–3248–0)

Event History Analysis. Kazuo Yamaguchi, 1991
Paper (0–8039–3324-X)

Meta-analytic Procedures for Social Research. Robert Rosenthal, 1991
Paper (0–8039–4246-X)

Research in Educational Settings. Geoffrey M. Maruyama and Stanley Deno, 1992
Paper (0–8039–4208–7)

Researching Persons with Mental Illness. Rosalind J. Dworkin, 1992
Cloth (0–8039–3603–6)
Paper (0–8039–3604–4)

Planning Ethically Responsible Research: a Guide for Students and Internal Review Boards. Joan E. Sieber, 1992
Paper (0–8039–3964–7)

Survey Research Methods (2nd edition). Floyd J. Fowler Jr., 1993
Cloth (0–8039–5048–9)
Paper (0–8039–5049–7)

Applied Research Design: a Practical Guide. Terry E. Hedrick, Leonard Bickman and Debra J. Rog, 1993
Cloth (0–8039–3233–2)
Paper (0–8039–3234–0)

Doing Urban Research. Gregory D. Andranovich and Gerry Riposa, 1993
Paper (0–8039–3989–2)

Secondary Research: Information Sources and Methods (2nd edition). David W. Stewart and Michael A. Kamins, 1993
Cloth (0–8039–5036–5)
Paper (0–8039–5037–3)

Telephone Survey Methods: Sampling, Selection, and Supervision (2nd edition). Paul J. Lavrakas, 1993

Cloth (0–8039–5306–2)
Paper (0–8039–5307–0)

Applications of Case Study Research.
Robert K. Yin, 1993
Cloth (0–8039–5118–3)
Paper (0–8039–5119–1)

Diagnosing Organizations: Methods,
Models, and Processes (2nd edition).
Michael I. Harrison, 1994
Cloth (0–8039–5644–4)
Paper (0–8039–5645–2)

Group Techniques for Idea Building
(2nd edition). Carl M. Moore, 1994
Cloth (0–8039–5642–8)
Paper (0–8039–5643–6)

Introduction to Facet Theory: Content
Design and Intrinsic Data Analysis in
Behavioral Research. Samuel Shye and
Dov Elizur with Michael Hoffman, 1994
Cloth (0–8039–5670–3)
Paper (0–8039–5671–1)

Graphing Data: Techniques for Display
and Analysis. Gary T. Henry 1994
Cloth (0–8039–5674–6)
Paper (0–8039–5675–4)

Research Methods in Special Education.
Donna M. Mertens and John
McLaughlin, 1994
Cloth (0–8039–4808–5)
Paper (0–8039–4809–3)

Case Study Research Design and
Methods (2nd edition). Robert K. Yin,
1994
Cloth (0–8039–5662–2)
Paper (0–8039–5663–0)

Improving Survey Questions: Design and
Evaluation. Floyd J. Fowler Jr., 1995
Cloth (0–8039–4582–5)
Paper (0–8039–4583–3)

Data Collection and Management: a
Practical Guide. Magda Stouthamer-
Loeber and Welmoet Bok van Kammen,
1995
Cloth (0–8039–5656–8)

Paper (0–8039–5657–6)

Mail Surveys: Improving the Quality.
Thomas W. Mangione, 1995
Cloth (0–8039–4662–7)
Paper (0–8039–4663–5)

Qualitative Research Design: an
Interactive Approach. Joseph A.
Maxwell, 1996
Cloth (0–8039–7328–4)
Paper (0–8039–7329–2)

Analyzing Costs, Procedures, Processes,
and Outcomes in Human Services: an
Introduction. Brian T. Yates, 1996
Cloth (0–8039–4785–2)
Paper (0–8039–4786–0)

Doing Legal Research: a Guide for
Social Scientists and Mental Health
Professionals. Roberta Morris, Bruce D.
Sales and Daniel W. Shuman, 1997
Cloth (0–8039–3428–9)
Paper (0–8039–3429–7)

Randomized Experiments for Planning
and Evaluation: a Practical Guide.
Robert F. Boruch, 1997
Cloth (0–8039–3509–9)
Paper (0–8039–3510–2)

Measuring Community Indicators: a
Systems Approach to Drug and Alcohol
Problems. Paul J. Gruenewald, Andrew J.
Treno, Gail Taff and Michael Klitzner,
1997
Cloth (0–7619–0684–3)
Paper (0–7619–0685–1)

Mixed Methodology: Combining
Qualitative and Quantitative Approaches.
Abbas Tashakkori and Charles Teddlie,
1998
Cloth (0–7619–0070–5)
Paper (0–7619–0071–3)

Narrative Research: Reading, Analysis
and Interpretation. Amia Lieblich, Rivka
Tuval-Mashiach and Tamar Zilber, 1998
Cloth (0–7619–1042–5)
Paper (0–7619–1043–3)

QUANTITATIVE APPLICATIONS IN
THE SOCIAL SCIENCES SERIES

Analysis of Ordinal Data. David K.
Hildebrand, James D. Laing and Howard
Rosenthal, 1970
Paper (0–8039–0795–8)

Analysis of Nominal Data (2nd edition).
H.T. Reynolds, 1977
Paper (0–8039–0653–6)

*Canonical Analysis and Factor
Comparison.* Mark S. Levine, 1977
Paper (0–8039–0655–2)

Causal Modeling (2nd edition). Herbert
B. Asher, 1977
Paper (0–8039–0654–4)

Cohort Analysis. Norval D. Glenn, 1977
Paper (0–8039–0794-X)

*Operations Research Methods: as
Applied to Political Science and the
Legal Process.* Stuart S. Nagel with
Marian Neef, 1977
Paper (0–8039–0651-X)

Tests of Significance 4. Ramon E.
Henkel, 1977
Paper (0–8039–0652–8)

Ecological Inference. Laura Irwin
Langbein and Allan J. Lichtman, 1978
Paper (0–8039–0941–1)

Multidimensional Scaling 11. Joseph B.
Kruskal and Myron Wish, 1978
Paper (0–8039–0940–3)

Analysis of Covariance. Albert R. Wildt
and Olli T. Ahtola, 1979
Paper (0–8039–1164–5)

*Factor Analysis: Statistical Methods and
Practical Issues.* Jae-On Kim and Charles
W. Mueller, 1979
Paper (0–8039–1166–1)

*Introduction to Factor Analysis: What it is
and How to do it.* Jae-On Kim and
Charles W. Mueller, 1979
Paper (0–8039–1165–3)

Multiple Indicators: an Introduction.
John L. Sullivan and Stanley Feldman,
1980
Paper (0–8039–1369–9)

Exploratory Data Analysis. Frederick
Hartwig and Brian E. Dearing, 1980
Paper (0–8039–1370–2)

Reliability & Validity. Edward G.
Carmines and Richard A. Zeller, 1980
Paper (0–8039–1371–0)

Analyzing Panel Data. Gregory B.
Markus, 1980
Paper (0–8039–1372–9)

Discriminant Analysis. William R.
Klecka, 1980
Paper (0–8039–1491–1)

Log-Linear Models. David Knoke, 1980
Paper (0–8039–1492-X)

Interrupted Time Series Analysis. David
McDowall, Richard McCleary, Errol E.
Meidinger and Richard A. Hay Jr., 1980
Paper (0–8039–1493–8)

Applied Regression: an Introduction.
Michael S. Lewis-Beck, 1980
Paper (0–8039–1494–6)

Research Designs. Paul E. Spector, 1981
Paper (0–8039–1709–0)

Unidimensional Scaling. John P. McIver
and Edward G. Carmines, 1981
Paper (0–8039–1736–8)

*Magnitude Scaling: Quantitative
Measurement of Opinions.* Milton Lodge,
1981
Paper (0–8039–1747–3)

Multiattribute Evaluation. Ward Edwards
and J. Robert Newman, 1982
Paper (0–8039–0095–3)

Dynamic Modeling: an Introduction.
R. Robert Huckfeldt, C.W. Kohfeld and
Thomas W. Likens, 1982
Paper (0–8039–0946–2)

Network Analysis. David Knoke and
James H. Kuklinski, 1982
Paper (0–8039–1914-X)

Interpreting and Using Regression.
Christopher H. Achen, 1982
Paper (0–8039–1915–8)

Test Item Bias. Steven J. Osterlind, 1983
Paper (0–8039–1989–1)

Mobility Tables. Michael Hout, 1983
Paper (0–8039–2056–3)

Measures of Association. Albert M.
Liebetrau, 1983
Paper (0–8039–1974–3)

*Confirmatory Factor Analysis: a Preface
to LISREL.* J. Scott Long, 1983
Paper (0–8039–2044-X)

*Covariance Structure Models: an
Introduction to LISREL.* J. Scott Long,
1983
Paper (0–8039–2045–8)

Introduction to Survey Sampling.
Graham Kalton, 1983
Paper (0–8039–2046–6)

Achievement Testing: Recent Advances.
Isaac I. Bejar, 1983
Paper (0–8039–2047–4)

Nonrecursive Causal Models. William D.
Berry, 1984
Paper (0–8039–2053–9)

Matrix Algebra: an Introduction.
Krishnan Namboodiri, 1984
Paper (0–8039–2052–0)

*Introduction to Applied Demography:
Data Sources and Estimation Techniques.*
Norfleet W. Rives Jr. and William J.
Serow, 1984
Paper (0–8039–2134–9)

*Game Theory: Concepts and
Applications.* Frank C. Zagare, 1984
Paper (0–8039–2050–4)

*Using Published Data: Errors and
Remedies.* Herbert Jacob, 1985
Paper (0–8039–2299-X)

Bayesian Statistical Inference. Gudmund
R. Iversen, 1985
Paper (0–8039–2328–7)

Cluster Analysis. Mark S. Aldenderfer

and Roger K. Blashfield, 1985
Paper (0–8039–2376–7)

*Linear Probability, Logit, and Probit
Models.* John H. Aldrich and Forrest D.
Nelson, 1985
Paper (0–8039–2133–0)

*Event History Analysis: Regression for
Longitudinal Event Data.* Paul D.
Allison, 1985
Paper (0–8039–2055–5)

*Canonical Correlation Analysis: Uses and
Interpretation.* Bruce Thompson, 1985
Paper (0–8039–2392–9)

Models for Innovation Diffusion. Vijay
Mahajan and Robert A. Peterson, 1985
Paper (0–8039–2136–5)

Multiple Regression in Practice. William
D. Berry and Stanley Feldman, 1985
Paper (0–8039–2054–7)

Stochastic Parameter Regression Models.
Paul Newbold and Theodore Bos, 1985
Paper (0–8039–2425–9)

Using Microcomputers in Research.
Thomas W. Madron, C. Neal Tate and
Robert G. Brookshire, 1985
Paper (0–8039–2457–7)

Secondary Analysis of Survey Data.
K. Jill Kiecolt and Laura E. Nathan,
1986
Paper (0–8039–2302–3)

Multivariate Analysis of Variance. James
H. Bray and Scott E. Maxwell, 1986
Paper (0–8039–2310–4)

The Logic of Causal Order. James A.
Davis, 1986
Paper (0–8039–2553–0)

*Introduction to Linear Goal
Programming.* James P. Ignizio, 1986
Paper (0–8039–2564–6)

*Understanding Regression Analysis: an
Introductory Guide.* Larry D. Schroeder,
David L. Sjoquist and Paula E. Stephan,
1986
Paper (0–8039–2758–4)

Randomized Response 58: a Method for Sensitive Surveys. James Alan Fox and Paul E. Tracy, 1986
Paper (0–8039–2309–0)

Meta-Analysis: Quantitative Methods for Research Synthesis. Fredric M. Wolf, 1986
Paper (0–8039–2756–8)

Linear Programming 60: an Introduction. Bruce R. Feiring, 1986
Paper (0–8039–2850–5)

Multiple Comparisons. Alan J. Klockars and Gilbert Sax, 1986
Paper (0–8039–2051–2)

Information Theory: Structural Models for Qualitative Data. Klaus Krippendorff, 1986
Paper (0–8039–2132–2)

Survey Questions: Handcrafting the Standardized Questionnaire. Jean M. Converse and Stanley Presser, 1986
Paper (0–8039–2743–6)

Latent Class Analysis. Allan L. McCutcheon, 1987
Paper (0–8039–2752–5)

Analysis of Variance (2nd edition). Gudmund R. Iversen and Helmut Norpoth, 1987
Paper (0–8039–3001–1)

Microcomputer Methods for Social Scientists (2nd edition). Edited by Philip A. Schrodt, 1987
Paper (0–8039–3043–7)

Three Way Scaling: a Guide to Multidimensional Scaling and Clustering. Phipps Arabie, Douglas Carroll and Wayne S. DeSarbo, 1987
Paper (0–8039–3068–2)

Q Methodology. Bruce McKeown, 1988
Paper (0–8039–2753–3)

Analyzing Decision Making: Metric Conjoint Analysis. Jordan J. Louviere, 1988
Paper (0–8039–2757–6)

Rasch Models for Measurement. David

Andrich, 1988
Paper (0–8039–2741–X)

Principal Components Analysis. George H. Dunteman, 1989
Paper (0–8039–3104–2)

Pooled Time Series Analysis. Lois W. Sayrs, 1989
Paper (0–8039–3160–3)

Analyzing Complex Survey Data. Eun Sul Lee, Ronald N. Forthofer and Ronald J. Lorimor, 1989
Paper (0–8039–3014–3)

Time Series Analysis: Regression Techniques (2nd edition). Charles W. Ostrom Jr., 1990
Paper (0–8039–3135–2)

Interaction Effects in Multiple Regression. James Jaccard, Robert Turrisi and Choi K. Wan, 1990
Paper (0–8039–3703–2)

Understanding Significance Testing. Lawrence B. Mohr, 1990
Paper (0–8039–3568–4)

Experimental Design and Analysis. Steven R. Brown and Lawrence E. Melamed, 1990
Paper (0–8039–3854–3)

Metric Scaling: Correspondence Analysis. Susan C. Weller and A. Kimball Romney, 1990
Paper (0–8039–3750–4)

Basic Content Analysis (2nd edition). Robert Philip Weber, 1990
Paper (0–8039–3863–2)

Longitudinal Research. Scott Menard, 1991
Paper (0–8039–3753–9)

Expert Systems. Robert A. Benfer, Edward E. Brent Jr. and Louanna Furbee, 1991
Paper (0–8039–4036-X)

Data Theory and Dimensional Analysis. William G. Jacoby, 1991
Paper (0–8039–4178–1)

Regression Diagnostics: an Introduction. John Fox, 1991
Paper (0–8039–3971-X)

Computer-assisted Interviewing. Willem E. Saris, 1991
Paper (0–8039–4066–1)

Contextual Analysis. Gudmund R. Iversen, 1991
Paper (0–8039–4272–9)

Summated Rating Scale Construction: an Introduction. Paul E. Spector, 1992
Paper (0–8039–4341–5)

Central Tendency and Variability. Herbert F. Weisberg, 1992
Paper (0–8039–4007–6)

ANOVA: Repeated Measures. Ellen R. Girden, 1992
Paper (0–8039–4257–5)

Processing Data: the Survey Example. Linda B. Bourque and Virginia A. Clark, 1992
Paper (0–8039–4741–0)

Logit Modeling: Practical Applications. Alfred DeMaris, 1992
Paper (0–8039–4377–6)

Analytic Mapping and Geographic Databases. G. David Garson and Robert S. Biggs, 1992
Paper (0–8039–4752–6)

Working with Archival Data: Studying Lives. Glen H. Elder Jr., Eliza K. Pavalko and Elizabeth C. Clipp, 1992
Paper (0–8039–4262–1)

Multiple Comparison Procedures. Larry E. Toothaker, 1992
Paper (0–8039–4177–3)

Nonparametric Statistics: an Introduction. Jean Dickinson Gibbons, 1992
Paper (0–8039–3951–5)

Nonparametric Measures of Association. Jean Dickinson Gibbons, 1993
Paper (0–8039–4664–3)

Understanding Regression Assumptions. William D. Berry, 1993
Paper (0–8039–4263-X)

Regression with Dummy Variables. Melissa A. Hardy, 1993
Paper (0–8039–5128–0)

Loglinear Models with Latent Variables. Jacques A. Hagenaars, 1993
Paper (0–8039–4310–5)

Bootstrapping: a Nonparametric Approach to Statistical Inference. Christopher Z. Mooney and Robert D. Duval, 1993
Paper (0–8039–5381-X)

Maximum Likelihood Estimation: Logic and Practice. Scott R. Eliason, 1993
Paper (0–8039–4107–2)

Ordinal Log-Linear Models. Masako Ishii-Kuntz, 1994
Paper (0–8039–4376–8)

Random Factors in ANOVA. Sally E. Jackson and Dale E. Brashers, 1994
Paper (0–8039–5090-X)

Univariate Tests for Time Series Models. Jeff B. Cromwell, Walter C. Labys and Michel Terraza, 1994
Paper (0 8039–4991-X)

Multivariate Tests for Time Series Models. Jeff B. Cromwell, Walter C. Labys, Michael J. Hannan and Michel Terraza, 1994
Paper (0–8039–5440–9)

Interpreting Probability Models: Logit, Probit, and Other Generalized Linear Models. Tim Futing Liao, 1994
Paper (0–8039–4999–5)

Typologies and Taxonomies: an Introduction to Classification Techniques. Kenneth D. Bailey, 1994
Paper (0–8039–5259–7)

Data Analysis: an Introduction. Michael S. Lewis-Beck, 1995
Paper (0–8039–5772–6)

Multiple Attribute Decision Making: an Introduction. K. Paul Yoon and Ching-Lai Hwang, 1995
Paper (0–8039–5486–7)

Causal Analysis with Panel Data. Steven E. Finkel, 1995
Paper (0–8039–3896–9)

Applied Logistic Regression Analysis. Scott Menard, 1995
Paper (0–8039–5757–2)

Chaos and Catastrophe Theories. Courtney Brown, 1995
Paper (0–8039–5847–1)

Basic Math for Social Scientists: Concepts. Timothy M. Hagle, 1995
Paper (0–8039–5875–7)

Basic Math for Social Scientists: Problems and Solutions. Timothy M. Hagle, 1996
Paper (0–8039–7285–7)

Calculus. Gudmund R. Iversen, 1996
Paper (0–8039–7110–9)

Regression Models: Censored, Sample Selected, or Truncated Data. Richard Breen, 1996
Paper (0–8039–5710–6)

Tree Models of Similarity and Association. James E. Corter, 1996
Paper (0–8039–5707–6)

Computational Modeling. Charles S. Taber and Richard John Timpone, 1996
Paper (0–8039–7270–9)

LISREL Approaches to Interaction Effects in Multiple Regression. James Jaccard and Choi K. Wan, 1996
Paper (0–8039–7179–6)

Analyzing Repeated Surveys. Glenn Firebaugh, 1997
Paper (0–8039–7398–5)

Monte Carlo Simulation. Christopher Z. Mooney, 1997
Paper (0–8039–5943–5)

Statistical Graphics for Univariate and Bivariate Data. William G. Jacoby, 1997
Paper (0–7619–0083–7)

Interaction Effects in Factorial Analysis of Variance. James Jaccard, 1998
Paper (0–7619–1221–5)

Odds Ratios in the Analysis of Contingency Tables. Tam[ac]as Rudas, 1998
Paper (0–7619–0362–3)

Statistical Graphics for Visualizing Multivariate Data. William G. Jacoby, 1998
Paper (0–7619–0899–4)

Applied Correspondence Analysis: an Introduction, Sten Erik Clausen, 1998
Paper (0–7619–1115–4)

Game Theory Topics: Incomplete Information, Repeated Games and N-Player Games. Evelyn C. Fink, Scott Gates and Brian D. Humes, 1998
Paper (0–7619–1016–6)

Social Choice: Theory and Research. Paul E. Johnson, 1998
Paper (0–7619–1406–4)

QUALITATIVE RESEARCH METHODS SERIES

Reliability and Validity in Qualitative Research. Jerome Kirk and Marc L. Miller, 1986
Paper (0–8039–2470–4)

Speaking of Ethnography. Michael H. Agar, 1986
Cloth (0–8039–2561–1)
Paper (0–8039–2492–5)

The Politics and Ethics of Fieldwork: Muddy Boots and Grubby Hands. Maurice Punch, 1986
Paper (0–8039–2517–4)

Linking Data. Nigel G. Fielding and Jane Fielding, 1986
Paper (0–8039–2518–2)

The Clinical Perspective in Fieldwork. Edgar H. Schein, 1987
Cloth (0–8039–2975–7)
Paper (0–8039–2976–5)

Membership Roles in Field Research.
Peter Adler, 1987
Cloth (0–8039–2760–6)
Paper (0–8039–2578–6)

Semiotics and Fieldwork. Peter K.
Manning, 1987
Cloth (0–8039–2761–4)
Paper (0–8039–2640–5)

Analyzing Field Reality. Jaber F.
Gubrium, 1988
Cloth (0–8039–3095-X)
Paper (0–8039–3096–8)

Gender Issues in Field Research. Carol
A.B. Warren, 1988
Paper (0–8039–3098–4)

Systematic Data Collection. Susan C.
Weller and A. Kimball Romney, 1988
Paper (0–8039–3074–7)

*Meta-Ethnography: Synthesizing
Qualitative Studies.* George W. Noblit
and R. Dwight Hare, 1988
Cloth (0–8039–3022–4)
Paper (0–8039–3023–2)

*Ethnostatistics: Qualitative Foundations
for Quantitative Research.* Robert P.
Gephart Jr., 1988
Cloth (0–8039–3025–9)
Paper (0–8039–3026–7)

The Long Interview. Grant McCracken,
1988
Cloth (0–8039–3352–5)
Paper (0–8039–3353–3)

*Microcomputer Applications in
Qualitative Research.* Bryan
Pfaffenberger, 1988
Paper (0–8039–3120–4)

*Knowing Children: Participant
Observation with Minors.* Gary Alan
Fine and Kent L. Sandstrom, 1988
Cloth (0–8039–3364–9)
Paper (0–8039–3365–7)

Interpretive Biography. Norman K.
Denzin, 1989
Cloth (0–8039–3358–4)
Paper (0–8039–3359–2)

Psychoanalytic Aspects of Fieldwork.
Jennifer C. Hunt, 1989
Cloth (0–8039–3472–6)
Paper (0–8039–3473–4)

Ethnographic Decision Tree Modeling.
C.H. Gladwin, 1989
Cloth (0–8039–3486–6)
Paper (0–8039–3487–4)

Writing up Qualitative Research. Harry F.
Wolcott, 1990
Cloth (0–8039–3792-X)
Paper (0–8039–3793–8)

*Writing Strategies: Reaching Diverse
Audiences.* Laurel Richardson, 1990
Cloth (0–8039–3521–8)
Paper (0–8039–3522–6)

Living the Ethnographic Life. Dan Rose,
1990
Cloth (0–8039–3998–1)
Paper (0–8039–3999-X)

Selecting Ethnographic Informants.
Edited by Jeffrey C. Johnson, 1991
Cloth (0–8039–3586–2)
Paper (0–8039–3587–0)

Analyzing Visual Data. Michael S. Ball
and Gregory W.H. Smith, 1992
Paper (0–8039–3435–1)

Understanding Ethnographic Texts. Paul
Atkinson, 1992
Cloth (0–8039–3936–1)
Paper (0–8039–3937-X)

Archival Strategies and Techniques.
Michael R. Hill, 1993
Cloth (0–8039–4824–7)
Paper (0–8039–4825–5)

Case Study Methods. Jacques Hamel,
Stephane Dufour and Dominic Fortin,
1993
Cloth (0–8039–5415–8)
Paper (0–8039–5416–6)

Doing Critical Ethnography, Jim
Thomas, 1993
Paper (0–8039–3923-X)

Ethnography in Organizations. Helen B. Schwartzman, 1993
Paper (0–8039–4379–2)

Secrecy and Fieldwork. Richard G. Mitchell Jr. 1994 (Cloth); 1993 (Paper).
Cloth (0–8039–4384–9)
Paper (0–8039–4385–7)

Narrative Analysis. Catherine Kohler Riessman, 1994 (Cloth); 1993 (Paper).
Cloth (0–8039–4753–4)
Paper (0–8039–4754–2)

Emotions and Fieldwork. Sherryl Kleinman and Martha A. Copp, 1994 (Cloth); 1993 (Paper).
Cloth (0–8039–4721–6)
Paper (0–8039–4722–4)

Strategies for Interpreting Qualitative Data. Martha S. Feldman, 1994
Cloth (0–8039–5915-X)
Paper (0–8039–5916–8)

Dangerous Fieldwork. Raymond M. Lee, 1994
Cloth (0–8039–5660–6)
Paper (0–8039–5661–4)

Conversation Analysis: the Study of Talk-in-Interaction. George Psathas, 1994
Paper (0–8039–5747–5)

Ethnomethodology. Alain Coulon, 1995
Cloth (0–8039–4776–3)
Paper (0–8039–4777–1)

The Active Interview. James A. Holstein and Jaber F. Gubrium, 1995
Cloth (0–8039–5894–3)
Paper (0–8039–5895–1)

Qualitative Media Analysis. David L. Altheide, 1996
Cloth (0–7619–0198–1)
Paper (0–7619–0199-X)

Studying Organizational Symbolism:

What, How, Why? Michael Owen Jones, 1996
Cloth (0–7619–0219–8)
Paper (0–7619–0220–1)

Insider/Outsider Team Research. Jean M. Bartunek and Meryl Reis Louis, 1996
Cloth (0–8039–7158–3)
Paper (0–8039–7159–1)

Working with Sensitizing Concepts: Analytical Field Research. Will C. van den Hoonaard, 1997
Cloth (0–7619–0206–6)
Paper (0–7619–0207–4)

Doing Team Ethnography: Warnings and Advice. Ken Erickson and Donald Stull, 1997
Cloth (0–7619–0666–5)
Paper (0–7619–0667–3)

Focus Groups as Qualitative Research (2nd edition). David L. Morgan, 1997
Cloth (0–7619–0342–9)
Paper (0–7619–0343–7)

A Narrative Approach to Organization Studies. Barbara Czarniawska, 1998
Cloth (0–7619–0662–2)
Paper (0–7619–0663–0)

The Life Story Interview. Robert Atkinson, 1998
Cloth (0–7619–0427–1)
Paper (0–7619–0428-X)

Employing Qualitative Methods in the Private Sector. Marilyn L. Mitchell, 1998
Cloth (0–8039–5980-X)
Paper (0–8039–5981–8)

The Ethnographer's Method. Alex Stewart, 1998
Cloth (0–7619–0393–3)
Paper (0–7619–0394–1)

APPENDIX D: SOURCES OF DEFINITIONS

'Selection of terms and definitions is difficult because of indistinct lines between methodological issues and philosophical terms and debates' (*Dictionary of Social Science Methods* 1983: vii).

Each definition included in this book has been obtained from existing literature, glossaries or dictionaries and readers will note the variety of sources. There are many different ones which could have been included, but the authors have chosen those which appeared to be the most clear and concise. However researchers, teachers and students may wish to use other definitions, depending upon their own research perspectives.

Each definition included in the list below may be found in the respective sections of the book. Please note that where 'References in this volume' are listed, full bibliographical details may be found on pages 330 to 331, otherwise its original source may be found in the item numbers listed.

Section number	Definition	Author(s)	Page in source text	Reference in this volume
2.3	Applied research	Polit & Hungler (1995)	636	References
	Basic research	Dictionary of Nursing Theory & Research	12	2.2.6
	Clinical research	Denzin & Lincoln	342 (adapted)	2.36.13
	Community health nursing research	Hockey	17	2.53.6
	Empirical research	Williamson	418	References
	Nursing research	Hockey, L.	17	2.53.6
	Research	Hockey, L.	17	2.53.6
	Research methodology	Abdellah & Levine	157	3.6.1
	Research-mindedness	Royal College of Nursing	not known	3.17.47
2.4	Research approaches	Abdellah & Levine	25	3.6.1
	Research processes	Treece & Treece	510	References
2.5	Concept	Polit & Hungler (1995)	638	References
	Conceptual framework	Denzin & Lincoln	440	2.36.13
	Constructivism	Schwandt	19	2.2.13
	Hermeneutics	The New International Webster's Comprehensive Dictionary	591	References

Section number	Definition	Author(s)	Page in source text	Reference in this volume
	Ontology	Reader's Digest Universal Dictionary	1083	References
	Operationalization	Baker	479	2.1.3
	Paradigm	Denzin & Lincoln	105	2.36.13
	Philosophy	Reader's Digest Universal Dictionary	1161	References
2.6	Epistemology	Dictionary of Nursing Theory & Research	51	2.2.6
	Human Becoming	Parse	171	2.6.30
	Praxis	Reader's Digest Universal Dictionary	1212	References
	Realism	Schwandt	133	2.2.13
2.7	Facet theory	Breakwell et al.	116	2.1.8
	Taxonomy	Reader's Digest Universal Dictionary	1551	References
	Theoretical [frameworks]	Dictionary of Social Science Methods	112	2.2.8
	Theoretical substruction	McQuiston & Campbell	117	2.7.16
	Theory	Dictionary of Nursing Theory & Research	170	2.2.6
2.8	Applied science	Dictionary of Nursing Theory & Research	157	2.2.6
	Basic science	Dictionary of Nursing Theory & Research	157	2.2.6
	Deductive reasoning	Dictionary of Nursing Theory & Research	64	2.2.6
	Inductive reasoning	Polit & Hungler (1995)	643	References
	Objectivity	Polit & Hungler (1995)	648	References
	Science	Dictionary of Nursing Theory & Research	157	2.2.6
	Scientific method	Williamson	424	References
2.9	Qualitative research	Bryman	94	2.9.4
	Quantitative research	Bryman	94	2.9.4
2.10	Feminist research	Dictionary of Nursing Theory & Research	65	2.2.6
2.11	New paradigm research	Reason & Rowan	Back cover	2.11.9
2.12	Literature review	Phillips, L.R.F.	149	2.95.17
	Systematic review	Droogan & Song	15	2.12.16
2.13	Replication	Williamson	423	References
2.14	Gatekeeper	Oliver	186	2.1.38
	Research protocol	Dictionary of Nursing Theory & Research	131	2.2.6

Section number	Definition	Author(s)	Page in source text	Reference in this volume
2.15	Collaborative research	The New International Webster's Comprehensive Dictionary	257	References
2.17	Anonymity	Baker	473	2.1.3
	Confidentiality	Williamson	416	References
	Covert research	Baker	474	2.1.3
	Deception	Medical Research Council of Canada	26	References
	Ethics	Williamson	418	References
	Informed consent	Dictionary of Nursing Theory & Research	89	2.2.6
	Institutional Review Boards	Polit & Hungler (1995)	643	References
	Research misconduct	Commission on Research Integrity	not known	References
2.18	Problem statement	Polit & Hungler (1995)	650	References
2.19	Construct	Williamson	416–17	References
	Dependent variable	Phillips, L.R.F.	456	2.95.17
	Extraneous variable	Williamson	419	References
	Independent variable	Phillips, L.R.F.	458	2.95.17
	Intervening variable	Baker	477	2.1.3
	Operational definition	Dictionary of Nursing Theory & Research	114	2.2.6
	Variable	Holm & Llewellyn	274	References
2.20	Alternative hypothesis	Dictionary of Nursing Theory & Research	4	2.2.6
	Hypothesis	Dictionary of Social Science Methods	91	2.2.8
	Null hypothesis	Baker	478	2.1.3
	Research objective	Bouma & Atkinson	48	2.1.6
2.21	Research design	Dictionary of Social Science Methods	72	2.2.8
2.22	Cluster sample	Williamson	171	References
	Convenience (accidental) sample	Williamson	171	References
	Population	Williamson	171	References
	Population element	Williamson	171	References
	Population stratum	Williamson	171	References
	Purposive sample	Williamson	172	References
	Quota sample	Williamson	172	References
	Sampling	Dictionary of Nursing Theory & Research	164	2.2.6
	Simple random sample	Williamson	172	References

Section number	Definition	Author(s)	Page in source text	Reference in this volume
	Snowball sample	Williamson	172	References
	Stratified random sample	Williamson	172	References
	Subject	Dictionary of Nursing Theory & Research	164	2.2.6
	Systematic random sample	Williamson	172	References
	Target population	Williamson	171	References
	Universe	Williamson	172	References
2.23	Pilot study	Dictionary of Social Science Methods	97	2.2.8
2.24	Inter-rater-(inter-observer) reliability	Polit & Hungler (1999)	705	References
	Intra-observer (rater) reliability	Litwin	83	2.52.15
	Reliability	Dictionary of Social Science Methods	96	2.2.8
	Split-half reliability	Leininger (1985)	68	References
	Test–retest reliability	Holm & Llewellyn	270	References
2.25	Concurrent validity	Polit & Hungler (1995)	638	References
	Construct validity	Leininger (1985)	69	References
	Content validity	Dictionary of Social Science Methods	21	2.2.8
	Convergent validity	Dictionary of Social Science Methods	23	2.2.8
	Criterion-related validity	Phillips, L.R.F.	454	2.95.17
	External validity	Phillips, L.R.F.	455	2.95.17
	Internal validity	Phillips, L.R.F.	457	2.95.17
	Member validation	Miller & Dingwall	41	2.36.40
	Qualitative validity	Leininger (1985)	68	References
	Predictive validity	Polit & Hungler (1995)	649	References
	Validity	Polit & Hungler (1995)	656	References
2.26	Data triangulation	Denzin & Lincoln	214	2.36.13
	Inter-disciplinary triangulation	Denzin & Lincoln	215	2.36.13
	Investigator triangulation	Denzin & Lincoln	215	2.36.13
	Methodological triangulation	Denzin & Lincoln	215	2.36.13
	Theory triangulation	Denzin & Lincoln	215	2.36.13
	Triangulation	Dictionary of Social Science Methods	102	2.2.8
2.27	Bias	Polit & Hungler (1995)	636	References

Section number	Definition	Author(s)	Page in source text	Reference in this volume
2.28	Generalizability	Dictionary of Social Science Methods	105	2.2.8
2.29	Control group	Phillips, L.R.F.	462	2.95.17
	Double-blind trial	Dictionary of Social Science Methods	34	2.2.8
	Experiment	Holm & Llewellyn	262	References
	Multi-centre trials	Abdellah & Levine	67	3.6.1
	Placebo effect	Dictionary of Social Science Methods	94	2.2.8
	Randomized clinical trial	Abdellah & Levine	76	3.6.1
2.34	Single-case design	Polgar & Thomas	84	References
2.35	Interrupted time-series designs	Woods & Catanzaro	564	References
	Non-equivalent control group	Woods & Catanzaro	564	References
	Quasi-experiment	Woods & Catanzaro	564	References
2.36	Field experiment	Baker	476	2.1.3
	Field notes	Polit & Hungler (1995)	642	References
	Field study	Polit & Hungler (1995)	642	References
	Field work	Dictionary of Nursing Theory & Research	69	2.2.6
	Naturalistic inquiry	Schwandt	101	2.2.13
	Qualitative research	Denzin & Lincoln	2	2.36.13
2.37	Action research	Dictionary of Social Science Methods	119	2.2.8
2.38	Atheoretical research	Phillips, L.R.F.	453	2.95.17
2.39	Case study	Polit & Hungler (1995)	636	References
2.40	Causal comparative	Dictionary of Nursing Theory & Research	20	2.2.6
	Correlational research	Polit & Hungler (1995)	638–9	References
2.41	Case control study	Dictionary of Nursing Theory & Research	17	2.2.6
	Epidemiological research	Dictionary of Nursing Theory & Research	50	2.2.6
2.42	Emic	Dictionary of Nursing Theory & Research	49	2.2.6
	Ethnography	Leininger (1985)	35	References
	Ethnology	Schwandt	44	2.2.13
	Ethnomethodology	Schwandt	44	2.2.13
	Ethnonursing	Leininger (1985)	38	References
	Ethnoscience	Leininger (1985)	237	References
	Ethology	Morse & Field	23	2.36.47
	Etic	Polit & Hungler (1995)	641	References
	Reflexivity	Schwandt	135–6	2.2.13

Section number	Definition	Author(s)	Page in source text	Reference in this volume
2.43	Evaluation research	Polit & Hungler (1995)	641	References
	Evidence-based medicine	Sackett et al.	2	2.43.33
	Outcomes research	Slater	245	2.43.35
2.44	Ex-post facto research	Baker	475	2.1.3
2.45	Dimensional analysis	Kools et al.	314	2.45.10
	Grounded theory	Polit & Hungler (1995)	643	References
	Heuristic research	Dictionary of Nursing Theory & Research	79–80	2.2.6
	Symbolic interaction	Lindlof	40	2.36.31
2.46	Historical research	Woods & Catanzaro	558	References
	Historiography	The New International Webster's Comprehensive Dictionary	599	References
	History	The New International Webster's Comprehensive Dictionary	599	References
2.47	Oral history	Baker	579	2.1.3
2.48	Cohort studies	Baker	474	2.1.3
	Developmental research	Williamson	418	References
	Longitudinal designs	Baker	477	2.1.3
2.49	Phenomenology	Woods & Catanzaro	563	References
2.50	Prescriptive theory	Woods & Catanzaro	563	References
2.51	Role play	The New International Webster's Comprehensive Dictionary	1968	References
	Simulation	The New International Webster's Comprehensive Dictionary	2122	References
2.52	Comparative survey	Treece & Treece	178–81	References
	Cross-cultural survey	Treece & Treece	178–81	References
	Cross-sectional survey	Treece & Treece	178–81	References
	Evaluation survey	Treece & Treece	178–81	References
	Field survey	Treece & Treece	178–81	References
	Long-term/ longitudinal survey	Treece & Treece	178–81	References
	Short-term survey	Treece & Treece	178–81	References
	Survey	Phillips, L.R.F.	464	2.95.17
2.53	Cross-cultural research	Brink	1–5	References

Section number	Definition	Author(s)	Page in source text	Reference in this volume
2.54	Criterion-referenced measures	Woods & Catanzaro	555	References
	Measurement	Woods & Catanzaro	560	References
	Norm-referenced measures	Woods & Catanzaro	562	References
	Outcome measures	Abdellah & Levine	25	3.6.1
2.55	Instrument	Polit & Hungler (1995)	643	References
2.64	Data	Polit & Hungler (1995)	639	References
	Data collection	Polit & Hungler (1995)	639	References
	Data set	Dictionary of Statistics & Methodology	61	2.2.10
	Database	Dictionary of Statistics & Methodology	59	2.2.10
	Primary source	Dictionary of Nursing Theory & Research	130	2.2.6
	Secondary source	Dictionary of Nursing Theory & Research	158	2.2.6
2.65	Critical incident	Flanagan (1954)	327–58	References
	Critical incident technique	Flanagan (1947)	not known	References
2.66	Consensus methods	Jones & Hunter	376	2.66 4
	Delphi technique	Dictionary of Nursing Theory & Research	41	2.2.6
2.67	Diaries	Field & Morse	85	References
2.68	Depth interview	Dictionary of Social Science Methods	62	2.2.8
	Exploratory interview	Dictionary of Social Science Methods	62	2.2.8
	Interview	Dictionary of Social Science Methods	62	2.2.8
	Interview schedule	Baker	477	2.1.3
	Pilot interview	Dictionary of Social Science Methods	62	2.2.8
	Semi-structured interview	Dictionary of Social Science Methods	62	2.2.8
	Standardized/ structured interview	Dictionary of Social Science Methods	62	References
	Transcript	Oliver	190	2.1.38
2.69	Focus group	Baker	476	2.1.3
2.70	Telephone interview	Seaman	433	References
2.71	Biographical method	Denzin (1989)	269	2.7.5
	Interpretive biography	Cresswell	232	2.36.11
	Life history	Polit & Hungler (1995)	645	References
	Self-report	Grady & Wallston	112	2.71.5

Section number	Definition	Author(s)	Page in source text	Reference in this volume
2.72	Non-participant observation	Seaman	434	References
	Observation	Seaman	434	References
	Participant observation	Seaman	434	References
2.73	Projective techniques	Dictionary of Social Science Methods	88	2.2.8
2.74	Q sort	Phillips, L.R.F.	462	2.95.17
2.75	Questionnaire	Holm & Llewellyn	270	References
2.76	Archival research	Baker	473	2.1.3
	Records	Treece & Treece	318	References
2.77	Personal construct	The Penguin Dictionary of Psychology	532	References
	Repertory grid	A Lexicon of Psychology, Psychiatry & Psychoanalysis	298	References
2.78	Conversation	Reader's Digest Universal Dictionary	347	References
	Narrative	The New International Webster's Comprehensive Dictionary	844	References
	Talk	Readers Digest Universal Dictionary	1543	References
2.79	Data analysis	Phillips, L.R.F.	455	2.95.17
	Non-parametric statistics	Portney & Watkins	687	2.29.38
	Parametric statistics	Portney & Watkins	688	2.29.38
	Raw data	Dictionary of Social Science Methods	92	2.2.8
2.81	Descriptive statistics	Dictionary of Social Science Methods	30	2.2.8
2.82	Inferential statistics	Phillips, L.R.F.	459	2.95.17
2.86	Constant comparison	Evidence-based Nursing	Inside back cover	(1998) 1(1) Glossary
	Qualitative analysis	Polit & Hungler (1995)	650	References
	Qualitative metasynthesis	Sandelowski	365–6	2.86.27
2.87	Exploratory data analysis	Dictionary of Nursing Theory & Research	61	2.2.6
	Quantitative data analysis	Polit & Hungler (1995)	651	References
2.88	Content analysis	Polit & Hungler (1995)	638	References
2.89	Contextual analysis	Polit & Hungler (1991)	535	References
	Contextualization	DePoy & Gitlin	296	2.1.22

Section number	Definition	Author(s)	Page in source text	Reference in this volume
	Discourse analysis	Schwandt	31	2.2.13
	Network analysis	Miller & Dingwall	119	2.36.40
	Semiotics	Denzin & Lincoln	466	2.36.13
2.90	Primary data analysis	Woods & Catanzaro	563	References
2.91	Secondary data analysis	Polit & Hungler (1995)	653	References
2.92	Meta-analysis	National Library of Medicine		http://www. nlm.nih. gov/m/ metaanal. htm/
2.95	Evaluating research findings	Phillips, L.R.F.	462	2.95.17
2.96	Research proposal	Abdellah & Levine (1994)	392	References
2.97	Plagiarism	Baker	479	2.1.3
	Research report	Polit & Hungler (1995)	652	References
2.98	Diffusion	Lomas	226–37	References
	Dissemination	Lomas	226–37	References
2.99	Abstract	Polit & Hungler (1995)	635	References
	Refereed journal	Polit & Hungler (1995)	651	References
2.101	Research utilization	Holm & Llewellyn	271	References
2.102	Implementing research findings	Phillips, L.R.F.	465	2.95.17
3.7	Journal club	Polit & Hungler (1995)	644	References
3.8	Research/practice gap	Phillips, L.R.F.	463	2.95.17
3.16	Research assistant	Williamson	423	References
3.18	Research supervisor	Williamson	423–4	References
3.23	Cross-disciplinary research	Epton et al.	9	3.23.3
	Multi- and inter-discplinary research	Epton et al.	9	3.23.3

KEY TO INDEXES

Author Index

Items in this book may be found by using either their individual numbers, as in the author index, or by page number, using the subject index and expanded contents list at the beginning. Items, particularly in Part 1, which have corporate authorship, e.g. bibliographies or directories, are not included individually in this index. They may best be found by consulting the expanded contents list and the individual sections.

In some instances authors have chosen not to use all their initials in works included in this book, and they are therefore treated separately in the index.

Key

*	original article or text
2.38	section number
2.38 eg	example relevant to section
2.38.1	individual item/cross-reference number

Subject Index

Items in this index have been generated from titles of books or articles, with occasional words from annotations for clarification, as titles are not always explicit. Because of the nature of this book it is not intended to be exhaustive so the main pages are featured, rather than each time a word appears in the text. Some entries include complete sections.

[Titles of individual literature reviews are included. A wide range is included in 2.12, with others in specific sections, in order so show a wide range of published reviews].

AUTHOR INDEX

Kilby, S. 1.8.47
Kim, E. 3.1.6
Kim, M.-I. 3.1.7, 3.1.8
Kimchi, J. 2.26.14
King, A. 2.16.16
King, C. 2.11.3
King, C.R. 2.99.32
King, G. 2.36.28
King, J. 2.15.13
King, K.C. 2.100.9
King, K.E. 2.10.19
King, L. 2.5.3
King, T. 2.85 eg
King's Fund Centre 3.4.13
Kingsland, S. 3.2.6, 3.2.7
Kinmonth, A.L. 2.14.39
Kipling, J. 2.16.6
Kipping, C. 2.86.16
Kirby, K.N. 2.84.19
Kirby, R.L. 2.90 eg
Kirby, S. 2.47.14
Kirchhoff, K.T. 2.102.25, 3.7.18,
  3.16.26, 3.16.32
Kirk, J. 2.24.8
Kirk, K. 2.4.5, 3.16.27
Kirkham, S.R. 2.6.42, 2.36.65,
  2.99.33
Kirkpatrick, H. 2.100.5
Kirk-Smith, M. 2.14.27, 2.43.19,
  2.75.10, 2.96 17
Kisilevsky, B.S. 2.101.33
Kitson, A. 2.12.32, 2.61.7, 2.98.10,
  2.101.12, 2.102.24, 3.9.16,
  3.20.14
Kit-Wai, C. 2.43 eg
Kitzinger, J. 2.69.10
Klakovich, M. 2.55.31
Kleiber, C. 2.102.36
Klein, D.F. 2.17.10
Kleinbeck, S.V.M. 2.40 eg
Kleinpell, R.M. 2.14.35, 2.70.9,
  2.86.19
Kleyman, P. 1.8.48
Knafl, K. 2.96.6
Knafl, K.A. 2.26.6, 2.26.15
Knapp, B.G. 2.80.12, 2.83.1
Knapp, T.R. 2.24.9, 2.25.5,
  2.79.14, 2.79.16, 2.80.13, 2.82.1
Knight, S. 2.101.13, 3.7.26, 3.23.7
Knight-Bohnhoff, K. 3.16.28
Koch, T. 2.5.13, 2.12.58, 2.36.29,
  2.43.20, 2.49.12, 2.54.10
Kogan, H. 2.50 eg
Kok, G. 2.17.116
Kokuyama, T. 2.13 eg
Kools, S. 2.45.10
Korenman, S.G. 2.17.3

Korn, K. 1.8.49, 1.8.50, 2.85.6
Korner-Bitensky, N. 2.70.7
Kortenbout, W. 2.69.4
Kory, L. 3.16.28
Koschnitzke, L. 2.14.41
Kosecoff, J. 2.52.18
Kosslyn, S.M. 2.94.4
Koyama, M. 2.43.21
Kozin, F. 2.58.18
Kraemer, L.G. 3.20.9
Kramer, J.J. 2.60.14, 2.60.19
Kramer, M. 2.13.6
Kramer, M.K. 2.7.3
Krantz, D.L. 2.9.12
Krippendorf, K. 2.88.6
Kristjanson, L.J. 2.101 eg
Kritzer, H.M. 2.89.11
Krosnick, J.A. 2.52.32
Krowchuk, H.K. 2.76.4
Krueger, J.C. 2.13.6
Krueger, R.A. 2.69.11, 2.69.16,
  2.69.19, 2.69.20, 2.69.21, 2.69.22
Krulik, T. 3.1.3
Krulwich, T.A. 2.17.4
Krusebrant, Å. 2.102.22
Kuhn, T.S. 2.6.23
Kulp, D. 2.27 cg
Kuzel, A. 2.15.5
Kvale, S. 2.68.18
Kyei, M.B. 3.7.19
Kyle, T.V. 2.12.33

La Schinger, H.K.S. 2.20.2
LaBruzza, A.L. 1.8.51
Lacey, E.A. 2.101.14, 3.17.30
Lackey, N.R. 2.23.2
Lai-Qwan, T. 2.43 cg
Lait, M.E. 2.12.34
Lake, D.G. 2.57.3
Lakeman, R. 2.85.7
Laker, S. 2.12.14
Lamb, G. 2.75.22
Lamb, M. 3.5.29
Lampard, R. 2.22.2
Lanara, V.A. 3.3.8
Lancaster, J. 2.15.10
Lancet 2.22.18, 3.7.20
Land, L. 2.12.35
Land, L.M. 2.69 eg
Landesman, C. 2.6.24
Lane, H. 2.39.4
Lane, S.D. 2.17.71
Lane, V. 2.79.15
Lang, N.M. 2.61.28
Lange, A. 2.55.55
Lange, I. 3.1.9
Lange, L.L. 2.76.7, 2.91.6

Langenbrunner, J.C. 2.92.8
Lars, L. 2.70.6
Larson, E. 2.22.19, 2.101.21, 3.6.4,
  3.17.24
Larsson, G. 2.55.70
Larsson, M. 2.55.70
Lasa, N.B. 2.92.27
Laschinger, H.K.S. 2.24.10,
  2.102.9
Lask, S. 2.11 eg
Lasus, H. 3.17.2
Lathlean, J. 2.17.72, 2.21.2, 2.48
  eg, 3.8.10
Lauffer, A. 3.13.14
Laugharne, C. 2.12.37, 2.42.25
Laurent, D. 2.58.8
Lauri, S. 3.3.9
Lauver, D. 2.79.16
Lauzon, S. 2.6.25
Lavrakas, P.J. 2.70.8
Layder, D. 2.36.30
Layman, E. 3.20.17
Lazega, A. 2.89.12
le Roux, B. 2.22.20
Lea, A. 2.55.68
Leatt, P. 2.21.3
Leddy, S.K. 2.14.28
Lee, P. 2.5.22
Lee, R.M. 2.14.29, 2.16.17,
  2.84.13, 2.84.14
Lee, V.I. 2.34.13
Lee, Y.Y. 2.99.34
Leedy, P.D. 2.1.30
Leeson, J. 2.41.11
LeFort, S.M. 2.87.14
Legat, M. 2.99.35
Leibenluft, E. 3.20.15
Leighton-Beck, L. 3.7.21
Leik, R.K. 2.87.15
Leininger, M. 2.42.26, 2.53.9,
  2.53.10
Leininger, M.M. 2.53.8
Leino-Kilpi, H. 3.3.15
LeLean, S.R. 3.4.14, 3.4.15, 3.4.16
Lenert, L.A. 2.85.14
Lengacher, C.A. 2.55.32
Lenz, E.R. 2.5.11, 2.5.15, 2.54.16,
  3.17.29, 3.17.31
Leong, F.T.L. 2.1.31
Lerheim, K. 2.8.9, 3.3.10, 3.3.11
Leske, J.S. 2.98.16
Leslie, L.A. 2.10.32
Lester, J.D. 2.97.19
Letherby, G. 2.71.18
Letts, L. 2.55.33
Leukefeld, C.G. 3.13.18, 3.13.19
Leung, K. 2.53.17

SUBJECT INDEX

Definitions and their page numbers are shown in **bold type**

Lecture Notes: Oncology

Lecture Notes
Oncology

Mark Bower
Professor of Oncology
Chelsea & Westminster Hospital and
Imperial College School of Medicine
London, UK

Jonathan Waxman
Professor of Oncology
Hammersmith Hospital
Imperial College School of Medicine
London, UK

Second Edition

WILEY-BLACKWELL
A John Wiley & Sons, Ltd., Publication

This edition first published 2010, © 2010 by Mark Bower and Jonathan Waxman
Previous editions: 2006

Blackwell Publishing was acquired by John Wiley & Sons in February 2007. Blackwell's publishing program has been merged with Wiley's global Scientific, Technical and Medical business to form Wiley-Blackwell.

Registered office: John Wiley & Sons Ltd, The Atrium, Southern Gate, Chichester, West Sussex, PO19 8SQ, UK

Editorial offices: 9600 Garsington Road, Oxford, OX4 2DQ, UK
The Atrium, Southern Gate, Chichester, West Sussex, PO19 8SQ, UK
111 River Street, Hoboken, NJ 07030-5774, USA

For details of our global editorial offices, for customer services and for information about how to apply for permission to reuse the copyright material in this book please see our website at www.wiley.com/wiley-blackwell

Library of Congress Cataloging-in-Publication Data

Bower, Mark.
  Lecture notes: Oncology / Mark Bower, Jonathan Waxman. – 2nd ed.
    p. cm.
  Other title: Oncology
  Includes index.
  ISBN 978-1-4051-9513-3 (pbk.)
1. Cancer–Outlines, syllabi, etc.   2. Oncology–Outlines, syllabi, etc.   I. Waxman, Jonathan.   II. Title.
III. Title: Oncology.
  [DNLM: 1. Neoplasms.   QZ 200 B786L 2010]
  RC254.5.B69 2010
  616.99′4–dc22

                                                                                      2010005587

A catalogue record for this book is available from the British Library.

Set in 8 on 12 pt Stone Serif by Toppan Best-set Premedia Limited
Printed in Singapore by Ho Printing Singapore Pte Ltd.

1   2010

Contents

Preface to the second edition

We are delighted that *Lecture Notes: Oncology* has progressed to a second edition, returning by popular demand with an updated format, enormous revisions and a few poor jokes.

The last decade has seen tremendous changes in oncology, with marvellous developments in targeted therapies, based on an understanding of the molecular biology of cancer. We are at a stage in oncology where death rates have fallen in many cancers, and where the survival for patients with metastatic disease has, in many instances, doubled. Cancer doctors used to proudly talk about curing a small minority of tumours such as lymphoma, leukaemia, choriocarcinoma and testicular cancer, but currently this shortlist of survivable cancers has increased, providing optimism in oncologists and delight in patients.

Oncology involves an understanding of the processes that lead to the development of malignant disease, and this understanding has led Medicine by its nose to the frontiers of science. These are exhilarating times to be an oncologist and we hope that the reader of this book enjoys our efforts to convey our excitement in oncology.

Mark Bower
Jonathan Waxman

Part 1

Introduction to Oncology

Chapter 1

What is cancer?

Cancer is not a single illness but a collection of many diseases that share common features. Cancer is widely viewed as a disease of genetic origin. It is caused by mutations of DNA and epigenetic changes that alter gene expression, which make a cell multiply uncontrollably. However, the description and definitions of cancer vary depending on the perspective as described below.

Epidemiological perspective

Cancer is a major cause of morbidity in the United Kingdom with around 289000 new cases diagnosed in 2005. There are more than 200 different types of cancer, but four of them (breast, lung, colorectal and prostate) account for over half of all new cases. Overall it is estimated that one in three people will develop some form of cancer during their lifetime. In the 30-year period 1976–2005 the overall age-standardized incidence rates for cancer increased by 35% in men and 16% in women but have remained fairly constant over the last decade (1996–2005). The cancers whose incidence is rising fastest in men are malignant melanoma, mesothelioma, prostate cancer and hepatocellular cancer, while in women they are mesothelioma, melanoma, endometrial cancer and oral cancer.

Cancer incidence refers to the number of new cancer cases arising in a specified period of time. Prevalence refers to the number of people who have received a diagnosis of cancer who are alive at any given time, some of whom will be cured and others will not. Therefore prevalence reflects both the incidence of cancer and its associated survival pattern. In 2008 approximately 3% of the population of the UK (around two million people) are alive having received a diagnosis of cancer. The single cancer that contributes most to the prevalence is breast cancer, with an estimated 550000 women alive who have had a diagnosis of breast cancer.

Sociological perspective

Patients with cancer adopt a medically sanctioned form of deviant behaviour described in the 1950s by Talcott Parsons as 'the sick role'. In order to be excused their usual duties and to not be considered responsible for their illness, patients are expected to seek professional advice and to adhere to treatments in order to get well. Medical practitioners are empowered to sanction their temporary absence from the workforce and family duties as well as to absolve them of blame. This behavioural model minimizes the impact of illness on society and reduces the secondary gain that the patient benefits from as a consequence of their illness. However, as Ivan Illich pointed out it also sets up physicians as agents of social control by

Lecture Notes: Oncology, 2nd edition. By M. Bower and J. Waxman. Published 2010 by Blackwell Publishing Ltd.

Table 1.1 The top cancer books (in the authors' opinion).

	Title	Author
1	Cancer Ward	Alexander Solzhenitsyn
2	A Very Easy Death	Simone de Beauvoir
3	Age of Iron	J. M. Coetzee
4	Cancer Vixen	Marisa Acocella Marchetto
5	One in Three	Adam Wishart
6	C: Because Cowards get Cancer, Too	John Diamond
7	Before I Say Goodbye	Ruth Picardie
8	Illness as Metaphor	Susan Sontag
9	The Black swan	Thomas Mann
10	Mom's Cancer	Brian Fies
11	Coda	Simon Gray
12	Cancer Tales	Nell Dunn

medicalizing health and contributing to iatrogenic illness – 'a medical nemesis'. Of all the common medical diagnoses, cancer probably carries the greatest stigma and is associated with the most fear. The many different ways in which cancer affects people has been explored in literature (Table 1.1).

Experimental perspective

In the laboratory, a number of characteristics define a cancer cell growing in culture. The four features listed below are used by scientists experimentally to confirm the malignant phenotype of cancer cells:

1. Cancer cells are clonal, having all derived from a single parent cell.
2. Cancer cells grow on soft agar, in the absence of growth factors.
3. Cancer cells cross artificial membranes in culture systems.
4. Cancer cells form tumours if injected into immunodeficient strains of mice (Box 1.1).

Histopathological perspective

Cancer is usually defined by various histopathological features, most notably invasion and metastasis, that are observed by gross pathological and microscopic examinations. Laminin staining of

Box 1.1: Onco-mice

Mice have been used as a laboratory model in cancer research for a century. In the 1930s, Sir Ernest Kennaway showed that polycyclic aromatic hydrocarbons were carcinogenic by inducing skin cancers in mice. In 1969 the first inbred mice were developed that were essentially genetically identical except for gender. These strains allowed the transfer of cells and tissues between mice without rejection as they are syngeneic (genetically identical). This has allowed the effects of experimental treatments on murine cancers to be evaluated in laboratory mice. Some inbred strains also spontaneously develop cancers (e.g. BALB/c mice frequently develop lung tumours) so that the effects of cancer prevention strategies can be studied. The development of immunodeficient mice allowed the transfer and study of human cancer cells in mice without the mice rejecting the xenograft (graft between different species). The first immunodeficient mice were 'nude mice', an inbred strain that lacks a thymus gland and T lymphocytes; they are hairless because of a mutation in a linked genetic locus. Subsequently, in 1983, even more immunodeficient SCID (severe combined immunodeficiency) mice were developed that lack both T and B cells. Genetically modified transgenic mice have been manufactured by knocking out specific genes ('knockout mice') or adding extra trans-genes, usually from different species ('transgenic mice'), to embryonic stem cells. These mice are used to elucidate the influence of individual genes on the phenotype. Finally, mice were the original source of monoclonal antibodies produced by immunizing inbred mice with the desired antigen and fusing spleen cells from the mouse with myeloma cells to yield hybridoma cells that produce monoclonal antibodies.

the basement membrane may assist the histopathologist in identifying local invasion by tumours that breach the basement membrane. In addition a number of microscopic features point to the diagnosis of cancer:

● Cancer cells differ morphologically from normal cells

● Tumour architecture is less organized than that of the parent tissue

● Cancer cells have increased nuclear DNA and nuclear:cytoplasmic ratio

● Cancer cells have hyperchromatic nuclei with coarsening of chromatin and wrinkled nuclear edges

- Cancer cells may be multinucleated or have macronucleoli
- Cancer cells may have numerous and bizarre mitotic figures

Cancers may be heterogenous with cells of varying sizes and orientation with respect to one another despite their clonal origin.

Molecular perspective

The molecular features that identify a cancer are described in 'Six steps to becoming a cancer' in Chapter 2. These six properties are:

1. Grow without a trigger (self-sufficiency in growth stimuli).
2. Don't stop growing (insensitivity to inhibitory stimuli).
3. Don't die (evasion of apoptosis).
4. Don't age (immortalization).
5. Feed themselves (neoangiogenesis).
6. Spread (invasion and metastasis).

How to read a histology report

The diagnosis of cancer is most commonly established following a histopathological report of a biopsy or tumour resection. A histopathological report should include both gross pathological features (tumour size and number and size of lymph nodes examined) and microscopic findings (tumour grade, architecture, mitotic rate, margin involvement and lymphovascular invasion). The grade and stage of a cancer are important prognostic factors that may influence therapy options (Box 1.2).

Box 1.2: Histopathology definitions

Quantitative changes: too small

Atrophy
Acquired shrinkage due to a decrease in the *size or number* of cells of a tissue, e.g. decrease in size of the ovaries after the menopause.

Quantitative changes: too big

Hypertrophy
Increase in the size of an organ or tissue due to an increase in the *size* of individual cells, e.g. pregnant uterus.

Hyperplasia
Increase in the *size* of an organ due to an increase in the *number* of cells, e.g. lactating breast.

Qualitative changes

Metaplasia
Replacement of one cell type in an organ by another. This implies changes in the differentiation programme and is usually a response to persistent injury. It is reversible so that removal of the source of injury results in reversion to the original cell type, e.g. squamous metaplasia of laryngeal respiratory epithelium in a smoker. Chronic irritation from smoking causes the normal columnar respiratory epithelium to be replaced by the more resilient squamous epithelium.

Dysplasia
Dysplastic changes are changes in cell type, as for metaplasia, that do not revert to normal once the injury is removed, e.g. cervical dysplasia initiated by human papillomavirus infection persists after eradication of the virus. Dysplasia is usually considered to be part of the spectrum of changes leading to neoplasia.

Invasion
The capacity to infiltrate the surrounding tissues and organs is a characteristic of cancer.

Metastasis
The ability to proliferate in distant parts of the body after tumour cells have been transported by lymph or blood or along body spaces.

Table 1.2 Histological features of benign and malignant tumours.

Features of malignancy	Features of benign tumours
Macroscopic features	
Invade and metastasize	Do not invade or metastasize
Rapid growth	Slow growing
Not clearly demarcated	Clearly demarcated from surrounding tissue
Surface often ulcerated and necrotic	Surface smooth
Cut surface heterogenous	Cut surface homogenous
Microscopic features	
Often high mitotic rate	Low mitotic rate
Nuclei pleomorphic and hyperchromatic	Nuclear morphology often normal
Abnormal mitoses	Mitotic figures normal

A histopathological definition of cancer: is it malignant or benign?

Malignancy is usually characterized by various behavioural features, most notably invasion and metastasis. However, the histopathologist may have to identify a cancer without this information. Cancers are composed of clonal cells (all are the progeny of a single cell) and have lost control of their tissue organization and architecture. In addition to the natural history, a number of physical properties help to distinguish between benign and malignant tumours (Table 1.2). However, there is no single histological feature that defines a cancer nor indeed that separates benign from malignant tumours. In general, benign tumours are rarely life-threatening but may cause health problems on account of their location (by pressure or obstruction of adjacent organs) or by overproduction of hormones. In contrast malignant tumours usually follow a progressive course and unless successfully treated are frequently fatal.

Is it *in situ* or invasive?

Invasive cancers extend into the surrounding stroma (see Plate 1.1). However tumours that exhibit all the microscopic features of cancers but do not breach the original basement membrane are termed *in situ* (non-invasive) cancers. Examples include *in situ* breast cancer confined to the mammary ducts (ductal carcinoma *in situ* or DCIS) or lobules (lobular carcinoma *in situ* or LCIS) (see Plate 1.2). Similar pre-invasive *in situ* cancers have been found in many organs (e.g. cervix, anus, prostate, bronchus) and are believed to represent a stage in the progression from dysplasia to cancer (see Plate 1.3).

Histopathologist's nomenclature: name that cancer

The histopathologists' lexicon often can be a tool for obfuscation, but follow a few simple rules and you can translate their lingo. The suffix -oma usually denotes a benign tumour (although it simply means 'swelling' and some -omas are not tumours, e.g. xanthoma). If a tumour is malignant the suffix -carcinoma (Greek for crab) is used for epithleial cancers or -sarcoma (Greek for flesh) for connective tissue cancers. The prefix is determined by the cells of origin of the tumour (e.g. adeno- for glandular epithelium), qualified by the tissue of origin (e.g. prostatic adenocarcinoma). There are numerous exceptions to this systematic nomenclature; for example leukaemias and lymphomas are malignant tumours of bone marrow and lymphoid tissue, respectively. As a general rule neoplasms are classified according to the type of normal tissue they most closely resemble. The four major categories are: epithelial, connective tissue, lymphoid and haemopoietic tissue, and germ cells (Tables 1.3–1.6). The latter arise in totipotential cells, and can develop into any cell type. Germ cell tumours contain a variety of different mature and/or immature tissues from different embryonic germ layers, and these are given names with the root terato- (Greek for monster). In addition, as with most fields of medicine where physicians try to leave their mark, there are a number of eponymous names (e.g. Hodgkin's disease). (Thomas Hodgkin (of Guy's Hospital) described seven cases in 1832 of the tumour that bears his name but re-examination in 1926 revealed that the diagnosis was inaccurate in four of the seven cases.)

Table 1.3 Nomenclature of epithelial tumours.

Epithelium	Benign tumour	Malignant tumour
Squamous	Squamous papilloma	Squamous carcinoma
Glandular	Adenoma	Adenocarcinoma
Transitional	Transitional papilloma	Transitional carcinoma
Liver	Hepatic adenoma	Hepatocellular carcinoma
Skin	Papilloma	Squamous cell carcinoma
		Basal cell carcinoma
Skin melanocyte	Naevus	Malignant melanoma

Table 1.4 Nomenclature of connective tissue tumours.

Tissue	Benign tumour	Malignant tumour
Bone	Osteoma	Osteosarcoma
Cartilage	Chondroma	Chondrosarcoma
Fat	Lipoma	Liposarcoma
Smooth muscle	Leiomyoma	Leiomyosarcoma
Striated muscle	Rhabdomyoma	Rhabdomyosarcoma
Blood vessel	Angioma	Angiosarcoma
Fibrous tissue	Fibroma	Fibrosarcoma

Table 1.5 Nomenclature of haematological tumours.

Tissue	Malignant tumour
Node lymphocyte	Lymphoma
Marrow lymphocyte	Lymphocytic leukaemia
Granulocyte	Myeloid leukaemia
Plasma cell	Myeloma

Table 1.6 Nomenclature of germ cell tumours.

Tissue	Benign tumour	Malignant tumour (male)	Malignant tumour (female)
Germ cell	Mature teratoma/dermoid cyst	Non-seminomatous germ cell tumour/malignant teratoma	Immature teratoma/embryonal carcinoma
	–	Seminoma	Dysgerminoma

Tumour grading

Tumours are graded according to the degree of tissue differentiation. Cancers that closely resemble their tissue of origin are graded as well differentiated cancers. Cancers that look nothing like the original tissue and have histological features of aggressive growth with high mitotic rates are graded as poorly differentiated cancers. The grade of a tumour is of prognostic significance.

In the case of breast cancer, the Scarff–Bloom–Richardson system is usually used to grade cancers based upon three features: the frequency of cell mitosis, tubule formation, and nuclear pleomorphism. Each of these features is assigned a score ranging from 1 to 3 (1 indicating slower cell growth and 3 indicating faster cell growth). The scores of each of the cells' features are then added together for a final sum that will range between 3 and 9. A tumour with a final sum of 3, 4 or 5 is considered a grade 1 tumour (well differentiated). A sum of 6 or 7 is considered a grade 2 tumour (moderately differentiated), and a sum of 8 or 9 is a grade 3 tumour (poorly differentiated). The five-year overall survival for grades 1, 2 and 3 are 95%, 75% and 50%, respectively.

In addition, pathologists may identify other features that relate to the natural behaviour of a tumour, such as lymphovascular invasion, which usually denotes a worse prognosis. The molecular properties of a cancer can also influence the biology, prognosis and treatment of a tumour. For example, the gene expression prolife of a breast cancer may be determined by gene expression microarray chip technology and the results assist clinicians in optimizing adjuvant therapy (see Plate 1.4).

Unknown primary identification (standard histological techniques)

Occasionally patients present with metastatic cancer without an obvious primary tumour site and, in addition to a careful clinical and radiological examination, the pathologist may provide a clue to the origins of the cancer. Most unknown primary cancers are adenocarcinoma (60%), and the remainder are poorly differentiated carcinomas (30%) and squamous cell carcinomas (5%). Light microscopy may provide pointers, for example the presence of melanin pigment favours melanoma, whilst mucin production is common in gastrointestinal, breast and lung cancers but less common in ovarian cancers and is rare in renal cell and thyroid cancers. Immunocytochemical staining of tissue samples can aid the pathologist in tissue identification. For example, the presence of oestrogen and progesterone receptors favours a diagnosis of breast cancer, whilst prostate-specific antigen and prostatic acid phosphatase staining points to prostatic adenocarcinoma. Similarly, cytokeratin expression patterns may provide helpful hints about the origin of metastatic cancers (Box 1.3 and see Plate 1.5). Cell surface immunophenotyping is a sophistication of immunocytochemistry that is frequently applied to haematological malignancies. The pattern of immunoglobulin, T-cell receptor and cluster designation (CD) antigen expression on the surface of lymphomas is helpful in their diagnosis and classification. Immunophenotyping can be achieved by immunohistochemical staining, immunofluorescent staining or flow cytometry.

Unknown primary identification (special histological techniques)

The study of intracellular organelles by electron microscopy may identify the cellular origin of a tumour; for example, the presence of melanosomes in melanomas and dense core neurosecretory granules in neuroendodermal tumours. Further laboratory techniques to aid diagnosis include molecular studies of DNA rearrangements that characterize malignancies. Monoclonal immunoglobulin gene rearrangements are present in B-cell malignancies and rearrangements of T-cell receptors occur in T-cell tumours. In addition, a number of chromosomal translocations involving the immunoglobulin genes (heavy chain on chromosome 14q32, light chains on 2p12 and 22q11) and T-cell receptor genes (TCRα on 14q11, TCRβ on 7q35, TCRγ on 7p15, TCRδ on 14q11) occur in malignancies arising from these cell types. For instance, low-grade follicular lymphomas rearrange the Bcl-2 gene on 18q21 (e.g. t(14;18) (q32;q21)), most Burkitt lymphomas rearrange the Myc gene on 8q24 (e.g. t(8;14)(q24;q32)) and most mantle cell lymphomas rearrange Bcl-1 on 11q13 (e.g. t(11;14)(q13;q32)). These rearrangements may be detected by karyotype analysis of mitotic chromosome preparations or by molecular techniques including Southern blotting and polymerase chain reaction (Box 1.4 and Table 1.7). Less commonly these same methods may assist the diagnosis of solid tumours that are associated with specific chromosomal abnormalities such as the i(12p) isochromosome found in germ cell tumours and the t(11;22)(q24;q12) translocation seen in Ewing's sarcoma and peripheral neuroectodermal tumours. In addition to translocations, gene amplification may be detected and may have prognostic

---

Box 1.3: Cytokeratins

Cytokeratins are intermediate filament proteins expressed in pairs comprising a type I (cytokeratins 9–20) and a type II (cytokeratins 1–8) cytokeratin. Different tissues express different pairs and immunocytochemical staining for cytokeratins can help identify the likely tissue origins of cancers cells. For example in disseminated peritoneal metastases, CK7 expression favours an ovarian origin, whilst lack of CK7 is more common in colorectal cancer (Figure 1.3).

Box 1.4: The language of chromosomes – karyotype nomenclature

Each arm of a chromosome is divided into one to four major regions, depending on chromosomal length; each band, positively or negatively stained, is given a number, which rises as the distance from the centromere increases. The normal male is designated as 46,XY and the normal female as 46,XX.

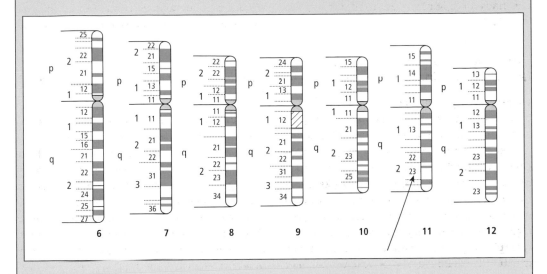

For example, 11q23 designates the chromosome (11), the long arm (q), the second region distal to the centromere (2) and the third band (3) in that region.

Polyploid
Cell with more than one complete chromosome set or with multiples of the basic number of chromosomes characteristic of the species; in humans this would be 69,92, etc.

Aneuploid
Individual with one or more chromosomes in addition or missing from the complete chromosome set; for example trisomy 21 (47,XX +21).

Deletion
The loss of a chromosome segment from a normal chromosome.

Duplication
An extra piece of chromosome segment which may be attached to the same homologous chromosome or transposed to another chromosome in the genome.

Inversion
A change in linear sequence of the genes in a chromosome that results in the reverse order of genes in a chromosome segment. Inversions may be pericentric (two breaks on either side of the centromere) or paracentric (both breaks on the same arm).

Isochromosome
breaks in one arm of a chromosome followed by duplication of the other arm of the chromosome to produce a chromosome with two arms that are both short (p) or both long (q) arms.

Translocations
Translocations are the result of the reciprocal exchange of terminal segments of non-homologous chromosomes.

Table 1.7 Examples of chromosomal abnormalities in cancers.

Chromosome defect	Karyotype	Tumour	Candidate gene
Monosomy	45,XY −22	Meningioma	NF2
Trisomy	47,XX +7	Papillary renal carcinoma	MET
Deletion	46,XY del(11)(p13)	Wilms' tumour	WT1
Duplication	46,XX dup(2)(p23-24)	Neuroblastoma	n-Myc
Inversion	46,XY inv(16)(p13q22)	Acute myeloid leukaemia (M4Eo)	MYH11/core-binding factor b
Isochromosome	47,XX i(12p)	Testicular germ cell tumour	
Translocation	46,XX t(9;22)(q34;q11)	Chronic myeloid leukaemia	bcr/abl

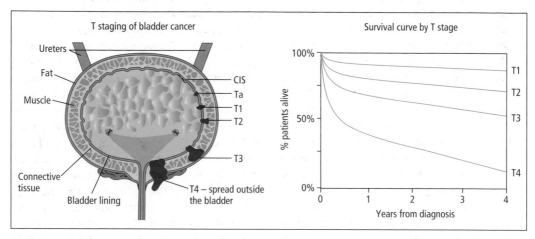

Figure 1.1 T-stage classification for bladder cancer and influence on survival. CIS, carcinoma *in situ*.

significance, e.g. the amplification of the n-Myc oncogene in neuroblastoma is an adverse prognostic variable.

How to stage a tumour

In addition to the histological grade of a tumour, an important criterion in treatment decisions and the major determinant of outcome is the extent of spread or stage of a cancer (Figure 1.1). Staging a tumour is essentially an anatomical exercise that uses a combination of clinical examination and radiology. A uniform staging system is employed for most tumour sites that is based upon the size of the primary **T**umour, the presence of regional lymph **N**odes and of distant **M**etastases. The details of this **TNM** classification vary between different

tumour sites. As always there are exceptions, including the staging system for lymphomas that was originally set out following a conference at the University of Michigan in Ann Arbour. It is known as the Ann Arbour Staging System and most radiologists assume that it is named after a person rather than a town, so this is a chance to score points at the X-ray meetings.

Radiology techniques

Staging depends to a large extent upon radiology and this is the most commonly used tool to evaluate the response of cancers to therapies. Anatomical imaging by plain films, computed tomography (CT), ultrasound and magnetic resonance imaging (MRI) are the standard methods. Using the correct terms impresses other clinicians and may make a trip to the radiology department less daunting for junior doctors requensting an investigation. X-rays measure radiodensity (radiolucency and radio-opacity) and ultrasound measures echogenicity and echoreflectivity, whilst CT scans report attenuation values measured in Hounsfield units and MRI reports signal intensity.

Computed tomography

CT scanning is the production of three-dimensional images using X-rays that have been directed through tissues and the images produced depend on the density of the tissues. CT was developed in the 1970s by Sir Godfrey Hounsfield and Allan McLeod Cormack who shared the Nobel Prize in 1979. The first CT scanner built at EMI Central Research Laboratories is said to have been funded by the success of the Beatles who were signed to the EMI label. CT measures the attenuation of different tissues to ionizing radiation and calculates a mean value for a volume of tissue known as a voxel. This is displayed on a two-dimensional image as a single pixel. The attenuation is calculated relative to water which has a Hounsfield unit (HU) value of 0, so high attenutation tissues have a positive HU value (e.g. bone +400 HU) and low attenuation tissues a negative HU value (e.g. fat −120 HU). Different window settings are used to look at different ranges of the Hounsfield greyscale. For example, in the bone windows setting the lungs will look uniformly black whilst in the lung windows the bones look uniformly white. Intravenous iodinated contrast agents improve the sensitivity and specificity of CT but are contraindicated in patients with asthma or allergies to contrast.

Magnetic resonance imaging

Unlike CT, MRI does not use ionizing radiation but instead a powerful magnetic field aligns the spin of protons, especially hydrogen atom protons, in water and fat. A radiofrequency pulse then energizes the protons and the gradual release of this energy from the protons as they relax back to their original magnetic alignment may be detected as radiofrequency signals. The signal intensity relates to the concentration of mobile hydrogen nuclei in tissues. T1 (longitudinal relaxation or spin-lattice) and T2 (transverse relaxation or spin-spin) relaxation time constants depend on the physical properties of the tissues. If you want to impress the neuroradiologists (not always a useful ploy in the authors' experience), water such as cerebrospinal fluid (CSF) is black (low signal intensity) on T1 images and white (high signal intensity) on T2 images (Figure 1.2). Whilst CT is a good tool to examine tissues composed of high atomic weight elements such as bone, MRI is better suited to non-calcified tissues. For similar reasons CT contrast agents usually are composed of high atomic number atoms such as iodine or barium, whilst MRI contrast agents such as gadolinium are paramagnets that have magnetic properties only in the presence of an externally applied magnetic field. MRI is generally superior for imaging the brain, whilst CT is better for solid tumours of the chest and abdomen as it is faster and generates fewer motion artifacts. MRI is also better suited to patients who may require many examinations because it does not carry the risks of ionizing radiation. MRI is, however, contraindicated in patients with metallic objects such as pacemakers *in situ* and it is also quite claustrophobic and noisy in the scanner.

Positron emission tomography

Positron emission tomography (PET) is a functional imaging modality that detects γ-rays emitted by positrons (positively charged electrons) emitting radionuclide tracers. Positrons have a short half-life and are generated by cyclotrons. Common positron-labelled radionuclides include fluorine (^{18}F), carbon (^{11}C), oxygen (^{15}O) and nitrogen (^{13}N). In oncology the most frequently used tracer is ^{18}F-fluorodeoxyglucose (FDG), a short half-life glucose analogue that is taken up into actively metabolizing cells including cancer cells and following intracellular phosphorylation is trapped in these cells. Hence the distribution in the body of

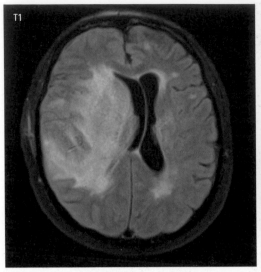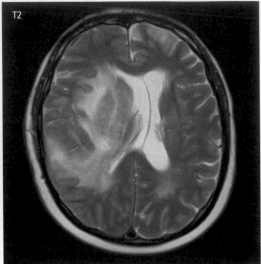

Figure 1.2 T1 and T2 MRI scan images of a primary cerebral lymphoma mass, showing a large right basal ganglia lesion with midline shift, compression of the right lateral ventricle and peritumoral oedema. In the T1 image the CSF is black (low attenuation) and the bone is white (high attenuation), whilst in the T2 image the CSF is white (high attenuation) and the bone is black (low attenuation).

FDG reflects glucose uptake within the body. This means that PET scanning may differentiate between residual masses and active disease in lymphoma. As a consequence FDG-PET scanning is used in both staging and monitoring cancer treatment (Figure 1.3 and see Plate 1.6).

Radio-isotope scanning

In addition to PET scanning other functional images may be used in the diagnosis and staging of specific cancers, using isotope-labelled radionuclide tracer elements (Table 1.8 and Figure 1.4). The isotope-labelled tracers that are used diagnostically may also be used therapeutically. Bone scintigraphy uses bisphosphonates labelled with ^{99}Tc and is more sensitive than X-rays for detecting metastases.

Performance status

In addition to the histological grade and the stage of a cancer, the general health of patients will determine how long they survive and may influence treatment decisions. Scales that measure the performance status or functional capacity of patients include the ECOG (Eastern Co-operative Oncology Group) grading system and the Karnovsky scale (Table 1.9). The performance status, however estimated, is an important prognostic indicator for almost all tumour types.

Prognosis: it's not cancer is it doc?

Although a very significant stigma is attached to the diagnosis of cancer, for most of the general population the fear outweighs the reality and comparison with other more palatable illnesses yield results that are not always expected (Table 1.10).

Cancer epidemiology

Epidemiology in UK

Cancer is now the commonest cause of death in the UK (if cardiovascular and cerebrovascular diseases are classed separately).
- One in three people in the UK will develop a cancer (289 000/year)
- One in four die of cancer (150 000/year).

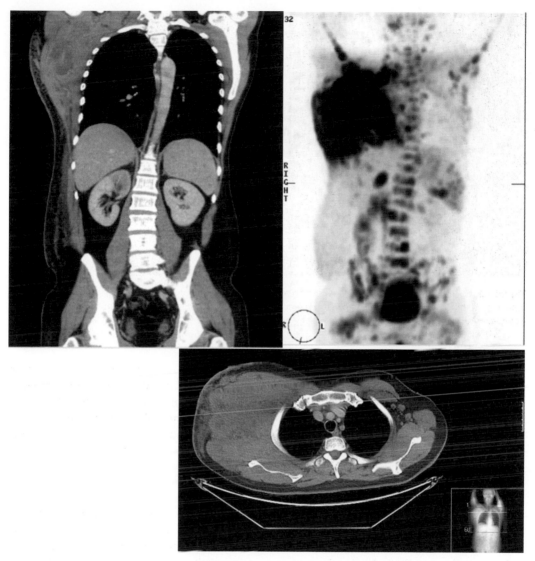

Figure 1.3 Coronal CT (top left), transverse CT (below) and FDG-PET (top right) scans demonstrating a huge right axillary and anterior chest wall mass due to Burkitt lymphoma. The FDG-PET also demonstrates extensive involvement of the other nodal groups, bones and right kidney upper pole (stage 4B).

Table 1.8 Commonly used isotopes in nuclear imaging in oncology.

Isotope	Half-life	Tracer	Oncological use
^{99}Tc (technetium)	6 hours	Methylene diphosphonate (MDP)	Bone scan
^{111}In (indium)	67 hours	Octreotide	Neuroendocrine tumours
^{131}I (iodine)	8 days	Sodium iodide	Thyroid cancer
^{131}I (iodine)	8 days	Meta-iodobenzylguanidine (MIBG)	Phaeochromocytoma neuroblastoma
^{67}Ga (gallium)	68 hours	Gallium citrate	Lymphoma

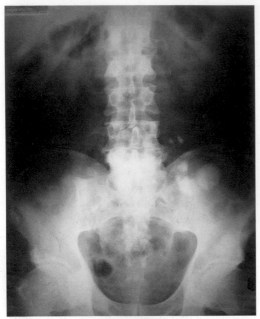

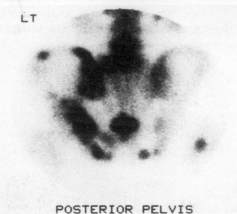

POSTERIOR PELVIS

Figure 1.4 Plain pelvic radiograph (above) and corresponding area of technetium pyrophosphate bone scan (below) of a patient with sclerotic bone metastases from prostate cancer.

The top ten cancers diagnosed in the UK excluding non-melanomatous skin cancers are shown in Table 1.11.

Global epidemiology

The incidence of different types of cancer varies geographically according to the risk factors and demographics of the local population (Figure 1.5). However, there is a general correlation between

Table 1.9 Functional capacity grading (ECOG) and Karnovsky performance scales.

ECOG functional capacity grading	
0	Asymptomatic
1	Symptomatic but fully ambulant
2	Symptomatic, ambulant >50% waking hours
3	Symptomatic, confined to bed >50% waking hours
4	Symptomatic, bedfast

Karnovsky performance status score (%)	
100	Normal; no complaints; no evidence of disease
90	Able to carry on normal activity; minor signs or symptoms
80	Normal activity with effort; some signs or symptoms
70	Care for self; unable to carry on normal activity or do active work
60	Requires occasional assistance, but able to care for most of needs
50	Requires considerable assistance and frequent medical care
40	Disabled; requires special care and assistance
30	Severely disabled; hospitalization indicated but death not imminent
20	Very sick; hospitalization necessary; active supportive treatment necessary
10	Moribund; fatal processes progressing rapidly

Table 1.10 Survival rates for various diseases.

	Myocardial infarction	Hodgkin's disease	Heart failure (NYHA III/IV)	Metastatic breast cancer
1-year survival rate	75%	90%	50%	60%
5-year survival rate	45%	85%	15%	20%

NYHA, New York Heart Association grading scale.

increasing wealth and increasing cancer incidence. This is attributable to tobacco use, diet and increased longevity in wealthy populations. There are intriguing exceptions, for example the Gulf states of Kuwait, Qatar, Bahrain, United Arab Emirates and Saudi Arabia have lower cancer incidences

Table 1.11 The 12 most common cancers diagnosed in UK.

Tumour	As percentage of all cancers diagnosed
Breast	15%
Lung	13%
Colorectal	13%
Prostate	12%
Non-Hodgkin's lymphoma	3.6%
Bladder	3.5%
Melanoma	3.3%
Stomach	2.7%
Oesophageal	2.7%
Pancreas	2.6%
Kidney	2.5%
Leukaemia	2.5%

than would be predicted from their per capita gross national product.

Cancer charities

Cancer charities

The UK has 640 cancer charities to counter the disease. Their expenditure increases awareness of cancer, improves diagnosis and treatment capability, and provides care for patients with the disease. The total income generated by the top 20 UK cancer charities in 2004 was £758m, and the average charitable efficiency was 64% providing £488m for spending on patients' care and research. The two largest UK cancer charities, the Imperial Cancer Research Fund (ICRF) and the Cancer Research Campaign (CRC) merged to form Cancer Research UK (CRUK) in 2002. CRUK is the largest volunteer-supported cancer research organization in the world, with 3000 scientists and an annual scientific spend of more than £339 million – raised almost entirely through public donations.

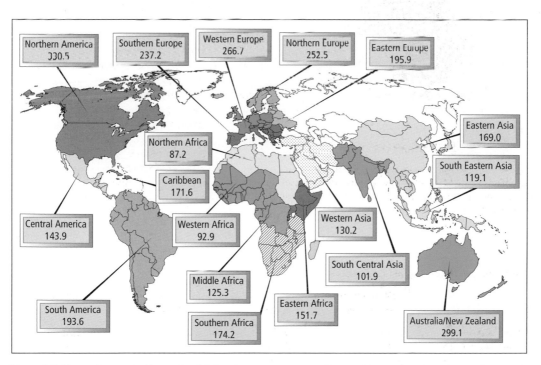

Figure 1.5 Figure of cancer incidences by global region.

Table 1.12 Rock star cancer deaths.

	Year of death	Age	Cause of death
Richard Wright (Pink Floyd)	2008	65	Cancer (type undisclosed)
Eartha Kitt	2008	81	Colon cancer
Johnny Ramone	2004	55	Prostate cancer
Little Eva	2003	60	Cervical cancer
George Harrison	2001	58	Non-small cell lung cancer
Joey Ramone	2001	49	Non-Hodgkin's lymphoma
Ian Dury	2000	58	Colorectal cancer
Dusty Springfield	1999	60	Breast cancer
Carl Wilson (Beach Boys)	1998	52	Lung cancer
Eva Cassidy	1996	33	Melanoma
Frank Zappa	1993	53	Prostate cancer
Freddy Mercury	1991	45	Kaposi's sarcoma
Mel Appleby (Mel & Kim)	1990	24	Spinal tumour
Bob Marley	1981	36	Melanoma

Cancer hospitals

Philanthropists and social reformers during the 19th century tried to provide free medical care for the poor. William Marsden, a young surgeon opened a dispensary for advice and medicines in 1828. His grandly named London General Institution for the Gratuitous Cure of Malignant Diseases – a simple four-storey house in one of the poorest parts of the city – was conceived as a hospital to which the only passport should be poverty and disease and where treatment was provided free of charge. The demand for Marsden's free services was overwhelming and by 1844 his dispensary, now called the Royal Free Hospital, was treating 30 000 patients a year. In 1846 when his wife died of cancer, Marsden opened a small house in Cannon Row, Westminster, for patients suffering from cancer. Within 10 years the institution moved to Fulham Road and became known as the Cancer Hospital, of which Marsden was the senior surgeon. The hospital was incorporated into the National Health Service in 1948 and renamed the Royal Marsden Hospital in 1954. Although other cancer hospitals have been established in Manchester (the Christie Hospital) and Glasgow (the Beatson Hospital), the Royal Marsden Hospital remains the most renown. With the recent emphasis on multidisciplinary approaches to cancer, single specialty hospitals are less in vogue and the majority of cancer departments are within large teaching hospitals.

Cancer celebrities

Celebrities influence public perceptions and behaviour inordinately and this is as true in oncology as elsewhere. Celebrities with cancer have contributed in three main ways: personal accounts bring patients' experiences into the limelight, reports of celebrity patients increase public awareness and may encourage health-seeking behaviour such as stopping smoking, and celebrity patients may support cancer charities and encourage donations. Prominent examples of patient's perspectives include John Diamond's account in *C: Because Cowards get Cancer, Too* and Ruth Picardie's *Before I Say Goodbye*, both moving accounts by accomplished journalists. Celebrity patients can influence the treatment choices that the public make. Following Nancy Reagan's mastectomy for localized breast cancer in 1987, there was a 25% fall in American women choosing breast-conserving surgery over mastectomy. Her husband's successful surgery for Dukes' B colon cancer whilst president in 1984 increased awareness and propelled the warning signs of colon cancer into the media. Similarly, the diagnosis and death from cervical cancer in 2009 of Jade Goody, a *Big Brother* celebrity, led to an increased uptake of cervical cancer screening especially amongst young women in the UK. Successful cancer treatment is often most widely publicized and no article describing Lance Armstrong's seven consecutive Tour de France cycling victories is complete without a mention of his treatment for metastatic non-seminomatous germ cell tumour and his two children conceived with stored sperm banked prior to chemotherapy.

Other celebrity patients have used their wealth and fame to establish and support charitable projects to support cancer research and treatment including Bob Champion, the steeple chase jockey treated for testicular cancer in the 1979, and Roy Castle, a lifelong non-smoker who was diagnosed with lung cancer in 1992. Of course, no one is immune to cancer; even rock stars whose deaths are more traditionally associated with suicide and substance abuse (Table 1.12).

Chapter 2

The scientific basis of cancer

Six steps to becoming a cancer

At a molecular level cancer cells are characterized by six acquired biological properties:

1. Self-sufficiency in growth stimuli (keep on doubling).

2. Insensitivity to inhibitory stimuli (don't stop doubling).

3. Evasion of apoptosis (don't die).

4. Immortalization (don't age).

5. Neoangiogenesis (feed themselves).

6. Invasion and metastasis (spread).

It is not certain, but probable, that all six features are necessary to a greater or lesser extent for a cell to posses malignant behaviour (Figure 2.1). Some single molecular changes in cancer cells may produce more than one of the six attributes (e.g. mutations of p53 may cause both avoidance of apoptosis and insensitivity to inhibitory stimuli). A number of mechanisms may contribute to the acquisition of these six properties, including genomic instability as a consequence of deficient DNA repair or loss of cell cycle arrest/death in response to DNA damage as well as epigenetic dysregulation of gene expression.

Lecture Notes: Oncology, 2nd edition. By M. Bower and J. Waxman. Published 2010 by Blackwell Publishing Ltd.

1. Autonomous growth signals

The instruction to a cell to grow and start dividing is communicated by extracellular growth factor ligands that bind to cell surface receptors. This usually results in the reversible phosphorylation of tyrosine, threonine or serine amino acid residues of the receptor. The transfer of these molecular switches from activated phosphorylated receptors to downstream signalling enzyme effectors and then to non-enzymatic second messengers in the cytoplasm and finally to nuclear transcription activators, is known as signal transduction (Figure 2.2). This cascade results in amplification of the initial stimulus. Cancers achieve self-sufficiency in growth factors and do not depend on these extracellular ligands for continued growth. The majority of dominant oncogenes act on this signal transduction mechanism by one of the following mechanisms:

• Overproducing growth factors, e.g. glioblastomas produce platelet-derived growth factor (PDGF)

• Overproducing growth factor receptors, e.g. epidermal growth factor receptor (EGFR/erbB) overexpression in breast cancers

• Mutations of the receptor or components of the signalling cascade that are constitutively active, e.g. mutations of Ras in lung and colonic cancers.

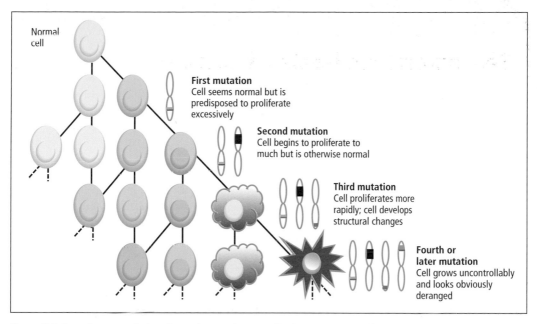

Figure 2.1 Stepwise accumulation of genetic mutations contributing to oncogenic phenotype.

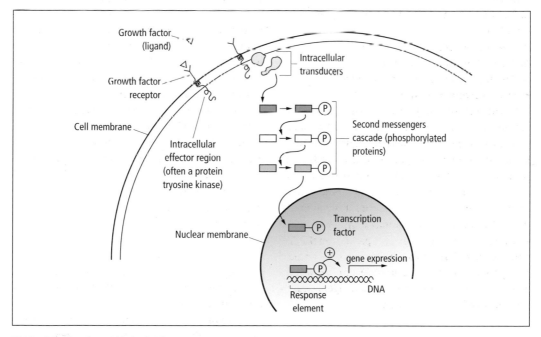

Figure 2.2 Signal transduction pathway.

2. Insensitivity to cell cycle checkpoints

Many normal cells grow throughout their lifespan and the co-ordination of their growth, differentiation, senescence and death is controlled by the cell cycle. Antiproliferative signals may be received by cells as soluble growth inhibitors or fixed inhibitors in the extracellular matrix. They act on the cell cycle clock (Box 2.1), most frequently arresting transit through G1 into S phase. Cancer cells ignore these stop signals.

The co-ordination of the cell cycle and its arrest at checkpoints in response to DNA damage is achieved by sequential activation of kinase enzymes that ultimately phosphorylate and dephosphorylate the retinoblastoma protein (Rb). Periodic activation of these cyclin–cyclin-dependent kinase (CDK) complexes drives the cell cycle

forward (Figure 2.3). Phosphorylation of Rb releases E2F, a transcription factor which is then able to promote the expression of a number of target genes resulting in cell proliferation. The brakes that balance this system are CDK inhibitors (CKIs). Interference in elements of the cell cycle regulatory process is a common theme in malignancy (see Table 2.2).

G1/S checkpoint

An important checkpoint or restriction point in the cell cycle occurs in G1 to ensure that errors in DNA are not replicated but instead are either repaired or that the cell dies by apoptosis. This is initiated by damaged DNA and is co-ordinated by p53, the gene that is probably most commonly mutated in cancers overall. Additional checkpoints are present in the S and G2 phases to allow cells to repair errors that occur during DNA duplication and thus prevent the propagation of these errors to daughter cells.

3. Evasion of apoptosis

Apoptosis is a pre-programmed sequence of cell suicide that occurs over 30–120 minutes. Apoptosis commences with condensation of cellular organelles and swelling of the endoplasmic reticulum. The plasma membrane remains intact but the cell breaks up into several membrane-bound apoptotic bodies, which are phagocytosed. Confining the process within the cell membrane reduces activation of both inflammatory and immune responses, so that programmed cell death does not cause autoimmune disease or inflammation. Amongst the molecules that control apoptosis are the Bcl-2 family that confusingly includes both pro-apoptosis members (e.g. Bax) and anti-apoptosis members (e.g. Bcl-2).

In mammalian cells two pathways initiate apoptosis (Figure 2.4):

1. **Intracellular triggers:** DNA damage leads via p53 to activation of pro-apoptotic members of the Bcl-2 family. This causes release of cytochrome c from mitochondria, which in turn activates the caspase (**c**leaves after **asp**artate prote**ase**) cascade.

> **Box 2.1: The cell cycle**
>
> There are five cell cycle phases:
> - **Quiescent phase (G0)**: Normal cells grown in culture will stop proliferating once they become confluent or are deprived of growth factors, and enter a quiescent state called G0. Most cells in normal tissue of adults are in a G0 state.
> - **First gap phase (G1)** (duration 10–14 hours): This occurs prior to DNA synthesis. Cells in G0 and G1 are receptive to growth signals but once they have passed a restriction point (R), are committed to DNA synthesis (S phase).
> - **Synthesis phase (S)** (duration 3–6 hours): During this phase DNA replication occurs and the cell becomes diploid.
> - **Second gap phase (G2)** (duration 2–4 hours): This occurs after DNA synthesis and before mitosis (M) and completion of the cell cycle.
> - **Mitosis (M)** (duration 1 hour).
>   Cell division completes the cell cycle.
>
>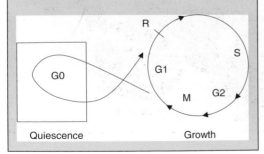

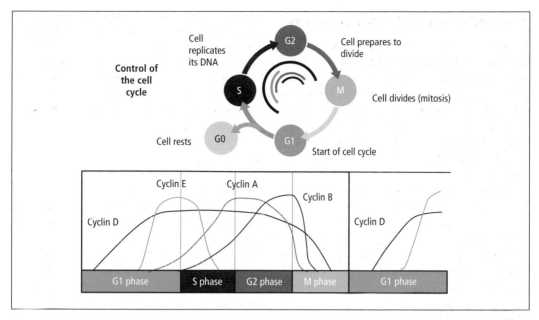

Figure 2.3 Oscillating levels of cyclins through the phases of the cell cycle.

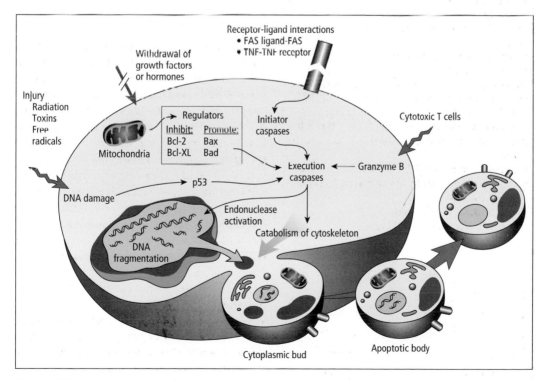

Figure 2.4 The apoptotic pathway.

2. **Extracellular triggers:** Binding of extracellular ligands to the cell surface death receptor superfamily (including CD95/Fas and tumour necrosis factor receptors) leads to a death-inducing cytoplasmic signalling complex that activates the caspase cascade.

Ultimately both pathways activate the caspase cascade, a series of protease enzymes that result in cell apoptosis. Evasion of this pathway is a prerequisite for malignant cell proliferation and a number of strategies to this end have been identified (see Table 2.2).

4. Immortalization

In culture, cells can divide a limited number of times, up to the 'Hayflick limit' (60–70 doublings in the case of human cells in culture), before the cell population enters crisis and dies off. This senescence is attributed to progressive telomere loss, which acts as a mitotic clock (Figure 2.5). Telomeres are the end segments of chromosomes and are made up of thousands of copies of a short 6 base pair sequence (TTAGGG). DNA replication always follows a 5′ to 3′ direction so that manufacturing the 3′ ends of the chromosomes cannot be achieved by DNA polymerases and each time a cell replicates its DNA ready for cell division, 50–100 base pairs are lost from the ends of chromosomes. Eventually the protective ends of chromosomes are eroded and end-to-end chromosomal fusions occur with karyotypic abnormalities and death of the affected cell.

Normal germ cells and cancer cells avoid this senescence, acquiring immortality in culture usually by upregulating the expression of human telomerase reverse transcriptase (hTERT) enzyme, which uses an RNA template and RNA-dependent DNA polymerase to add the 6 base pair sequence back onto the ends of chromosomes to compensate for the bases lost during DNA replication (see Table 2.2). Dyskeratosis congenita is an inherited condition, characterized by many abnormalities, including premature ageing and an increased risk of skin and gut cancers. It is due to mutations of components of the telomerase complex including the telomerase RNA and dyskerin.

5. Angiogenesis

All tissues including cancers require a supply of oxygen and nutrients. For cancers to grow larger

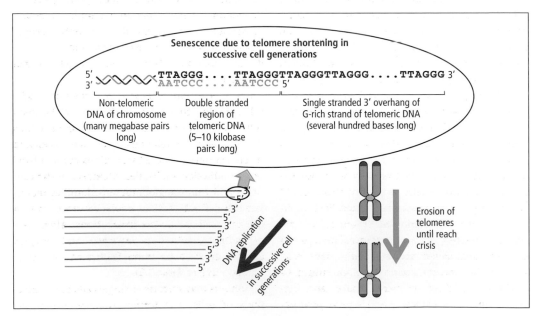

Figure 2.5 With every round of cell replication the chromosomes become shorter due to loss of the telomere repeats. Eventually this encroaches on the non-telomeric DNA of the chromosome and the cell enters crisis and dies.

Table 2.1 The angiogenic switch of angiogenic factors and inhibitors.

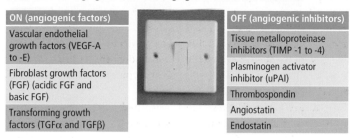

ON (angiogenic factors)		OFF (angiogenic inhibitors)
Vascular endothelial growth factors (VEGF-A to -E)		Tissue metalloproteinase inhibitors (TIMP -1 to -4)
Fibroblast growth factors (FGF) (acidic FGF and basic FGF)		Plasminogen activator inhibitor (uPAI)
		Thrombospondin
Transforming growth factors (TGFα and TGFβ)		Angiostatin
		Endostatin

than about 0.4 mm in diameter, a new blood supply is needed to deliver these. The growth of new blood vessels from pre-existing vasculature is termed angiogenesis. The 'angiogenic switch' denotes the ability of tumours to recruit new blood vessels by producing growth factors and is necessary for tumour growth and metastasis. Angiogenesis is determined by the relative balance of angiogenesis promoters and inhibitors (Table 2.1).

Vascular endothelial growth factors (VEGF-A to -E) are a family of growth factor homodimers that act via one of three plasma membrane receptors (VEGFR 1 to -3) on endothelial cells. Overproduction of VEGF and/or FGF (fibroblast growth factor) is a common theme in many tumours (see Table 2.2). Angiogenesis may be measured microscopically as microvessel density in an area of tumour, or by assays of angiogenic factors. These measures are of prognostic significance in several human tumours. Angiogenesis is becoming a major focus of anticancer drug development. It is an attractive target for several reasons. Angiogenesis is a normal process in growth and development but is quiescent in adult life except during wound healing and menstruation, so side effects are predicted to be minimal. As the target will be normal endothelial cells without any genetic instability, there should be little capacity to acquire resistance. Each capillary supplies a large number of tumour cells, so the effects should be magnified in terms of tumour cell kill. Anti-angiogenic agents should have easy access to their target through the blood stream. In combination, these elements make anti-angiogenic therapies attractive and several pharmaceutical companies have invested heavily in attempts to develop these agents. Bevacizumab is a monoclonal antibody that binds VEGF; it was originally licensed for use in colon cancer and is also a valuable treatment for age-related macular degeneration, which is caused by retinal vessel proliferation.

6. Invasion and metastasis

The properties of tissue invasion and metastatic spread are the histopathological hallmarks of malignant cancers that discriminate them from benign (see Plate 2.1). A number of sequential steps have been identified in the process of metastatic spread of cancers:

1. Motility and invasion from the primary site.
2. Embolism and circulation in lymph or blood.
3. Arrest in a distant vascular or lymphatic capillary and adherence to the endothelium.
4. Extravasation into the target organ parenchyma.

Central to many of these steps is the role of cell–cell adhesion that controls the contact between cells, and cell–extracellular matrix connections that influence the relationship between a cell and its environment. These interactions are regulated by cell adhesion molecules. Members of the cadherin and immunoglobulin superfamilies modulate cell–cell interactions whilst integrins control cell–extracellular matrix interactions. Alterations of cadherin, adhesion molecule and integrin expression are a common feature of metastatic cancer cells (see Table 2.2).

Tumours may migrate as single cells or as collections of cells. The former strategy is used by lymphoma and small cell lung cancer cells. It requires changes in integrins that mediate the

Box 2.2: How cancers metastasize: routes and destinations

Routes of metastasis

Breast cancer cells that leave a primary tumour in blood vessels will be carried in the blood first through the heart and then to the capillary beds of the lungs. Some cancer cells might form metastases in the lung (Figure 2.6) whilst others pass through the lung to enter the systemic arterial system, where they are transported to remote organs, such as bone. By contrast, colon cancer cells will be taken by the hepatoportal circulatory system first to the liver. There is no direct flow from the lymphatic system to other organs, so cancer cells within it – for example, melanoma cells – must enter the venous system to be transported to distant organs. Rarely, routes other than blood and lymphatic vessels are used in metastasis. Transcoelomic spread across the abdominal cavity occurs for gastric tumours that metastasize to the ovaries (known as Krukenberg tumours). Spread within the cerebrospinal fluid is thought to be responsible for the metastasis of medulloblastoma up and down the spinal column.

Where cancers metastasise

Certain cancers tend to metastasize to particular organs and this cannot be accounted for by blood flow alone. The basis for this tissue tropism has been found to relate to chemokine and chemokine receptor expression. Breast cancer cells express high levels of the CXCR4 chemokine receptor. Lung tissue expresses high levels of a soluble ligand for the CXCR4 receptor. Therefore, breast cancer cells that are taken to the lung find a strong chemokine receptor 'match', which may lead to chemokine-mediated signal activation. By contrast, in other organs where breast cancers less commonly metastasize, there are low levels of the ligand.

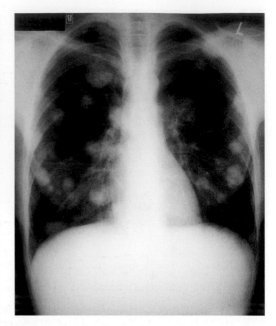

Figure 2.6 Plain chest radiograph showing multiple rounded metastases of varying sizes in a man with a metastatic testicular non-seminomatous germ cell tumour. Other tumours that commonly metastasize to the lungs include lung, breast, renal and thyroid cancers and sarcomas.

Figure 2.7). A number of mechanisms are in place to prevent cells acquiring all six properties, including efficient mechanisms to correct errors in DNA and to eradicate cells with extensive DNA damage. In fact, DNA mutation is facilitated in cancer cells by error-prone DNA replication (mutator phenotype), including deficient DNA repair leading to genetic instability, and uncoupling of the DNA damage cell cycle arrest/apoptosis response.

cell–extracellular matrix interaction and matrix-degrading proteases. Metastatic migration as clumps of cancer cells is common for most epithelial tumours. In addition, this needs changes in cell–cell adhesion through cadherins and other adhesion receptors, as well as cell–cell communication via gap junctions.

How to acquire the six capabilities

Cancer is a somatic genetic disease caused by DNA mutations and epigenetic changes (Table 2.2 and

Genome instability

DNA damage or mutation will normally result in cell cycle arrest followed by DNA repair or apoptosis. Interference in this process may occur either by deficient DNA damage recognition and repair, or abnormal gatekeeping of the cell cycle arrest/apoptosis response. This will result in the uncorrected accumulation of a large number of genetic abnormalities, which is referred to as 'genomic instability'. It is thought that this allows cells to acquire

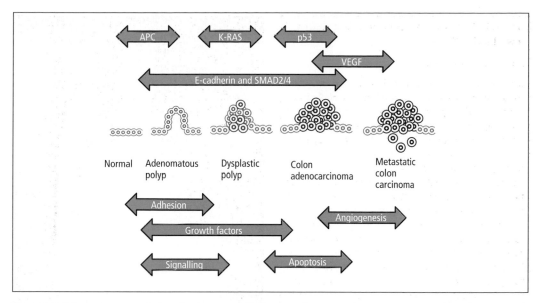

Figure 2.7 Schematic representation of colon cancer development from normal mucosa to metastatic carcinoma associated with stepwise acquisition of oncogenic mutations. APC, adenomatous polyposis coli gene; K-RAS, Kirsten-rat sarcoma viral oncogene homologue; p53, tumour protein 53 (TP53); SMAD, *Homo sapiens* homologue of *Drosophila* protein MAD (mothers against decapentaplegic); VEGF, vascular endothelial growth factor.

Table 2.2 Examples of the six features and their molecular basis in cancers.

Feature	Colorectal cancer	Glioma	Head and neck squamous cancer
1. Growth factor independence	K-Ras mutation	EGFR amplification or mutation NF1 loss	EGFR mutation
2. Over-riding inhibitory signals	SMAD2/SMAD4 mutation	CDK4/p16 mutation	Cyclin D amplification p16 and p21 mutation
3. Evasion of apoptosis	p53 mutation	p53 mutation/MDM2 overexpression	p53 mutation
4. Immortalization	hTERT re-expression	hTERT re-expression	hTERT re-expression
5. Angiogenesis	VEGF expression	PDGF/PDGFR overexpression	Nitric oxide pathway activation of VEGF
6. Invasion and metastasis	APC, inactivate E-cadherin	Cathepsin D, MMP-2 and -9 and UPA overexpression	Cathepsin D, MMP-1, -2 and -9 overexpression

APC, adenomatous polyposis coli gene; EGFR, endothelial growth factor receptor; hTERT, human telomerase reverse transcriptase; MMP, matrix metalloproteinase; PDGF, platelet-derived growth factor; PDGFR, platelet-derived growth factor receptor; VEGF, vascular endothelial growth factor; UPA, urokinase-type plasminogen activator.

the six capabilities that characterize the cancer cell phenotype and physiology.

DNA repair

Environmental damage to DNA occurs commonly and eukoryotes have developed several techniques for repairing both double strand and single strand errors in DNA.

1. Repair of double strand breaks in DNA:
   - homologous recombination using the sister chromatid as a template
   - non-homologous end joining (NHEJ).
2. Repair of single strand mutations in DNA:
   - nucleotide excision repair (NER) for bulky lesions
   - mismatch repair (MMR) for single mispaired bases and short deletions
   - base excision repair (BER) for alkylated bases.

Hereditary mutations of the enzymes involved in DNA repair will predispose to malignancy as they confer genome instability (Table 2.3).

DNA damage recognition

Another group of enzymes are required to recognize damaged DNA, leading to cell cycle arrest to allow DNA repair to be completed before the damage is replicated and passed on to the progeny cells. A number of cancer-predisposing syndromes are associated with inherited mutations of these enzymes. Examples include p53, whose inactiva-tion is an early step in the development of many cancers. Patients with the Li–Fraumeni syndrome carry one mutant germline p53 allele and are at high risk for the development of sarcomas, leukae-mia and cancers of the breast, brain, and adrenal glands.

Epigenetic changes

Most of the discussion above about the molecular mechanisms of malignancy has described somatic and occasional germline mutations of DNA that lead to aberrant proteins that in turn contribute to oncogenesis. This argument follows the central dogma of molecular biology introduced by Francis Crick in the late 1950s that stated that information flows in a unidirectional course from DNA sequence via RNA sequence to protein sequence. Although there are recognized exceptions to the central dogma, such as retroviruses and prions, it remains broadly true. However, some inheritable changes in phenotype or gene expression arise by mechanisms other than changes in the sequence of DNA bases. These inheritable changes passed on from a cell to her daughters are called epigenetic changes and perhaps the most obvious of these is cell differentiation.

The term epigenetics was introduced by the British developmental biologist Conrad Hal Wad-dington in 1942 as a metaphor for cell differentia-tion and development from a progenitor stem cell. Waddington likened differentiation to a marble

Table 2.3 Table of hereditary DNA repair syndromes.

DNA repair mechanism	Example of defect of DNA repair	Examples of cancers associated with defects
Homologous (sister chromatid) repair	BRCA1 (herediatry breast and ovarian cancer)	Breast and ovarian cancers
Non-homologous end joining (NHEJ)	XRCC4 (X-ray repair complementing defect gene) (lethal)	None (lethal defect)
Nucleotide excision repair (NER)	XP (xeroderma pigmentosa)	Skin cancers, leukaemia and melanoma
Mismatch repair (MMR)	MSH and MLH (hereditary non-polyposis colon cancer)	Colon, endometrium, ovarian, pancreatic and gastric cancers
Base excision repair (BER)	MYH (hereditary non-polyposis colon cancer)	Colon cancers

rolling down a landscape of hills and valleys to reach a final destination. The destination (cell fate) was determined by the landscape (epigenetics) and the marble could not travel back to the top (terminal differentiation). Today the term refers to modification of DNA and chromatin that influences gene transcription, alteration of post-transcriptional RNA and finally to protein degradation.

DNA methylation

Perhaps the most recognized epigenetic modification of DNA is nucleotide base methylation, typically the addition of a methyl group to the cytosine pyrimidine ring. In vertebrates, DNA methylation usually occurs in a CpG dinucleotide. Unmethylated CpGs are grouped in clusters called 'CpG islands' that occur in the 5' regulatory regions of many genes. DNA methylation of CpG islands inhibits gene transcription by impeding the binding of transcriptional proteins and by binding methyl-CpG-binding domain (MBDs) proteins. MBD proteins recruit additional proteins, such as histone deacetylases, that modify histones to form compact, inactive chromatin termed silent chromatin. Since epigenetic changes such as DNA methylation are inherited during cell replication, maintenance of the pattern of DNA methylation is required following each cycle of DNA replication and this is achieved by DNA methyltransferases using the conserved DNA strand as the template (Figure 2.8). DNA methylation of tumour suppressor genes has been found to be a common mechanism of epigenetic gene silencing in cancers.

Chromatin modification

Chromatin is composed of DNA and proteins, chiefly the histone proteins around which the DNA is wound. There are six classes of histones organized into core histones (H2A, H2B, H3 and H4) and linker histones (H1 and H5). The core histones, which are highly conserved through nature, share N-terminal amino acid sequences that are the sites for post-transcriptional modification, for example acetylation and methylation. These histone modifications alter the binding of the DNA to the nucleosome, and modify RNA polymerase activity and hence gene expression. In general, tightly bound DNA is less expressed. Numerous enzymes have been identified that are involved with the modification of histone protein leading to alterations of chromatin structure and regulation of gene expression. These include histone methyltransferase (HMT) and histone acetyltransferase (HAT); other enzymes catalyze the removal of these modifications including histone deacetylase (HDAC) (Figure 2.9). Acetylation of histone tails reduces their binding affinity for DNA, allowing access for RNA polymerase and enhancing gene transcription. HDAC, therefore, by reversing histone tail residue acetylation suppresses gene expression, including tumour suppressor gene expression contributing to oncogenesis. A number

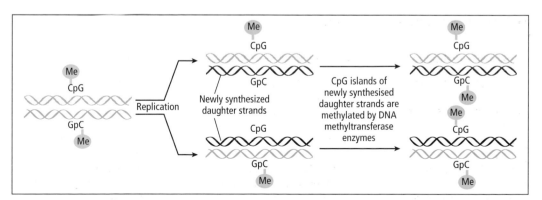

Figure 2.8 DNA methylation is passed on during cell replication to progeny cells by DNA methyltransferase enzymes that methylate CpG islands. CpG refers to the DNA dinucleotide sequence CG joined by the phosphate backbone of DNA.

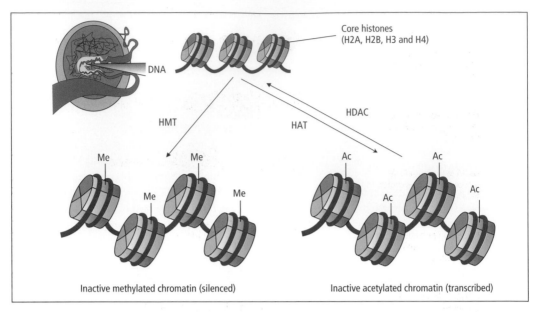

Figure 2.9 Mechanism of chromatin modification. Ac, acetyl; HAT, histone acetyltransferase; HDAC, histone deacetylase; HMT, histone methyltransferase; Me, methyl.

of HDAC inhibitors have been studied including valproate and more recently vorinostat or suberoylanilide hydroxamic acid (SAHA), which is licensed for the management of cutaneous T-cell non-Hodgkin's lymphoma.

RNA interference

Post-translational interference of messenger RNA (mRNA) transcripts can also modify the expression of genes without altering the DNA sequence. Two types of small RNA molecules, microRNA (miRNA) and small interfering RNA (siRNA), can bind to specific complementary sequences of RNA or DNA and either increase or decrease their activity, for example by preventing an mRNA from producing a protein (Figure 2.10). RNA interference was originally identified in petunia plants. Botantists attempting to produce darker and darker petunia flowers inserted additional genes of an enzyme that catalyzes pigment synthesis. However, the transgenic plants produced white or variegated white flowers and this was subsequently found to be due to post-transcriptional inhibition of gene expression brought about by rapid mRNA degrada-

tion. The eventual explanation of this gene silencing phenomenon was identified in *Caenorhabditis elegans* by Craig Mello and Andrew Fire in 1998 who demonstrated that double stranded RNA caused the gene silencing. They called this RNAi (RNA interference) and won the Nobel Prize in 2006 for this work. Both the role of RNAi in the epigenetic generation of cancers and the potential of RNAi as a therapeutic approach are the focus of fevered research.

Protein degradation

A further form of epigenetic modification that contributes to the cellular phenotype is the destruction of proteins chiefly by proteosomes. Proteins are tagged for degradation by a small protein called ubiquitin and this reaction is catalyzed by enzymes including the product of the gene disrupted in Von Hippel–Lindau syndrome and Fanconi's anaemia. At least four ubiquitin molecules attach to the condemned protein, in a process called polyubiquitination, and the protein then moves to a proteasome, where the proteolysis occurs (Figure 2.11). Epigenetic regulation of protein degradation

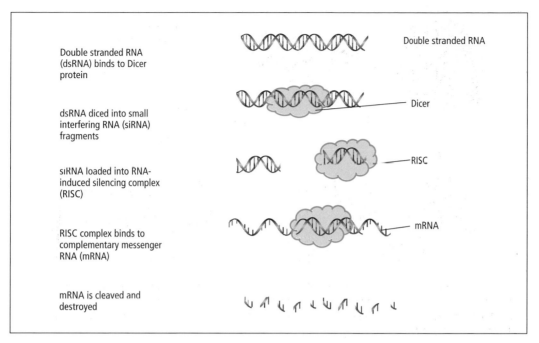

Figure 2.10 Mechanism of RNA interference.

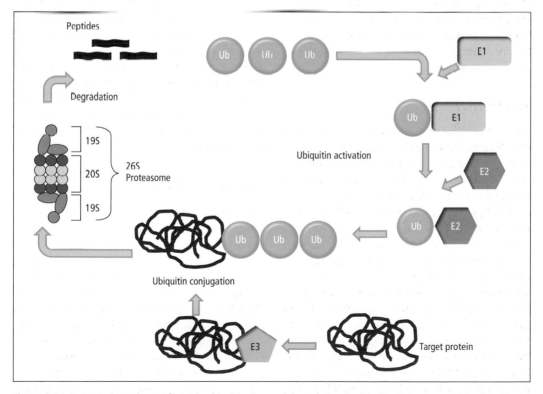

Figure 2.11 Proteosome pathway of protein ubiquitination and degradation. E, ubiquitination enzymes; Ub, ubiquitin.

could contribute to oncogenesis in a variety of ways. Gankyrin, a component of the proteosome is overexpressed in hepatocellular cancers. Bortezomib, a new treatment for myeloma, acts by inhibiting proteosome function.

Genetic causes of cancer

The causes of cancer may be usefully divided into genetic and environmental factors. The genetic factors are either germline mutations that are present in every cell of the body or somatic alterations only found in the tumour cells. Germline mutations may be either inherited, in which case they follow a familial pattern, or may be new sporadic mutations that neither parent has. Some of the germline mutations have been outlined as mutator phenotypes (DNA repair and damage recognition genes) above. Other germline cancer-predisposing mutations occur in tumour suppressor genes and oncogenes.

Oncogenes

The first clue to the identification of specific genes involved in the development of cancer came from the study of tumour viruses. Although cancer is generally not an infectious disease, some animal leukaemias, lymphomas and solid tumours, particularly sarcomas, can be caused by viruses. Oncogenes were identified following the discovery by Peyton Rous in 1911 that sarcomas could be induced in healthy chickens by injecting them with a cell-free extract of the tumour of a sick chicken. This was due to transmission of Rous sarcoma virus (RSV), an oncogenic retrovirus with just four genes:

- *gag* (group-specific antigen), which encodes the capsid protein
- *pol* (polymerase), which encodes the reverse transcriptase
- *env* (envelope), which encodes the envelope protein
- *src*, which encodes a tyrosine kinase.

It is the *src* gene that is necessary for cell transformation and is therefore an oncogene – literally a gene capable of causing cancer. In the late 1970s

Harold Varmus and Michael Bishop discovered that a homologous proto-oncogene (c-SRC) is present in the normal mammalian genome (the human *src* locus is on chromosome 20q12-q13) and has been hijacked by the retrovirus. The prefix v- denotes a viral sequence and the prefix c- a cellular sequence. In 1956, 55 years after his discovery of RSV and at the age of 87, Peyton Rous was (finally) awarded a Nobel Prize, whilst Bishop and Varmus only waited 10 years from their discovery to the award of their Nobel Prize in 1989. Around 50 oncogenes have been identified by their presence in transforming retroviruses (e.g. erbB, H-RAS, JUN) and further oncogenes have been discovered by positional cloning of chromosomal translocations (e.g. Bcl-2, BCR-ABL) and by transfection studies (e.g. N-RAS, RET). Most oncogenes contribute to cancer's autonomy in growth factors, either as plasma membrane receptors (e.g. RET, PTCH), signal transduction pathways (e.g. PTEN, NF1 and 2, VHL) or transcription factors (e.g. c-MYC, WT1) (Table 2.4).

Tumour suppressor genes

In contrast to oncogenes, tumour suppressor genes act as cell cycle brakes, slowing the proliferation of cells, and mutations in these genes also contribute to cancer. Germline mutations of tumour suppressor genes behave as autosomal-dominant familial cancer predispositions. Tumour suppressor genes require the loss of both functional alleles to support a cancer (unlike oncogenes where one mutant allele suffices). In 1971 Alfred Knudson proposed the two hit model of tumour suppression to account for the differences between familial and sporadic retinoblastoma in children. In familial cases, tumours arose at a younger age and were more frequently bilateral. Knudson hypothesized that these children had inherited one defective retinoblastoma gene allele, followed by loss of the function of the second allele in the cancer cells through a somatic mutation (see Plate 2.3). Tumour suppressor genes, like oncogenes, also involve a variety of functional categories, including cell cycle regulation (e.g. p53, Rb), DNA repair and maintenance (e.g. BRCA1 and 2, MLH1, MSH2), as

Table 2.4 Table of hereditary cancer predisposition syndromes.

Syndrome	Malignancies	Inheritance	Gene	Function
Breast/ovarian	Breast, ovarian, colon, prostate	AD	BRCA1	Genome integrity
		AD	BRCA2	
Cowden	Breast, thyroid, gastrointestinal, pancreas	AD	PTEN	Signal transduction (tyrosine phosphatase)
Li–Fraumeni	Sarcoma, breast, osteosarcoma, leukaemia, glioma, adrenocortical	AD	p53	Genome integrity
Familial polyposis coli	Colon, upper gastrointestinal	AD	APC	Cell adhesion
Hereditary non-polyposis colon cancer (Lynch type II)	Colon, endometrium, ovarian, pancreatic, gastric	AD	MSH2	DNA mismatch repair
		AD	MLH1	
		AD	PMS1	
		AD	PMS2	
MEN 1 (multiple endocrine neoplasia 1)	Pancreatic islet cell, pituitary adenoma	AD	MEN1	Transcription repressor
MEN 2 (multiple endocrine neoplasia 2)	Medullary thyroid, phaeochromocytoma	AD	RET	Signal transduction (receptor tyrosine kinase)
Neurofibromatosis 1 (see Plate 2.2)	Neurofibrosarcoma, phaeochromocytoma, optic glioma	AD	NF1	Signal transduction (regulates GTPases)
Neurofibromatosis 2	Vestibular schwannoma	AD	NF2	Cell adhesion
von Hippel–Lindau	Haemangioblastoma of retina and central nervous system, renal cell, phaeochromocytoma	AD	VHL	Ubiquination
Retinoblastoma	Retinoblastoma, osteosarcoma	AD	RB1	Cell cycle regulation
Xeroderma pigmentosa	Skin, leukaemia, melanoma	AR	XPA	DNA nucleotide excision repair
		AR	XPC	
		AR	XPD	
		AR	XPF	
Gorlin	Basal cell skin, brain	AD	PTCH	Signal transduction (repressor of hedgehog signalling)

AD, autosomal dominant; AR, autosomal recessive; GTPase, guanosine triphosphatase.

well as signal transduction (e.g. NF1, PTEN) and cell adhesion (e.g. APC) (Table 2.3).

Environmental causes of cancer

The multitude of environmental factors that are associated with the development of malignancy may be usefully divided into:
- Physical (radiation)
- Chemical (chemical carcinogens)
- Biological (infections).

Radiation

The major physical carcinogen is radiation. Radiation is ubiquitous and may either be ionizing (e.g. γ-rays from cosmic radiation and isotope decay, α-particles from radon, X-rays from medical imaging) or non-ionizing (e.g. ultraviolet (UV) light from the sun, microwave and radiofrequency radiation from mobile phones, electromagnetic fields from electricity generators and pylons, ultrasound radiation from imaging). Ionizing radiation ejects electrons from atoms yielding an ion pair and requires 10–15 eV (electronvolts). Ionizing radiation may be either electromagnetic (X-rays, γ-rays) or particulate (α-particles, neutrons). Non-ionizing radiation does not yield an ion pair but can still excite electrons resulting in chemical change.

Ultraviolet radiation

UV radiation is subdivided into three wavelength bands:
- UVA (313–400 nm)
- UVB (290–315 nm)
- UVC (220–290 nm).

UVC has the most potent effects on DNA, which absorbs most strongly at 254 nm. However, UVC is quickly absorbed in air and hence UVB is considered to be the greater environmental hazard. Most UV radiation is absorbed by atmospheric ozone in the stratosphere and this ozone layer is being depleted in part due to chlorine in chlorofluorocarbons (CFCs), resulting in increasing UV exposure levels. One of the major lesions induced in DNA by UV radiation is the thymidine dimer, a covalent bonding of adjacent thymidine residues on the same DNA strand. This causes local distortion of the double helix which is repaired by the nucleotide excision repair (NER) pathway. The seven identified xeroderma pigmentosa genes encode essential components that undertake NER and hence xeroderma pigmentosa predisposes to UV-induced skin malignancies. Melanin pigment in the skin normally absorbs UV radiation, thus protecting the skin. Basal cell and squamous cell skin cancers increase with cumulative UV exposure, whilst the relationship is less straightforward for melanoma. The evidence for an association with cancer for other forms of non-ionizing radiation (microwave, radiofrequency, ultrasound and electromagnetic radiation) is weak and inconsistent.

Ionizing radiation

Natural sources
Exposure to natural sources of ionizing radiation varies in different populations. Higher altitude and further latitude from the equator are both associated with higher cosmic radiation exposure. In addition, various regions have higher natural background levels from radon. Radon is a colourless, odourless gas formed from decay as part of the uranium-238 series. The radon-222 isotope, along with a number of its progeny, is an α-particle emitter. Radon gas levels are normally quoted in Bq/m^3 (1 becquerel (Bq) is one decay per second) and the average indoor levels in the UK are about 20 Bq/m^3. Local geology (igneous granite) with high levels of uranium produces high levels of radon in soil gas, but for it to escape to the surface the soil must be highly porous. In the UK, radon levels are particularly high in Devon and Cornwall, Derbyshire and Northamptonshire. From the results of eight case–control studies, it is believed that radon exposure accounts for a small fraction of lung cancers with a 14% increased risk for a person living for 30 years in a house with levels of 150 Bq/m^3.

Nuclear warfare
Most of the information on the induction of cancers by ionizing radiation comes from exposed populations, including Japanese people exposed to atomic bombs at Hiroshima (Little Boy was a uranium-235-enriched bomb) and Nagasaki (Fat Man was a plutonium-239 bomb). The estimated populations of the two cities at the time of bombing was 560 000 and approximately 200 000 people died within the first few months of the acute effects of blast, burns and radiation exposure (Table 2.5).

Table 2.5 How atomic bombs kill.

Timing	Effect
1–2 hours	Radiation sickness (acute nausea and vomiting)
2–10 days	Denuded intestinal epithelium (intractable diarrhoea, gastrointestinal haemorrhage, septicaemia)
7–21 days	Pancytopenia (neutropenic sepsis, haemorrhage)
3–10 years	Acute myeloid leukaemia
10–50 years	Solid tumours (breast, bone, thyroid, lung, gastrointestinal, ovary, skin)

Table 2.6 Cancer deaths in the hibakusha (survivors of Hiroshima and Nagasaki atomic bombs).

	Total number of deaths	Estimated number of deaths due to radiation	Percentage of deaths attributable to radiation
Leukaemia	176	89	51%
Solid tumours	4687	339	7%
Total	4863	428	9%

Box 2.3: Chernobyl

On 26 April 1986, nuclear reactor number 4 at Chernobyl exploded in the world's worst nuclear accident. Over 10^{19} Bq of radioactive isotopes were released, including 5.2×10^{18} Bq of β-emitting isotopes of iodine that concentrate in the thyroid gland. An increase in thyroid cancer in children was first reported in 1990 but an excess of other tumours has not (yet?) been reported. Fallout from Chernobyl affected millions of people living within a few hundred kilometres of the reactor and caused a 30–100-fold increase in the incidence of thyroid cancer, especially in children. The younger the child at exposure, the greater the risk is. The increase so far is almost entirely papillary carcinoma of the thyroid and the dominant subtype has solid papillary morphology. At a molecular level, these tumours show rearrangement of the RET oncogene by inversion or translocation with partner genes to yield constitutively active c-RET tyrosine kinases.

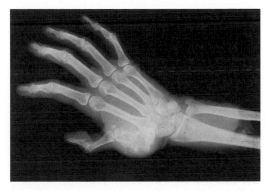

Figure 2.12 Osteosarcoma of the first metacarpal 15 years after radiotherapy for arthritis (no longer used). This radiograph shows cortical destruction, a soft tissue mass, with internal calcification and periosteal reaction.

The Radiation Effects Research Foundation has followed 86 000 survivors or hibakusha, and, up to 1990, 7827 had died of cancer. The excess risk of leukaemia was seen especially in those exposed as children and was highest during the first 10 years after the bombing. However, the excess risk of solid tumours occurred later and still persists (Table 2.6).

Medical radiation

The hazards of medical ionizing radiation may be difficult to determine as ionizing radiation-induced tumours are not identifiable by a particular signature DNA mutation (unlike the thymidine dimers induced by UV radiation). Some tissues, such as breast, thyroid and bone marrow, are more susceptible to the carcinogenic effects of ionizing radiation, although tumours have been described in every organ site following radiation exposure

(Figure 2.12). Well-described examples of iatrogenic tumours include acute leukaemias induced by radiation treatment for ankylosing spondylitis prescribed in the late 1930s in the UK. Similarly, 20 000 Israelis received radiation for *Tinea capitis* (ringworm) in the 1950s, and by the 1980s there was a significantly increased risk of meningioma. Similar increases in tumours have been observed in patients treated with radiotherapy, including men treated for prostate cancer, women treated for cervical cancers and Hodgkin's disease survivors. Diagnostic imaging radiation doses are shown in Table 2.7.

Occupational radiation

The first victims of occupational exposure to radiation included Marie Curie and her daughter Irène Joliot-Curie (also a Nobel laureate), who both died of leukaemia. In the 1920s, watch dials were hand painted with radium-based luminous paint. The female radium dial painters often licked their paint brushes to give them a sharp point and

Table 2.7 Diagnostic imaging radiation doses.

Imaging procedure	Radiation dose	Equivalent to natural background radiation for:
Chest X-ray	0.02 mSv	3 days
Chest CT scan	8 mSv	3.6 years
Abdominal CT scan	10 mSv	4.5 years
Intravenous urogram	2.5 mSv	14 months
Brain CT scan	2.3 mSv	1 year
Mammogram	0.7 mSv	3 months

Box 2.4: Units of radiotherapy

The becquerel (Bq) is the SI unit of radioactivity and 1 Bq is equivalent to one nuclear decay per second. It is named after Henri Becquerel who shared the Nobel Prize with Marie and Pierre Curie for the discovery of radioactivity. The Hiroshima bomb produced 8×10^{24} Bq.

The gray (Gy) is the SI unit of absorbed radiation dose for ionizing radiation. One gray is the absorption of 1 joule (J) of ionizing radiation by 1 kg of matter, usually human tissue. It is named after Hal Gray, a British pioneer of radiation biology and physics who also established the Gray Laboratories at Mount Vernon Hospital.

The sievert (Sv) is the SI unit of radioactive dose equivalence and reflects the biological effects in tissue of radiation rather than its physical attributes. The equivalent dose will depend on the absorbed dose (measured in grays) as well as the type of radiation, as well as the time and volume and part of body irradiated. It is named after Rolf Sievert, a Swedish medical physicist. A dose of 3 Sv will lead to a lethal dose (LD) 50/30, or death in 50% of cases within 30 days, and over 6 Sv survival is very unusual.

---

ingested the radium. Up to 3% of these women subsequently developed osteosarcomas after a latency of 5–10 years. These 'radium girls' successfully sued their employer and this litigation resulted in the introduction of industrial safety standards and health and safety regulations at work. Similarly, pitchblende (uranium oxide) and uranium miners in Czechoslovakia, Sweden, Newfoundland and Colorado who have been exposed to radon are at increased risk of lung cancers.

Chemical carcinogenesis

Cancer is essentially a genetic disease arising from mutations of genes that affect the control of normal cell function (proto-oncogenes and tumour suppressor genes) or from polymorphic genes that govern enzyme systems that activate or detoxify environmental carcinogens (phase I and phase II enzyme reactions). Carcinogenic mutations can arise in several ways: genotoxic environmental factors (e.g. radiation and many chemical carcinogens), spontaneous DNA aberrations occurring during normal cell replication, or hereditary germline mutations. Chemical carcinogenesis was shown to be a multistep process following studies in the 1940s using PAHs (polycyclic aromatic hydrocarbons) and a murine skin cancer model system. This identified three steps – initiation, promotion and progression – that involve separate biological processes. Chemical carcinogens may operate at any or all three stages. The minority of chemical carcinogens act directly on DNA (e.g. alkylating agents), whilst the majority are procarcinogens that require metabolic activation to the ultimate carcinogen forms. Many ultimate carcinogens are potent electrophiles, capable of accepting electrons (e.g. epoxides derived from polycyclic hydrocarbons, vinyl chloride and aflatoxins, the *N*-hydroxylated metabolites of azo dyes, and the alkyldiazonium ions derived from nitrosamines).

Initiation

The key feature of initiation is the need for cell replication without repair of the chemically induced DNA damage. Initiation is irreversible, usually involves simple DNA mutations that are 'fixed' by cell division, and results in no morphological changes to the cells. Single exposure to a carcinogen may be sufficient for initiation. For example, aflatoxin B1 is one of a family of mycotoxin contaminants of food crops such as grain and groundnuts (peanuts). It is produced by *Aspergillus flavus*, which favours hot and humid conditions and is therefore most likely to contaminate food in Africa and Asia. Aflatoxin B1 is oxidized by hepatic P450 microsomal enzymes into aflatoxin B1 2,3-epoxide, which binds to DNA bases forming mutagenic adducts that preferentially induce GC to TA transversions. These transversions have been identified frequently in codon 249 of the p53 gene in hepatocellular carcinomas in patients from southern Africa and China who are exposed to high levels of aflatoxin B1 and may also have hepatitis B virus infection.

Promotion

Promotion is a reversible process requiring multiple exposures to the carcinogen, usually with a dose–response threshold. Promotion does not usually involve DNA mutations (non-genotoxic carcinogenesis) but provides a chemically mediated selective growth advantage. Thus, promotion results in the clonal expansion of cells. In the 1940s it was noted that 5% of mice treated with penzpyrene developed tumours but this figure rose to 80% when croton oil was added. Croton oil alone, however, produced no tumours. Subsequently, it was found that tetradecanoylphorbol acetate (TPA), a natural component of croton oil (from the seeds of *Croton tiglium*, a tree cultivated in India that resemble castor seeds), interacts with the protein kinase c signal pathway, stimulating growth and thus acting as a promoter. TPA is the most widely used tumour promoter in cellular experimental models of oncogenesis. Similarly, oestrogens are believed to act as carcinogenic promoters. Indeed, transplacental diethylstilboestrol (DES) was shown to induce vaginal clear cell adenocarcinomas in young women whose mothers had been treated with DES during pregnancy.

Progression

Progression is an irreversible step that results in morphologically identifiable cellular changes and frequently involves multiple complex DNA changes, such as chromosomal alterations. Progression and the accumulation of multiple genetic abnormalities that characterize cancer cells may occur spontaneously or may be driven by chemical carcinogens. Since individual cells may acquire these genetic changes, progression leads to heterogeneity of the cell population. Ultimately some cells will acquire a mutator phenotype and the six genetic attributes that characterize a cancer cell.

Diet and cancer

A role for dietary constituents has been described for a number of cancers and the evidence for some of these relationships is more robust than for others. Alcohol intake has been convincingly associated with an increased risk of oral, oesophageal and hepatic cancers. In contrast, dietary fat was believed to play an important role in breast cancer development based on animal studies, migrant studies and a few case–control trials. This led to great enthusiasm for reduced dietary fat intake to reduce the incidence of breast cancer. However, results from large prospective studies have failed to confirm a strong relationship between dietary fat intake and breast cancer. Two paths may contribute to dietary carcinogenesis. Firstly, foodstuffs may include dietary genotoxins formed by contaminating moulds, products of storage or fermentation of food, products of cooking and food additives (e.g. aflatoxin contamination of food). Secondly, endogenous genotoxins, such as reactive oxygen species, may be formed and higher calorific intake may yield more genotoxins.

Carcinogenic infections

The association between infection and cancer is usually attributed to Peyton Rous, who described the acellular transmission of sarcoma between chickens in 1911. However, six years earlier, Goebel had reported a link between bladder tumours and bilharzia (schistosomiasis). It is estimated that 15% of cancers globally are attributable to infections (11% viruses, 4% bacteria and 0.1% helminths) (Table 2.8).

Oncogenic human DNA viruses

Human papillomavirus (HPV)
The papillomaviruses are non-enveloped, icosahedral, double stranded DNA viruses. Around 100

Box 2.5: A brief epidemiological history of smoking and cancer

Tobacco was one of the 'gifts' from the New World to the Old along with syphilis and potatoes. Nicotine is named after Jean Nicot, a 15th century French ambassador to Lisbon, who was a great advocate of smoking and who in 1559 sent tobacco to Catherine de Medici, the then Queen of France. Tobacco was subsequently introduced to England by Sir Walter Raleigh in 1586. Smoking was actively encouraged amongst soldiers in the Thirty Years War, Napoleonic campaigns, Crimean War and, most notably, the First World War. Smoking reduces fear and anxiety and suppresses appetite and these were deemed beneficial to soldiers.

Early epidemiological links with non-lung cancers

In 1761, John Hill, a London doctor, wrote up several cases of nasal cancer amongst heavy tobacco snuff users and, in 1795, Thomas van Soemmering suggested a link between pipe smoking and lip cancer. The American Civil War Yankee general and later USA president, Ulysses S. Grant died in 1885 of throat cancer and this was attributed to his cigars. In an early cohort study in the 1920s, Dr R. Abbe observed that, of 90 patients with oral cancer, 89 were smokers.

Epidemiological links with lung cancer

In 1939, Dr Franz Muller of the University of Cologne performed what is generally recognized as the earliest case–control study of smoking, which showed that a very high proportion of lung cancer patients were heavy smokers. However, the results were dismissed as unreliable because Hitler was a fanatical antismoker. Shortly after the Second World War, Austin Bradford Hill, Edward Kennaway, Percy Stock and Richard Doll set out to investigate links between smoking and lung cancer, at a time when 90% of adult males in the UK smoked, using a case–control dose–response strategy. Their case–control study was performed in 1948 in 20 London hospitals, interviewing two controls with gastric or colonic cancer as controls for each lung cancer patient. In all analyses, there was a dose–response relationship between the number of cigarettes smoked and the risk of lung cancer. This was published in 1950 in the *British Medical Journal*.

In 1951, Doll and Hill set up a prospective cohort study of 60 000 doctors on the medical register who were recruited via a letter in the *BMJ*; 40 000 replies were received and, in the following 2.5 years, there were 789 deaths, including 36 from lung cancer. There was a significant increase in the risk of lung cancer with increased tobacco consumption (see table below). However, they noted that the only two doctors who definitely died of smoking had died after setting fire to their beds whilst smoking in bed! This relationship was maintained in a 1993 update of the original cohort, which now includes 20 000 deaths (883 from lung cancer), and the relative risk for smoking >25 g tobacco a day was 20-fold.

	N	Tobacco 1 g/day	Tobacco 15 g/day	Tobacco >25 g/day
Lung cancer deaths	36	0.4/10 000	0.6/10 000	1.1/10 000
All deaths	789	13/10 000	13/10 000	16/10 000

Similar findings were reported in the early 1950s in the USA by Ernst Wynder, a medical student, and Evarts Graham, a thoracic surgeon, who, in 1950, published 'Tobacco smoking as a possible etiologic factor in bronchiogenic carcinoma: a study of 684 proven cases' in the *Journal of the American Medical Association*. Evarts, a chain smoker, did not take enough heed of his own findings and himself died of lung cancer.

genotypes have been identified and >30 of these infect the female genital tract. Some genotypes are associated with benign lesions, such as warts (e.g. HPV-6 and -11), whilst others are known as high-risk genotypes and are associated with invasive cancer (e.g. HPV-16, -18, -31, -33, -45, -51, -52, -58 and -59) (Table 2.9). The prevalence of infection varies between populations but is 20–30% in women aged 20–25 years and declines to 5–10% in women over 40 years old. HPV is sexually transmitted and the main determinant of infection is the number of sexual partners. Most infections are cleared spontaneously but a small proportion persist and are believed to be the origin of cervical dysplasia and invasive cancers. Latent infection is associated with cervical intraepithelial neoplasia

Table 2.8 Cancers attributed to infection.

Infection	Cancer	Number of cancer cases worldwide per year
RNA viruses		
Human T-cell leukaemia virus	Leukaemia	3000
HIV (and Epstein–Barr virus)	Non-Hodgkin's lymphoma	9000
HIV (and human herpesvirus 8)	Kaposi's sarcoma	45000
Hepatitis C virus	Hepatocellular cancer	110000
DNA viruses		
Human papillomavirus	Cervical cancer	360000
Hepatitis B virus	Hepatocellular cancer	230000
Epstein–Barr virus	Burkitt lymphoma, Hodgkin's disease, nasopharyngeal cancer	100000
Bacteria		
Helicobacter pylori	Gastric cancer, gastric lymphoma	350000
Helminths		
Schistosoma haematobium	Bladder cancer	10000
Liver flukes	Cholangiocarcinoma	1000

HIV, human immunodeficiency virus.

Table 2.9 Human papillomavirus genotypes and associated conditions.

Human disease	HPV genotype
Skin warts	HPV-1, 2, 3, -7 and -10
Epidermodysplasia verruciformis	HPV-5, -8, -17 and -20
Anogenital warts: exophytic condylomas	HPV-6 and -11
Anogenital warts: flat condylomas	HPV-16, -18, 31, 33, -42 and -43
Respiratory tract papillomas	HPV-6 and -11
Conjunctival papillomatosis	HPV-6 and -11
Focal epithelial hyperplasia	HPV-13 and -32

(CIN), which is graded 1 to 3 according to the severity of cytological changes. The histological equivalents of these lesions are called squamous intraepithelial lesions, which may be low or high grade. Over 99% of invasive cervical cancers have detectable HPV DNA present and HPV can transform cells in culture. The molecular basis of papillomavirus-induced neoplasia is attributed to two viral oncogenes, E6 and E7. HPV E6 inactivates p53 and E7 degrades Rb protein. High-risk HPV geno-

types have also been associated with anal, penile, vaginal and vulval cancers. In addition HPV is thought to play a role in the development of a number of other malignancies, including head and neck cancers, conjunctival squamous cancers, oesophageal cancers and possibly cutaneous squamous cell cancers.

Studies have suggested that the detection of HPV in the cervix may be more sensitive for detecting CIN than conventional cytological screening. Prophylactic HPV vaccines that induce neutralizing antibodies may prevent infection and the associated malignancies. Most of the vaccines have used virus-like particles constructed of major capsid proteins without viral DNA or enzymes present. A nationwide HPV vaccination programme for teenage girls was started in UK in 2008.

Hepatitis B virus (HBV)

Hepatitis B virus is a double stranded DNA virus that includes a single stranded DNA region of variable length. The virus possesses a DNA-dependent DNA polymerase as well as a reverse transcriptase and replicates via an RNA intermediate. HBV has three main antigens: the 'Australian antigen' is

37

Table 2.10 Serological markers of hepatitis B virus infection.

	HBsAg	HBeAg	Anti-HBe	Anti-HBs	Anti-HBc	Anti-HBc IgM
Acute infection	+	+/−	+/−	−	+	+++
Highly infectious carrier	+++	+	−	−	+	−
Low infectious carrier	+	−	+	−	+	−
Past infection	−	−	+	+	+	−
Past immunization	−	−	−	+	−	−

associated with the surface (HBsAg), the 'core antigen' (HBcAg) is internal, and the 'e antigen' (HBeAg) is part of the same capsid polypeptide as HBcAg. All of these antigens elicit specific antibodies and are used diagnostically (Table 2.10).

Hepatitis B is one of the most common infections worldwide with two billion people having been infected and 300–350 million chronic carriers. Hepatitis B is the ninth most common cause of death worldwide. Acute hepatitis B infection may be associated with extrahepatic immune-mediated manifestations and 1–4% of patients develop a fulminant form. Following acute infection, up to 10% will develop chronic hepatitis, either chronic persistent hepatitis, which is asymptomatic with modest elevation of transaminases and little fibrosis, or chronic active hepatitis, which causes jaundice and cirrhosis and is associated with a 100× increased risk of hepatocellular cancer 15–60 years after infection. It is uncertain how hepatitis B leads to cancer, although the X protein of hepatitis B may interact with p53 causing disruption of the cell cycle control, or the virus may act indirectly by causing increased hepatic cell turnover associated with cirrhosis.

Although treatment with α-interferon and antiviral agents (e.g. lamivudine, tenofovir, telbivudine, entecavir, adefovir) may lead to clearance of hepatitis B in chronic infection, recombinant subunit vaccines have been available since the early 1980s. The introduction of a mass immunization programme in Taiwan has been associated with a dramatic reduction in liver cancer in children.

Epstein–Barr virus (EPV)

Epstein–Barr virus (or HHV-4, human herpesvirus 4) is a ubiquitous double stranded DNA gamma-

Table 2.11 Diseases associated with Epstein–Barr virus infection.

Non-malignant
Infectious mononucleosis
X-linked lymphoproliferative syndrome (Duncan's syndrome)
Oral hairy leukoplakia

Malignant
Burkitt lymphoma
Nasopharyngeal cancer
Post-transplant lymphoproliferative disorder
Hodgkin's disease
Primary cerebral lymphoma
Primary effusion lymphoma (with HHV8)
Leiomyosarcoma in children with HIV
Nasal T/NK non-Hodgkin's lymphoma

herpesvirus. It was first identified by Epstein and his colleagues by electron microscopy of a cell line derived from a patient with Burkitt lymphoma in 1964. Burkitt lymphoma had been described only a few years earlier in 1956 by Dennis Burkitt, a surgeon working in Uganda. The subsequent finding that EBV was the cause of infectious mononucleosis arose serendipitously when a laboratory technician in Philadelphia developed mononucleosis and was found to have acquired antibodies to EBV. EBV infects over 90% of the world's population, is transmitted orally and, in normal adults, from 1 to 50 B lymphocytes per million are infected by latent EBV. A carcinogenic role for EBV has been confirmed for several types of lymphoma (Burkitt lymphoma, Hodgkin's disease and immunosuppression-associated non-Hodgkin's lymphoma) and nasopharyngeal cancer (Table 2.11). EBV is estimated to be responsible for 100 000 cancers per year in the world.

Primary infection of epithelial cells by EBV is associated with the infection of some resting B lymphocytes. The majority of infected B cells have latent virus with a small percentage undergoing spontaneous activation to lytic infection. During lytic infection EBV replicates in the cell and when the progeny virions are released the host cell is destroyed. In contrast, during latent infection there is neither virus replication nor host cell destruction. Most infected B lymphocytes have latent virus expressing at most ten of the >80 genes of EBV. The roles of these latent genes include maintenance of the episomal virus DNA, growth and transformation of B cells and evasion of the host immune system. A number of these latent genes are thought to contribute to the oncogenicity of EBV. For example LMP-1 (latent membrane protein 1) mimics a constitutively activated receptor for tumour necrosis factor (TNF), and BHRF1 and BALF1 are viral homologues of the anti-apoptotic protein bcl-2 that leads to evasion of programmed cell death. Thus, in contrast to retroviruses, which generally possess a single oncogene, EBV uses a number of genes that contribute to the steps towards cancer.

Human herpesvirus 8 (HHV-8/KSHV)

Kaposi's sarcoma (KS) was originally described over a century ago and four forms have subsequently been recognized. The first is classic KS and is usually found on the lower legs of elderly men of Mediterranean or Jewish descent without any immunosuppression. A second form, endemic or African KS, is found in all age groups in sub-Saharan Africa, where even before the HIV epidemic it was as common as colorectal cancer is in Europe. A third form associated with iatrogenic immunosuppression was recognized in patients who had received an allogeneic organ transplant. The fourth and most common form of the disease is associated with AIDS (acquired immune deficiency syndrome). All forms of KS are associated with HHV-8 (also known as Kaposi sarcoma herpesvirus, KSHV), which was identified in 1994. In addition, this virus is most prevalent in the populations at risk of KS. HHV-8 is also implicated in the pathogenesis of two rare lymphoproliferative diseases, primary effusion lymphoma and multicentric Castleman's disease (see Plate 2.4). Like EBV, HHV-8 includes a number of cellular gene homologues that are thought to contribute to its oncogenic potential.

Oncogenic human RNA viruses

Hepatitis C virus (HCV)

Hepatitis C virus was identified in 1989 as the cause of transfusion-acquired non-A non-B hepatitis by Houghton, Choo and Kuo. HCV is a single stranded RNA virus belonging to the flavivirus genus along with yellow fever and dengue. The prevalence of HCV varies geographically from 1–1.5% in Europe and the USA to 3.5% in Africa, and transmission is chiefly parenteral, particularly by blood transfusion prior to the introduction of blood product screening. In contrast to HBV, 85% develop persistent HCV and 65% progress to chronic liver disease including hepatocellular cancer for which the relative risk is 20-fold (Table 2.12). The oncogenic mechanism for HCV remains unclear. Unlike retroviruses, there is no evidence of genome integration but cancer is preceded by cirrhosis and it is hypothesized that the virus induces

Table 2.12 Comparison of HIV and hepatitis B and C viruses.

	HCV	HBV	HIV
Global prevalence	3%	35%	0.5%
Global prevalence	170 million	1.2 billion	36.1 million
Chronic infection rate	2.30%	6%	0.5%
Chronic infection	129 million	350 million	36.1 million
Deaths per year	476000	1.2 million	2.8 million
Annual death rate	0.40%	0.49%	7.80%

a cycle of inflammation, repair and regeneration and thus indirectly contributes to the formation of cancer. There are at least six genotypes of HCV and the diagnosis is usually made by enzyme immunoassay for anti-HCV antibodies and confirmed by polymerase chain reaction (PCR) for HCV RNA. Treatment with pegylated interferon and ribavarin leads to clearance of the virus in 40–60% depending in part upon the HCV genotype. Promising specific protease and polymerase inhibitors are in late phase trials for HCV.

Human T-cell leukaemia virus type 1 (HTLV-1)

HTLV-1 is the main cause of adult T-cell leukaemia/lymphoma, a malignancy characterized by hypercalcaemia, lymphadenopathy, hepatosplenomegaly and myelosuppression. It is associated with a particularly poor prognosis and occurs almost exclusively in areas where HTLV-1 is endemic, such as the Caribbean, Japan and West Africa or in immigrants from these regions and their offspring. HTLV-1 is also associated with tropical spastic paraparesis and uveitis. HTLV-1 is an enveloped retrovirus that integrates into the host cellular genome. The virus is able to immortalize human T lymphocytes and this property is attributable to a specific viral oncogene, *tax*. Tax is a trans-activating transcription factor that can also lead to repression of transcription. Adult T-cell leukaemia/lymphoma develops in 2–5% of HTLV-1 infected people and is commoner in those infected at a younger age.

Oncogenic bacteria

Helicobacter pylori

Helicobacter pylori is a spiral, flagellated, Gram-negative bacteria that colonizes the human gastrointestinal tract. It causes gastritis leading to peptic ulceration, although many infections are asymptomatic. The discovery of *H. pylori* and the recognition of its place in the pathogenesis of peptic ulcer disease are chiefly due to Barry Marshall, who, in order to prove his point, swallowed a solution of the organism and developed acute gastritis 1 week later. It is believed that half of the world population is chronically infected with *H. pylori*. Prospective sero-epidemiological data suggest that *H. pylori* infection is associated with a two to four-fold increase in the risk of gastric cancer as well as an increase in gastric low-grade mucosa-associated lymphoid tissue (MALT) lymphoma. As with the hepatitis viruses, the mechanism of oncogenesis is obscure but is believed to be an indirect result of chronic inflammation and consequential epithelial cell proliferation. The combination of two antibiotics with either a bismuth preparation or a proton pump inhibitor for 14 days eradicates *H. pylori* in 80% patients. However, re-infection is common, *H. pylori* is very prevalent and the time interval between *H. pylori* infection and gastric cancer is thought to be several decades. For these reasons, it may prove very difficult to assess the value of eradication interventions in reducing cancer risk.

Oncogenic helminths

Schistosomes

Schistosomes are parasitic blood flukes or flatworms (platyhelminths) belonging to the trematode class whose intermediate hosts are snails. Three species infect humans: *Schistosoma haematobium*, *Schistosoma mansoni* and *Schistosoma japonica*. Humans are infected by contact with fresh water where the parasite cercaria form penetrates the skin. It is estimated that 200 million people are infected with schistosomes (Table 2.13). Acute infection may produce swimmer's itch dermatitis and tropical pulmonary eosinophilia, although most people remain asymptomatic. The development of adult worms, days to weeks after infection, may cause Katayama fever, a systemic illness of fevers, rigors, myalgia, lymphadenopathy and hepatosplenomegaly. Chronic infection leads to granuloma formation at sites of egg deposition, in the bladder for *S. haematobium* and in the bowel and liver for *S. mansoni* and *S. japonica*. The late sequelae include squamous cell carcinoma of the bladder in the case of *S. haematobium* and probably hepatocellular cancer with *S. japonica*. A single oral dose of praziquantel resolves the infection.

Table 2.13 Global distribution of schistosomiasis.

Species	Geographical distribution	Number of humans infected
Schistosoma haematobium	North Africa, Middle East, sub-Saharan Africa	114 million
Schistosoma mansoni	Sub-Saharan Africa, Middle East, Brazil	83 million
Schistosoma japonica	China, the Philippines, Indonesia	1.5 million

Table 2.14 Global distribution of liver fluke infection.

Species	Geographical distribution	Number of humans infected
Opisthorchis viverrini	Northern Thailand, Laos	9 million
Opisthorchis felineus	Kazakhastan, Ukraine	1.5 million
Clonorchis sinensis	China, Korea, Taiwan, Vietnam	7 million

Liver flukes

Three species of food-borne liver flukes of the trematode class cause illness in humans. Infection is acquired by eating raw or undercooked freshwater fish and the flukes migrate to the biliary tree and mature in the intrahepatic bile ducts. There are two intermediate hosts in the life cycle – snails and fish. As many as 17 million people are estimated to be infected (Table 2.14). Cholangiocarcinoma has been recognized as a complication of chronic infection and case–control studies have found a five-fold increased risk with liver fluke infection. The oncogenic mechanism is again unclear although chronic inflammation is believed to play a role. The antihelminth drug praziquantel is the treatment of choice.

Worldwide contributions to cancer

The current world population is six billion and the global burden of cancer is estimated to be 10 million new cases and six million deaths annually. Projections for 2020, when the global population is estimated to have risen to eight billion, are 20 million new cases and 12 million deaths annually. Tobacco contributes to three million cases of cancer (chiefly lung, head and neck, bladder), diet to an estimated three million cases (upper gastrointestinal, colorectal) and infection to a further 1.5 million cases (cervical, stomach, liver, bladder and lymphomas) globally. Prevention by tobacco control, dietary advice and affordable food, and infection control and immunization could have a major impact in reducing the global burden of cancer. The differences in outcome for tumours between the developed and the developing worlds are most marked for the rare but curable cancers where access to therapy dramatically improves survival (e.g. acute leukaemias, Hodgkin's disease and testicular cancers). Small differences are recorded where screening programmes aimed at early detection are effective (e.g. cervical and breast cancers), whilst there are little differences in outcome in the common tumours where prevention has a major role (e.g. lung, stomach and liver cancers). These observations have led to a World Health

Table 2.15 WHO cancer priority ladder.

1. Tobacco control
2. Infection control
3. Curable cancer programme
4. Early detection programme
5. Effective pain control
6. Sample cancer registry
7. Healthy eating programme
8. Referral guidelines
9. Clinical care guidelines
10. Nurse education
11. National cancer network
12. Clinical evaluation unit
13. Platform technology focus for region
14. Clinical research programme
15. Basic research programme
16. International aid programme

Organization (WHO) list of priorities to reduce global cancer, that starts not with scientific research or expensive chemotherapy, but with tobacco and infection control (Table 2.15). In an optimistic scenario the implementation of these priorities could reduce the estimated cancer incidence of 20 million in 2020 to 15 million and could reduce the expected mortality of 12 million to 6 million.

Chapter 3

The principles of cancer treatment

Appropriate care

The care of people with cancer requires careful deliberation and consultation with the patient. The appropriate care will depend upon the prognosis, the effectiveness and toxicity of any therapy, and finally, most importantly, on the patient's wishes. To empower patients to participate in this decision-making process requires them to be fully informed and the clear delivery of this information is essential. A number of resources are available to supplement the information divulged by clinicians to their patients. These include a number of web-based resources as well as patient information leaflets published by charities including Macmillan Cancerbackup and individual tumour-type patient groups such as Breast Cancer Breakthrough. It is increasingly appreciated that the management of patients with cancer requires a multidisciplinary approach involving a team of professionals including surgeons, clinical and medical oncologists, palliative care physicians, radiologists, histopathologists, specialist oncology and palliative care nurses, clinical psychologists, counsellors, dieticians, occupational therapists, physiotherapists, social workers and clinical geneticists.

The aims of therapy should be clearly identified before embarking on a course of treatment. Treat-

ment may either be curative, aiming to prolong the quantity of life, or palliative, aiming to improve the quality of life. When considering the management of individual tumour types, the maxim that prevention is better than cure should be recalled. Cancer prevention and screening are essential if the global burden of malignancy is to be minimized.

During the last quarter of the 20th century, the role of chemotherapy, radiotherapy and endocrine therapy after primary surgery for localized breast cancer was recognized. These additional treatments are defined as adjuvant therapies. Thus adjuvant therapy is treatment after the primary tumour has been removed surgically and in the absence of detectable residual disease. Whilst large clinical trials demonstrated the advantages of adjuvant therapy to a population of women with breast cancer, the benefits for an individual woman are not measurable. In part for this reason and with a view to facilitating surgery, oncologists developed neoadjuvant treatments. Neoadjuvant therapy, usually chemotherapy or endocrine therapy, is delivered prior to surgery or radiotherapy to downsize the tumour, thus demonstrating the sensitivity of the tumour and potentially reducing the extent of the surgical resection or radiation field.

Surgical oncology

Surgery has six major roles in the management of people with cancer:

Lecture Notes: Oncology, 2nd edition. By M. Bower and J. Waxman. Published 2010 by Blackwell Publishing Ltd.

1. Cancer prevention.
2. Cancer diagnosis and staging.
3. Treating cancer.
4. Management of oncological emergencies.
5. Palliation of cancer symptoms.
6. Surgical reconstruction following cancer therapy.

Surgical oncology is the oldest discipline for the management of cancer and originates with attempts at curative resections. Surgical oncology enjoyed a golden era at the end of the 19th century and early 20th century prior to the First World War (Table 3.1). Subsequent advances in surgical oncology included the development of endocrine surgery for metastatic disease. Surgical hormone ablation was pioneered by George Beatson, a Glaswegian surgeon who gave his name to Scotland's largest cancer centre for the management of breast cancer over 100 years ago (Table 3.2).

Table 3.1 Landmarks in radical surgical oncology.

Year	Surgeon	Operation
1881	Albert Billroth	Subtotal gastrectomy
1890	William Halsted	Radical mastectomy
1897	Carl Schlatter	Total gastrectomy
1898	Johann von Mikulicz	Oesophagogastrectomy
1900	Ernest Wertheim	Radical hysterectomy
1906	W. Ernest Miles	Abdominoperineal excision of rectum
1913	Franz Torek	Oesophagectomy
1913	Wilfred Trotter	Partial pharyngectomy
1933	Evarts Graham	Pneumonectomy
1935	A. O. Whipple	Pancreaticoduodenectomy

Table 3.2 Landmarks in endocrine surgery for advanced cancer.

Year	Surgeon	Operation
1896	George Beatson	Oophrectomy for breast cancer
1941	Charles Huggins and Clarence Hodges	Orchidectomy for prostate cancer
1951	Rolf Luft and Herbert Olivecrona	Hypophysectomy for breast cancer
1952	Charles Huggins and D. M. Bergenstal	Adrenalectomy for breast cancer

Surgical cancer prophylaxis

The prevention of cancer by surgery has expanded greatly in recent years with the identification of individuals at high risk of developing malignancies because they have inherited germline genetic mutations associated with cancer predisposition. However, perhaps the most widespread example of surgical cancer prevention is the role of orchiopexy in the management of undescended testes. Undescended testes are the most common birth defect of the male genitalia, affecting up to 3% of live births. Although in many cases the testes will descend to the scrotum during the first year of life, undescended testes are associated with a 4–40-fold increased risk of malignancy, especially testicular seminoma. Orchiopexy, surgey to move the undescended testis into the scrotum, has been shown to reduce infertility although it remains controversial whether it also reduces the risk of malignancy. Nevertheless, it certainly makes the detection of testicular tumours easier to recognize and diagnose at an earlier stage. Familial adenomatous polyposis (FAP) is an autosomal dominant disorder characterized by the development of multiple polyps in the colon which may undergo transformation to malignant tumours. Most patients with FAP will develop a colonic cancer by the age of 40 years old, so prophylactic colectomy is generally recommended before the age of 25 years. Similarly, risk-reducing prophylactic mastectomy may be advocated for women with inherited mutations of BRCA genes (Table 3.3).

Table 3.3 Prophylactic surgery.

Indication	Prophylactic operation
Cryptorchidism	Orchiopexy
Polyposis coli/chronic ulcerative colitis	Colectomy
Familial medullary thyroid cancer (MEN 2 and 3)	Thyroidectomy
Familial breast cancer (BRCA 1 and 2)	Mastectomy
Familial ovarian cancer (BRCA 1 and 2)	Oophrectomy

BRCA, breast cancer; MEN, multiple endocrine neoplasia.

Surgical diagnosis and staging of cancer

Oncological diagnosis hinges on histopathology, and surgeons play a major role along with interventional radiologists in obtaining tissue specimens. Whilst aspiration cytology and fine-needle biopsies can be undertaken radiologically or endoscopically, more extensive incision or excision biopsies require surgical involvement. Careful specimen orientation and inking prior to histological sectioning may be required to assess the status of tumour margins. The optimal surgical approach and biopsy technique for tumour sampling must take into account concerns about contaminating new tissue planes with cancer cells that could jeopardize subsequent therapy. For example, thoracoscopic pleural biopsy of mesothelioma may result in needle-track metastases along the path of surgical instrumentation. The risk of this surgical spread of the cancer is reduced in mesothelioma by postoperative radiotherapy to the biopsy track. Surgery had a major role in the staging of tumours prior to the development of improved radiological techniques and a staging laparotomy was routine care in the management of Hodgkin's disease until the late 1980s. Surgical staging retains a role in the management of ovarian epithelial cancer and the surgical placement of radio-opaque titanium clips (that are non-ferrous and thus safe in the magnetic resonance imaging (MRI) scanner) may guide postoperative radiotherapy in some tumours.

Surgical treatment of cancer

The surgical treatment of cancer includes definitive curative surgery (with or without adjuvant treatments), debulking operations, metastasectomy and endocrine ablation surgery for advanced disease, although the later is largely historical as pharmacological hormone manipulations have taken over most of this role. It is really important to avoid unnecessary surgery in patients with extensive unresectable cancer whilst ensuring that patients with potentially curative tumours are not denied surgery. The treatment of cancer by multidisciplinary teams including radiologists, pathologists, physicians and surgeons is designed to ensure the right patients have the right operations at the right time. For example, this approach aims to guarantee that patients who are candidates for neoadjuvant down-staging therapy prior to surgery are not wheeled straight into the operating theatre. Most early curative surgery aimed to remove tumours *en bloc*, that is with the draining lymph nodes. In recent times surgeons have developed the use of more conservative function-preserving operations. Examples of the latter include wide local excision rather than mastectomy and partial nephron-sparing nephrectomy rather than radical nephrectomy for small renal tumours. A further development in surgery for skin tumours was introduced by Dr Frederic Mohs when he was still a medical student at the University of Wisconsin-Madison. Mohs' surgery for skin tumours involves the sectioning and mapping of surgical margins during the operation to ensure completeness of tumour resection. Instead of using a breadknife and the pathologist looking at each slice, the Mohs' technique is like a vegetable peeler with the pathologist examining each peeling for involvement during the surgery. Whilst this is a more laborious technique, it is especially valuable for tumours at specific anatomical sites such as the eyelids and in recurrent disease.

Debulking operations that do not result in complete surgical removal of the tumour are not always futile. They can provide important clinical benefits in selected tumour types including ovarian cancer and primary brain tumours and are usually followed by either chemotherapy or radiotherapy. Debulking surgery forms part of the treatment algorithm in several uncommon tumours such as thymomas and pseudomyxoma peritonei. Mucin secretion into the abdominal cavity by mucinous adenocarcinomas most commonly arising in the appendix is the usual cause of pseudomyxoma peritonei. The term 'myxoma' is derived from the Greek for mucin but the etymology of the medical terms myxoma and pseudomyxoma seem to have got mixed up. Myxomas are benign, pedunculated connective tissue tumours usually arising in the atria of the heart and are not mucinous, whilst pseudomyxoma peritonei fills the abdominal cavity with true jelly-like mucin.

The surgical resection of secondary deposits may seem perverse since the presence of metastases implies systemic dissemination of the cancer. Nevertheless, surgical oncologists have embraced this approach enthusiastically, mainly on the basis of relatively weak evidence from uncontrolled retrospective series that have been interpreted as demonstrating a survival benefit. The resection of lung, liver and brain metastases has become a part of the routine treatment strategy for a number of types of cancer. The most common indication for surgical metastasectomy is for hepatic secondaries from colorectal cancer. The rationale for this approach is based upon reported five-year survivals of around 30% in patients undergoing surgery compared to around 10% in those who received chemotherapy. However, there are no randomixed controlled studies that support hepatic metastasectomy and the case series are inevitably confounded by selection and reporting bias. Similarly, pulmonary metastasectomy has been widely adopted for osteogenic sarcomas, soft tissue sarcomas, renal cell tumours and melanomas and cerebral metastasectomy has also been advocated in a similar spectrum of malignancies. In contrast to metastasectomy, the surgical resection of residual masses following the completion of chemotherapy forms part of the multidisciplinary treatment of advanced non-seminomatous germ cell tumours to remove residual differentiated teratoma that could relapse at a later date. Finally, surgical endocrine ablation is nowadays rarely indicated for metastatic cancer although surgical castration is occasionally performed for advanced prostate cancer.

Surgery for oncological emergencies

Surgery has an important role in the optimal management of oncological emergencies, in particular metastatic spinal cord compression where rapid surgical decompression reduces neurological disability (see Cord compression in Chapter 46). Surgical decompression and spinal column stabilization should be offered to patients with a good prognosis and needs to be undertaken as swiftly as possible, preferably before patients lose the ability to walk. The optimal neurosurgical approach will depend upon the anatomical site of compression and the stability of the spine. If spinal metastases involve the vertebral body or threaten spinal stability, posterior decompression should always be accompanied by internal fixation with or without bone grafting.

Surgical palliation of cancer

The palliation of tumour-associated obstruction, fluid accumulation and bleeding may require surgical intervention, although the placement of shunts and stents is now more frequently undertaken by endoscopists and interventional radiologists. Plastic or metal stents are used to relieve obstruction of the bowel, oesophagus, bronchial tree, biliary ducts and ureters, and even patients with advanced malignancy benefit. Diathermy or laser coagulation of tumour-related haemorrhage similarly is a valuable palliative intervention which can often be undertaken endoscopically. Surgical relief of bowel obstruction may be indicated when stenting is not feasible but usually requires either colostomy or ileostomy depending upon the level of the obstruction. Fistulae are abnormal passageways connecting two epithelial-lined organs not normally connected and include rectovaginal, enterovaginal, colovesical and vesicovaginal or combinations of these. Fistulae may be either related to locally advanced disease or may be a consequence of radiotherapy. Fistula surgery is complex and demanding, requiring surgical expertise and often prolonged recovery, so it is usually reserved for cancer patients in remission. The surgical placement of shunts to prevent the reaccumulation of ascites (usually peritoneal–venous shunts, e.g. Leveen shunt) and pleural effusions (usually pleuroperitoneal shunts, e.g. Denver shunt) may be indicated for symptom palliation. Surgical oncologists may also be called upon to perform surgery for ulcerating and necrotic locally advanced cancers such as toilet mastectomy for fungating breast tumours. Orthopaedic surgeons frequently operate on pathological bone metastases either as a form of secondary prevention or following pathological fractures. Internal fixation of bones with lytic metastases are especially important in weight-bearing bones with large deposits occupying more than half the bone cortex that are at a high risk of fracturing. Surgeons thus have an important role in the palliation of symptoms in advanced malignancy and their input into the multidisciplinary team should not be seen as just to establish the diagnosis and surgically resect curable cancers.

Surgical reconstruction following cancer therapy

The aggressive treatment of bulky tumours often leaves major residual defects and, in combination with plastic surgeons, the discipline of surgical oncology has developed reconstructive surgery to reduce some of the effects of tumour resections. Plastic surgeons have developed a reconstructive ladder of increasingly complex wound management to deal with some of these residual deficits (Table 3.4). Reconstructive surgery is not, however, the exclusive responsibility of plastic surgeons. For example, orthopaedic surgeons have developed sophisticated procedures for limb reconstruction following sarcoma surgery using bone grafts and prostheses. Maxillofacial surgeons reconstruct mandibles with free-flap fibula transplants following surgery for oral cavity cancers. ENT surgeons medialize vocal cords with silicon injection to overcome the hoarse voice associated with recurrent laryngeal nerve palsy caused by mediastinal tumours. Breast reconstruction following mastectomy often involves the insertion of a tissue expander that is progressively injected with saline

Table 3.4 Reconstructive ladder of increasingly complex wound management coined by plastic surgeons.

1. Healing by secondary intent
2. Primary closure
3. Delayed primary closure
4. Split thickness graft
5. Full thickness skin graft
6. Tissue expansion
7. Random pattern graft
8. Pedicled flap
9. Free flap with vascular microsurgery

over the ensuing weeks until a suitable size and shape has been achieved, when it may be replaced by a more permanent implant. The second most common breast reconstruction procedure involves flaps of tissues from other parts of the body such as the back, abdomen, buttocks or thigh. These flaps may be pedicled, leaving the original blood supply, or may be free flaps with vascular microsurgery to connect to a new blood supply. A latissimus dorsi muscle flap can be performed without significant loss of function and retaining its original blood supply. Abdominal flaps usually take tissue from the lower abdomen, for example the TRAM (transverse rectus abdominis myocutaneous) flap which leaves the abdominal wall weakened. More recent abdominal flaps attempt to retain abdominal wall strength by using a muscle-sparing DIEP (deep inferior epigastric perforator) flap or SIEA (superficial inferior epigastric artery) flap. These require greater microsurgical skill. Other autologous tissue donor sites for breast reconstruction include SGAP (superior gluteal artery perforator) and IGAP (inferior gluteal artery perforator) flaps from the buttocks.

Radiotherapy

Radiotherapy involves the use of high-energy ionizing radiation to cause DNA damage and ultimately cell death. The damage induced by ionizing radiation may be lethal or sub-lethal to the tumour cells. In sub-lethal cell injury, damage to cellular proteins and organelles causes microscopic changes in the cell characterized down the microscope by swelling of mitochondria and endoplasmic reticulum and cloudiness of the cytoplasm known as hydropic degeneration. Cells may repair sub-lethal damage by removing damaged proteins and organelles by a cell stress response and autophagy and replace them with newly synthesized components. In contrast, lethal damage results in either cell necrosis or apoptosis.

Ionizing radiation acts by ejecting an electron from an atom to yield an ion pair. This may lead to direct damage to DNA via molecular excitation or indirectly via the hydrolysis of water into free radicals with an open electron shell configuration

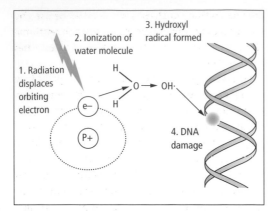

Figure 3.1 How radiation damages DNA.

characterized by the presence of an unpaired electron (Figure 3.1). These free radicals are highly reactive, usually short-lived chemicals such as the neutrally charged hydroxyl radical (OH·) derived from water which has an *in vivo* half-life of about 10^{-9} seconds. The other common free radical formed from water is superoxide (O_2^-) with one unpaired electron, which is responsible for the 'oxidative burst' or oxygen-dependent intracellular killing of ingested bacteria by phagocytes and is detoxified by the enzyme superoxide dismutase.

The dose of radiotherapy is defined as the amount of energy deposited in tissues and is measured in Grays (Gy) after Hal Gray, a British pioneer of radiation biology and physics who also established the Gray Laboratories at Mount Vernon Hospital. One Gray is the dose absorbed when 1 J (joule) is deposited in 1 kg of tissue. Each Gray per cell causes approximately 10 000 damaged DNA bases, 1000 damaged deoxyribose sugars, 1000 single strand breaks, 40 double strand breaks, 150 DNA–protein cross-links and 30 DNA–DNA cross-links. Radiation can have an effect at any point in the cell cycle, although it is only at the time of mitosis that cell death occurs. Therefore, there can be a time lag of days, weeks or even months between the radiotherapy and the full effects of the treatment becoming manifest. Typical radiotherapy doses for solid epithelial tumours are 60–80 Gy. This is delivered as multiple fractions over time for several reasons. Dose fractionation allows normal cells to recover from sub-lethal damage between

fractions, whilst tumour cells are less efficient at repairing damage. Dose fractionation also ensures that tumour cells in different phases of the cell cycle are exposed to radiation since it causes greatest damage in the G2 and M phases. The exact scheduling and fractionation of radiotherapy varies but in general doses of around 2 Gy are delivered on a daily basis five days a week. In some circumstances more frequent dosing has been shown to be more efficacious but is of course more demanding on resources. For example, CHART (continuous hyperfractionated accelerated radiotherapy) involves radiotherapy delivered three times a day, every day of the week, usually for a fortnight.

Radiotherapy utilizes X-rays, electron beams and β- or γ-radiation produced by radioactive isotopes. X-rays are produced when a high-energy electron beam that is produced by heating an electrode in a vacuum, strikes matter. The energy of X-rays can be changed by altering the voltage input to the cathode of the X-ray tube that accelerates the electrons. Diagnostic radiology uses low-voltage equipment (e.g. 50 kV), producing X-rays of longer wavelength that are less penetrating. Therapeutic X-rays are produced by higher voltage machines (30–50 MeV) producing shorter wavelength, more penetrating X-rays.

Radiotherapy is delivered in three ways: external beam radiotherapy, brachytherapy and radioisotope therapy. External beam radiotherapy involves the use of isotope sources or linear accelerators to deliver radiation from a distance. In the case of brachytherapy, the radioactive source is a solid radioactive nuclide emitting γ-rays which is placed within the tumour or closely applied to the tumour. Finally, radioactive isotopes that are preferentially taken up in the target organ may be administered orally or intravenously; for example, oral iodine-131 is given for the treatment of thyroid tumours and intravenous strontium-89 in palliative treatment of bone metastasis.

External beam radiotherapy

Superficial voltage machines operate at 50–150 kV and their energy does not penetrate more than

1 cm below the surface of the skin. They are used chiefly to treat superficial skin cancers. Orthovoltage machines that yield X-rays of 200–300 kV energy penetrate to a depth of 3 cm. Metastases in bones close to the skin surface (ribs, sacrum) are frequently treated on these machines. Megavoltage radiotherapy machines usually use a cobalt-60 source that produces X-rays of 1.25 MeV on decaying to nickel-60. The cobalt-60 sources are contained within a protective lead shield and an adjustable window in this shield allows regulation of the γ-ray beam. However, there is considerable scatter of the beam, limiting the focus, and the relatively short half-life of the cobalt source means that it needs to be replaced every three to four years and that treatment times may become prolonged as the cobalt nears the replacement date. It is

speculated that cobalt-60 sources could be used by terrorists to produce a 'dirty' bomb, a conventional explosive device to which radioactive material has been added.

Megavoltage machines have been replaced by linear accelerators that produce a high-energy electron beam by accelerating electrons down a cylindrical waveguide before they bombard a fixed target, resulting in a high-intensity electron beam (4–20 MeV) with greater penetration and less scatter. The advantages of this electron beam over X-rays lie in the penetration and decay characteristics that allow an electron beam to deliver its high energy to deep-seated tumours whilst sparing normal tissues in its pathway (Figure 3.2).

The accurate shaping of the radiation field to encompass the cancer but minimize damage to

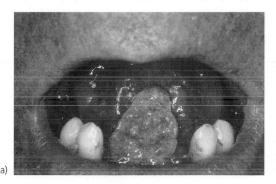
(a)

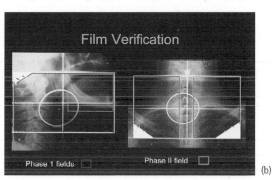
(b)

(c)

Figure 3.2 (a) Squamous cell cancer of the oral cavity. (b) Radiological verification of the radiotherapy fields. (c) The planned radiotherapy fields.

normal tissues really began with the introduction of the multileaf collimator composed of over 100 metal leaves, 5 mm thick and each aligned parallel to the radiation field. As each leaf may be moved independently to block part of the field, the resulting radiation field may be shaped and sculpted to suit the target. A further refinement of this process, known as intensity-modulated radiotherapy (IMRT), involves moving the multileaf collimator during the dose so that another level of fine tuning of the field can be achieved (Figure 3.3). One more recent development is image-guided radiation therapy (IGRT) that links the carefully shaped field with a continuous image of the patient. This process can overcome, for example, movement artefacts generated by the patient (hopefully still) breathing.

Brachytherapy

Brachytherapy employs sealed radionuclide sources that are implanted directly into a tumour or body cavity to deliver localized radiotherapy (Table 3.5). Examples of bachytherapy include radioactive iridium-192 needles or wires implanted into tumours of the breast, tongue and floor of the mouth. Sealed caesium-137 radioactive sources may also be placed into the vagina or rectum to treat cancers of the vagina, cervix, lower uterus, rectum or anus. Brachytherapy seeds are increasingly being used to treat localized prostate cancer (Figure 3.4). The major disadvantage of brachytherapy is the risk to staff handling the radioactive sources and caring for the patients. The radioactivity exposure of all staff involved with brachytherapy must be monitored. Another method used to reduce exposure is to place inactive source holders while the patient is anaesthetized, and once they have been correctly located (as determined by X-ray) the patient is allowed to recover from the procedure. With the patient in a shielded room, the live radioactive source is then introduced, either manually or by remote control using a selectron. This routine is termed manual or remote

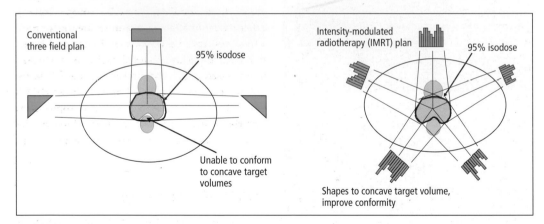

Figure 3.3 Comparison of conventional and intensity-modulated radiotherapy planning.

Table 3.5 Radionuclides used for brachytherapy.

Source	Half-life	Mean X-ray energy	Form
Cobalt-60	5.3 years	1.25 MeV	Pellets (beads, tubes, needles)
Caesium-137	30 years	0.66 MeV	Tubes, needles
Iridium-92	74 days	0.37 MeV	Wires, hairpins, cylinders
Iodine-125	60 days	0.03 MeV	Grains, seeds

Table 3.6 Table of systemically administered radionuclides used in oncology.

Radioisotope	Decay	Uses in oncology
Iodine-131	Beta: 192 keV Gamma: 364 keV Half-life: 8 days β- and γ-emitter	Used in treating thyroid cancer and in imaging the thyroid gland
Phosphorus-32	1.71 MeV Half-life: 14 days β-emitter	Used in the treatment of polycythemia vera
Rhenium-188	2.12 MeV Half-life: 17 hours β-emitter	Used to irradiate coronary arteries via an angioplasty balloon and in relieving the pain of bone metastases
Samarium-153	Beta: 825 keV Gamma: 103 keV Half-life: 47 hours β- and γ-emitter	Used in relieving the pain of bone metastases
Strontium-89	1.481 MeV Half-life: 50 days β-emitter	Used in relieving the pain of bone metastases

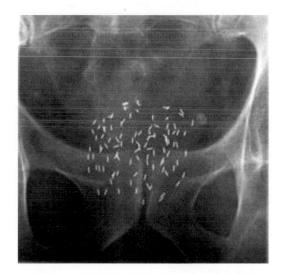

Figure 3.4 Prostate brachytherapy seeds *in situ* seen on pelvic X-ray.

after-loading and is frequently used for tumours of the upper vagina, cervix and endometrium.

Radioisotope therapy

Radioactive isotopes can be given by mouth or injection and are taken up by a particular tissue where they remain. Radioisotope therapy can only be used where a tumour is in a tissue that will preferentially accumulate a specific isotope, leaving other tissues unaffected. Examples are the thyroid, which will take up radioactive iodine and bone, that naturally accumulates phosphorus or will take up bone-seeking radiochemicals such as rhenium-186 hydroxyethylidine diphosphate (^{186}Re-HEDP) (Table 3.6). A disadvantage with this approach is that the source cannot be recovered, limiting the degree of control over the total exposure to radiation.

Toxicity of radiotherapy

External beam radiotherapy is usually given as repeated daily dose fractions rather than as a single large dose of radiotherapy, which would lead to severe damage to the normal tissues. Even with fractionation, normal tissues have a maximum tolerated dose as indicated in Table 3.7. The area to be irradiated is referred to as the radiation field. This is marked out on the skin before treatment and such markings often persist after treatment as tattooed dots. These radiotherapy tattoos are assiduously sought by clinical medical exam candidates but in

Table 3.7 Table of normal tissue tolerance of radiotherapy.

Tissue	Radiation effect	Dosage
Testis	Sterility	0.2 Gy
Eye	Cataract	10 Gy
Lung	Pneumonitis	20 Gy
Kidney	Nephritis	25 Gy
Liver	Hepatitis	30 Gy
Central nervous system	Necrosis	50 Gy
Gastrointestinal tract	Ulceration, haemorrhage	60 Gy

real life most patients will tell you that they have had radiotherapy if you ask them nicely. In general, radiation-related side effects occur within the field of treatment although a few systemic manifestations such as fatigue and nausea may occur. The toxicity of radiotherapy increases with both the volume of tissue irradiated and the dose given. The transient side effects that develop during treatment tend to reflect the acute damage to normal healthy tissue. Careful planning of the beam size and shielding of surrounding tissue, ensuring that radiation fields give effective tumour eradication with an acceptable level of toxicity, is, therefore, a prerequisite of successful therapy.

Radiotherapy-related side effects can be usefully divided into early and late toxicities (Table 3.8). Early toxicity occurs in hours to weeks and includes both systemic effects such as nausea, lethargy and

myelosuppression (when a large volume of bone marrow is within the treated area, for example whole femur or pelvis radiation). Localized skin toxicity is a common early side effect that may be local erythema progressing to ulceration and desquamation in the more severe cases. Other early side effects depend on the anatomy of the radiotherapy field, e.g. alopecia with cranial irradiation (see Plate 3.1), oropharyngeal mucositis with head and neck radiotherapy, and diarrhoea, proctitis and cystitis with pelvic fields. These early reactions occur in tissues that are rapidly dividing and are usually present during or shortly after the course of radiotherapy and in most cases are reversible. Late side effects may take months or years to manifest themselves and once again depend upon the site being irradiated. These late tissue reactions occur when slowly dividing cells attempt division and are less frequently reversible. In some cases the effects are believed to be mediated by fibrosis of the vascular endothelium. Examples of late reactions include necrosis in the central nervous system leading to transverse myelitis and paralysis with spinal cord radiation fields, radiation-induced nephritis and osteomyelitis. Finally, radiotherapy is carcinogenic and may induce secondary tumours.

Radiosensitivity and radioresistance

Tumour resistance to radiotherapy appears to be an intrinsic property of that cancer, rather than an

Table 3.8 Table of adverse early and late reactions to radiotherapy.

Timing	Tissue	Reaction
Early reactions	Skin	Dermatitis
	Oral mucosa	Stomatitis
	Bladder	Cystitis
	Oesophagus	Oesophagitis
	Bowel	Diarrhoea, ulceration
	Bone marrow	Myelosuppression
Late reactions	Central nervous system	Necrosis
	Kidney	Nephritis
	Liver	Hepatitis
	Lung	Pneumonitis and fibrosis
	Vascular endothelium	Fibrosis

acquired attribute selected for by treatment, as in the case of chemotherapy. Indeed the radiation sensitivities of many types of tumour are relatively predictable. The response of tissues both malignant and normal to fractionated radiation depends upon the '5 Rs':

- Repair
- Reassortment
- Repopulation
- Reoxygenation
- Radiosensitivity.

In this context, repair is recovery from sub-lethal damage and is dependent on DNA repair mechanisms. Reassortment refers to the cell cycle phase of the tumour cells. Cells in G2 and M phases are most susceptible to radiotherapy and so after a first dose cells in G1 and S will make up a greater proportion of the live tumour cells. Depending on the timing of the subsequent fraction of radiotherapy these cells may have progressed or 'reassorted' to G2 and M phases with increased sensitivity. Repopulation is the ability of tumour cells to grow and divide between doses of radiotherapy; this is a particular problem with prolonged fractionation and delayed fractions. Hypoxic cells are relatively radioresistant and after the first fractions of radiotherapy, the death of sensitive cells reduces the competition for oxygen in the tumour and cells that were hypoxic previously become reoxygenated and hence more susceptible to radiation. Different cell lineages are more or less radiosensitive and these differences are in part intrinsic and independent of environmental factors. Amongst the factors that influence the radiosensitivity of tumours are the DNA repair genes, the production of free radical scavenging molecules (e.g. glutathione-S-transferases, superoxide dismutases, glutathione peroxidase), genes controlling apoptosis and cell cycle regulatory genes.

Chemotherapy

Drug discovery

The origins of chemotherapy for cancer lie in the use of biological warfare during the First World War, most hauntingly described in Wilfred Owen's poem 'Dulce et decorum est'. Following the extensive use of chlorine gas in trench warfare, the German army first released mustard gas at Ypres on the night of 12–13 July 1917. Mustard gas had been synthesized in 1854 by Victor Meyer and was noted to be a vesicant in 1887. As a weapon of mass destruction, mustard gas or Yperite as it was then known, had the advantages over chlorine of requiring smaller doses, being almost odourless and remaining active in the soil for weeks. The British gas casualties from 1914–1918 reveal the greater fatalities with mustard gas. Mustard gas exposure causes a severe blistering rash and conjunctivitis followed by meyelosuppression after around four days. During the Second World War the only use of mustard gas resulted in an own goal when the Luftwaffe sunk the USS *John Harvey* off Bari harbour in southern Italy in 1943. The ship was carrying 2000 M47A1 bombs containing a total of 100 tonnes of mustard gas and the American sailors who survived developed conjunctivitis and skin blistering followed by a steep fall in their white cell counts, as documented by the naval surgeon Colonel Stewart Alexander. Meanwhile at Yale University, Alfred Gilman and Louis Goodman were using the closely related nitrogen mustard (mechlorethamine) initially in murine lymphoma models. In 1944 the first patient with lymphosarcoma (high-grade non-Hodgkin's lymphoma) was treated and although Mr J. D., a 48-year-old silversmith, achieved a temporary remission of his tumour, he later died of bone marrow failure.

The subsequent development of chemotherapy following this fortuitous finding as a by-product of biological warfare, owes much to luck and trial and error rather than design. One serendipitous discovery was made by Barnett Rosenberg, a physicist at Michigan State University in 1965. He studied the effects of electric currents on *Escherichia coli* using platinum electrodes in a water bath and found that they stopped dividing but not growing, leading to bacteria up to 300 times longer than normal. This was found to be due to cisplatin, a product from the platinum electrodes, which was interfering with DNA replication. By the end of the 1960s a number of cytotoxic drugs from natural sources had been identified. In 1971 President Nixon, losing a war in Vietnam, declared war on cancer, signing the Cancer Act and establishing a drug discovery programme at the National Cancer Institute (NCI). This project trawled though thousands of natural chemicals in search of potential cytotoxic agents. It was not until the 1990s that rational drug design targeting known tumour-related features emerged. Examples of this include trastuzumab, a monoclonal antibody raised against erbB2/neu/Her-2 in breast cancer, and imatinib, which inhibits the adenosine triphosphate (ATP) binding site of brc-abl fusion protein kinase in chronic myeloid leukaemia.

Mechanisms of cytotoxic drug

Amongst the many classifications of cytotoxic agents is a functional classification of cytotoxics (Table 3.9).

Alkylating agents

Alkylating agents transfer an alkyl group to purine (adenine and guanine) bases of DNA. Bifunctional alkylating agents form covalent bonds between two different bases resulting in interstand or intrastrand cross-links, whilst monofunctional alkylating agents cannot form cross-links but cause adducts. Both forms of DNA alteration inhibit DNA synthesis, so alkyating agents act chiefly during the S phase of the cell cycle. Bifunctional agents can act on more than one base and are more cytotoxic, whilst monofunctional agents are more mutagenic and carcinogenic. One of the mechanisms of tumour resistance to alkylating agents is enzymatic removal of alkyl groups from purine bases and enhanced repair of cross-links.

Antimetabolites

Antimetabolites are structurally similar to natural compounds and in general interfere with cellular enzymes. These agents inhibit the metabolism (usually synthesis) of compounds necessary for DNA, RNA or protein synthesis. They include: (1) purine analogues, (2) pyrimidine analogues, (3) folic acid analogues, and (4) others, e.g. hydroxyu-

rea. Most antimetabolites have their greatest activity during the S phase.

Intercalating agents

Intercalating agents disrupt the steric integrity of the DNA double helix. The exact mechanisms of this action remain uncertain although anthracycline antibiotics intercalate into the DNA major groove between base pairs of the DNA double helix and this action is non-covalent with no base sequence specificity. Platinum agents also intercalate and form intrastrand links similar to those formed by alkylating agents.

Spindle poisons

Antimicrotubule drugs can be divided into two groups, those that stabilize microtubules by inhibiting depolymerization (e.g. taxanes) and those that are depolymerizing agents that inhibit polymerization of tubulin (e.g. vinca alkaloids). Spindle poisons inhibit the mitotic spindle function and therefore act in the M phase of the cell cycle. Tubulin exists as α-tubulin and β-tubulin monomers in dynamic equilibrium with tubulin polymers, or microtubules. Resistance to spindle poisons may occur by mutations of β-tubulin and these point mutations do not confer cross-resistance between taxanes and vincas. An early spindle cell poison included colchicine used for acute gout, familial Mediterranean fever and rarely psoriasis. Although colchicine, like vincas causes depolymerization, it binds to a distinct site and is not used as a cytotoxic.

Topoisomerase inhibitors

Topoisomerases prevent DNA strands from becoming tangled by cutting DNA and allowing it to wind or unwind. There are two mammalian classes of topoisomerases: topoisomerase I breaks single strands of DNA, whilst topoisomerase II breaks both strands of DNA. Topoisomerase I inhibitors act by inhibiting the re-ligation step of the nicking–closing reaction trapping topoisomerase I in a covalent complex with DNA. Topoisomerase I

Table 3.9 A functional classification of cytotoxics.

Functional group	Chemical group	Examples
Alkylating agents	Nitrogen mustards	Chlorambucil
		Cyclophosphamide
		Melphalan
	Nitrosoureas	BCNU (carmustine)
		CCNU (lomustine)
		Streptozotocin
	Tetrazine compounds	Dacarbazine
		Temozolomide
	Aziridines	Mitomycin C
		Thiotepa
	Methane sulphonic esters	Busulphan
Antimetabolites	Purine analogues	6-Mercaptopurine
		6-Thioguanine
	Pyrimidine analogues	Cytarabine
		Gemcytabine
	Dihydrofolate reductase inhibitors	Methotrexate
		Ralitexed
	Thymidylate synthetase inhibitors	5-Fluorouracil
	Ribonucleotide reductase inhibitors	Hydroxyurea
Intercalating agents	Platins	Cisplatin
		Carboplatin
		Oxaliplatin
	Antibiotics	Doxorubicin
	Anthracyclins	Daunorubicin
	Anthraquinones	Mitoxantrone
	Others	Bleomycin
		Mitomycin C
		Actinomycin D
Spindle cell poisons	Vinca alkaloids	Vincristine
		Vinblastine
		Vinorelbine
	Taxanes	Paclitaxel
		Docetaxel
Topoisomerase inhibitors	Topoisomerase I inhibitors: camptothecins	Topotecan
		Irinotecan
	Topoisomerase II inhibitors: epipodophylotoxins	Etoposide
		Teniposide

inhibitors act in the S phase and belong to the camptothecin group. Camptothecin was discovered by the NCI screening of plant-derived compounds and was isolated from a Chinese small tree *Camptotheca acuminata*. Topoisomerase II is inhibited both DNA intercalators (e.g. anthracyclines) and by non-intercalators (e.g. epipodophyllotoxins).

Chemotherapy resistance

The major obstacle to successful cures with chemotherapy is the development of drug resistance by tumours. Indeed the intrinsic resistance of some tumour cell types accounts, in part, for the variable sensitivity of different cancers to chemotherapy (Table 3.10). In some circumstances drug

Table 3.10 Sensitivity and curability of selected cancers treated with chemotherapy.

Chemosensitivity	Tumour
Sensitive and curable	Leukaemias
	Lymphomas
	Germ cell tumours
	Childhood tumours
Sensitive and normally	Small cell lung cancer
incurable (radical palliation)	Myeloma
Moderately sensitive	Breast cancer
(palliation or adjuvant	Colorectal cancer
treatments)	Ovarian cancer
	Bladder cancer
Low sensitivity (chemotherapy	Kidney cancer
of limited use)	Melanoma
	Adult brain tumours
	Prostate cancer

resistance is to a single drug only, whilst in other cases there is cross-resistance between different drugs. The latter mechanism is due to the expression of molecular efflux pumps in tumour cell membranes. The most commonly found pump in multiresistant tumour cells is P-glycoprotein (Pgp) or the multidrug resistance protein (MDR). This transmembrane protein pumps natural toxins out of cells (including most chemotherapy agents) and is normally present in selected cells of the body such as renal proximal tubule cells, the apical mucosal cells of the colon and the canilicular surface of hepatocytes. Overexpression of Pgp/ MDR by cancer cells confers a survival advantage in the presence of chemotherapy by inducing tumour resistance.

Cytotoxic-specific drug resistance can be achieved by a number of mechanisms including efficient repair of DNA, reduced drug uptake, increased drug efflux, decreased intracellular activation of the drug, increased intracellular inactivation of the drug, activation of biochemical pathways that bypass the pathway being blocked by the cytotoxic drug, and finally compensation for blocked enzyme pathways by increased enzyme production. An example of the last form of drug-specific resistance occurs with methotrexate, an antifolate antimetabolite that inhibits dihydrofolate reduct-

ase (DHFR). The first ever cancer cures with chemotherapy alone were reported with methotrexate for choriocarcinoma in 1963. In resistant tumour cells there is amplification of the DHFR gene with many thousands of copies of the gene leading to higher levels of DHFR to overcome the inhibitory actions of methotrexate.

How chemotherapy is used

Cytotoxic drugs are rarely used as single agents but are usually administered in combinations in an attempt to improve treatment efficacy by reducing the development of drug resistance, based on similar principles in the management of infectious diseases such as tuberculosis. A number of considerations are applied to the design of chemotherapy combinations. Only drugs that have proven activity as single agents should be included and preference should be given to drugs with non-overlapping toxicities and different modes of action. Cycles or pulses of chemotherapy given intermittently are designed to allow for recovery of normal tissues between doses without enabling the tumour cells to repopulate. Although this goal is frequently desirable, in recent years a number of continuous infusion chemotherapy regimens have been developed. The importance of a good acronym for a chemotherapy regimen should not be underestimated. No single regimen has remained the gold standard of care for as long as the CHOP regimen for non-Hodgkin's lymphoma, easily seeing off competition from the likes of ProMACE-CytaBOM. With greater experience of the benefits and disadvantages of chemotherapy, its safety has improved and the indications for its use have expanded. As with radiotherapy and endocrine treatments chemotherapy is increasingly used in an adjuvant context (Table 3.11).

In some circumstances chemotherapy resistance may be overcome by escalating the dose of cytotoxic drugs. In many circumstances the dose-limiting toxicity (DLT) of chemotherapy is myelosuppression and if this can be avoided doses may be doubled or more before reaching the next DLT, which is often mucosal damage. Autologous (from the patient him/herself) and allogeneic

Table 3.11 Cancers effectively treated by neoadjuvant and adjuvant chemotherapy.

Therapy	Tumour
Cancers effectively treated by neoadjuvant chemotherapy	Soft tissue sarcoma Osteosarcoma Locally advanced breast cancer
Cancers effectively treated by adjuvant chemotherapy	Wilms' tumour Osteosarcoma Breast cancer Colorectal cancer

(from a donor) bone marrow transplantation was developed to this end. Prior to high-dose chemotherapy, progenitor stem cells are harvested either from multiple bone marrow aspirations (bone marrow transplant or BMT) or now more often from peripheral blood following growth factor stimulation (peripheral blood stem cell transplant or PBSCT). These stem cells are immature haematopoietic cells capable of repopulating the bone marrow. The patient then receives the conditioning high-dose chemotherapy and/or radiotherapy and subsequently the stem cells are re-infused as a transfusion. This approach has an appreciable mortality of 20–50% in the case of allogeneic BMT and of 5% with autologous PBSCT. However, stem cell transplantation has a defined role in the management of a number of malignancies (Table 3.12).

Side effects of chemotherapy

The main actions of chemotherapy are focused on killing rapidly dividing cancer cells and hence many of their toxicities arise because of the effects on normal cells with high rates of turnover. Indeed the side effects of chemotherapy may be divided into the predictable toxicities that are common, often dose related and usually related to the mechanism of action of the drug. In contrast idiosyncratic side effects are usually rarer, unrelated to dose or mechanism of action but tend to be drug specific. The predictable effects of chemotherapy on fast dividing normal cells (bone marrow, gastrointestinal tract epithelium, hair follicles, spermatogonia) will be a consequence of inhibition of cell division and are especially found with cell cycle phase-specific cytotoxics. In contrast the side effects on slow-growing cell types will occur most frequently with drugs that are not cell cycle specific such as the alkylating agents that introduce DNA mutations into these cells resulting in secondary leukaemias and other tumours.

The side effects of chemotherapy may be divided into three time groups, immediate effects that occur within hours, delayed effects that occur within days, weeks or months but are generally manifested whilst the full course of chemotherapy treatment is on-going, and late effects that occur

Table 3.12 Cancers effectively treated by high-dose chemotherapy and stem cell transplantation.

Disease	Stage	Transplant	Approx. 5-year disease-free survival
CML	Stable phase	Allogeneic	30%
ALL	Second remission	Allogeneic/autologous	40%
AML	First remission	Allogeneic/autologous	50%
High-grade non-Hodgkin's lymphoma	Responsive relapse	Autologous	45%
Hodgkin's disease	Responsive relapse	Autologous	45%
Neuroblastoma	High risk first line	Allogeneic/autologous	50%
Neuroblastoma	Relapsed	Allogeneic/autologous	25%
Non-seminomatous germ cell tumour	Responsive relapse	Autologous	50%
Myeloma	First line	Allogeneic/autologous	30%

ALL, acute lymphoblastic leukaemia; AML, acute myeloid leukaemia; CML, chronic myeloid leukaemia.

months, years or decades after the chemotherapy has ceased. The top five side effects ranked by patients according to severity are nausea, fatigue, hair loss, concern about the effects on friends and family and finally vomiting. The immediate toxicities include nausea and vomiting, anaphylaxis, extravasation and tumour lysis. The delayed side effects are the most abundant and include alopecia, myelosuppression, stomatitis and the majority of the unpredictable toxicities. The late effects of chemotherapy include infertility and secondary malignancies.

Early side effects

Nausea and vomiting

Vomiting is a central reflex initiated in the vomiting centre of the medulla that co-ordinates the contraction of the diaphragm and abdominal muscles with relaxation of the cardiac sphincter and the muscles of the throat. There are four inputs into the vomiting centre: the labyrinths (e.g. motion sickness), the higher cortical centres (e.g. fear, anticipation), the vagus nerve sensory input from the gastrointestinal tract particularly the small bowel, and finally the chemoreceptor trigger zone (CTZ). The CTZ is located in the area postrema adjacent to the fourth ventricle where the blood–brain barrier is relatively deficient and chemicals in the blood and cerebrospinal fluid (CSF) are sensed, stimulating the vomiting centre. The different inputs to the vomiting centre rely on different neurotransmitters and this can be exploited pharmacologically in the control of symptoms (Figure 3.5). Chemotherapy chiefly acts on the gastrointestinal tract causing serotonin (5-hydroxytryptamine, 5HT) release and acting via the afferent vagus nerve. It also stimulates the chemoreceptor trigger zone which employs

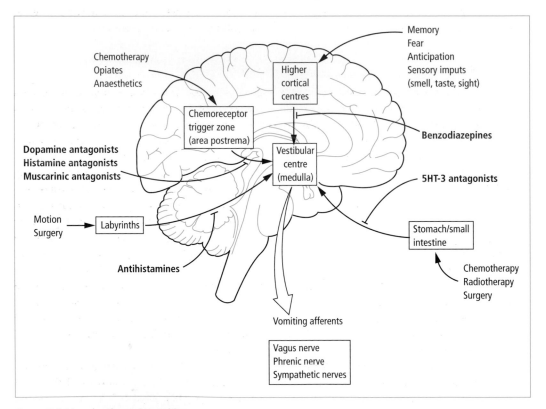

Figure 3.5 Neural pathways in vomiting.

dopaminergic and muscarinic pathways. Occasionally anticipatory vomiting is problematic and this acts through the higher cortical centres using γ-aminobutyric acid (GABA) neurotransmission. In contrast, the labyrinthine pathways utilize histamine-1 receptors and motion sickness is often successfully controlled with antihistamines.

The likelihood of being sick with chemotherapy depends upon the emetogenicity of the cytotoxics used as well as host-related factors. Cisplatin and mustine are amongst the most emetogenic whilst vinca alkaloids rarely cause nausea. Younger age, women, patients who have been sick previously with chemotherapy, and patients with a low alcohol intake are all more likely to suffer with chemotherapy-induced vomiting. Acute vomiting within six hours of chemotherapy is best controlled by a combination of steroids and 5HT-3 receptor antagonists. Delayed vomiting occurring up to five days after the chemotherapy is best treated with steroids and dopamine antagonists. Anticipatory vomiting that occurs prior to receiving chemotherapy is treated with benzodiazepines.

Anaphylaxis

As with all medicines, anaphylaxis may occur with chemotherapy and the most common culprits are taxanes and asparaginase. The incidence of hypersensitivity with paclitaxel is so high that routine prophylaxis with steroids and antihistamines (H1 and H2) is administered to all patients receiving paclitaxel.

Extravasation

Extravasation is the inadvertent administration of chemotherapy into subcutaneous tissue. This leads to pain, erythema, inflammation and discomfort, which if unrecognized and untreated can lead to tissue necrosis with the possibility of serious sequelae. The position, size and age of the cannulation site are the factors that have the greatest bearing on the likelihood of problems occurring (Figure 3.6) and the experience of the specialist administering the chemotherapy is crucial in this aspect. The likelihood of damage occurring is determined by the

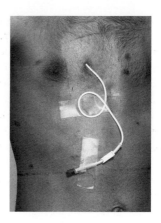

Figure 3.6 A patient with a Hickman line, a skin-tunnelled, long-term silicon catheter with a dacron cuff about 2 cm above the exit site that acts as a barrier to micro-organisms and prevents catheter dislodgment. Hickman lines are used for continuous infusional chemotherapy or for patients with poor venous access. Hickman lines are placed in the radiology department using ultrasound guidance or in theatres under general anaesthetic.

cytotoxic drug, with anthracyclines being especially likely to cause severe injury.

Tumour lysis

The rapid cytolysis of a large volume of cancer cells at the start of chemotherapy occasionally results in the tumour lysis syndrome or metabolic chaos. The destruction of tumour DNA leads to hyperuricaemia from the breakdown of nucleotide bases. The cytolysis causes hyperkalaemia by releaseing intracellular potassium and the breakdown of proteins and DNA causes hyperphosphataemia and secondary hypocalcaemia. Acute renal failure may be a consequence of the high levels of urate and phosphate, whilst the high levels of potassium may lead to cardiac arrthymias. Tumour lysis only really occurs with acute leukaemias and high-grade lymphomas including Burkitt lymphoma. Bulky tumours, poor renal function and high levels of urate before chemotherapy increase the risk of tumour lysis.

Uric acid is soluble at physiological pH but precipitates in the acidic environment of the renal tubules, leading to crystallization in the collecting ducts and ureters, leading to obstructive uropathy.

Similarly calcium phosphate is precipitated in the renal tubules and microvasculature producing nephrocalcinosis. The most important issue in the management of tumour lysis is its prevention by a combination of hyperhydaration, allopurinol and urinary alkalinization to pH >7 with sodium bicarbonate to reduce urate precipitation in the renal tubules. Allopurinol is an inhibitor of xanthine oxidase, the enzyme that catalyzes the conversion of soluble xanthine (a product of purine catabolism) to uric acid. The treatment of established tumour lysis is an oncological emergency. The majority of patients who develop tumour lysis have chemosensitive tumours and are receiving potentially curative treatment. These patients should be considered candidates for urgent haemodialysis. A relatively new addition to the treatment is recombinant urate oxidase (rasburicase) which converts insoluble urate to soluble allantoin (Figure 3.7).

Delayed side effects (predictable)

The main predictable delayed side effects of chemotherapy are alopecia, bone marrow suppression and gastrointestinal mucositis.

Alopecia and onychodystrophy

Hair loss with chemotherapy is both drug and dose dependent and is related to the frequency of cycle repetition. Long-term therapy may result in loss of pubic, axillary and facial hair in addition to scalp hair. The loss of scalp hair often occurs in an acute

episode while washing, usually two to six weeks after starting chemotherapy. It should be emphasized to patients that alopecia from chemotherapy is reversible, with hair regrowth beginning one to two months after completing chemotherapy. The hair may regrow a lighter or darker colour and is often curlier initially. Doxorubicin and cyclophosphamide are the commonest culprits. Patients should be offered wigs available on the NHS. Scalp cooling (below 22°C) may reduce alopecia by causing vasoconstriction and reducing circulation to hair follicles. The pharmacokinetic profiles of cytotoxics dictate that scalp cooling is only effective for anthracyclines. Concerns have been raised over the potential risk of developing scalp and cerebral metastases due to reduced drug circulation to these sites with scalp cooling. Along with alopecia, a frequent complication of chemotherapy is onychodystrophy or nail changes other than colour changes that usually make the nails brittle and prone to shedding (onycholysis) as well as fungal infection (onychomycosis). A common physical sign in patients who have received cyclical chemotherapy are Beau lines, horizontal grooves or lines on the nail plate that indicate cycles of arrested nail growth with chemotherapy cycles (see Plate 3.2).

Myelotoxicity of chemotherapy

The myelosuppressive effects of chemotherapy may affect the circulating red cells, white cells and platelets and the manifestations in these three series are in part related to their circulatory lifespans. In circulation the half-life of an erythro-

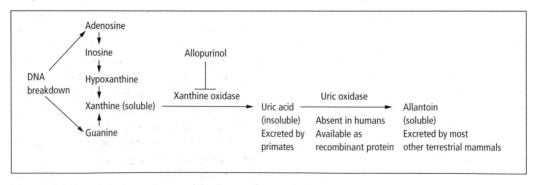

Figure 3.7 Purine catabolism pathway and the therapy of tumour lysis.

cyte is 120 days, of a leucocyte is six to eight hours and of a platelet is seven days.

There is a significant risk of severe myelosuppression if chemotherapy is initiated when the total white cell count is $<3.0 \times 10^9/l$ (or the neutrophil count is $<1.5 \times 10^9/l$) and/or the platelet count is $<150 \times 10^9/l$. These values are the usual cut-offs for administering a cycle of chemotherapy, however it may be given at lower values in patients with haematological malignancies or if supportive therapy is anticipated and when non-myelosuppressive regimens are employed. Myelosuppression is the dose-limiting toxicity for many cytotoxic agents; the main exceptions are vincristine, bleomycin, streptozotocin and asparaginase, which do not cause myelosuppression.

Thus anaemia is rarely a dose-limiting toxicity but is generally cumulative over successive cycles of chemotherapy. Anaemia is most troublesome with cisplatin since the nephrotoxicity of this agent may decrease erythropoietin production from the kidneys in response to anaemia. The symptoms of anaemia include fatigue, lethargy and exertional dyspnoea with haemoglobin levels in the range 8–10g/dl. Reduced exercise capacity progresses to dyspnoea and tachycardia at rest and complications including cerebrovascular (e.g. transient ischaemic attacks) and cardiovascular (e.g. angina) ischaemia as the haemoglobin falls below 8g/dl. The management of chemotherapy-induced anaemia is with transfusion and in the case of cisplatin-induced anaemia, at least, erythropoietin may be beneficial (Box 3.1).

Neutropenia (neutrophil count $<1.0 \times 10^9/l$) is the commonest dose-limiting toxicity of chemotherapy and is a frequent cause of treatment delays and dose reductions. Neutropenia is most often manifest as infection (Figure 3.8) and neutropenic sepsis is a medical emergency, which if left untreated is potentially fatal. It is frequently overlooked by untrained medical staff and delays in starting intravenous antibiotics can be fatal. Neutropenic sepsis is defined as a fever of 38.0°C or higher for at least two hours when the neutrophil count is below $1.0 \times 10^9/l$.

The treatment of neutropenic sepsis includes a thorough clinical history and physical examina-

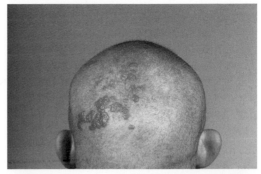
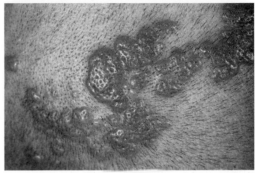

Figure 3.8 Herpes zoster scalp (with close up below): herpes zoster of left C2 distribution erupting as an opportunistic infection during a course of chemotherapy for Hodgkin's disease.

tion to identify possible sources of infection. Initial management must include resuscitation measures for shock if present. An infection screen should be performed, including blood cultures from peripheral veins as well as from any central access catheters, a urine sample for microscopy and culture, a chest X-ray and a throat swab for culture. Treatment should not be delayed awaiting the results of cultures. The most common organisms associated with neutropenic sepsis are common bacterial pathogens. Empirical antibiotic treatment should be instituted with broad-spectrum bactericidal antibiotics and policies will be dictated by local antibiotic resistance patterns. The most common initial treatment regimens are a parenteral combination of an aminoglycoside with either a cephalosporin or a broad-spectrum penicillin. Alternatively, monotherapy with a cephalosporin may be used. If there is no response within 36–48 hours, the antibiotic regimen should be reviewed

Box 3.1: Haematopoietic growth factors

The proliferation and maturation of blood cell lineages is determined by haemopoietic growth factors (Figure 3.9) or colony-stimulating factors (CSFs). Bone marrow stromal cells produce many of these growth factors. Recombinant haemopoietic growth factors are administered to ameliorate chemotherapy-induced cytopenias. They are given parenterally to avoid proteolytic degradation in the gastrointestinal tract.

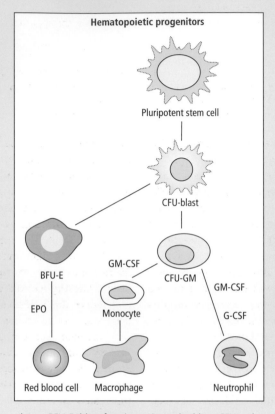

Figure 3.9 Haematopoetic pathway. BFU-E, blast-forming unit, erythroblast; CFU, colony-forming unit; CFU-GM, colony-forming unit, granulocyte–macrophage; EPO, erythropoietin; G-CSF, granulocyte colony-stimulating factor; GM-CSF, granulocyte–macrophage colony-stimulating factor.

Erythropoietin

This growth factor is naturally produced by the kidney in response to hypoxia and stimulates red cell proliferation. It may be overproduced in renal cell carcinoma leading to paraneoplastic polycythemia. As well as its role in the treatment of anaemia of chronic renal failure, erythropoietin may be used to treat cytotoxic-induced anaemia, particularly where cisplatin is implicated.

Granulocyte colony-stimulating factor (G-CSF)

G-CSF is a lineage-restricted growth factor promoting granulocyte differentiation whilst granulocyte–macrophage CSF (GM-CSF) is multifunctional, affecting granulocytes, monocytes, megakaryocytes and erythroid precursors but not basophils. Both CSFs are used in the treatment of chemotherapy- and radiotherapy-related neutropenia. Evidence-based guidelines are available that describe the rational use of G-CSF in four circumstances:

(continued on p. 63)

(continued)
1. Primary prophylaxis (i.e. with the first cycle of chemotherapy): not routinely used, occasionally used for pre-existing neutropenia, e.g. due to marrow infiltration.
2. Secondary prophylaxis: only for curable tumours with proven importance of maintaining dose intensity (germ cell tumours, choriocarcinoma, lymphoma).
3. Febrile neutropenia: data do not support routine G-CSF usage, but indicate use in the presence of pneumonia, hypotension, multiorgan failure and fungal infection.
4. Peripheral blood stem cell mobilization prior to harvesting for high-dose therapy and stem cell rescue.

Thrombopoietin (TPO)

TPO is constitutively produced by the liver and kidneys and acts on many stages of megakaryocyte growth and differentiation. It has yet to become incorporated into routine clinical use. Interleukin-11 however also raises platelet counts following chemotherapy and has been licensed for this indication in the USA.

---

in the light of culture results, and consideration given to adding antifungal cover (e.g. amphotericin B). For patients with severe neutropenic sepsis as defined by hypotension, pneumonia or multiorgan failure, granulocyte colony-stimulating factor (G-CSF) should be administered. Following an episode of neutropenic sepsis consideration should be given to reducing the chemotherapy dosage in subsequent cycles, or if dose intensity has been shown to influence the outcome (e.g. germ cell tumours, Hodgkin's disease) secondary prophylaxis with G-CSF to reduce the duration of neutropenia should be considered (Box 3.1).

Thrombocytopenia is a common side effect of chemotherapy, particularly with carboplatin, that rarely causes clinical manifestations unless it is severe. Although petechiae and bruising may occur, major haemorrhage is very rare unless the platelet count falls below 20×10^9/l. At platelet counts below 10×10^9/l there is an appreciable risk of gastrointestinal or cerebral haemorrhage and prophylactic administration of pooled platelets is warranted. Growth factor support for thrombocytopenia is currently investigational only (Box 3.1) and chemotherapy dose delays and reductions may be necessary following low platelet nadir counts.

Gastrointestinal tract mucositis

Mucositis is a frequent delayed side effect of chemotherapy occurring in 40–50% of patients, and is even more common in patients receiving chemo-

radiotherapy or radiotherapy alone for head and neck cancers. It is thought that chemotherapy and radiotherapy damage basal epithelial cells in the intestinal mucosa leading to apoptosis, atrophy and ulceration. Once ulceration occurs, bacterial and fungal infection and activation of macrophages leads to further inflammation. Mucositis is associated with significant morbidity and mortality risk, and chemotherapy dose reductions and delays. Sucking ice lollies during chemotherapy may reduce the incidence of mucositis with some cytotoxics by a mechanism analogous to the cold cap treatment for the prevention of alopecia. Various 'magic mouthwashes' (usually a mild local anaesthetic and antiseptic combination) may provide symptomatic relief from mucositis. The time course of mucositis closely resembles that of neutropenia, typically occurring 7–14 days after the administration of chemotherapy. Recent developments in the management of mucositis also hint at comparisons with the investigational study of keratinocyte growth factors as treatment for mucositis. In a few cases specific antidotes reduce the incidence of mucositis, such as folinic acid rescue after methotrexate.

Delayed side effects (idiosyncratic)

Many delayed side effects of chemotherapy are drug specific and are not immediately predictable from their mechanisms of action. The organs most frequently affected include the skin, nerves, heart, lungs and blood vessels.

Dermatological side effects

Dermatological complications include the already mentioned acute complications of extravasation and anaphylaxis as well as idiosyncratic delayed toxicities. These include hyperpigmentation, which occurs commonly with 5-fluorouracil and bleomycin and may follow the lines of the veins into which the chemotherapy has been administered. A hand and foot syndrome of painful redness, scaling or shedding of the skin of the palms and soles may occur with continuous infusions of 5-fluorouracil chemotherapy and also with liposomal anthracycline chemotherapy. In the latter case, the cytotoxics are delivered in a liposome to dramatically prolong their half-life, mimicking the pharmacokinetics of a continuous infusion regimen. A third unusual dermatological side effect of chemotherapy is radiation recall, an erythematous reaction of skin in the area of a previous radiation field. Indeed this may occur even when the radiation treatment was decades earlier and is most commonly seen with gemcitabine chemotherapy.

Cardiological side effects

Acute arrythmias can occur during chemotherapy infusions or shortly thereafter and this rare occurrence happens most frequently with taxanes. Similarly, 5-fluorouracil rarely precipitates chest pain and acute myocardial infarction, pericarditis and cardiac shock. However, the most common cardiotoxicity of chemotherapy is a dose-related dilated cardiomyopathy seen with anthracyclines. This usually presents with heart failure within 8 months of the last anthracycline dose. Diuretics improve symptoms and the early use of an angiotensin-converting enzyme inhibitor can increase the left ventricular ejection fraction, improving prognosis which, however, remains poor. This side effect limits the total cumulative dosage of anthracyclines that can be administered. The maximum cumulative lifetime doses of the anthracyclines have been established although cardiomyopathy may be seen at lower total doses.

Neurological side effects

Although only a few cytotoxics penetrate the cerebrospinal fluid, many cytotoxics cause neurotoxicity. Peripheral neuropathy, the most frequent neurotoxicity of chemotherapy, is commonly seen with vinca alkaloids, taxanes and platinum derivatives. The longest nerves are most affected so it presents as a symmetrical sensory loss over the feet and hands. This may progress to worsening paraesthesia, loss of tendon reflexes and eventually motor loss. Features usually slowly improve over several months following cessation of chemotherapy, although residual deficits may persist indefinitely. The same cytotoxics may be responsible for an autonomic neuropathy leading to abdominal pain, constipation, paralytic ileus, urinary retention, bradycardia and postural hypotension. Acute encephalopathy most commonly is associated with ifosfamide and symptoms include confusion, agitation, seizures, somnolence and coma. Cerebellar toxicity may follow cytarabine therapy and 5-fluorouracil. Cisplatin-induced ototoxicity is characterized by the progressive loss of high-tone hearing and tinnitus.

The inadvertent intrathecal administration of vinca alkaloids is fatal and this catastrophic clinical error has arisen because of confusion of the drug with a cytotoxic agent intended to be given intrathecally (usually methotrexate). Five such incidents have occurred in NHS hospitals in the past decade, representing an estimated rate of about three per 100 000 intrathecal chemotherapy treatments and recently resulting in the jailing of a junior doctor. A number of strict guidelines surrounding the administration of intrathecal chemotherapy are now in place to prevent this occurrence.

Pulmonary side effects

Chronic pulmonary toxicity and fibrosis occurs with a number of cytotoxics and the outcome is generally poor. Bleomycin is the most common culprit and the risk increases with dose. The cardinal symptom of drug-induced pulmonary toxicity is dyspnoea associated with non-productive cough,

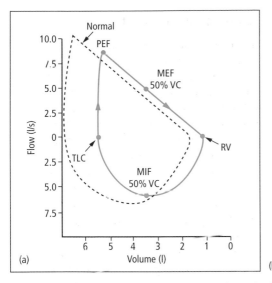

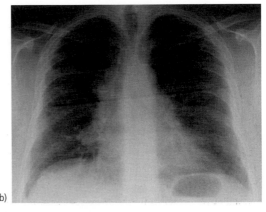

Figure 3.10 (a) Lung flow loop and (b) chest radiograph of a 35-year-old man treated with combination chemotherapy including bleomycin for advanced germ cell tumour of the testis. The chest radiograph demonstrates diffuse interstitial shadowing most prominent in the lower zones. The lung flow loop shows a restrictive deficit typical of bleomycin fibrosis. MEF, mid expiratory flow; MIF, mid inspiratory flow; PEF, peak expiratory flow; RV, residual volume; TLC, total lung capacity; VC, vital capacity.

fatigue, fever and malaise. Symptoms usually develop over several weeks to months. The chest X-ray classically shows reticulonodular infiltration at the bases and occasionally pleural effusions (Figure 3.10a). Lung function tests demonstrate a reduced diffusing capacity for carbon monoxide and restrictive ventilatory defects (Figure 3.10b). The usual treatment is with corticosteroids although there is little to support this and the mortality is high.

Hepatic side effects

Many cytotoxics cause elevated serum transaminases and bilirubin, and fatty infiltration and cholestasis may occur as the toxic effect progresses. Hepatic veno-occlusive disease (VOD) results from the blockage of venous outflow in the small centrilobular hepatic vessels following damage to cells in the area of the liver surrounding the central vein. This rare side effect occurs with high-dose chemotherapy often as part of stem cell transplantation. The clinical features are painful hepatomegaly, ascites, peripheral oedema, marked elevations in

serum enzymes and bilirubin, and hepatic encephalopathy. The onset is often abrupt, occurring during the first post-transplant week, and the clinical course is fatal in up to 50%.

Late side effects

Gonadal side effects

Chemotherapy causes a variety of toxic effects on male and female gonads leading to infertility. Moreover, cytotoxic drugs given during pregnancy may have teratogenic effects on the fetus. If fertility is maintained or restored, there are concerns about the heritability of the cancer and at least a theoretical risk of mutagenic alterations to germ cells.

Adult male gonadal toxicity

Male germ cells lie within the seminiferous epithelium and include stem spermatogonia, differentiating spermatogonia, spermatocytes, spermatids and sperm. The differentiating spermatogonia actively proliferate and are therefore highly susceptible to cytotoxic agents. In contrast, the Leydig cells, which are in the interstitium and produce androgens, and the Sertoli cells, which provide support and regulatory factors to the germ cells, do not proliferate in adults and so survive most cytotoxic therapies. Because later stage germ cells (spermatocytes onwards) do not proliferate they are not susceptible to chemotherapy – sperm counts do not fall immediately on starting chemotherapy, but may take two to three months to decline; although minor falls in testosterone production may occur, only testicular radiation will produce significant testosterone deficiency. Men due to start chemotherapy should be offered sperm storage in order to enable them to father children in the future. Modern developments in *in vitro* fertilization are particularly relevant to the cancer patient. For those patients who were considered to be unsuitable for semen storage and remain azoospermic post treatment, the technique of intracytoplasmic sperm injection (ICSI) may be appropriate. Just remember, only one sperm is required to fertilize one ovum.

Adult female gonadal toxicity

In women, unlike men, the germ cells do not proliferate whereas the somatic cells do and this accounts for the different gonadal toxicity of chemotherapy in women and men. Female germ cells proliferate before birth as oogonia that arrest at the oocyte stage. At birth, a woman has 1 million oocytes, which are reduced to 300000 at puberty. Oocytes are progressively lost by atresia, development and ovulation, until almost all are lost and menopause is reached. The interval from recruitment of primordial follicles to ovulation is 82 days and when cytotoxics destroy maturing follicles, temporary amenorrhea results. However, if the number of remaining primordial follicles falls below the minimum number necessary for menstrual cyclicity, irreversible ovarian failure occurs with permanent amenorrhea. This accounts for the increased risk of chemotherapy-induced menopause in older patients. Permanent ovarian failure is often accompanied by vasomotor symptoms, whilst temporary amenorrhoea, which may last up

to 5 years after chemotherapy, is usually asymptomatic. As in men, alkylating agents are the major culprits causing permanent gonadal failure in women. At present ovum storage remains an unreliable method for routine usage and requires ovarian stimulation prior to egg harvesting, which introduces a delay prior to starting chemotherapy and is relatively contraindicated in breast cancer. The storage of fertilized eggs (embryos) is more successful. The Roman Catholic Church opposes all forms of *in vitro* fertilization and under the papacy of Benedict XVI has condemned the practice in the 2008 magisterial instruction *Dignitas Personae*.

Teratogenicity of chemotherapy

Many cytotoxics are teratogenic in murine models although data in humans are thankfully limited. All alkylating agents are teratogenic with limited information suggesting a significant risk of malformed infants if exposed in the first trimester but no increased risk during the second and third trimesters. Methotrexate is, of course, a potent abortifactant during early pregnancy. No clear evidence is available to support the timing of pregnancy following chemotherapy although most clinicians advise a two to five-year gap before pregnancy

Carcinogenicity of chemotherapy

Many cytotoxic agents are genotoxic and this accounts for their antitumour activity but also carries the risk of inducing cancers; alkylating agents are the most potent carcinogens in this group (Table 3.13). The risk of induced malignancies depends not only on the cytotoxics administered but also on the initial cancer diagnosis, with greatest risks in patients with Hodgkin's disease where the second malignancy rate is 10–15% after 15 years. Two forms of secondary acute leukaemia following chemotherapy are widely recognized. Alkylating agents are carcinogenic with acute leukaemias occurring in up to 5% three to five years after exposure and associated with chromosome

Table 3.13 Table of carcinogenic medicines.

Carcinogenic drug	Associated tumour
Cytotoxics (especially alkylating agents and topoisomerase II inhibitors)	Acute myeloid leukaemia
Cyclophosphamide	Bladder cancer
Immunosuppression	Kaposi's sarcoma, post-transplantation lymphoproliferation
Oestrogens (unopposed)	Endometrial cancer
Oestrogens (transplacental)	Vaginal adenocarcinoma
Oral contraceptive pill	Hepatic adenoma
Androgenic anabolic steroids	Hepatocellular carcinoma
Phenacetin	Renal pelvis transitional cell cancer
Chloramphenicol	Acute leukaemia
Phenytoin	Lymphoma, neuroblastoma

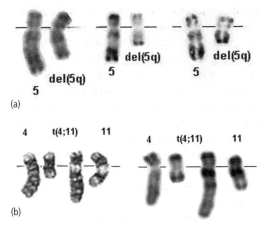

Figure 3.11 Chromosome translocation in secondary leukaemia. Partial karyotypes from patients with secondary acute leukaemia follow chemotherapy. (a) Deletions on the long arm of chromosome 5 are characteristic of alkylating agent-related secondary acute myeloid leukaemias that typically arise three to five years after chemotherapy and may be preceded by myelodysplasia. (b) The t(4:11) reciprocal chromosomal translocation commonly found in acute leukaemias that occur two to three years after chemotherapy with topoisomerase II inhibitors.

5q or 7 deletions (Figure 3.11a). Survival after secondary acute myeloid leukaemia (AML) is poor, usually only a few months. There is also an increased incidence of solid tumours after alkylating agents. Secondary acute leukaemia also occurs in patients treated with topoisomerase II inhibitors (Figure 3.11b). These leukaemias occur early, two to three years after therapy, and are associated with translocations of 11q23 (MLL gene) or 21q22 (AML1 gene). Data on the development of secondary solid tumours are less clear although cyclophosphamide is linked to a four-fold relative risk of bladder cancer and appears to be related to cumulative dose. Antimetabolites are generally not thought to be carcinogenic.

There is something quite horrible about the development of second cancers after curative treatment of a first cancer and for this reason effort has been expended in developing alternative treatment programmes that are not associated with increased cancer risk. The development of second cancers used to be a problem of particular poignancy in patients with Hodgkin's disease. This tumour commonly occurs in younger people who are returned to a normal life expectancy until the unpleasantness of their presentation with a second cancer. The alternative programme, which is in current use for the treatment of Hodgkin's disease, is called ABVD. This was originally introduced by a group of Italians, whose pronouncements about the effectiveness of ABVD chemotherapy were regarded with some scepticism by the medical community. However a randomized trial organized in North America showed that the Italians were right.

Psychiatric dysfunction

It is generally thought that patients who have cancer would tend to be more depressed than the population without malignancy. However, this is far from the truth. So far from the truth that it is a completely incorrect view. There is no difference in the incidence of mental illness in people affected with cancer than in a normal population. There is controversy around the association between pre-morbid psychiatric conditions and the development of cancer. The only malignancy in which there has been shown to be an association is breast cancer, where early work described a link between pre-morbid depression and breast cancer. The link is slight. Patients with cancer go through a series of mental changes around the time of their diagnosis. Each of these stages may be protracted, even to the extent that the patient remains unable to grow beyond that particular phase. These symptoms are symptoms of a grief response as seen in many other situations. Initially patients deal with malignancy by denial. They next move to a grief response, progressing from there to acceptance of their own situations.

Delayed side effects in children

Growth disorders in children

Both growth disorders and mental changes are problems that come chiefly as a result of the use of radiotherapy in childhood. Irradiation of the chest in the treatment of Hodgkin's disease is associated with destruction of the growing plates of the vertebrae and ribs, and dysmorphic appearance in later life. For this reason treatment with spinal radiotherapy is generally avoided in leukaemia and lymphoma occurring in childhood, with chemotherapy the preferred option.

Mental change in children

Cerebral radiotherapy given as part of prophylaxis for central nervous system recurrence of leukaemia may also cause significant problems. These problems are not generally of growth or of hormonal function, as the pituitary is relatively resistant to radiation. However personality defects are described with increased incidence, as are global loss of cerebral function manifesting as a less than expected IQ, personality change and occasionally fits. Although relatively resistant to radiation therapy, pituitary function can be damaged with loss of the gonadotrophs leading to failure to achieve puberty. Loss of thyroid-stimulating hormone (TSH) production occurs with high dosage radiotherapy and loss of posterior pituitary

function with even higher dosages of radiation therapy.

Gonadal toxicity in children

The germinal epithelium in the prepubertal testis does not appear to be any more resistant to cytotoxic therapy than in the adult and the sterilizing effects of chemotherapy on prepubertal boys may be predicted from data in adults. In contrast prepubertal girls are less susceptible to ovarian failure than adult women. Most chemotherapy regimens do not cause failure of pubertal development and menarche.

Endocrine therapy

Endocrine therapy (or hormonal manipulation) is an important part of managing cancers whose growth is dependent on hormones, namely, breast and prostate cancers. The aims of endocrine therapy for cancer are to reduce the circulating levels of hormones or block their actions on the cancers. The origins of endocrine therapy for breast and prostate cancer come from surgical oophrectomy and orchidectomy.

Breast cancer

In order to grow, many breast cancers that produce oestrogen receptors rely on supplies of oestrogen (Figure 3.12). Luteinizing hormone-releasing hormone (LHRH) agonists such as goserelin cause downregulation of pituitary LHRH receptors and, via a decrease in LH/FSH (luteinizing hormone/follicle-stimulating hormone), to a reduced plasma oestradiol. This is used in the neoadjuvant, adjuvant and palliative setting in premenopausal women. Tamoxifen binds to oestrogen receptors and prevents oestradiol binding. It is used in the neoadjuvant, adjuvant and palliative setting in postmenopausal women. Aromatase inhibitors, such as anastrozole, bind and inhibit aromatase enzyme in peripheral tissues including adipose tissue, which converts androstenedione and testosterone and other androgens into oestradiol and oestrone. This is the major source of oestradiol synthesis in postmenopausal women. They are used in

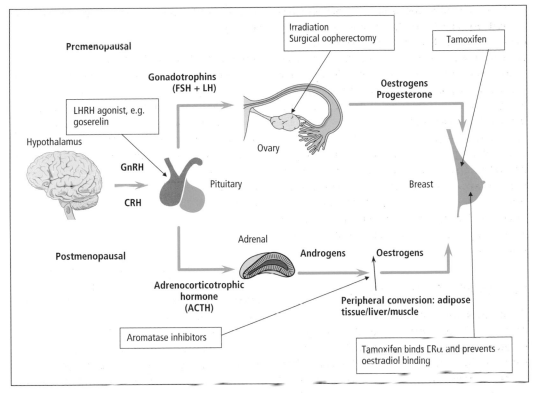

Figure 3.13 Hypothalamic–pituitary–gonadal axis in women and potential therapeutic interventions. CRH, corticotrophin-releasing hormone; ERα, oestrogen receptor α; FSH, follicle-stimulating hormone; LH, luteinizing hormone; LHRH, luteinizing hormone-releasing hormone; GnRH, gonadotrophin-releasing hormone.

the palliative setting for women whose disease progresses on tamoxifen. All the above drugs can cause menopausal symptoms, namely hot flushes, sweats and vaginal dryness. Specific and important adverse effects of tamoxifen are thromboembolic disease and uterine carcinoma.

Prostate cancer

The growth of prostatic carcinoma is under the control of androgens, hence the aim of hormonal therapy is to reduce testosterone levels or prevent it binding to the androgen receptor. LHRH agonists cause downregulation of pituitary LHRH receptors and via a decrease in LH to a reduced serum testosterone and tissue dehydrotestosterone (Figure 3.13). The adverse effects are impotence, loss of libido, gynaecomastia and hot flushes.

Tumour flare, an increase in tumour size which can cause symptoms such as increase in bone pain and spinal cord compression, can occur with the initial use of these drugs, due to an initial increase in testosterone. Therefore an anti-androgen such as bicalutamide, cyproterone and flutamide should be prescribed for a few weeks before LHRH agonists to prevent this happening. Anti-androgens act by blocking and preventing testosterone from attaching to the receptors in prostate cancer cells (Figure 3.13). The adverse effects of anti-androgens are hepatotoxcity, gynaecomastia, diarrhoea and abdominal pain. Combined androgen blockade (or maximal androgen blockade) is a term used to describe the use of an LHRH agonist and androgen receptor antagonist together. These agents are used alone or in combination for either locally advanced or metastatic prostate cancer.

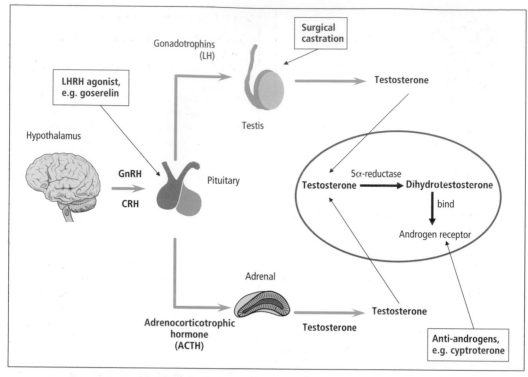

Figure 3.13 Site of actions of LHRH agonists and anti-androgens on the hypothalamic–pituitary–testis axis. CRH, cortico-trophin-releasing hormone; LH, luteinizing hormone; LHRH, luteinizing hormone-releasing hormone; GnRH, gonado-trophin-releasing hormone.

Immunological therapy

As far back as the 1700s, it was recorded that certain infectious diseases could exert a beneficial thera-peutic effect upon malignancy. Most prominent among the clinicians aiming to take advantage of these observations was a New York surgeon, William B. Coley. He used a bacterial vaccine to treat inoperable cancers and in 1893 reported high cure rates. Although a central role for the immune system in the surveillance and eradication of tumours has been postulated since then, immuno-therapy has only a minor place in the treatment of cancers. Support for any role of immunity in the control of cancer comes from a number of observa-tions. For some malignancies, a dense infiltration of lymphocytes in the tumour imparts a better prognosis. Cultivating and re-infusing these tumour-infiltrating lymphocytes occasionally results in some regression of the tumour. Con-

versely, people with immunodeficiencies have higher rates of cancers, however in general these tumours are less common cancers that are caused by oncogenic viruses. Both passive and active spe-cific immunotherapy and non-specific immuno-therapy have a limited role in the management of cancer.

Passive specific immunotherapy

Passive immunotherapy with monoclonal anti-bodies is an established treatment for breast cancer and non-Hodgkin's lymphoma. Monoclonal anti-bodies are produced by a single clone of B cells and may be humanized to reduce their immunogenic-ity. In 1975, Georges Kohler and Cesar Milstein developed a procedure to fuse myeloma cells with B-lymphocyte cells from the spleen of immunized mice. These fused hybridoma cell clones retained the ever-living characteristics of myeloma cells and

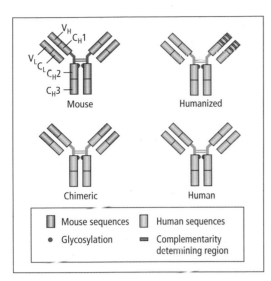

Figure 3.14 Nomenclature and structure of chimeric and humanized monoclonal antibodies.

Box 3.2: Name that antibody

Common suffix for all monoclonal antibodies:
  -mab
  Suffix sub-stem denotes the origin of the antibody:

-o-	mouse	ibritumomab, sulesomab
-xi-	chimeric	cetuximab, infliximab
-zu-	humanized	bevacizumab, trastuzumab
-u-	human	adalimumab

  Suffix sub-sub-stem denotes disease or therapeutic area:

-anib-	angiogenesis inhibitor	ranibizumab
-ci-	cardiovascular	abciximab, bevacizumab
-le(s)-	inflammatory lesions	sulesomab
-li-	immunomodulator	infliximab, omalizumab
-tu-	tumour	cetuximab, trastuzumab
-vi-	viral	palivizumab

However, there are inconsistencies. For example, bevacizumab, which according to the sub-stem -ci- was perhaps originally expected to be used in cardiovascular disease, is used to treat patients with colorectal cancer and macular degeneration; bevacizumab, cetuximab and ranibizumab all inhibit angiogenesis but have different sub-stems.

the ability to secrete monoclonal antibodies against the antigen that the mouse was immunized with. Milstein and Kohler shared the 1984 Nobel Prize with Niels Jerne for this work. Cesar Milstein had left his native Argentina for Cambridge in 1963 following the military coup that deposed the moderate President Frondizi. He joins a long list of distinguished British Nobel laureates in physiology and medicine who arrived in Britain as political asylum seekers, including Max Perutz (discoverer of the structure of haemoglobin), Hans Krebs (who described the citric acid cycle) and Ernst Chain (who, with Florey, developed the clinical application of Fleming's discovery of penicillin).

Several monoclonal antibodies are currently widely used in oncology and have been genetically modified to reduce the murine origins to prevent the development of host antibodies against the mouse sequences of the antibodies (Figure 3.14), for example rituximab and trastuzumab (Box 3.2). Rituximab is a chimeric monoclonal antibody directed against CD20, a protein expressed on pre-B and mature B cells. This is non-specific as it will ablate both normal and malignant B cells. However, the normal cells are subsequently regenerated by the bone marrow from normal stem cells. It is effective in low-grade and follicular non-Hodg-

kin's lymphoma. Trastuzumab is a humanized monoclonal antibody directed against human epidermal growth factor receptor 2 (HER2), which is overexpressed in 30% of breast cancers and is associated with a poorer prognosis. It is used in metastatic breast cancer that is HER2 positive. Both these drugs can cause flu-like symptoms on infusion, such as chills and pyrexia. In addition, trastuzumab has been noted to be cardiotoxic, especially when given with anthracyclines.

Active specific immunotherapy

Active cellular immunotherapy involves the harvesting and *ex vivo* activation (in the test tube) of lymphokine-activated killer (LAK) cells (cytokine primed immune cells) and is an experimental treatment for renal cancers and melanoma. Other trial active immunotherapies include tumour vaccines and this technology is most often studied in the tumour types where occasional spontaneous regressions have been documented.

Non-specific immunotherapy

Global stimulation of the host cellular immune system in order to promote tumour rejection was probably the basis of Coley's adjuvant therapy. This has been replaced with the use of bacillus Calmette–Guerin (BCG), which is administered intravesically (via a catheter into the bladder) to prevent recurrence of superficial bladder cancers, and interferons and intereukins.

Interferon

There are three human interferons:
- Interferon alpha (IFN-α) produced by leukocytes
- Interferon beta (IFN-β) produced by fibroblasts
- Interferon gamma (IFN-γ) produced by T lymphocytes.

IFN-α is licensed for use currently and may act by enhancing the expression of human leucocyte antigen (HLA) antigens by tumour cells leading to increased recognition and lysis by cytotoxic T cells and natural killer cells. Only IFN-α is used in the treatment of cancers, including hairy cell leukaemia, chronic myeloid leukaemia, melanoma, renal cell cancer and Kaposi's sarcoma. The adverse effects of IFN-α are flu-like symptoms, fatigue and myelosuppression.

Interleukin-2

Interleukin-2 (IL-2) is a cytokine produced predominantly by activated CD4+ helper T lymphocytes that have been stimulated by antigen. It acts via a cell surface receptor expressed also on activated T cells thus behaving as an autocrine growth factor. In response to IL-2, CD4+ helper T cells are capable of differentiating from an initial common state (T_H0) into one of two apparently distinct types called T_H1 and T_H2. The T_H1 pathway

is essentially cell-mediated immunity, with the activation of macrophages, natural killer cells, cytotoxic T cells and a prolonged inflammatory response. The T_H2 pathway is essentially a humoral pathway, with the production of cytokines, which promote B-cell growth and the production of antibodies. IL-2 causes the growth and proliferation of activated T cells thus expanding tumouricidal LAK cells and may be used to treat melanoma and renal cell cancers. The adverse effects of IL-2 are fluid retention, multiorgan dysfunction and bone marrow and hepatic toxicity.

Protein kinase inhibitor therapy

Protein kinase enzymes phosphorylate the amino acid residues of their substrates, usually tyrosine, serine or threonine. The human genome includes about 500 protein kinases and perhaps 30% of all human proteins may be modified by phosphorylation, which may result in functional changes. Phosphorylation of substrate proteins may alter their enzyme activity, cellular location or association with other proteins and this is especially important in cellular pathways such as signal transduction that are dysregulated in cancer cells. Protein kinase inihibitors are a relatively new and rapidly expanding class of drugs used in cancer treatment and include both monoclonal antibodies (-mabs) and small molecules (-nibs) (Table 3.14). In general, nibs target tyrosine kinase domains whilst mabs target the ligand-binding domains of receptors. Many of these novel agents have been developed using knowledge of the biology of tumours to target specific pathways in cancer cells. It was anticipated that this would have the added benefit of minimizing toxicity although some unexpected side effects have emerged such as the cardiotoxicity of trastuzumab.

Clinical trials

As new cytotoxic drugs are developed and other novel agents are found it is essential to evaluate their potential in a structured fashion in clinical trials. A stepwise progression has been introduced that includes three phases of clinical trials. Phase I

Table 3.14 Table showing the common protein kinase inihitors used in oncology.

Name	Target	Class	Clincal uses
Bevacizumab	VEGF	Monoclonal antibody	Colon cancer and NSCLC
Cetuximab	EGFR	Monoclonal antibody	Colon cancer and head and neck cancer
Dasatinib	BCR/ABL	Small molecule	CML
Erlotinib	EGFR	Small molecule	NSCLC
Gefitinib	EGFR	Small molecule	NSCLC
Imatinib	BCR/ABL	Small molecule	CML and GIST
Lapatinib	EGFR and Her2	Small molecule	Breast cancer
Sorafenib	Multiple target kinases	Small molecule	Kidney cancer and liver cancer
Sunitinib	Multiple target kinases	Small molecule	Kidney caner and GIST
Trastuzumab	Her2	Monoclonal antibody	Breast cancer

BCR/ABL, breakpoint cluster region/Abelson murine leukaemia viral oncogene homologue; CML, chronic myeloid leukaemia; EGFR, epidermal growth factor receptor; GIST, gastrointestinal stromal tumour; NSCLC, non-small cell lung cancer; VEGF, vascular endothelial growth factor.

trials determine the toxicity, including the dose-limiting toxicities and the dose scheduling of a new agent. They enrol a small number of patients with resistant tumours. Phase II studies are designed to identify promising tumour types using the dosing regimens established from the phase I trials. Phase III trials are larger randomized comparisons that allocate patients either to the new treatment or the established standard therapy. In all phases of clinical trials evaluations of response and toxicity are according to well-established standards. The side effects are measured using the Common Toxicity Criteria scale that rates the severity of side effects on a four point scale. The response to treatment is assessed using the RECIST (response evaluation criteria in solid tumours) criteria which are largely radiological and clinical measurements of the tumour size before and after treatment. A complete response is defined as the complete disappearance of all known disease, whilst a partial response roughly equates to a greater than 50% reduction in the size of measurable lesions with no new ones appearing. Although there is considerable debate as to whether these response criteria are appropriate for some of the novel therapies such as anti-angiogenic treatments, they are currently necessary for licensing approval of cancer drugs. The aims of clinical trials of a new agent include proving that it works, obtaining a license from the Food and Drug Administration (FDA) in the USA and the European Medicines Evaluation Agency (EMEA) as well as making money. In most cases all the goals are complementary, however there are examples from the biotechnology boom of the 1990s where making money appeared to be the sole objective and venture capitalists made fortunes without a drug ever achieving clinical use or benefiting any patients.

Randomized clinical trials are needed to establish evidence-based treatment protocols as well as determining the value of new agents. Large clinical trials are a major focus of clinical activity in oncology and patients are actively encouraged to participate in studies. The principles that underlie clinical trial management are outlined within Box 3.3.

Palliative care

Although it is widely held that palliative care is only offered when there is no chance of cure, this attitude risks denying patients adequate analgesia and supportive care irrespective of their prognosis. The concept that palliative care to provide optimal symptom control and enhanced quality of life should only be available to those patients with advanced disease is ridiculous. The integration of palliative care into the early management of patients with cancer is recognized as benefiting

Box 3.3: Does it work?

The value of a diagnostic test in clinical medicine depends upon whether the result means what you think it does and nowhere is this more relevant than in screening tests. The usefulness depends upon three factors, the sensitivity and specificity of the test and the population prevalence of the condition.

Sensitivity
The sensitivity of a test is the ability of a test to pick up a condition:
- Sensitivity = number of true cases detected/all true cases.
  A test that is 95% sensitive will detect 95% of all cases (or, put another way, miss 5% of cases).

Specificity
The specificity of a test is the probability that a negative test is a true negative:
- Specificity = number of true negatives detected/all true negatives.
  A 75% specificity means that 75% of all negative tests are true negatives, or conversely that 25% of negative tests are actually positive for a condition.

Usefulness
The practical usefulness of a test in a given population can be summarized using:
- Positive predictive value (the chance that a positive will be a true positive in that population) = true cases detected/all positive test results (true positives and false postitives)
- Negative predictive value (the chance that a negative will be a true negative in that population) = true negative results/all negative test results (true negatives and false negatives).

Prevalence and incidence
- Prevalence = frequency of a condition in the community at a given point in time (e.g. the prevalence of cancer in children in the USA is one in 330 children <19 years)
- Incidence = frequency of a disease occurring over a period in time (e.g. the incidence of breast cancer in England in 1998 was 131/100 000 females).

Running a trial

Ethics
The Declaration of Helsinki outlines an international basis of ethical clinical research. It describes the rights of patients including the right to abstain from a study, access to adequate information about both potential benefits and hazards of involvement, the right to withdraw from the trial at any time and finally the desirability of giving written informed consent prior to enrolment. In the UK, research trials must be submitted to research ethics committees for review.

Trial design
- Phase I trials determine the relationship between toxicity and dose schedules of treatment
- Phase II trials identify tumour types for which the treatment appears promising
- Phase III trials assess the efficacy of treatment compared to standard treatment including toxicity.

Randomization
Proper randomization should ensure unbiased comparisons. It achieves control for both known and unknown confounding factors.

Control
Controlled trials compare a 'new' test therapy with an existing treatment – either active or placebo.

Blinding
In double blinded trials neither the patient nor the doctor knows which treatment is being administered.

(continued on p. 75)

(continued)

Sample size

The number of patients (sample size) required in a trial will depend on the number of events (deaths or relapses) predicted in each arm and the difference that you wish to be able to demonstrate between the two arms of the trial. If you wish to detect a small difference between the two groups, more patients are needed.

Analysis

Intention to treat analysis compares outcomes between all patients originally allocated one treatment with all patients allocated to the other treatment.

Endpoints

Clinical trial endpoints include overall survival duration, disease-free survival, time to disease progression, response rate, quality of life measures, adverse effects and treatment toxicity. The efficacy of treatment may be measured using the response evaluation criteria in solid tumours (RECIST) criteria, which evaluate response in terms of radiological and clinical tumour shrinkage. The definitions broadly are:

- Complete response: disappearance of all known disease
- Partial response: >50% reduction in measurable lesions and no new lesions
- Stable disease: lesions unchanged (<50% smaller or <25% larger)
- Progressive disease: new lesions or measurable lesions >25% larger.

CTC toxicity scales

Grading scales exist to compare the side effects of treatments in trials including the common toxicity criteria (CTC).

Interpreting the results

Evidence-based medicine

Over the last two decades there have been numerous advances in evidence processing, including the production of streamlined guides to aid critical appraisal of the literature, evidence-based abstraction services, online and other forms of electronic literature searching, growing numbers of high-quality systematic reviews, and frequently updated textbooks in paper and electronic formats. All these initiatives have contributed to the emergence of evidence-based medicine as the optimal framework for clinical management.

Meta-analysis

Combining published data into a meta-analysis to provide an evidence base for clinical management is widely advocated. A meta-analysis may provide a more precise, less biased and more complete assessment of the available information than individual studies. However, the preferential publication of striking results in small studies and non-publication of larger negative studies ('publication bias') may skew meta-analyses. Thus the reliability of a meta-analysis depends on the quality and quantity of the data that go into it.

Bias

Bias in a study is a design flaw that results in an inevitable likelihood that the wrong result may be obtained. Bias cannot be controlled for at the analysis stage.

Potential biases in screening for cancer

Screening should reduce mortality but the following should be considered:

1. *Lead time bias*: the diagnosis of disease is made earlier in the screened group, resulting in an apparent increase in survival time, although the time of death is the same in both groups.

(continued on p. 76)

(continued)

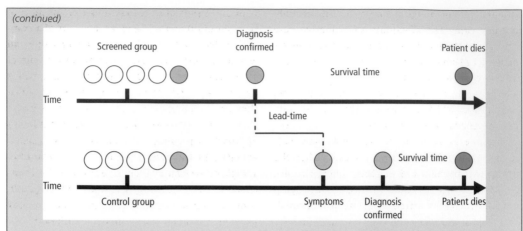

2. *Lag time bias*: the probability of detecting disease is related to the growth rate of the tumour. Aggressive, rapidly growing tumours have a short potential screening period. More slowly growing tumours have a longer potential screening period and are more likely to be detected when they are asymptomatic, causing an apparent improvement in survival.

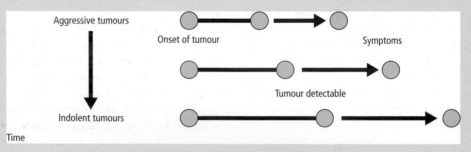

3. *Overdiagnosis bias*: The detection of very slow growing tumours in the screened group produces an apparent increase in the number of cases. In contrast these indolent tumours may remain silent in the control population as they may never cause symptoms. In this diagram, two patients in the control group died with undiagnosed cancer that did not affect their natural lifespan.

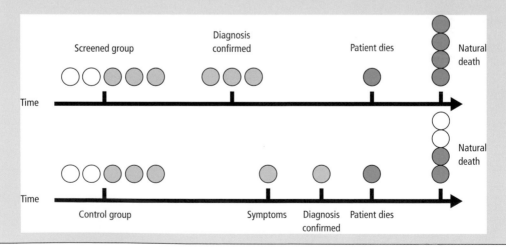

patients and encouraging a more holistic attitude to their care. The discipline of palliative care throughout the globe owes much to the pioneering work of Dame Cecily Saunders. She started life as a nurse during the Second World War and subsequently worked as a social worker before training in medicine, which she viewed then as the only route to change the care of the dying. She advocated above all else listening to patients as the best way to care for them. In 1967 she established the first hospice in the world, St Christopher's Hospice in London, in order to meet the needs of the dying patient, which are so often left unmet in a hospital. The hospice movement developed a comprehensive approach to dealing with the variety of symptoms experienced by patients with progressive debilitating illness including promoting the safe use of opiate analgesia. This attitude has been developed to deliver whole person care and to view the patient not in isolation but as part of a social unit that includes also family and friends.

Pain is the most feared and most common symptom of advanced malignancy and emotional, spiritual and psychological components may intensify physical pain. In Mother Teresa's Home for the Dying, the homeless of Kolkata (formerly Calcutta) were denied any analgesia other than aspirin and often suffered unnecessarily with great pain in the pursuit of austere religion. The relief of pain should therefore be viewed as part of a comprehensive pattern of care encompassing all aspects of suffering. The physical component of pain cannot be treated in isolation, nor can a patient's anxieties be effectively addressed whilst they are suffering physically. It is obvious under these circumstances that a multidisciplinary approach is required. In addition to pain relief, expertise in the management of other common symptoms is essential including constipation, diarrhoea, nausea, vomiting, dyspnoea and fatigue. In some circumstances surgery or radiotherapy may provide valuable symptomatic palliation, for example for the relief of spinal cord compression. Moreover in selected circumstances palliative chemotherapy is indicated even if the term seems to be a clinical oxymoron.

The delivery of palliative care until recently has been hospice based. However, the hospice concept has now extended to both the acute hospital and community settings, where specialist teams work in partnership with primary care teams in the delivery of palliative care. Community-based palliative care may enable patients to die at home or at least remain at home for as long as possible, which has long been known to be the favoured option of most patients.

Chapter 4

Cancer and people

Social and psychological aspects of cancer

Psychological carcinogenic risk factors

There is a great deal of speculation and anecdotal evidence connecting psychological factors and both the risk of developing cancer and its prognosis. Much of the research on the relationship between stressful life experiences and the onset of cancer has been poorly designed. However, the few well-conducted trials have failed to establish a link. A large study of women with newly diagnosed breast cancer found that women who have a severely stressful life experience in the year before the diagnosis or in the five years afterwards, do not seem to be at increased risk of developing a recurrence of the disease. Moreover, a meta-analysis addressed the influence of psychological coping strategies (including fighting spirit, helplessness/ hopelessness, denial and avoidance) on cancer survival and recurrence. This meta-analysis found that there was little consistent evidence that psychological coping styles play an important part in survival from or recurrence of cancer.

Lecture Notes: Oncology, 2nd edition. By M. Bower and J. Waxman. Published 2010 by Blackwell Publishing Ltd.

Psychological distress in cancer patients

Psychological distress is frequent in patients with cancer and is often overlooked or even deliberately neglected by clinicians. However, over the last few decades, more oncologists have appreciated that psychological distress and psychiatric disorders such as anxiety, depression and delirium (in hospitalized patients) are frequent co-morbid conditions. Increasingly, the outcome measures in clinical trials of new therapies have included quality of life evaluation and not just assessed survival endpoints. A number of factors have been found to be associated with an increased risk of psychological distress in patients with cancer (Table 4.1). Clinical features of anxiety include anorexia, fatigue, loss of libido, weight loss, anhedonia, insomnia and suicidal ideation. Many of these key symptoms are at times attributed to the cancer and as few as one-third of cancer patients who might benefit from antidepressants are prescribed them.

As well as pharmacological treatments, psychological interventions are frequently employed in the care of people with cancer. These interventions have a positive effect on psychological morbidity and functional adjustment and may ameliorate disease and treatment-related symptoms. The most useful psychological intervention appears to be a group of treatments termed cognitive-behavioural psychotherapy. These include behaviour therapy,

Table 4.1 Factors increasing the risk of psychological morbidity in cancer patients.

History of mood disorder
History of alcohol or drug misuse
Cancer or its treatment associated with visible deformity
Younger age
Poor social support
Low expectation of successful treatment outcome

Table 4.2 Top tips for communicating with patients.

Clarify patient's statements
Use open questioning (not leading)
Note verbal and non-verbal clues
Enquire about patient's psychosocial problems (e.g. depression)
Keep patients to the point
Prevent needless repetition
Provide verbal and visual encouragement
Obtain precise information
Use brief questions
Avoid jargon

behaviour modification and cognitive therapy in various combinations. In behavioural therapy, a formal analysis of the patient's problem leads to an individualized programme of techniques aimed at changing their behaviour. Cognitive therapies explore how thoughts influence feelings and behaviour and aim to modify thought processes directly. These therapies consist of identifying maladaptive thought patterns (such as hopelessness in depression) and teaching patients to recognize and challenge these. Probably the most widely employed psychosocial intervention for cancer patients is supportive counselling that along with information and patient education empowers patients.

Psychosocial problems in cancer survivors

Even after successful curative treatment of cancer, patients continue to suffer psychological morbidity. The psychological sequelae in cancer survivors may relate to the illness and its treatment as well as family and personal issues. The majority of children who survive cancer cope well with long-term adjustment although adults generally fare less well. Three well-recognized scenarios in this context are:
• The Lazarus syndrome (difficulty with returning to normal life)
• The Damocles syndrome (fear of recurrence and terror of minor symptoms)
• The survivor syndrome (guilt about surviving where others have died).

Cancer survivors also suffer social problems including financial difficulties, particularly with insurance and mortgages. They have also been found to have greater problems in obtaining employment and keeping jobs and these may be compounded by frequent follow-up clinic visits.

Breaking bad news

Medical students have identified breaking bad news as their greatest fear in terms of communicating with patients, and in the first half of the 20th century it was routine practice to hide the diagnosis from patients with cancer. It is uncertain whether this was a paternalistic policy to protect the patient or because physicians avoided a difficult task that many found unpleasant (and one that might lead them to question their practices). Although many students believe that good communication skills are innate, it is clear that like so many things the techniques can be taught and learnt (Table 4.2). The way in which the diagnosis is communicated to patients is an important determinant of subsequent psychological stress and, even if patients recall little of the conversation that followed, they state that the competence of the doctor at breaking bad news is critical to establishing trust. Why do doctors fear breaking bad news? Obviously the information causes pain and distress to patients and their relatives, making us feel uncomfortable. We fear being blamed and provoking an emotional reaction. Breaking bad news reminds us of our own mortality and fears of our own death. Finally, we often worry about being unable to answer a patient's difficult questions since we never know what the future holds for either our patients or ourselves. Breaking bad news to patients should not involve protecting them from the truth but rather imparting the information in a sensitive manner at the patient's own pace.

Breaking bad news to patients requires preparation and this aspect is very often overlooked. The setting for these discussions should be quiet, comfortable and confidential so that the whole ward does not eavesdrop and so that your bleep and mobile phone do not constantly intrude. An adequate period of time (at least 30 minutes) should be set aside and the patient should be asked if she/he wants someone else present. The conversation should open with a question to find out how much the patient already knows. An open question such as 'What have you already been told about your illness?' can reveal not only what has been said and how much has been understood but also the emotional state of the patient ('I'm so terrified it's cancer'). This opening gambit frequently takes care of much of the hard work for you ('I think it's cancer but the doctors do seem to want to say'). Under these circumstances the diagnosis can be confirmed in an empathetic fashion. If this initial question does not open up a useful avenue, a warning shot should be fired off ('I have the results of your biopsy and I'm afraid that the news is not good'). Following this warning shot, wait for the patient to respond and check if the patient wants to be told more. This cycle of warning shot, pause and checking should be repeated when elaborating on details of the diagnosis and treatment options. In this way the patient determines how much information is delivered. Certainly long monologues are overwhelming and confusing and it is hopeless and insensitive to use this opportunity to try and teach pathophysiology. Learning to identify and acknowledge a patient's reaction is essential to breaking bad news. In general, prognostication with respect to 'how long have I got Doc?' and the quoting of five-year-mortality statistics are rarely helpful. Few doctors can explain the implications of skewed distributions, medians and confidence intervals, let alone in a way that is accessible to patients. Many patients will ask for these predictions hoping for reassurance. In these circumstances it is always easier to give false reassurance but the temptation must be resisted as you will not be doing your patient a favour in the long run. After answering the patient's enquiries, it should be possible to synthesize their concerns and medical issues into a concrete plan. Even in the bleakest of situations setting short-term achievable plans leaves the patient with a goal for the future and hope. The plan should include an explicit arrangement for following up the conversation and a method for the patient to contact you if something arises before the next planned visit.

Coping strategies

Increased interaction and empathy with cancer patients has costs to health care professionals that need to be appreciated and addressed. Improved communications brings health care professionals closer to the patient and may increase feelings of inadequacy when faced with insoluble issues and of failure when patients die. Health care professionals dealing with dying patients and their families risk burn-out and although the medical profession is notoriously resistant to external help, a team spirit, adequate training through communication workshops and peer support are important elements in coping with these emotional stresses. Another technique that is frequently employed is distancing, which may protect the doctors from their feelings but often reduces their compassion and their capacity to care for patients. Although the burden of caring for people with cancer falls most heavily on doctors and nurses, other staff members may also be affected. Indeed, when patients are dying their distress and that of their care givers trickles down to everyone in the clinic or ward.

Medical burn-out

The depletion of physical and mental resources induced by excessive striving to reach an often unrealistic work-related goal is termed burn-out. Burn-out of staff working in cancer care is common and victims often describe themselves as workaholics. The Maslach burn-out inventory is a tool that measures burn-out and a quarter of consultant oncologists in the UK have scores that denote this. The consequences of medical burn-out include emotional exhaustion leading to psychological detachment from patients and the sensation that little is being achieved in terms of personal accomplishment. This may account for the high frequency of experienced oncologists changing roles in their 50s, taking on management positions or jobs with cancer charities or immersing themselves increasingly in research rather than patient contact.

Unconventional treatments

The unmet emotional needs of patients have been held responsible for the increasing use of unconventional treatments for cancer. The void that patients may feel at a vulnerable stage in their lives may be filled with complementary treatments, alternative therapies or quackery.

Complementary and alternative therapies

According to the Cochrane Project, complementary and alternative medicine (CAM) is a broad

domain of healing resources that encompasses all health systems, modalities and practices and their accompanying theories and beliefs, other than those intrinsic to the politically dominant health system of a particular society or culture in a given historical period. Thus, whilst orthodox medicine is politically dominant, CAM practices outside this system and is, for the most part, isolated from the universities and hospitals where health care is taught and delivered. As some CAM disciplines (e.g. acupuncture) become increasingly incorporated into conventional medicine they therefore loose their 'alternative' status. Indeed it is this co-operation of health systems that led to the introduction of the term 'complementary medicine' rather than the title 'alternative medicine'.

Every year around 20% of the population in the UK use CAM and this is interpreted as a measure of disillusion with conventional medicine. In contrast, the prevalence of use in the USA is 40% and in Germany is >60%. There is a prolonged history in Germany of CAM use and indeed Samuel Hahnemann (1755–1843), who first described homoeopathy (Box 4.1), was a German physician. The pantheon of complementary and alternative therapies includes alternative therapies with

---

Box 4.1: Homoeopathy – does it work?

The underlying principle of homoeopathic medicine is the use of extremely low-dose preparations prescribed according to the belief that like should be cured with like (readers may wish to refer to the Mitchell and Webb sketch 'Homeopathic A&E' on youtube). Treatments are chosen according to the symptoms that they elicit when administered to healthy people. Since raw onions cause crying, stinging eyes and a runny nose, *Allium cepa* (derived from onions) is used as a homoeopathic remedy for hayfever. The most notorious experimental trial that attempted to explain the mechanism of action of homoeopathy was undertaken by Jacques Benveniste. He hypothesized that water had the ability to remember solutes that had been dissolved in it after finding that very dilute solutions of allergens could elicit basophil responses. In a show trial experiment, the then editor of *Nature* Sir John Maddox brought a team of independent referees to observe the experiments in Benveniste's laboratory. The observers included James Randi, a magician and investigator of the paranormal, and under his scrutiny Benveniste's team were unable to repeat the findings. Since that failure, Benveniste has continued to pursue the storage of memory in water, claiming to be able to store an electronic record in water that can be transferred back into an email format. These claims have been met with even greater scepticism and have earned him an unprecedented second IgNobel Prize.

Despite these claims the most widely believed theory of the mechanism of homoeopathy remains a placebo effect and more effort has been focused on establishing the efficacy of homoeopathy. A meta-analysis, published in the *Lancet*, examined over 100 randomized, placebo-controlled trials and found a significant odds ratio of 2.45 in favour of homoeopathy. Homoeopathic medicines can be purchased over the counter at chemists and health stores. In contrast to other forms of CAM, homoeopathy is supported by the NHS through both the National Homoeopathic Hospital in London and the fact that homoeopathic remedies may be prescribed on the NHS by any doctor registered with the General Medical Council.

Box 4.2: Acupuncture

Acupuncture originated over 2000 years ago in China. It was used by William Osler, the celebrated Canadian-born physician who was both Chief of Staff at Johns Hopkins University and subsequently Regius Professor of Medicine at Oxford University at the start of the 20th century. The recent resurgence in popularity of acupuncture dates from President Nixon's visit to China in the 1970s. The stimulation of acupuncture points by fine needles is intended to control the Qi energy circulating between organs along channels or meridians. The 12 main meridians correspond to the 12 major functions or 'organs' of the body and acupuncture points are located along these meridians. The analgesic actions of acupuncture may be explained by a conventional physiological gating model and acupuncture is known to release endogenous opioids. There is convincing evidence supporting the value of acupuncture in the management of both nausea and acute pain. The evidence base for the use of acupuncture in chronic pain is less secure and current evidence suggests that it is unlikely to be of benefit for obesity, smoking cessation and tinnitus. For most other conditions the available evidence is insufficient to guide clinical decisions. Acupuncture appears to be a relatively safe treatment in the hands of suitably qualified practitioners, with serious adverse events being extremely rare. It has been estimated that 1 million acupuncture treatments are given on the NHS in England each year, at an estimated cost of £26 million, equivalent to all other complementary therapies combined. A further 2 million acupuncture treatments are given in the private sector annually.

Box 4.3: Herbalism

The most widely used herbalism in the UK is Chinese and derives from the Daoist concepts of balancing the yin and yang elements of Qi energy. The revenue from herbal products in the UK exceeds £40 million per year. Perhaps the most familiar example of herbal medicine is the use of St John's wort (*Hypericum perforatum*) for treating mild to moderate depression. Systematic reviews of randomized controlled trials confirm its efficacy over placebo and its equivalence to amitryptilline with fewer side effects. St John's wort is, however, not free of side effects and has important drug interactions caused by inducing hepatic microsomal enzymes. Other more severe toxicities have been described with herbal medicines including rapidly progressive interstitial renal fibrosis in several women after taking Chinese herbs containing powdered extracts of *Stephania tetrandra* prescribed by a slimming clinic.

recognized professional bodies (e.g. acupuncture (Box 4.2), chiropractic, herbal medicine (Box 4.3), homoeopathy, osteopathy), complementary therapies (e.g. Alexander technique, aromatherapy, Bach and other flower extracts, body work therapies including massage, counselling stress therapy, hypnotherapy, meditation, reflexology, shiatsu, healing, Maharishi Ayurvedic medicine, nutritional medicine, yoga), alternative therapies that lack professional organization but have established and traditional systems of health care (e.g. anthro-

posophical medicine, Ayurvedic medicine, Chinese herbal medicine, Eastern medicine (Tibb), naturopathy, traditional Chinese medicine) and, finally, there are other 'new age' alternative disciplines (e.g. crystal therapy, dowsing, iridology, kinesiology, radionics).

Many doctors remain concerned about the use of complementary and alternative medicines. These concerns may be based on a number of factors including that patients may be seen by unqualified practitioners, may risk delayed or missed diagnosis, may decline or stop conventional therapies, may waste money on ineffective therapies and may experience dangerous adverse effects from treatment. Moreover, the scientific academic training in medicine leads many doctors to question the value of those therapies where a plausible mechanism of action is not available. At present practitioners of CAM in the UK are free to practice as they wish without clear regulation; greater co-operation and respect between conventional doctors and complementary therapists would improve patient care.

Quackery

The word quack is supposedly derived from 'quacksalver', a 17th century variant spelling of quicksilver or mercury, which was used in certain remedies that the public came to recognize as

---

Box 4.4: The Luigi Di Bella cure

This treatment is named after its proponent, Professor Luigi Di Bella (1912–2003), a retired physiologist who lived in Modena. It is based on a combination of somatostatin, vitamins, retinoids, melatonin and bromocriptine. ACTH (adreno-corticotrophic hormone) and low doses of the oral chemotherapeutic agents cyclophosphamide and hydroxyurea are sometimes also included. It was claimed that the treatment stimulated the body's self-healing properties without damaging healthy cells. No scientific rationale or supportive experimental evidence was provided, and despite claims to have cured thousands of patients no clinical results were published in peer-reviewed scientific journals. In December 1997 a judge in the southern Italian city of Maglie ruled that the health authority should fund this treatment for a patient and this pattern was followed elsewhere. Although the initial child died of cancer, unprecedented public interest in the unconventional therapy led to public demonstrations with the right-wing media in Italy championing the cause. The socialist Italian government under considerable pressure decided to carry out phase II open-label studies in several cancer centres. Scrutiny of Di Bella's own clinical records of 3076 patients revealed that 50% lacked evidence that the patient had cancer and a further 30% had no follow-up data. Adequate data were available for just 248 patients of whom 244 had in addition received conventional treatments for their tumours. These findings rattled Di Bella's credibility and in October 1998 the findings of the first clinical trial were published in the *British Medical Journal*. Of 386 patients, just three had shown a partial response. The findings, however, failed to shake Di Bella's confidence. He accused drug companies of conspiring against him, and suggested that the results were sabotaged by mainstream doctors. Even in 2003, some 3000 patients receive Di Bella-based cancer treatments paid for by three Italian regional health services.

---

harmful. Pseudoscience uses the language and authority of science without recognizing its methods. It produces claims that cannot be proven or refuted and often poses as the victim ('scientists are suppressing the truth'). A quack may reasonably be defined as a pseudoscientist who is selling something, and a charlatan as a cynical pseudoscientist who knows he or she is deceiving the public. It is a sorry monument to human greed and stupidity that more money is spent on health frauds every year than on medical research. Quacks are convincing because they tell people what they want to hear. Moreover it is almost impossible for the cancer quack to fail. When a patient deteriorates, the cancer quack resorts to lines such as 'if only you had come to me sooner'. However, we should appreciate that quacks can teach us a great deal whilst we retain an honest and informed practice of medicine. Their popularity is attributed to their patience and ability to listen carefully and show both interest and affection. As well as this, quacks encourage patients to take an active role in their health care thus empowering them. The internet appears to have made cancer quackery even easier. Whilst much health information on the web is evidence based and of high quality, the open access has also been abused. Entrepreneurs have recognized the value of the web as a free-for-all market and have used it to promote fraudulent cancer treatments ranging from £100 a pound shark cartilage powder (Box 4.5) to 'The Zapper', a 9 volt electrical device for zapping away cancers.

Euthanasia

Euthanasia is the intentional killing by act or omission of a dependent human being for his or her alleged benefit. The term assisted suicide is used when someone provides an individual with the information, guidance and means to take his or her own life with the intention that they will be used for this purpose. Although active euthanasia remains illegal in the UK it was legalized in Australia's Northern Territory in 1995, but this bill was overturned by the Australian parliament in 1997. In 1998 Oregan state, USA, legalized assisted suicide following a ballot of the population. There were 129 deaths under Oregon's Physician Assisted Suicide Act between 1998 and 2002. Euthanasia was legalized in 2000 in Holland and in 2002 in Belgium. A survey published in 1994 showed that half of a mixture of hospital consultants and general practitioners in England had been asked by a patient to take active steps to hasten death, and that a third of those asked had complied with the patient's request. The reason people choose

---

Box 4.5: Shark cartilage

In 1993, William Lane a marine biologist and entrepreneur published a book entitled *Sharks Don't Get Cancer* following the discovery that some species of sharks have lower than predicted rates of cancer. This was followed by a prime-time television documentary focusing on a Cuban study of 29 cancer patients who received shark cartilage preparations. This resulted in patients clambering for sharks' cartilage and a consequent devastation of North American shark populations. According to the National Marine Fisheries Service 'the Atlantic shark … is severely over-capitalized' and it is estimated that over 200 000 sharks are killed in American waters just for their cartilage every month. The powdered cartilage has modest anti-angiogenic activity *in vitro*, however oral administration results in the digestion of these proteins prior to absorption. An open-label phase II clinical trial, which was in part funded by shark cartilage manufacturers, found not a single responder amongst 58 patients although both nausea and vomiting were reported. Cartilage Technologies subsequently announced that it would support no additional research on shark cartilage as a cancer remedy. It is, however, intriguing that squalamine, an aminosterol antibiotic isolated from shark livers, inhibits angiogenesis and suppresses the growth of tumour xenografts in animal models. Squalamine is easily synthesized without the need to fish for sharks and is under clinical trial investigation in age-related macular degeneration as well as solid tumours.

---

euthanasia is mostly out of fear of losing autonomy and/or bowel/bladder control, and an increasing proportion of the British public wishes to allow euthanasia for patients in certain incurable disease scenarios.

Ethics

Four principles underpin medical ethics: respect for autonomy, non-maleficence, beneficence and justice. In health care decisions, respect for autonomy means that the patient is allowed to act intentionally, with understanding and without controlling influences. This is the basis of informed consent. The principle of non-maleficence requires that we do not intentionally cause harm or injury to a patient, either through acts of commission or omission. In common language this is avoiding negligence and is based on Hippocrates' (460–377 BC) original decree 'primum non nocere'. The principle of beneficence is the duty of health care professionals to provide benefit to patients and prevent harm befalling them. These duties apply not only to the individual patient but to society as a whole, and therein frequently lies the problem. In practice, double effect reasoning, first attributed to Thomas Aquinas (1224–1274), may apply when an action has two outcomes – one good and one bad – and allows a lesser harm for a greater good.

Justice in health care terms is defined as fairness in distribution of care particularly when allocating scarce resources. A number of political doctrines interpret this differently. Karl Marx (1818–1883), of course, believed in egalitarianism 'from each according to his abilities, to each according to his needs'. Modern health care is rarely provided on this basis but rather on a system that distributes care according to a number of factors including need, effort, contribution, merit and free-market exchanges. Utilitarian philosophers, on the other hand, advocate a system that balances benefit between the collective public and the individual.

Perhaps the most interesting example of the rationing of health care is the Oregon health plan. The Oregon health plan was set up in 1987 with the aim of serving more low-income people using federal funds through a system that prioritizes heath care. An extensive list of more than 700 physical health, dental, drug dependency and mental health services was drawn up and their priority publicly debated in order to reflect a consensus of social values of Oregonians. The list of 587 approved procedures went into operation in 1994. The innovation that most sharply and controversially characterizes this systematic approach is its commitment to providing a standard health benefit based on ranking the effectiveness and value of all medical treatments. To determine which conditions are to be covered, Oregon's Health Services Commission ranks diagnoses from the most important (treatment has the greatest impact on health status) to the least important. This prioritization introduces a transparent approach to health care rationing and was originally designed to use the savings achieved to extend coverage to more people. Moreover it requires public involvement in health policies and incorporates public values into the rankings. The top five ranked items were the diagnosis and treatment of head injury, insulin-dependent diabetes mellitus, peritonitis, acute glomerulonephritis (including dialysis) and pneumothorax. At the cut-off cusp, medical treatment of contact and atopic dermatitis and symptomatic urticaria are covered, as is repair of damaged knee ligaments, but the treatment of sexual dysfunction with psychotherapy or medical and surgical approaches does not make the cut, nor does the medical treatment of chronic anal fissure nor complex dental prostheses. The Oregon Health Services Commission also excluded treatment for hepatocellular cancer and widely disseminated cancer.

Sociology of oncology

Inequalities in health are not confined to the marked differences between wealthy and poor nations but are recapitulated within countries, such as the UK. Eight tube stations on the Jubilee tube line separate Westminster from Canning Town in Newham and the life expectancy of a child born in Westminster exceeds that of a child born in Newham by six years – almost one year lost for each stop travelled. How much of this disparity is attributable to differences in health care is uncertain, even in a state health monopoly that is free at the point of delivery. Certainly, Marxist health analysts such as Howard Waitzkin propose that doc-

tor–patient encounters reproduce the dominant ideologies of wider society and that medicine is a tool for social control. Modern medicine stands accused of serving the interests of capital and of ensuring that people adhere to the norms of behaviour. Many oncological health inequalities are behavioural and medicine has branded these as self-inflicted, for example tobacco use and diet. Similar arguments have accused medicine of gender discrimination. Women are greater users of health care because they live longer and because of the medicalization of reproductive health. It is also worth noting that the only national cancer screening programmes are for women (mammogram and cervical smears). Medicine has a long history of reinforcing a subordinate role for women in society leading to both radical and reformist responses from the feminist movement. Equivalent oncological responses would be the alternative medicine movement, which wishes to overthrow the current practice of oncology, and complementary medicine, which wishes to change cancer medicine from within, encouraging the adoption of a wider vision and a more holistic approach.

The use of metaphors in cancer medicine has been attacked by both Susan Sontag and John Diamond, who use their personal experiences of cancer to describe the negative implications of these metaphors. Many of these metaphors are bellicose, 'the fight against cancer' belittles the patient as 'a victim'. The use of these figures of speech may render cancer socially as well as physically devastating and 'losing the battle against cancer' denigrates a patient's role in society.

Part 2

Types of Cancer

Chapter 5

Breast cancer

Diseases of the breast, including tumours, have been attracting medical interest for more than 5000 years. The earliest written records of breast cancer are in the Edwin Smith papyrus, from ancient Egyptian civilizations of 3000 to 2500 BC. Hard and cold lumps were recognized as tumours, whilst abscesses were hot. The next major advances in the management of breast cancer occurred during the golden age of surgery at the end of the 19th century, following advances in antisepsis and anaesthesia. William Halsted in Baltimore described radical mastectomy in 1894. Moreover, in an early example of surgical audit, he reported a local recurrence rate in 50 women of only 6%. The next major advance in the management of breast cancer occurred in 1896 with the development of surgical oophrectomy as a treatment strategy for advanced breast cancer, which was pioneered by George Beatson in Glasgow (the Beatson Institute for Cancer Research in that city is named after him). Geoffrey Keynes, the brother of Maynard, and an expert in the watercolours of William Blake, developed lumpectomy and radiotherapy as a breast conservation measure in the 1930s whilst appointed as surgeon at St Bartholomew's Hospital in London. In the 1960s and 1970s the radical women's movements in Europe and America took breast cancer as a campaigning point, and their

campaigns led to increased focus on breast cancer treatment and research. Copying the AIDS awareness red ribbons, breast cancer activists adopted pink ribbons and now there are a rainbow of different cancer ribbons. These campaigns directly led on to improvements in screening strategies, and screening programmes were introduced without a significant evidence base for efficacy and against the views of the medical establishment. As a consequence of increased screening, the survival rates of breast cancer have risen steadily over the last 30 years. A list of five-year survival of breast cancer patients by stage of disease can be found in Table 5.1. Breast cancer patients were largely viewed as the property of the surgeons. In the United Kingdom in the last few years central governmental directives have led to multidisciplinary working. This has directly led to a decrease in the use of mutilating surgery, and an increase in the use of adjuvant treatments.

Epidemiology

Breast cancer is a common disease. According to the most recent figures, 45 500 women are affected annually and 11 750 die in England and Wales as a result of this condition. The likelihood of the development of breast cancer is affected by a positive family history of breast cancer, increasing age, diet, social class and nulliparity. Breast cancer risk increases with age, plateauing during the menopausal years of 45–55. Women are at increased risk

Lecture Notes: Oncology, 2nd edition. By M. Bower and J. Waxman. Published 2010 by Blackwell Publishing Ltd.

Table 5.1 Five-year survival of women with breast cancer by stage of disease.

Tumour stage	Stage definition	5-year survival
Stage I	Tumour <2 cm, no nodes	88%
Stage II	Tumour 2–5 cm and/or moveable axillary nodes	69%
Stage III	Chest wall or skin fixation and/or fixed axillary nodes	43%
Stage IV	Metastases	12%

from breast cancer from non-vegetarian diets; it is not clear what the reason for this should be. Women who are more than two standard deviations above average height and weight are at a greater risk from breast cancer, as are women of social classes I and II. There is a protective effect of a full-term pregnancy, provided the pregnancy is achieved prior to the woman's 30th birthday. There is a minor protective effect of having more than five pregnancies, but probably no protective effect from breast feeding. A late menopause correlates with an increased risk of breast cancer, but there is little evidence that an early menarche predicates for increased risk. Oestrogen-only hormone replacement therapy (HRT), as well as combined oestrogen and progestogen HRT, increase the risk of breast cancer in proportion to the duration of HRT administration. Both the oral contraceptive pill and alcohol and coffee consumption have been linked to breast cancer, but the associations are controversial.

A family history of breast cancer is a very important risk factor for breast cancer. If more than two first-degree relatives are affected, the risk to other female family members increases by a factor of two. There are clear links between breast cancer and other cancers, with associations between ovarian and endometrial cancer, and colonic tumours. There are four relatively common genes that lead to an increased risk of breast cancer and these are: BRCA1 and 2, CHEK2 and FGFR2. Prevalence and penetrance of mutions in these genes are variables reported and lead to a lifetime risk of breast cancer of greater than 80% and up to 60% of ovarian cancer. BRCA1 has been located to chromosome 17q21 and is a tumour suppressor gene, the product of which is involved in cell cycle regulation. The BRCA product binds with Rad51, a major protein of 3418 amino acids, which is involved in sensing and directing the molecular response to double stranded DNA damage.

The detected incidence of breast cancer is increasing in England and Wales, almost certainly as a result of the introduction of the screening programme. Death rates have fallen by nearly 30% over the last 15 years and survival chance has increased from 65% to almost 80%. Survival rates have increased to those seen in the United States. They are almost certainly due to the successes of the screening programme, which has led to the earlier detection of tumours at an earlier stage, with the resultant better prognosis. There are also contributions to this fall in mortality rate from an increased use of adjuvant chemotherapy and hormonal therapy. This contribution to a fall in mortality rates is likely to be in the range 4–7%.

Presentation

Women with breast cancer generally present to their clinicians with a lump in their breast. On average, there is a delay of approximately three months between the woman first noting the mass in her breast and her seeing a hospital clinician. Alternative sources of referral are from breast screening programmes, where mammographic detection leads to diagnosis of a previously unnoted breast lump. As a result of governmental concerns over the care of patients with breast cancer, the investigation and treatment of this disease has been prioritized. Patients in whom this condition is suspected ought to be seen in 'outpatients' within two weeks of receipt of the referral letter.

Outpatient diagnosis

The current standard is for women to be seen in a multidisciplinary setting that offers a 'one-stop shop' for diagnosis. Surgeons, with a special interest in breast cancer are located in a clinic with oncologists, with access to same-day cytology and imaging services. A careful history should be obtained from the patient prior to examination when seen in outpatients. The mass may be thought to be benign or malignant. Benign lumps are more likely in younger women and tend to be painful, enlarging before menstruation. Malignant lumps tend to be more common in older women and are generally painless: only 30% of malignant breast lumps are painful, and just 10% of lumps seen in new patients are malignant.

Diagnosis is by clinical, mammographic (Figure 5.1), ultrasonographic, cytological and histological means. After clinical examination, mammography, that is, a soft tissue X-ray of the breast, aspiration cytology, which is removal of cells by means of a needle and syringe, and core biopsy should be performed to further assess the significance of the breast lump. In a younger woman, ultrasonogra-

phy rather than mammography is the radiological investigation of choice. If there is confirmed malignancy, all women should then proceed to surgery within two weeks of diagnosis, as recommended by government guidelines (Figure 5.2 and see Plate 5.1).

Staging and grading

There are two main pathological variants of breast cancer, ductal and lobular, and these are both graded as given in Table 5.2. This grading was first described by Bloom and Richardson, and bears their eponyms. This grading scheme depends upon the degree of tumour tubule formation, the mitotic activity and the nuclear pleomorphism of the tumour. As one might expect, poorly differentiated tumours have a worse prognosis than moderately differentiated ones, which in turn have a worse prognosis than well differentiated breast cancer. There may be pre-invasive changes, and these are

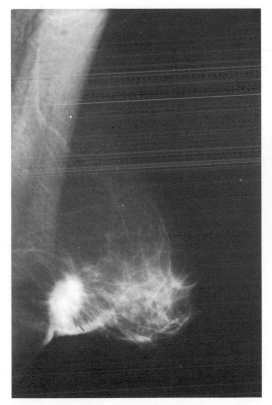

Figure 5.1 Lateral view of a breast mammogram showing a large, dense, speculated mass highly suggestive of breast cancer.

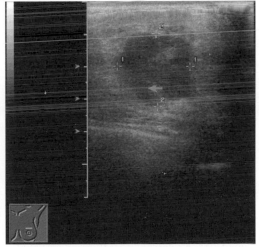

Figure 5.2 Breast ultrasound showing large, echo-dense, irregular, primary breast cancer lesion.

Table 5.2 Breast cancer grading and prognosis.

Grade	5-year survival
G1 Well differentiated	95%
G2 Moderately differentiated	75%
G3 Poorly differentiated	50%

Table 5.3 TNM staging of breast cancer.

T stage (primary tumour)	N stage (nodal status)	M stage (metastatic status)
T0 No detectable primary tumour	N0 No nodes involved	M0 No metastases
T1 Tumour less than 2 cm	N1 Mobile axillary nodes	M1 Spread to distant organs
T2 Tumour measuring between 2 and 5 cm	N2 Fixed axillary nodes	
T3 Tumour measuring greater than 5 cm	N3 Involved supra- or infraclavicular nodes	
T4 Tumour of any size extending into skin or chest wall		

described as either ductal (DCIS) or lobular carcinoma *in situ* (LCIS). LCIS are additionally graded according to their microscopic features (see Plates 1.1 and 1.2).

Stage is defined according to the classification of the Union Internationale Contre Le Cancer (UICC), which is updated every 10 years or so (Table 5.3). The subscript 'P' denotes a pathological staging following surgery. There are many other staging systems.

Treatment

Surgery

Surgery for breast cancer depends upon the clinical stage of the disease. If the mass is less than 5 cm in size and not fixed, the preferred treatment is removal of the lump, which is termed 'lumpectomy'. Axillary lymph node dissection was conventionally performed, but now this has largely been replaced by sentinel lymph node biopsy which, if positive, may then be followed by an axillary clearance. The reason for this is that if the nodes are affected by a cancer, there is an advantage in this group of women to adjuvant chemotherapy. In the 'node-negative' woman there is a very much smaller advantage to adjuvant chemotherapy. In an older woman there may be an argument against routine axillary dissection. The reason for this is that adjuvant treatment with chemotherapy within this group of women is not dictated by lymph node status, because the advantage is much smaller than in younger women and the toxicity of the treatment outweighs these

modest gains. It is clear, however, that knowledge of the axillary nodal status does provide some prognostic information.

For a woman whose tumour measures 5–10 cm in size, the preferred surgical option is mastectomy, that is removal of the breast with axillary dissection. For more advanced breast cancer, the value of surgical treatment is much more contentious, and elderly women may be treated with hormonal therapy alone if the breast cancer expresses oestrogen receptors and/or progesterone receptors. In a younger woman, neoadjuvant chemotherapy may be given in the first instance, to reduce the size of the tumour, and this may be then followed by surgery and radiotherapy. There is a major role for reconstructive surgery and this may be carried out at the time of primary surgery or at a later date upon completion of adjuvant radiotherapy or chemotherapy. The psychological gain is tremendous and needs to be considered in older as well as younger women, for breasts are considered valued personal property in older just as much as in younger women.

Adjuvant radiotherapy

After lumpectomy, radiotherapy is given to the breast. This is done in order to reduce the risk of local recurrence of the tumour. Without radiation this risk is between 40% and 60%; whereas with radiation, the risk is reduced to approximately 4–6%, which is the same as that for more radical surgical procedures. Radiotherapy is generally given over a six-week period and requires daily attendance at hospital. The side effects of radiation include tiredness and burning of the skin, which is generally mild. More serious consequences of radiation are seen only rarely and include damage to the brachial nerve plexus and, with more old-fashioned treatment machines and plans, damage to the coronary blood vessels. Rarely, a second cancer, such as an angiosarcoma, may follow at the site of radiotherapy treatment.

Adjuvant hormonal therapy

Treatment with tamoxifen has been shown to have an advantage in terms of disease-free and overall survival in both pre- and postmenopausal women and is now given routinely to this group of patients. It is usually recommended that treatment should extend for five years. There is no advantage to adjuvant tamoxifen in oestrogen receptor-negative tumours. There have been changes in our understanding of the oestrogen receptor. Two different classes of oestrogen receptor (ER), described as α and β, have been identified. Tamoxifen is a selective ERα-antagonist, which in turn has effects on the progesterone receptor. In postmenopausal women, recent studies suggest that a newer group of drugs, the aromatase inhibitors, may be even more effective than tamoxifen as adjuvant therapy. The current standard is to give sequential therapy with tamoxifen and then an aromatase inhibitor. Treatment is given for a total of five years. Approximately 10% of circulating oestrogens derive from adrenal precursors, such as androstenedione, through the action of aromatase enzymes. The aromatase inhibitors block this action, limiting the synthesis of oestrone and oestrone sulphate produced by a second series of enzymes; the sulphatase system (Figure 5.3). Use of aromatase inhibitors is associated with osteoporosis. There have been reports of cases of endometrial carcinoma associated with the use of tamoxifen. The estimated risk is one case per 20 000 women per year of use.

Adjuvant chemotherapy and receptor targeting therapy

Adjuvant chemotherapy has a significant place in the management of breast cancer. Although chem-

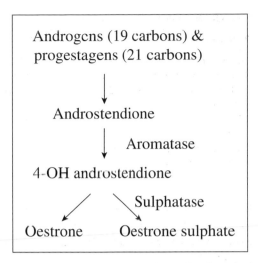

Figure 5.3 Peripheral oestrogen (18 carbons) synthesis pathway.

otherapy using the CMF (cyclophosphamide, methotrexate, 5-fluorouracil (5FU)) programme was the regimen first shown to be of benefit, and is widely used. A large international study showed that more intensive therapy using the FEC (5FU, epirubicin, cyclophosphamide) regimen is more effective than CMF. There has been recent interest in the use of taxane chemotherapy given in the adjuvant setting, with the possibility that survival may be further improved. Third generation adjuvant chemotherapy combining alternating FEC and taxane based treatment are now considered to be the standard. There is no evidence whatsoever that intensifying adjuvant therapy any further using, for example, high-dose treatments with bone marrow or peripheral blood stem cell support, improves the disease-free interval or the overall survival. About a quarter of breast cancers express the epidermal growth factor receptor 2 (EGFR2), also known as Her-2/neu, and c-erbB-2. This is the target for the monocloncal antibody trastuzumab (Herceptin). For patients with Her-2 receptor-positive tumours, treatment with adjuvant trastuzumab may be considered. Treatment is conventionally given for periods of 12–18 months. The advantage to treatment with trastuzumab is small, but is recommended in the context of the 60–70% five-year survival chance that patients with Her-2 strongly positive tumours have. The toxicity of treatment with trastuzumab is significant, and particularly of note are the direct cardiac effects that may manifest as heart failure.

Treatment of metastatic breast cancer

The treatment of metastatic breast cancer depends very much upon the age of the patient and the sites of metastasis. It is only rarely curable, and so life quality issues are immediately important. When we described this point to one patient, she replied: 'my dear, it's death quality issues that bother me'. In older women whose metastases are in the skin or bone, the preferred treatment option is hormonal therapy, provided that the tumour expresses oestrogen and/or progestogen receptor positivity. The agent of first choice is tamoxifen because of its lack of toxicity and efficacy. Approximately 70% of women aged 70 respond to this therapy. In a premenopausal woman, hormonal therapy is generally less effective, and at the age of 30, just 10% of patients overall will respond to treatment at all. But oophorectomy, (that is, removal of the ovaries by either radiotherapeutic, surgical or medical means), is generally the first therapeutic stratagem. Surgical oophorectomy is unnecessary, given that an equivalence of effect is provided by the use of medical treatment with an LHRH (luteinizing hormone receptor hormone) agonist. How much easier is it to provide a simple three-monthly depot injection than to expose a woman to laparoscopy and surgical oophorectomy. Radiotherapy is not a particularly successful way of causing gonadal failure. Ovaries are relatively radiotherapy resistant, and the conventional dosages of radiotherapy given to sterilize may not sterilize a younger woman, and certainly will not lead to an instant reduction in circulating ovarian steroid hormones.

In both pre- and postmenopausal women, radiation treatment is very effective in controlling bone pain. The addition of regular bisphosphonate therapy both relieves bone pain and reduces skeletal events such as fractures and spinal cord compression. If lungs or liver are affected, then chemotherapy is required. Overall, between 40%

and 60% of patients respond to chemotherapy, and this response is for a median duration of one year. The median survival of women with metastatic breast cancer ranges between 18 and 24 months, with 5–10% alive after five years. It should be noted that there are patients with very prolonged survival, and these include those women who have, for example, single sites of metastatic disease.

High-dose chemotherapy

Breast cancer responds to chemotherapy, but often after responding, patients relapse and die. There have been attempts to maximize response rates by intensifying chemotherapy. High-dose treatments were popular in the early 1980s. Response rates were found to be higher than for conventional treatment; toxicity, however, was significantly worse, and death rates reached 20% as a result of the side effects of treatment. Even more significantly, patients who responded and survived the toxicity, later relapsed, and the median duration of response was no better than that expected with conventional treatment.

In the 1990s, there was an increase in the numbers of patients receiving high-dose therapy for breast cancer. This was possible as a result of the improvement in supportive therapy, principally bone marrow rescue, either with stem cells or with marrow. Mortality has decreased and now is 5% in the best centres. Overall, there has been no significant improvement in the expectation for survival for patients with metastatic breast cancer, and only 20% of patients are alive two years after the transplantation. It has been recently argued that the relatively good results of intensive therapy reported in early studies are entirely the result of the selection of good-prognosis patients for treatment with high-dose therapy, and that the same effects could be achieved with less intensive, conventional therapy. It may be the case that early intensive therapy given as adjuvant treatment to patients with poor-risk tumours will lead to improved survival, but this has not been shown in any randomized study.

Carcinoma *in situ*

Carcinoma *in situ*, diagnosed by excision biopsy will progress to invasive cancer in 40% of patients over five years. Treatment with adjuvant radiotherapy will limit this progression rate to 1–4% per annum. An alternative to radiation therapy is mastectomy. Both radiotherapy and mastectomy are equally effective in local disease control. Lobular carcinoma *in situ* is associated with bilaterality, and mirror biopsy is recommended of the contralateral breast.

Paget's disease of the nipple

This is an eczematous condition of the nipple, associated in 80% of cases with an underlying ductal carcinoma, and in about 20% of cases with underlying ductal carcinoma *in situ*.

New treatment

Further hormonal therapies are also likely to become available with interest in the development of sulphatase inhibitors (Figure 5.3). Poor-prognosis breast cancer highly expresses EGFR. Therapy with gefitinib may be effective in these tumours. mTOR is a component of the P13K/Akt signalling pathway that mediates cell growth and prolifera-

tion. Inhibitors of this pathway, such as temsirolimus, have been shown to have activity in breast cancer.

Triple negative breast cancer, which is breast cancers ER, PR and HER2 negative, constitutes about 15% of all breast cancers and has an aggressive natural history. These triple negative tumours are highly sensitive to chemotherapy with DNA-damaging agents such as cisplatin, and the effects of these drugs can be potentiated by the use of PARP inhibitors which disable DNA base excision repair. In early clinical trials these agents have shown a highly significant improvement in response rates and overall survival.

Angiogenesis inhibitors, such as bevacizumab, have also been shown to have an effect in breast cancer, but this is likely to be of minor significance. Targeted therapies, in which an antibody to HER2+ or EGFR+ is tagged to a cytotoxic agent, have provided a way of delivering targeted chemotherapy to breast cancer, and have led, in a small randomized clinical trial, to have some efficacy, as have agents capable of inhibiting the tyrosine kinase linked to HER1 and -2 activation.

So, it is clear that there is hope that breast cancer will become a curable cancer within the next 10 years. There has been progress in the identification of susceptibility genes for breast cancer, and it is hoped that targeted therapy will lead to progress.

Chapter 6

Central nervous system cancers

The first recognized resection of a primary brain tumour was performed in 1884 by Rickman Godlee in collaboration with the Westminster Hospital neurologist Alexander Bennett. It should be remembered that the removal of the cerebral cortex tumour was performed before any diagnostic imaging was available, but even then the surgeon knew to operate on the contralateral side to the clinical signs! There are about 4500 people diagnosed with a brain tumour each year in the UK. That is the equivalent to an incidence of about seven in every 100 000 people each year. Brain tumours are slightly more common in men than in women. A further 300 children are diagnosed with central nervous system tumours in the UK each year.

Scientists use animal models to study genetics, development and oncogenesis and the most common models are mice (see onco-mice in Chapter 1), fruit flies (*Drosophila*) and nematode worms (*Caenorhabditis elegans*). However, fish have also turned out to be useful subjects – in particular zebrafish (*Danio rerio*), which are tropical freshwater minnows with five horizontal stripes running from their mouth to caudal fin. Zebrafish are the vertebrate model for studying the genetics of embryonic development because the embryos are transparent and the genome sequence is known

and can readily be modified by knockouts. A less well known fish model of cancer is the damselfish (*Pomacentrus partitus*) that lives on coral reefs and has several vertical stripes. Deb and Flo in *Finding Nemo* are damselfish, so that is an excuse to watch it again. Damselfish neurofibromatosis is a naturally occurring, neoplastic disease of these fish that consists of multiple neurofibromata and neurofibrosarcomas. It has been proposed as an animal model for neurofibromatosis type 1 in humans. However, whilst von Recklinghausen's neurofibromatosis type 1 is vertically transmitted as an autosomal dominant trait, damselfish neurofibromatosis is transmitted horizontally between fish and is thought to be due to an oncogenic retrovirus named damselfish neurofibromatosis virus (DNFV).

Epidemiology

Metastases to the brain are about ten times more common than primary brain tumours. The most common primary tumour sites amongst patients with brain metastases are lung, breast, melanoma and kidney. In addition, nasopharyngeal cancers may directly extend through the skull foramina. Meningeal metastases occur with leukaemia and lymphoma, breast and small cell lung cancers, and from medulloblastoma and ependymal glioma as a route of spread. Primary tumours of the central nervous system (CNS) account for 2–5% of all

Lecture Notes: Oncology, 2nd edition. By M. Bower and J. Waxman. Published 2010 by Blackwell Publishing Ltd.

cancers, and 2% of cancer deaths. Fewer than 20% of CNS cancers occur in the spinal cord. There appears to be a modest increase in the incidence of primary brain tumours over the last two decades, particularly amongst the elderly. A more dramatic rise in the incidence of primary CNS lymphomas is attributable to the AIDS epidemic.

Aetiology

Although the cause of most adult brain tumours is not established, a number of inherited phakomatoses are associated with brain tumours. Phakomatoses are a group of familial conditions with unique cutaneous and neurological manifestations and dysplasias of a number of organ systems. They include neurofibromatosis (von Recklinghausen's disease), tuberous sclerosis (Bourneville's disease), von Hippel–Lindau disease (cerebroretinal angiomatosis), Sturge–Weber syndrome (ezcephalotrigeminal angiomatosis), Osler–Rendu–Weber syndrome and Fabry's disease (angiokeratoma corporis diffusum). The first three of these are associated with brain tumours; von Recklinghausen's neurofibromatosis with cranial and root schwannomas, meningiomas, ependymomas and optic gliomas (see Plate 2.2); tuberous sclerosis with gliomas and ependymomas; and von Hippel–Lindau disease with cerebellar and retinal haemagioblastoma (Table 6.1). In addition, an increased incidence of brain tumours is a feature of Gorlin's basal naevus syndrome (medulloblastoma), Turcot syndrome (gliomas) and Li–Fraumeni syndrome (glioma). High-dose ionizing radiation to the head region administered in the past for benign conditions such as scalp tinea capitis fungal infection (ringworm) increases the risk of nerve sheath tumours, gliomas and meningiomas. There is much public concern that low-frequency non-ionizing electromagnetic fields such as those emitted by 60 Hz power cables may increase the risk of brain tumours, but there is no consistent evidence to support this hypothesis. Similarly, despite scares, there is no evidence to support an association with wireless radiofrequency devices such as mobile phones. This joins the long list of things that cause cancer according to the *Daily Mail*. It includes Facebook, deodorant, hair dye, talcum powder, mouthwash, tooth whitener, oral sex, chips and chocolate.

Pathology

Primary nervous system tumours may be glial tumours, non-glial tumours or primary cerebral non-Hodgkin's lymphoma. As you will recall from embryology, the early embryo has three distinct germ layers of cells; the innermost endoderm that gives rise to the digestive organs, lungs and bladder, the middle layer or mesoderm that gives rise to the muscles, skeleton and blood system, and the outer layer or ectoderm that gives rise to the skin and nervous system. Neuroectodermal tumours are classified on the basis of the predominant cell type and include all neoplasms with either central or peripheral nervous system-derived cell origins. After embryonic development ceases, neurons do not divide, but glial cells retain the ability to proliferate throughout life and thus most adult neurological tumours are derived from glial cells and are named gliomas. Seventy percent of primary brain tumours in adults are supratentorial, situated above the tentorium cerebelli, the tent of dura mater that lies between the cerebellum and the interior portion of the occipital lobes. In contrast primary brain tumours in children are usually located below the tentorium (Table 6.2).

Gliomas account for 50% of brain tumours and are divided into grade I (non-infiltrating pilocytic astrocytoma), grade II (well to moderately differentiated astrocytoma), grade III (anaplastic astrocytoma) and grade IV (glioblastoma multiforme). The prognosis deteriorates with rising tumour grade. Other glial tumours include ependymomas, that arise from ependymal cells, usually lining the fourth ventricle, and oligodendrogliomas that arise from oligodendroglia. In the peripheral nervous system, neurofibromata and schwannomas are the most frequent glial tumours. Medulloblastoma is a glial tumour of childhood usually arising in the cerebellum, which may be related to primitive neuroectodermal tumours elsewhere in the CNS. Non-glial brain tumours include pineal parenchymal tumours, extragonal germ cell

Table 6.1 Phakomatoses associated with brain tumours.

Condition	Inheritance and genetics	Cutaneous manifestations	Eye	Nervous system	Brain tumours
Von Recklinghausen's neurofibromatosis (NF-1)	Autosomal dominant NF-1 gene (encodes neurofibromin that regulates GTPases in signal transduction)	Café au lait macules, axillary freckles	Lisch nodules (pigmented iris hamartomas)	Neurofibromata	Schwann cell tumours of spinal and cranial nerves, meningiomas, ependymomas, optic gliomas
Acoustic neurofibromatosis (NF-2)	Autosomal dominant NF-2 gene (encodes Merlin protein involved in cell adhesion)	Café au lait macules less common than in NF-1	Presenile cataracts	Bilateral acoustic neuromas Neurofibromata	Schwann cell tumours of spinal and cranial nerves, meningiomas, astrocytomas, ependymomas, optic gliomas
Tuberous sclerosis	Autosomal dominant TSC1 gene (encodes hamartin protein) and TSC2 gene (encodes tuberin protein)	Adenoma sebaceum, Shagreen patches, subungual fibromata, café au lait spots		Seizures, mental retardation	Giant cell astrocytoma of the foramen of Munro, gliomas, ependymomas
Von Hippel–Lindau	Autosomal dominant VHL gene (encodes VHL protein involved in ubiquination)	Skin hamartomas	Retinal angiomas		Cerebellar haemagioblastomas, ependymomas, phaeochromocytoma

Table 6.2 Brain tumours by age and site.

Adult	Child
Supratentorial	
Metastases	Craniopharyngioma
Glioma	Pinealoma
Meningioma	Optic glioma
Pituitary tumour	
Infratentorial	
Metastases	Medulloblastoma
Acoustic neuroma	Cerebellar astrocytoma
Cerebellar	Ependymoma of
haemangioblastoma	fourth ventricle

Table 6.3 Common presentation of brain tumours by site.

Tumour site	Common presentations
Frontal	Personality change
	Contralateral motor signs
	Dysphasia (dominant hemisphere)
Parietal	Contralateral sensory signs
	Visual field defects (optic radiation)
	Neglect
Occipital	Homonymous hemianopia
Temporal	Memory and behavioural disturbances
Posterior fossa	Raised intracranial pressure
	Ataxia and nystagmus
	Cranial nerve lesions

tumours, craniopharyngiomas, meningiomas and choroid plexus tumours. Meningioma is the commonest non-glial tumour and constitutes 15% of brain tumours. The majority of spinal axis tumours in adults are extradural, metastatic carcinoma, lymphoma or sarcoma. Primary spinal cord tumours include extradural meningiomas (26%), schwannomas (29%), intramedullary ependymomas (13%) and astrocytomas (13%).

Presentation

Glial tumours

Glial tumours may produce both generalized and focal effects, and these will reflect the site of the tumour and the speed of its growth. General symptoms from the mass effect, increased intracranial pressure, oedema, midline shift and herniation syndromes are all seen, including progressive altered mental state and personality, headaches, seizures and papilloedema. Focal symptoms depend upon the location of the tumour (Table 6.3). Although seizures are a feature of up to half of all glial tumours, fewer than 10% of first fits are due to tumours and only 20% of supratentorial tumours present with fits.

Meningioma

These tumours, which are more common in women, present as slowly growing masses produc-

ing headaches, seizures, motor and sensory symptoms and cranial neuropathies, depending on their site (Table 6.4 and see Plate 6.1). Meningiomas are some of the few tumours that produce characteristic changes on plain skull X-rays with bone erosion, calcification and hyperostosis.

Spinal axis tumours

For spinal axis tumours, the proportion of tumour sites is 50% thoracic, 30% lumbosacral and 20% cervical or foramen magnum. These tumours present with radicular symptoms due to nerve root infiltration, syringomyelic disturbance (dissociated sensory loss of pain and temperature sensation) due to central destruction by intramedullary tumours, or sensorimotor dysfunction (limb weakness and a sensory level) due to cord compression.

Investigation and staging

Neuroradiology has developed into the most important investigation in patients with suspected brain tumours, following the introduction of computed tomography (CT) in the mid-1970s by Geoffrey Hounsfield and magnetic resonance imaging (MRI) in the 1980s. Newer techniques, such as positron emission tomography (PET), single photon emission computerized tomography (SPECT) and functional MRI have also found roles in the diagnosis and management of patients with brain tumours. MRI with gadolinium enhancement

Table 6.4 Clinical features of meningiomas by site.

Tumour site	Clinical features
Parasagittal falx	Progressive spastic weakness
	Numbness of legs
Olfactory groove	Anosmia
	Visual loss
	Papilloedema (Foster–Kennedy syndrome)
	Frontal lobe syndrome
Sella turcica	Visual field loss
Sphenoid ridge	Cavernous sinus syndrome (medial)
	Exophthalmos and visual loss (middle)
	Temporal bone swelling and skull deformity (lateral)
Posterior fossa (foramen magnum, tentorium)	Hydrocephalus (tentorium)
	Gait ataxia and cranial neuropathies
	V, VII, VIII, IX and X (cerebellopontine angle)
	Suboccipital pain, ipsilateral arm and leg weakness (foramen magnum)

Parasagittal meningioma

Tentorial meningioma

Sphenoid ridge meningioma

Olfactory groove meningioma

Foramen magnum meningioma

Sella turcica meningioma

is the imaging technique of choice with advantages over CT particularly for posterior fossa tumours and non-enhancing low-grade gliomas (see figures in Chapter 1). PET with fluorodeoxyglucose-18, which accumulates in metabolically active tissues, may help to differentiate tumour recurrence from radiation necrosis (see Plate 6.1). Stereotactic biopsy is required to confirm the diagnosis, although occasionally tumours are diagnosed on clinical evidence, because biopsy might be hazardous, as in brain stem gliomas, for example.

Treatment

Some gliomas are curable by surgery alone and some by surgery and radiotherapy; the remainder require surgery, radiotherapy and chemotherapy, and these tumours are rarely curable. Surgical removal should be as complete as possible within the constraints of preserving neurological function. Radiation can increase the cure rate or prolong disease-free survival in high-grade gliomas and may also be useful symptomatic therapy in patients with low-grade glioma, who relapse after initial therapy with surgery alone (Figure 6.1). Chemotherapy with nitrosurea or temozolomide may prolong disease-free survival in patients with oligodendrogliomas and high-grade gliomas, although its high toxicity may not always merit this approach.

Therapy of meningiomas is surgical resection, which may be repeated at relapse. Radiotherapy reduces relapse rates and should be considered for high-grade meningiomas or incompletely resected tumours. Relapse rates are 7% at five years if completely resected and 35–60% if incompletely resected.

Unlike with other brain tumours, surgical resection does not have a useful role in primary cerebral lymphomas. In immunocompetent patients, the combination of chemotherapy and radiotherapy produces median survivals of 40 months. In contrast, in the immunocompromised patients, especially those with HIV infection, the prognosis is far worse, with a median survival of under three months. Palliative radiotherapy or best supportive care are the appropriate treatment options here.

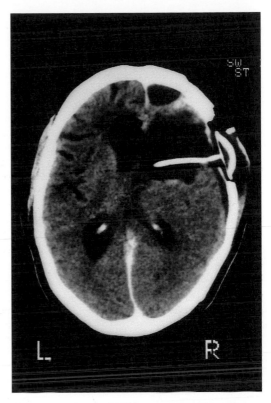

Figure 6.1 CT scan showing a patient with an Omaya shunt (a closed cerebrospinal fluid (CSF) shunt joining the lateral ventricle with a reservoir below the scalp) in place that is leaking, resulting in air seen in the right anterior brain and fluid accumulating around the shunt site. Omaya shunts may be placed to relieve non-communicating hydrocephalus caused by obstruction to CSF flow within the ventricular system, or to administer intrathecal chemotherapy.

Complications of treatment

Early complications of cranial radiotherapy which occur in the first three to four months are due to reversible damage to myelin-producing oligodendrocytes. This recovers spontaneously after three to six months. It causes somnolence or exacerbation of existing symptoms in the brain and Lhermitte's sign (shooting numbness or paraesthesia precipitated by neck flexion) in the cord. Late complications include radiation necrosis, causing irreversible deficits due to vessel damage. This may mimic disease recurrence, is radiation dose related and occurs in up to 15% of patients, with the

Table 6.5 Five-year survival rates of adult patients with brain tumours.

Tumour	5-year survival
Grade I glioma (cerebellar)	90–100%
Grade I glioma (other sites)	50–60%
Grade II (astrocytoma)	16–46%
Grade III (anaplastic astrocytoma)	10–30%
Grade IV (glioblastoma multiforme)	1–10%
Oligodendroglioma	50–80%
Meningioma	70–80%

highest frequency in children also receiving chemotherapy. SPECT and PET scanning may differentiate radionecrosis and relapse.

Prognosis

The prognosis of glial tumours depends upon the histology, the grade and size of the tumour, on the age and performance status of the patient and on the duration of the symptoms. The median survival for anaplastic astrocytoma is 18 months, and for glioblastoma multiforme is 10–12 months. Meningiomas, if completely resected, are usually cured, and the median survival is over 10 years.

New treatment

The treatment of brain tumours may well improve in the next 5–10 years. The most important recent advance has been with the use of adjuvant chemotherapy. It is hoped that the application of temozolamide, which crosses the blood–brain barrier, to radiotherapy for high-grade glioma will dramatically improve survival chances. Many high-grade gliomas express receptors for cErbB2/neu. Targeted antibody therapy delivered intravascularly may lead to further improvements in survival. Another recent advance is the use of biodegradable wafers implanted with chemotherapy that may be inserted at the time of surgery.

Newer radiotherapy delivery techniques that have been pioneered in the treatment of brain tumours include both gammaknife and cyberknife treatments, which have caught the attention and interest of the gently dozing neurosurgeon in the multidisciplinary team. Gammaknife radiotherapy is delivered by 201 cobalt-60 sources arranged in a ring in a helmet that is bolted to the patient's skull. Cyberknife radiotherapy uses a linear accelerator to deliver radiotherapy via a robotic arm that is linked to an image guidance system. Cyberknife radiotherapy does not need a skull frame because the real-time image linking means that if the patient moves, the robotic arm also moves so that the radiotherapy dose is delivered to the correct site.

Gene therapy has been adopted for trials in gliomas with viral vectors being administered either into the blood or directly into the tumour by surgeons. The genetically modified viral vectors may be non-replicating viruses that deliver a transgene that causes an anticancer effect, or replicating oncolytic viruses that directly lyse cancer cells by replicating. Gliomas are a good model to try these methods because they are pretty much the only cells dividing in the brain (apart from microglia and endothelial cells).

Chapter 7

Gastrointestinal cancers

Gastrointestinal malignancies have been attributed an important role in the history of Europe. Ferrante I of Arragon, the then King of Naples, was mummified and embalmed, following his death in 1494 and placed in a wooden sarcophagus at the Abbey of San Domenico Maggiore, Naples. In 1996, an autopsy was performed which revealed a large pelvic mass, and polymerase chain reaction (PCR) identified a mutation of the RAS oncogene, suggesting a colonic primary cancer. In 1821, Napoleon Bonaparte, the former Emperor of France, died in exile at Longwood House, St Helena. His health had been declining over a number of months with abdominal pain, weakness and vomiting, which he attributed to mistreatment by his English captors. An autopsy performed following his death concluded that the cause of death was stomach cancer; and indeed, there was a strong history of stomach cancer in his family, although

longstanding *Helicobacter pylori* infection may have contributed. Nineteen years later, Napoleon's grave was opened, and his body was returned to Paris to be finally interred in the magnificent tomb at the church of the Invalides, where it rests today. A popular alternative hypothesis proposed that his death was a consequence of chronic arsenic poisoning by his captors.

The gastrointestinal tract is one of the most frequent sites of cancer, and Table 7.1 shows the registration data for the most common tumours of the digestive system for southeast England in 2001 and the five-year survivals.

Gastrointestinal cancers include oesophageal cancer, gastric cancer, hepatobiliary cancer, pancreatic cancer and colorectal cancer, and these will be dealt with in more detail in the following five chapters.

Table 7.1 Gastrointestinal cancer registration data for southeast England for 2005

Tumour	Percentage of registrations		Rank of registration		Lifetime chance of cancer 1995–2005		Change in ASR		5-year
	Male	Female	Male	Female	Male	Female	Male	Female	Male
Oesophagus	3.4%	1.9%	7th	13th	1 in 75	1 in 95	+8.7%	−1.8%	8%
Gastric	3.6%	2.0%	6th	10th	1 in 44	1 in 86	−30%	−31%	13%
Pancreas	2.6%	2.7%	11th	8th	1 in 96	1 in 95	−2.0%	+5.1%	3%
Colorectal	14%	12%	3rd	2nd	1 in 18	1 in 20	−2.4%	−5.5%	46%

ASR, age-standardized rate.

Lecture Notes: Oncology, 2nd edition. By M. Bower and J. Waxman. Published 2010 by Blackwell Publishing Ltd.

Chapter 8

Oesophageal cancer

Epidemiology and pathogenesis

Cancer of the oesophagus is a relatively uncommon cancer in the UK, but the incidence is rising, at least in men (see Table 7.1). Worldwide, oesophageal cancer is the sixth most common cause of death from cancer. One-third are adenocarcinoma of the distal oesophagus and two-thirds are squamous cell cancers, with 15% in the upper, 45% in the mid and 40% in the lower portions of the oesophagus. Tobacco is a major risk factor for both histological types of oesophageal cancer, but the two types otherwise vary not only in their histology and anatomical distribution but also in their risk factors. Chronic irritation appears to be a major precipitant of squamous cell cancer and may be caused by alcohol, caustic injury, radiotherapy or achalasia. The Plummer–Vinson syndrome (also known as Patterson–Kelly–Brown syndrome) of chronic iron deficiency anaemia, dysphagia and oesophageal web is associated with squamous cell cancer of the oesophagus, particularly in impoverished populations. Tylosis is an autosomal dominant abnormality, characterized by hyperkeratosis (skin thickening) of the palms and soles. It carries a 95% risk of squamous cell cancer of the oesophagus by the age of 70. In contrast, the major precipi-

tant of oesophageal adenocarcinoma appears to be gastro-oesophageal reflux disease (GORD). Related markers of reflux, such as hiatus hernia, obesity, frequent antacid and histamine H2 blockers, are also associated with an increased risk. Barrett's oesophagus (named after Norman Barrett, a thoracic surgeon at St Thomas' Hospital, London) develops in 5–8% of adults with reflux leading to metaplasia of the normal squamous epithelium of the lower oesophagus to columnar epithelium, which may become dysplastic. The annual rate of transformation to oesophageal adenocarcinoma is 0.5%, which is a hundred times greater than the normal risk. Over the last three decades, there has been a radical shift in the histology of oesophageal cancer in the industrialized world, with a marked decline in squamous cell cancers and a rise in adenocarcinomas. Adenocarcinomas are thought to take their origin from the stomach. Where they occur at the junction of the stomach and oesophagus, they are classified as carcinomas of the gastro-oesophageal junction, as the intelligent reader of this book might have concluded independently of the authors of this book. This may reflect alterations in the number of smokers and in the obesity and nutrition of patients.

Prevention

Half of all cases of oesophageal cancer could be prevented by giving up smoking, drinking less alcohol

Lecture Notes: Oncology, 2nd edition. By M. Bower and J. Waxman. Published 2010 by Blackwell Publishing Ltd.

and improving diet, substituting fresh fruit and vegetables for poorly preserved, high salt foods contaminated with nitrosamine carcinogens or microbial toxins. Endoscopic surveillance is recommended every two to five years for patients with Barrett's oesophagus but the evidence that screening is effective is absent. Low-grade dysplasia requires aggressive antireflux management, whilst multifocal or high-grade dysplasia should be treated by surgical resection.

Presentation

Patients present with dysphagia or odynophagia, weight loss and, less frequently, with haematemesis. At the time of diagnosis, more than half of the patients will have locally advanced, unresectable disease or metastases present. Left supraclavicular lymphadenopathy (Virchow's node), hepatomegaly and pleural effusion are common features of metastatic dissemination. The diagnosis is usually confirmed by upper gastrointestinal endoscopy and barium studies (Figure 8.1).

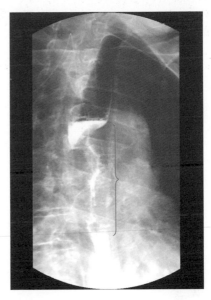

Figure 8.1 Oesophageal cancer. Gastrograffin swallow image showing a long tight stricture of the distal third of the oesophagus with shouldering that encroaches on the gastro-oesophageal junction. This malignant stricture was due to adenocarcinoma of the oesophagus.

Staging and grading

Although CT staging is most helpful in defining operability, additional information can be obtained from using endoscopic ultrasound. This allows the surgeon to have a better view as to the extent of the resection that is required.

Treatment

Only 40% of patients will have localized disease at presentation and are candidates for oesophagectomy with or without postoperative adjuvant chemoradiation. Surgery has a 5–20% mortality rate and may be complicated early by anastomotic

Table 8.1 Five-year survival rates of patients with oesophageal cancer, according to stage at presentation.

Stage	T stage (local tumour)	N stage (nodal status)	M stage (metastatic status)	5-year survival
0	Tis	N0	M0	>95%
I	T1	N0	M0	50–80%
IIA	T2–3	N0	M0	30–40%
IIB	T1–2	N1	M0	10–30%
III	T3–4	N0–1	M0	10–15%
IV	Any T	Any N	M1	<2%

Tis, carcinoma *in situ*; T1, invasion of lamina propria; T2, invasion of muscularis propria; T3, invasion of adventitia; T4, invasion of adjacent structures.

leaks, and later by strictures, reflux and motility disorders. At diagnosis, 25% of patients will have local extension and are treated with palliative radiotherapy, which may cause oesophageal perforation and haemorrhage, pneumonitis and pulmonary fibrosis, as well as transverse myelitis. The remaining 35% of patients will have metastases at presentation and are usually treated symptomatically. Although cancer of the oesophagus is sensitive to chemotherapy, the duration of response is typically short and may be measured in weeks. Cisplatin-based combination regimens have higher response rates, but this may be offset by their greater toxicity. Adjuvant chemoradiotherapy, either prior to surgery (neoadjuvant), or following resection, has yet to be proven as being beneficial. Over the last 30 years, there have been a large number of trials that investigated the benefit of chemotherapy given in the adjuvant setting for carcinoma that had arisen at the junction of the oesophagus and stomach. Until a short time ago, no benefit had been shown, but recent trials have led to the consensus that chemotherapy is probably of benefit in the adjuvant setting, though this benefit is small.

Prognosis

The five-year survival of patients with oesophageal cancer according to stage at presentation is detailed in Table 8.1.

New treatment

As we write, sadly, there are no new therapies that these authors know of for oesophageal cancer.

Chapter 9

Gastric cancer

Epidemiology and pathogenesis

Gastric cancer is the sixth most common malignancy in the UK and constitutes approximately 5% of all cancers. The male to female ratio is 1.5 to 1. In 2005 nearly 8000 people were diagnosed with stomach cancer in the UK and 5200 died of stomach cancer. The average age at presentation is 65 years. The survival for gastric cancer has tripled over the last 25 years but currently only 13% of patients are alive five years after diagnosis. Surprisingly, gastric cancer is the second most common cause of cancer deaths worldwide with 900 000 new diagnoses in 2002. There are extreme geographical variations, with the incidence being five times higher in Japan than in the US.

The incidence of gastric cancer has fallen in the industrialized world over the last few decades. This is particularly the case for distal tumours of the stomach. It had been thought that one of the reasons for the decrease in the West is better food preservation. The reducing agents used to preserve food are thought to reduce the availability of free radicals within the stomach, a major cause of carcinogenesis, but this has not been proven in prospective studies. There is contradictory evidence for a protective benefit from fruit and vegetable intake, and also from the use of non-steroidal anti-inflammatory drugs.

In 1926 the Nobel Prize for medicine was awarded to a Dane, Dr Johannes Fibiger, who had described a nematode worm that he called *Spiroptera carcinoma*, which caused stomach cancers in rats that he caught in an infested sugar refinery. It was subsequently shown that the cancers were in fact only metaplasia and that the cause was vitamin A deficiency. Although Fibiger has been branded a fibber, it turns out that chronic infection is the cause of most human gastric cancers. The single most common cause of gastric cancer is infection with *Helicobacter pylori*: probably the most common chronic bacterial infection in man. This bacterium colonizes over half of the world's population. Infection is usually acquired in childhood and in the absence of antibiotic therapy persists for the life of the host. How *H. pylori* causes gastric cancer remains unclear. Strains that have CagA genes are more oncogenic and the products of these genes regulate protein secretion by epithelial cells. In addition, chronic *H. pylori* infection leads to the local production of inflammatory cytokines that are also thought to be involved in oncogenesis. Infection by *H. pylori* explains the aetiology of cancers developing in patients with atrophic gastritis. *Helicobacter* infection is more common in patients with gastric cancer than in 'controls', in particularly in younger patients.

Lecture Notes: Oncology, 2nd edition. By M. Bower and J. Waxman. Published 2010 by Blackwell Publishing Ltd.

Presentation

Patients with gastric cancer generally present to their general practitioner with symptoms of abdominal pain. Classically, the pain is epigastric and worse with meals. The differential diagnosis includes benign peptic ulceration. The routine prescription of protein pump inhibitors, without investigation by endoscopy, may lead to late diagnosis and the presence of advanced disease at diagnosis. Because the symptoms of gastric cancer are very similar to those of peptic ulceration, and because peptic ulceration is very common and not necessarily routinely investigated, early diagnosis of gastric cancer in the West presents a difficult problem. Fewer than 2% of patients with first time dyspepsia will have gastric cancer but the risk is greater in people over 55 years and those with dysphagia, vomiting, weight loss, anorexia or symptoms of gastrointestinal bleeding. Walk-in endoscopy clinics, however, are becoming much more widely available in the UK, and it is hoped that they will impact upon survival figures for gastric cancer.

Outpatient diagnosis

After initial assessment, which should include a full blood count, liver function tests and chest X-ray, more specialized investigations should be undertaken. These should include endoscopy with biopsy, ultrasonography and CT imaging of the abdomen and chest. There have been advances in endoscopic ultrasound that have allowed improvements in local staging of gastric tumours. These improvements are such that mucosal invasion can be distinguished from submucosal invasion. Twenty years ago, the vast majority of patients with gastric cancer presented with inoperable disease. Currently, approximately 50% of tumours are operable at the time of presentation although only 20% are curative resections.

Staging and pathology

The TNM staging system is widely used for staging gastric cancer, with the 'p' prefix denoting pathological confirmation of the staging. Ninety-five percent of all gastric tumours are adenocarcinomas. The remainder are squamous cell cancers and lymphomas. Small cell cancers are reported only rarely.

Treatment

Surgery

The only significant chance for a cure rests with surgery. Laparoscopic staging is carried out prior to definitive laparotomy. There is considerable debate concerning the operative procedures of first choice. Older retrospective data suggested that survival was improved with total gastrectomy compared with subtotal gastrectomy. Randomized trials, however, have since shown equivalent survival, with lesser complications for subtotal gastrectomy for carcinoma of the antrum, compared with total gastrectomy. One recent randomized study showed equal five-year survival of patients with either subtotal or total gastrectomy with lymphadenectomy. The operative mortality in the UK varies from 5% to 14% and is related to the number of these operations performed by the surgeon. Surgical developments have been led by the Japanese, who have to deal with the highest incidence of carcinoma of the stomach in the world. The current recommendation by the Japanese Society for Research in Gastric Cancer is for extensive lymphadenectomy, which involves the removal of the lymphatic chains along the coeliac axis and hepatic and splenic arteries. This sort of dissection also has the advantage of allowing more accurate staging for gastric cancer and has been associated with improved survival. For early-stage disease, advances in endoscopic techniques have led to curative mucosal resection techniques equivalent to subtotal gastrectomy, with clear evidence of reduced morbidity. Tumours of the gastro-oesophageal junction are increasing in the West and are treated surgically by subtotal resection of the oesophagus, along with the cardia and gastric fundus.

Adjuvant treatment

In 30 years of adjuvant therapy investigation, no significant role for adjuvant radiation or chemotherapy had been found. Despite this, active trial work continued with the hope of improving prognosis and recent trials have shown a benefit to adjuvant treatment. These benefits continue to be debated. However, neoadjuvant chemotherapy prior to surgery using ECF (epirubicin, cisplatin and infusional 5-fluorouracil (5FU)) or ECX (epirubicin, cisplatin, capecitabine) has been found to improve survival in patients with operable gastric cancer.

Treatment of metastatic or locally inoperable gastric cancer

Patients with inoperable local disease or metastases may be treated with chemotherapy. Over the years, many treatment programmes have been introduced, and the majority have contained 5FU. There is uncertainty as to whether or not combination therapy offers benefit. The response rates are higher but overall survival is similar for combination chemotherapy compared with single-agent 5FU treatment. In the 1970s, there was considerable enthusiasm following the introduction of a combination therapy containing 5FU, adriamycin (doxorubicin) and mitomycin C. This treatment schedule, known as the 'FAM regimen', was initially reported as leading to responses in 40% of patients, with a median duration of response of approximately nine months. Randomized trials have since shown that the same order of response can be obtained with single-agent 5FU, with the same expectations of survival. In recent times, there has been considerable support for combination chemotherapy using epirubicin and cisplatin with either continuous infusion 5FU (ECF) or its oral prodrug capecitabine (ECX). Initially, a 70% response rate was reported, and the median survival of patients responding was seven months. The programme is well tolerated and offers patients reasonable quality of life.

Survival

In the West, more than two-thirds of patients present with advanced tumours. The median survival of patients with advanced local disease or metastatic tumour is approximately six months.

Improving survival in gastric cancer

Patients with early gastric cancer have very good chances of survival, which can be in excess of 90%. For early-stage disease, surgery can be minimal, with advances in endoscopy, endoscopic ultrasonography and endoscopic surgery providing great improvements in limiting the morbidity of interventional therapies. Significant improvements have been seen in Japan as a result of the widescale implementation of screening endoscopy. In Japan, up to 40% of patients are found to have early-stage tumours, which contrasts with the situation in the West. One can only conclude that more widespread availability of endoscopic screening and earlier referral by GPs remains the only significant chance for improved survival. The development of effective therapies based upon any understanding of the biological basis of this tumour group seems to be a distant possibility at this point.

Chapter 10

Hepatobiliary cancer

Epidemiology and pathogenesis

Hepatobiliary cancer is the sixth most common malignant tumour in the world. The highest incidences are seen in South East Asia. In the United Kingdom, hepatobiliary cancer is relatively uncommon. There are approximately 3200 men and women registered with the condition each year, and sadly 3200 deaths. Generally, there are more women than men affected by these tumours. Liver cancer is divided into four main groups of tumour: hepatocellular cancer, which accounts for 75% of this group, and is more common in men than women; biliary tree cancers, also known as cholangiocarcinomas, which account for over 25%; and the rare hepatoblastomas and angiosarcomas which account for 1–2% of all liver cancers.

Hepatocellular cancer is associated with chronic infection with hepatitis B virus (HBV) infection. This is prevalent in up to 15% of males in certain populations. The lifetime risk of developing a tumour is 40% in this group of men. An epidemiological study of 22 707 Taiwanese male government employees followed over 10 years found that the relative risk of liver cancer was 98 for men with HBV. To put this risk into context, the relative risk for lung cancer amongst smokers is around 17. How HBV causes liver cancer is uncertain. The HBV

genome does include a weak oncogene HBX. However, since the greatest risk is amongst those with chronic infection it is thought that the constant proliferation of hepatocytes caused by the need to replace virus-damaged cells and the chronic inflammatory response in the liver are the main culprits. Support for this hypothesis also comes from hepatitis C virus (HCV) induced liver cancer. HBV and HCV are very different viruses genetically but both cause similar chronic infection and inflammation of the liver and both are associated with a high risk of liver cancer. In terms of the model for chemical carcinogenesis these viruses appear to act as tumour promoters rather than initiators. This is supported by synergism in risk between chronic HBV infection and mutagens such as aflatoxin B1. Aflatoxin B1 is derived from *Aspergillus fumigatus* which commonly infects foods such as peanuts that are stored in damp conditions and which causes mutation of p53. In one study from China the relative risk of liver cancer in people with HBV was 7, in those exposed to aflatoxin was 3, but in those exposed to both HBV and aflatoxin was 60. Hepatocellular cancers are also associated with alcoholism and other hepatitides causing cirrhosis such as haemochromatosis and acute and chronic hepatic porphyrias (acute intermittent porphyria, porphyria cutanea tarda, hereditary coproporphyria and variagate porphyria).

There is great interest in the role of the hepatitis-causing viruses in the aetiology of hepatocellular

Lecture Notes: Oncology, 2nd edition. By M. Bower and J. Waxman. Published 2010 by Blackwell Publishing Ltd.

cancer, and this is for three reasons. Firstly, a vaccine based on the surface antigen envelope protein of HBV (HBVsAg) protects against the acquisition of HBV. The widespread introduction f this vaccine in Taiwan has been shown to reduce the risk of hepatocellular cancer in children and a similar protection in adults is likely. Secondly, antiviral therapy against hepatitis B that is effective at lowering HBV titres may reduce the risk of liver cancer amongst people with chronic HBV. Similarly interferon-based therapy for chronic HCV may also reduce the risk of hepatocellular cancer in chronically infected individuals. Finally, screening people with chronic HCV and HBV may reduce the mortality of liver cancer by diagnosing patients earlier with surgically resectable disease. Liver ultrasound and serum α-fetoprotein (AFP) screening should be performed every six months in patients with chronic HBV or HCV. There are significant concerns with regard to the increasing infection rates with hepatitis C in Europe. It is thought that the risk of developing hepatobiliary cancer in the presence of chronic hepatitis C infection is even greater than that associated with hepatitis B infection.

The aetiology of hepatoblastoma is not known. Hepatic angiosarcoma is associated with exposure to polyvinyl choride (PVC) monomer. The mechanism for this is not clear, and the development of this tumour does not always occur in those men and women who have the heaviest exposure to PVC, as for example in those workers involved in autoclave cleaning in chemical works. When workers exposed to PVC are examined for their lifetime risk of developing angiosarcoma this is overall clearly four times higher than in the general population. Where there is a coincident HBV infection, the risk increases 25-fold compared with the general population. PVC exposure is also associated with the development of brain and lung tumours.

Tumours of the biliary tree are divided into intrahepatic bile duct cancers (which are treated in the same way as hepatocellular cancers), perihilar cholangiocarcinomas (also known as Klatskin tumours) that occur at the bifurcation of the left and right hepatic ducts, and extrahepatic cholangiocarcinomas and gall-bladder cancers (Figures 10.1 and 10.2). They are seen at increased frequency in patients with ulcerative colitis and primary sclerosing cholangitis. In South East Asia, where these tumours are common, they are seen in association with biliary infestation with liver flukes (Clonorchis sinensis and Opisthorchis viverrini).

Presentation

Patients with hepatobiliary cancer generally present with advanced disease. Typical presentations are with jaundice, liver pain and weight loss.

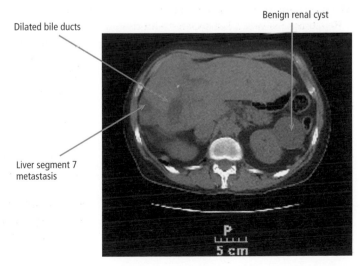

Dilated bile ducts

Benign renal cyst

Liver segment 7 metastasis

Figure 10.1 CT scan demonstrating intrahepatic dilated bile ducts that were due to cholangiocarcinoma. There is also a low attenuation metastasis in segment 7 of the liver and an incidental (benign) renal cyst.

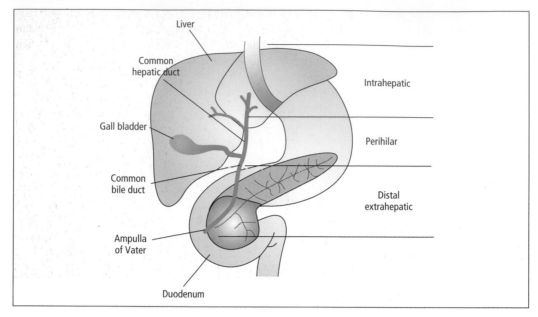

Figure 10.2 Anatomy of biliary tract cancers.

A patient with a suspected diagnosis of hepatobiliary cancer should be referred to the appropriate surgical unit for investigation. The management of these conditions is very complex and should only be in centres of excellence with highly specialized surgical units, who achieve significantly better results.

Standard investigations for patients with hepatocellular cancer should include blood counts, liver function tests, renal function tests, chest X-rays, ultrasound assessment and CT imaging. Ultrasonography has developed considerably over the last decade, and these technical improvements have been matched by improved standards in endoscopic assessment of the patient. Hepatobiliary cancers are associated with raised serum levels of AFP, which is characteristically raised to many thousands of ng/ml. In patients with cirrhosis, who may have AFP levels raised to a few hundreds of ng/ml, increasing levels are clues to the development of hepatobiliary cancer. CEA and CA199 are useful markers in the monitoring of hepatobiliary tumours.

Characteristically, patients with these tumours will commonly present with jaundice, and this presentation requires external stenting to stabilize the patient, enable investigations to take place and surgery to be considered. After staging, histological confirmation of the presence of a tumour should be obtained by percutaneous endoscopic retrograde cholangiopancreatography (ERCP) with needle aspiration or brush cytology or by liver biopsy.

Staging and grading

Hepatobiliary tumours are described as well, moderately or poorly differentiated. Staging for hepatic and billiary tract tumours is according to the TNM classification.

Treatment

Liver resection is the only treatment that offers a chance for cure for liver cancer. Surgery is limited by the degree of spread of the tumour and the presence or absence of background cirrhosis. The aim of surgery generally is to remove the lobe of the liver containing the tumour. It may be possible for patients with hepatobiliary cancer to be treated by

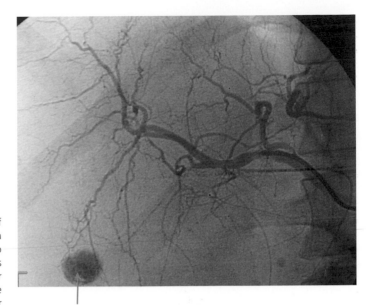

Figure 10.3 Selective angiography of the right hepatic artery showing a small area of hypervascularity due to hepatocellular carcinoma. As this was inoperable (there were four other lesions in different segments of the liver), it was treated by transcatheter arterial chemoembolization (TACE).

Hepatocellular carcinoma

liver transplantation and, if this is the case, the chance of survival increases dramatically. It is estimated that just 10% of patients with liver cancers have operable tumours. When curative-surgery is not possible, hepatic embolization, sclerotherapy and chemotherapy may be appropriate (Figure 10.3). Tumours of the biliary tree are chemosensitive and very, very rarely operable. Similar treatment programmes are used in this condition as in hepatocellular cancer. Major problems have come for patients as a result of obstruction of the biliary tree, and this is actively treated by percutaneous or endoscopic stenting. This leads to relief of obstruction and to a useful, though limited, extension of life. Tumour embolization is now a much more commonly used procedure. Transcatheter arterial chemoembolization is performed, where a mixture of chemotherapy, with radio-opaque contrast and an embolic agent, is injected into the right or left hepatic artery (see Figure 10.2). Other approaches include radiofrequency ablation, which uses high-frequency radiowaves to heat up and destroy tumours, using electrodes inserted into the tumour under image guidance. A third treatment for localized unresectable tumours is percutaneous ethanol injection.

Table 10.1 Five-year survival rates of patients with hepatic and biliary tract cancers.

Tumour	5-year survival
Hepatocellular cancer	5%
Gall bladder cancer	5%
Cholangiocarcinoma	5%
Periampullary cholangiocarcinoma	50%

Prognosis

Five-year survival for patients with operable liver cancer is in the order of 33% when management involves partial liver resection. The five-year survival of patients transplanted is 80%. The median survival of patients who are not treated with curative intent is six to seven months (Table 10.1). The median survival of patients in the Far East is much poorer, and the vast majority die within two to three months of diagnosis.

New treatment

We have great hope that mortality from liver tumours will decrease significantly in the next few years. The reason for this is the development of effective campaigns for vaccination against hepatitis B. However, there is considerable concern in Europe that the rising prevalence of hepatitis C, for which no vaccine is available, will lead to a rise in deaths from this condition.

There have been major changes over the last few years in our understanding of the molecular basis for hepatobiliary cancer, with the identification of cell surface receptors for VEGFR (vascular endothelial growth factor receptor) and EGFR (epidermal growth factor receptor). Treatments targeting these receptors and pioneered for patients with renal cell cancer have been found to be effective in hepatobiliary cancer. Responses are seen to sunitinib and sorafenib, but the use and value of these agents, though clear, has been, as ever, stymied by the action of the National Institute for Health and Clinical Excellence (NICE) in the UK. This action by NICE seems particularly bizarre in the context of a clear evidence base demonstrating a doubling of survival time with sorafenib in a large phase III clinical trial.

Chapter 11

Pancreatic cancer

Epidemiology and pathogenesis

Carcinoma of the pancreas has increased in incidence over the last decade. It is the tenth most common cancer, and is now the fifth most frequent cause of cancer deaths. There is an equal incidence between the sexes, and annually in the UK there are about 7700 deaths. It is very sad to note that registration figures virtually equal mortality rates. There is an increased risk of developing pancreatic cancer with age. In the 1980s it was suggested that excessive coffee consumption predisposed to the development of cancer of the pancreas, but this has subsequently been refuted. Smoking is also associated with an increased risk of this disease of between two- and five-fold. Diabetes, obesity and chronic pancreatitis all increase the risk of pancreatic cancer. Pancreatic exocrine cancers constitute well over 90% of all pancreatic malignancies and are adenocarcinomas. Pancreatic adenocarcinoma is believed to arise from ductal epithelial cells that progress through stages of pancreatic intraepithelial neoplasia with the sequential accumulation of somatic mutations in several genes including the oncogene K-RAS and the tumour suppressor genes P53, P16/CDKN2A and SMAD4/DPC4. Pancreatic adenocarcinoma cells

express a wide variety of receptors that are potential therapeutic targets including epidermal growth factor (EGF) receptors, vascular endothelial growth factor (VEGF) receptors and insulin-like growth factor (IGF) receptors. Pancreatic adenocarcinoma also expresses a wide variety of hormone receptors, and these include receptors for somatostatin, gonadotrophin-releasing hormone, steroid hormones, insulin-like growth factors and VEGFs. It should be emphasized that these receptors are present in carcinomas, and that they are not present in the unusual secretory endocrine pancreatic tumours. The rare endocrine tumours of the pancreas are known as islet cell tumours or nesidioblastomas and include gastrinomas, insulinomas and pancreatic carcinoids. These tumours may be functional or non-secretory.

Presentation

Patients with carcinoma of the pancreas present with many different symptoms. These include abdominal and back pain, weight loss, anorexia and fatigue. In many patients the disease is asymptomatic, until they present with obstructive jaundice. Other, less common presentations include superficial venous thrombosis (Trousseau's sign), a palpable gall bladder in the presence of obstructive jaundice (Courvoisier's law states that this is unlikely to be due to gall stones) and diabetes. Because of the anatomical position of the tumour,

Lecture Notes: Oncology, 2nd edition. By M. Bower and J. Waxman. Published 2010 by Blackwell Publishing Ltd.

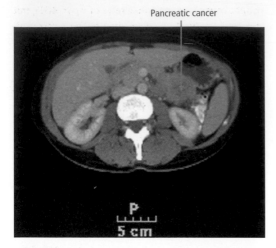

Pancreatic cancer

P
⌞⌞⌞⌞⌟
5 cm

Figure 11.1 CT scan of a mass in the tail and body of the pancreas showing a low attenuation centre suggesting central necrosis of an adenocarcinoma of the pancreas.

late presentation is very common. The patient with a suspected diagnosis of pancreatic cancer should be referred by his or her GP to a general surgeon or a gastroenterologist and be seen in outpatients within two weeks of receipt of the GP's letter of referral. The clinician should organize a number of tests, which include full blood count, renal and liver function tests, a chest X-ray and a CT scan of the abdomen (Figure 11.1). Abdominal ultrasonography is also helpful but endoscopic ultrasound (EUS) is probably the most valuable diagnostic test when coupled with percutaneous needle biopsy. The measurement of serum levels of the carbohydrate antigen tumour marker CA19-9 is less helpful in the diagnosis of cancer of the pancreas as it may be elevated in most causes of obstructive jaundice (false positive) and may be normal in patients with pancreatic cancer (false negative). CA19-9 is, however, useful in monitoring cancer of the pancreas in patients with raised levels at diagnosis.

Investigation of the patient with pancreatic cancer is aimed at establishing the diagnosis and defining operability. After the initial tests have been carried out, the patient should proceed to EUS or, if not available, endoscopic retrograde cholangiopancreatography (ERCP). At ERCP, cytology specimens may be obtained from brush-

ings, suction of the pancreatic duct or biopsy. ERCP is more invasive than other diagnostic imaging modalities and carries a significant complication rate so it is usually reserved for patients with biliary obstruction who require stenting. A failure to obtain a diagnosis by endoscopy should be followed by further investigation. Fine needle aspiration cytology under CT scan is usually successful at obtaining a tissue diagnosis.

Staging and grading

As with other cancers, numerous different staging systems are used including the TNM classification. The group staging system is summarized below:

- Stage I: cancer confined to the pancreas (T1N0M0 if <2 cm, T2N0M0 if >2 cm)
- Stage II: cancer has grown into the adjacent duodenum or bile duct but not spread to the lymph nodes (T3N0M0)
- Stage III: cancer has spread to the lymph nodes with (T3N1M0) or without (T1–2N1M0) direct tumour extension
- Stage IVA: cancer has invaded into the stomach, spleen, colon or nearby large blood vessels, and lymph nodes may (T4N1M0) or may not (T4N0M0) be involved
- Stage IVB: there is spread to distant organs by metastases (T1–4N0–1M1).

The vast majority of pancreatic cancers are exocrine adenocarcinomas of ductal origin and they are graded as either well, moderately or poorly differentiated tumours. The tiny minority of endocrine tumours are classified according to the products that they secrete.

Treatment

There is considerable nihilism attached, quite reasonably, to the treatment of a patient with pancreatic cancer. The initial management consists of relieving symptoms of pain and obstructive jaundice. For less than 20% of patients is there any hope for operability, as defined by imaging. No attempt should be made to proceed to surgery until the jaundice has completely resolved. Jaundice is dealt with by relief of biliary obstruction, either by endoscopic stenting or by percutaneous transhepatic stenting of the biliary system. Pain may be relieved by the use of opiates or may resolve with the relief of biliary obstruction. At laparotomy, just 30% of those 20% of patients with radiologically operable disease turns out to have surgically operable tumours.

Pancreatic surgery requires a considerable degree of specialization and should not be carried out outside of the setting of a specialist treatment centre. The reason for this is simple: specialist centres achieve better survival rates and lower morbidity and mortality rates. The operation of choice is Whipple's procedure, and this involves removal of the distal half of the stomach (antrectomy), gall bladder (cholecystectomy), distal common bile duct (choledochectomy), head of the pancreas, duodenum and proximal jejunum, and regional lymph nodes. Reconstruction consists of attaching the pancreas to the jejunum (pancreaticojejunostomy), the common bile duct to the jejunum (choledochojejunostomy), and the stomach to the jejunum (gastrojejunostomy), to allow bile, digestive juices and food to flow! There are modifications of this procedure, such as the pylorus-conserving pancreaticoduodenectomy, that are associated with less postoperative morbidity and equivalent efficacy.

Thirty years ago, surgery for pancreatic cancer was associated with a very high morbidity of approximately 25%. This has fallen in specialist centres to 5%, with the expectation that 20% of patients with operable disease will survive five years. Ampullary carcinomas of the pancreas generally present with early-stage disease because of their anatomical position. These tumours are associated with better prognoses than cancers of the rest of the pancreas. There is no role whatsoever for adjuvant chemotherapy or radiotherapy.

Treatment of inoperable disease

Patients with inoperable pancreatic cancer have a poor prognosis and the treatment of this condition is palliative. The median survival is four to six months. Active treatment with chemotherapy may be advised. The most successful chemotherapy programmes have response rates of up to 40%, but the median duration of survival of these responding patients is just one month longer than might be expected without active treatment. Because pancreatic cancer is relatively common, a number of chemotherapy agents have been tried for this condition. The consensus view is that combination therapy using the more active agents, such as anthracyclines and taxanes, offers little benefit. The more drugs that are combined, the more toxicity, without an improvement in survival. The current consensus view is that single-agent gemcitabine probably offers as good an opportunity for disease palliation as does any combination regimen, although in practice it is often combined with cisplatin. Gemcitabine is easy to administer and has little toxicity. Quality of life issues are paramount in this condition because of the poor prognosis for inoperable disease.

An alternative approach to the management of pancreatic cancer is to treat symptoms. This is managed by stenting to relieve jaundice and by coeliac axis block. This procedure blocks the pain fibres originating from the pancreas and ensures good quality of life. The technique requires skill and is relatively well tolerated.

Prognosis

The outlook for patients with operable pancreatic cancer is unfortunately not particularly good, with a 20% chance of five-year survival. The outlook for those patients with locally advanced or metastatic disease is very poor, with a median survival of three to four months. It is for this reason that there is such an emphasis upon quality of life in pancreatic cancer, rather than on the prospects for cure.

New treatment

The expression by pancreatic cancer cells of numerous receptors and the poor results with systemic chemotherapy has led to strategies targeting these receptors. Epidermal growth factor receptor inhibitors including the protein kinase inhibitor erlotinib and the monoclonal antibody cetuximab have been studied with limited success. The VEGF pathway has also been targeted with the anti-VEGF monoclonal antibody bevacizumab and receptor tyrosine kinase inhibitors of VEGF receptors including sorafenib. Again the results have disappointed. The IGF pathway that is activated in pancreatic and other cancers is a novel target for therapeutic strategies and monoclonal antibodies targeting both the ligand (IGF1 and IGF2) and the receptor (IGF receptor 1, IGFR1) are under investigation along with receptor tyrosine kinase inhibitors of IGFR1.

The transfer of suicide genes to tumour cells by retroviral vectors has also been applied in pancreatic cancer cell lines. This approach is known as gene-directed enzyme prodrug therapy (GDEPT). The adenovirus vector that was used carried the herpes simplex virus thymidine kinase gene that phosphorylates the prodrug ganciclovir into deox-

yGTP that is incorporated into replicating DNA causing strand termination. This GDEPT strategy inhibited gene expression and cell growth of pancreatic cancer cell lines. The technique has been extensively modified with different viral vectors as well as different enzyme and prodrug combinations.

Pancreatic endocrine tumours

This is a fascinating group of tumours, interesting not only because of their biology, but also because patients with these tumours are expected to do well. Pancreatic endocrine tumours include carcinoids, insulinomas, glucagonomas, gastrinomas and Vipomas. The bizarre constellation of symptoms produced by carcinoids are well known even to medical students, as are the gastrointestinal

Table 11.1 Cinical manifestations of secretory endocrine tumours.

Tumour	Major feature	Minor feature	Common sites	Percentage malignant	MEN associated
Insulinoma	Neuroglycopenia (confusion, fits)	Permanent neurological deficits	Pancreas (β-cells)	10%	10%
Gastrinoma (Zollinger–Elison syndrome)	Peptic ulceration	Diarrhoea, weight loss, malabsorption, dumping	Pancreas Duodenum	40–60%	25%
Vipoma (Werner–Morrison syndrome)	Watery diarrhoea, hypokalaemia, achlorhydria	Hypercalcaemia, hyperglycaemia, hypomagnesaemia	Pancreas, neuroblastoma, SCLC, phaeochromocytoma	40%	<5%
Glucagonoma	Migratory necrolyic erythema, mild diabetes mellitus, muscle wasting, anaemia	Diarrhoea, thromboembolism stomatitis, hypoaminoacidaemia, encephalitis	Pancreas (α-cells)	60%	<5%
Somatostatinoma	Diabetes mellitus, cholelithiasis, steatorrhoea, malabsorption	Anaemia, diarrhea, weight loss, hypoglycaemia	Pancreas (β-cells)	66%	Case reports only

MEN, multiple endocrine neoplasia; SCLC, small cell lung cancer.

symptoms resulting from Vipomas, and the hypo- and hyperglycaemia from insulinomas and glucagonomas respectively (Table 11.1). Old school general physicians will expect that every medical student reading this book will be able to recount the ten skin conditions associated with carcinoid tumours, as well as describe the reasons for the effects of this tumour on the heart. They will take delight in quizzing you on their ward rounds so we suggest that you google them if there is an inpatient with carcinoid on your ward.

These endocrine malignancies are associated with enormously long natural histories, which may date back over decades.

The major treatment options for pancreatic endocrine tumours include octreotide to decrease hormonal secretion, and chemoembolization to reduce the symptoms that result from tumour bulk. Octreotide is an octapeptide mimic of somatostatin that inhibits the secretion of a whole host of peptide hormones including gastrin, glucagon, growth hormone, insulin, pancreatic polypeptide (PP) and vasoactive intestinal polypeptide (VIP). Octreotide also reduces pancreatic and intestinal fluid secretion, hence its use in the management of malignant bowel obstruction. Octreotide has a median period of effect of one year in carcinoids, but leads to no clinical evidence of disease regression. Interferon may also lead to a reduction in secretory symptoms of carcinoid tumours. Where symptoms are significant and octreotide has failed, embolization is considered, both to the primary site and to hepatic metastases. Embolization is a significant enterprise and is associated in even the best centres with mortality rates of 3–5%. It should therefore be considered with great care before it is undertaken.

There has been considerable debate as to whether or not interferon causes a reduction in tumour mass. The balance of the evidence is in favour of interferon having a minor effect in reducing tumour bulk.

Chapter 12

Colorectal cancer

Epidemiology and pathogenesis

Colorectal cancer is a major cause of morbidity in the West. Each year in the UK approximately 37 500 people are diagnosed with colorectal cancer and 16 000 die of the disease. The incidence has risen modestly over the last quarter of a century and the five-year overall survival has doubled over the same time interval. In the 1960s and 1970s, there was increasing recognition of the possibility of a dietary basis to colorectal cancer. The disease was thought to be uncommon in the developing world, whilst the high red meat and low fibre diet and obesity in the more developed market economies were seen to be responsible for a higher incidence of colorectal cancer. Certainly the EPIC (European Prospective Investigation into Cancer and Nutrition) study revealed a 55% increase in risk for each 100 g/day increase in red meat consumption. This risk with red meat is supported by three meta-analyses that revealed significant, although smaller, risks. High fibre diets increase the transit time of the stool and decrease the colorectal epithelial exposure to carcinogens within the stool. The EPIC study also demonstrated a modest 20% reduction (mainly of left-sided colon cancers) in risk amongst the highest fibre eaters. However, this association has not been confirmed in meta-analyses despite the constant advise to eat five fruits (or vegetables) a day. Nevertheless, the authors suggest that you do not tell young children this information as the reactions of their mothers is wholly unpredictable. Aspirin has been shown to have a protective effect against colorectal cancer, and epidemiological studies of prolonged aspirin use have shown a consistent reduction of up to 50% in the risk of colorectal cancers. This decrease in risk is thought to be due to the inhibitory effect of aspirin on cyclooxygenase-2, which is an enzyme found in high concentrations in colorectal tissue and promotes the growth of polyps. In randomized studies, aspirin has been shown to reduce the incidence of adenomatous polyps in patients screened after the excision of a primary colorectal tumour. There has, however, only been one single randomized trial of aspirin prophylaxis, which has shown no evidence for a reduction in colorectal cancer incidence and the toxicity, especially the risk of gastrointestinal haemorrhage, means that it is premature to recommend aspirin as chemoprevention. Patients with both Crohn's disease and ulcerative colitis are at risk from developing colonic tumours, and this risk rises to nearly 40% after 20 years follow-up.

Up to 20% of patients with colorectal cancer have a family history of colorectal cancer. There are two significant familial causes for colorectal cancer: familial adenomatous polyposis (FAP) and hereditary non-polyposis colorectal cancer (HNPCC). FAP is an autosomal dominant condi-

Lecture Notes: Oncology, 2nd edition. By M. Bower and J. Waxman. Published 2010 by Blackwell Publishing Ltd.

tion that accounts for 1% of all colorectal cancer. The gene for FAP was mapped to chromosome 5q21 in 1987 and the responsible gene APC was cloned in 1991. All patients with FAP develop colorectal cancer by the age of 40 years, so prophylactic colectomy is offered to teenagers with FAP. HNPCC, or Lynch syndrome, is responsible for 2–5% of colorectal cancers. HNPPC is characterized by colorectal cancers occurring at an early age and they are often sited in the right side of the colon. In addition, HNPCC is associated with endometrial carcinoma, and gastric, renal, ureteric and central nervous system malignancies. In this condition, the genetic abnormalities include microsatellite instability and mutated mismatch-repair genes (most frequently hMSH2 and hMLH1). In the vast majority of non-inherited colorectal malignancy, the molecular changes consist of a sequential accumulation of mutations in genes including p53, and deletion of the colorectal gene (DCC), K-Ras and APC.

Presentation

Patients with colorectal tumours present to their general practitioners with a history of altered bowel habit and rectal bleeding. This may also be accompanied by weight loss and abdominal pains.

These symptoms are suggestive of malignancy, and accordingly an urgent referral should be made to a specialist bowel surgeon. The patient should be seen within two weeks of receipt of the general practitioner's referral letter.

Outpatient diagnosis

In outpatients, the surgeon should take a full history from the patient and examine him or her. This should include a rectal examination, which may show the patient to have melaena. Proctoscopy and sigmoidoscopy should be performed in the outpatient setting. Blood tests should be organized, which should include a full blood count, renal function and liver function tests. A chest X-ray should be carried out and a barium enema or colonoscopy arranged as an outpatient procedure. The barium enema may show narrowing of the colon. In malignancy, this narrowing is typical and has the appearance of an apple core (Figure 12.1). Endoscopy may show a stenosing lesion or a polyp. Biopsies should be taken of the suspicious area.

Staging and grading

The tumour should be examined histologically. It is described as being either well, moderately or

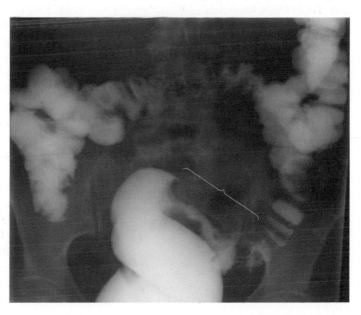

Figure 12.1 Barium enema investigation showing irregular stricture of the sigmoid colon with shouldering giving an apple core appearance typical of sigmoid colon cancer.

Table 12.1 TNM staging of colorectal cancer.

T stage (primary tumour)	N stage (nodal status)	M stage (metastatic status)
T0 No evidence of primary tumour	N0 No nodes	M0 No distant metastases
T1 Tumour invades submucosa	N1 Metastasis in 1–3 pericolic nodes	M1 Distant metastases
T2 Tumour invades muscularis	N2 Metastasis in 4 or more pericolic nodes	
T3 Tumour invades through the muscularis	N3 Metastasis in any lymph node	
T4 Tumour perforates the peritoneum		

poorly differentiated. The original staging system for colorectal cancer was reported by Cuthbert Esquire Dukes, a British pathologist, in 1932. With various modifications this system is still in use today. A Dukes' stage is given, and this reflects the degree of invasion of the tumour. Dukes' stage A is specified when a tumour is confined to the mucosa. Dukes' stage B is a tumour that perforates the serosa, and Dukes' stage C is given when lymph nodes are affected. Tumours of the colon are, furthermore, divided according to their anatomical sub-sites. These are the appendix, caecum, ascending colon, hepatic flexure, transverse colon, splenic flexure, descending colon and sigmoid colon. Finally, the tumour can be staged according to the TNM clinical classification system (Table 12.1).

Treatment

The suspicion of malignancy having been raised, the patient should be worked up for surgery including an assessment of operability by CT scanning. The CT scan will show whether or not there are enlarged lymph nodes within the abdomen and will define the possibility of further spread involving the liver. If there is no gross evidence of dissemination, the patient should be admitted to hospital for colectomy or an abdominoperitoneal resection. Removal of the primary is still considered in the presence of metastatic disease, to reduce the risk of perforation or obstruction.

The surgical plan depends upon the experience and practice of the clinician. There have been considerable developments in the area of laparoscopic surgery. If the patient is therefore considered to be an appropriate candidate, a laparoscopic colectomy might be performed. The results of rectal surgery are critically surgeon dependent, and much better results are obtained in centres where the surgeon specializes in this procedure.

Surgery for colonic cancer

At operation, a midline incision should be performed and the abdominal contents inspected. The tumour should be mobilized and removed together with a good margin of normal tissue. The tumour should be inspected and frozen sections performed, to ensure that the resection edges of the apparently normal gut contain no tumour. An end-to-end anastomosis is then made. If the patient is found to have three to five liver metastases at operation, these should be resected at an appropriate time, as successful resection is associated with a good prognosis and the possibility of cure. If there are more metastases, no operative action should be taken. Extensive resection of the lymph nodes should be performed, providing histopathological information which affects the patient's management.

Surgery for rectal cancers

The surgery that is performed depends upon the site of the carcinoma and a preoperative assessment of operability. Tumours of the upper and middle third of the rectum are treated by anterior resection. In this procedure, the rectum is mobilized from the sacral hollow, and the tumour is removed together with an adequate margin of normal tissue. This normal margin ranges between

2 and 5 cm. The mesorectum and lateral pararectal tissue should be removed. Lesions of the lower third of the rectum are treated by abdominoperineal resection, which requires a permanent colostomy. The rectum is mobilized, and the peritoneum at the base of the bladder or posterior vagina is incised. The lateral ligaments are divided and the anus excised. The quality of surgery in rectal cancer is critically important. Extensive lymphadenectomy is associated with significantly improved chances for survival.

Complications of surgery

A neurogenic bladder is very common after pelvic surgery but will usually recover within 10 days. Ureteric tears or transections may complicate surgery, but only rarely so. Sexual dysfunction in males is inevitable, and the most common problems are retrograde ejaculation and erectile impotence. Change in sexual function in women has not been assessed. Surgery is complicated by a mortality rate of 1–2%.

Adjuvant treatment for colonic cancer

Following recovery from surgery, no additional treatment is recommended for patients with Dukes' stage A disease. The value of adjuvant chemotherapy for Dukes' B disease remains controversial. This is because no major advantage has been shown for adjuvant chemotherapy within this group of patients. Patients with Dukes' C tumours, however, should receive adjuvant chemotherapy. The reason for this is that there is a survival advantage in this group of patients. Treatment should be with a 5-fluorouracil (5FU)-containing programme. There is considerable contention as to which is the optimal treatment schedule. In the late 1980s and early 1990s, the use of levamisole was prevalent, but treatment with this agent is no longer recommended. At present we have a plethora of agents that are active in metastatic colorectal cancer. The current problem is to know which agent or combination of agents are the most effective in prolonging survival in the adjuvant setting. The active agents, oxaliplatin, capecitabine, iri-

notecan and bevacizumab, which are all of benefit in this disease, may be considered with or without a 5FU and folinic acid-containing adjuvant treatment programme. Current recommendations are for treatment with 5FU, which may be administered intravenously, or as the oral analogue of 5FU, capecitabine. The patient might also be offered an oral combination chemotherapy regimen with the acronym UFT, containing tegafur and uracil. Treatment may be given in combination with folinic acid and irinotecan in the FOLFIRI regimen, or with folinic acid and oxaliplatin in the FOLFOX regimen.

Adjuvant treatment for rectal cancer

Patients with rectal cancer may receive preoperative radiotherapy. This has been shown to limit pelvic recurrence. It is disputed whether adjuvant radiotherapy improves survival. Alternatively, after the patient has recovered from surgery, he or she may receive pelvic radiotherapy. This has been shown in randomized studies to decrease the risk of pelvic recurrence by 5–10%. Patients with more advanced tumours (T3 and T4) may be treated with adjuvant chemoradiotherapy prior to surgery, in addition to radiotherapy. There is increased postoperative morbidity with chemotherapy given in conjunction with radiotherapy.

Management of metastatic disease

In the situation where there are limited metastases from colorectal cancer, consideration is given to the possibility of curative surgical treatment. If the patient is fit, and there are three to five hepatic metastases or less than three pulmonary metastases, resection may be considered to be appropriate. If surgery is successful, then the prognosis is relatively good, with survival chances ranging up to 40% at five years.

Generally, however, metastatic colorectal carcinoma has a poor prognosis, and the current recommendation for appropriate treatment is with 5FU-based regimens and radiotherapy. There is debate as to whether or not the addition of folinic acid is of an advantage to the patient. The current consensus is that there is a benefit at least in terms of remission rates, although no consensus has been reached regarding survival. The treatment regimen of first choice was called the 'De Gramont regimen' and includes fortnightly 5FU and folinic acid given for six months. A host of new treatments have recently become available for patients with colorectal cancer. The most commonly used chemotherapy regimens are FOLFOX and FOLFIRI. The addition of irinotecan and oxaliplatin to 5FU in these regimens has improved median survival from 9 to 18 months. Recently the addition of bevacizumab, a humanized monoclonal antibody against vascular endothelial growth factor (VEGF), to both the FOLFOX and FOLFIRI regimens has led to a further modest improvement in survival. Cetuximab, a partially humanized monoclonal antibody against the epidermal growth factor receptor (EGFR), and panitumumab, a fully humanized antibody against EGFR, have both been shown to prolong survival in patients with metastatic colon cancer that lack mutations in K-Ras. As a result of the use of these agents, survival in metastatic colorectal cancer has been extended from 18 months to almost 2 years. In this context, the cost of treatment becomes a significant political issue but, amongst the discussion on the politics of cancer care, little attention seems to be paid to the cost of not treating the patient. Dying from metastatic colorectal cancer without drug treatment is an expensive process, and the authors of this chapter are not merely considering financial cost when we make this statement.

Screening

It is estimated that there may be a genetic predisposition to colorectal cancer in more than 20% of patients with these tumours. In the vast majority of colorectal cases there is, however, at present no direct evidence of there being a genetic risk. Patients with a risk of developing colorectal tumours can be stratified as having low, low–moderate, moderate, moderate–high or high risk of developing malignancy. The criteria for proceeding to screening for these patients are defined as in Table 12.2.

Table 12.2 Screening scheme for colorectal cancer.

Risk	Action	Age
Low risk		
1 relative >45 years *or*	Reassure: no colonoscopy	
2 relatives >70 years		
Low–moderate risk		
2 first-degree relatives, average age 60–70 years	Single colonoscopy	Aged 55 years
Moderate risk		
2 first-degree relatives, average age 50–60 years	5-yearly colonoscopy	Aged 35–65 years or starting
1 first-degree relative <45 years		5 years before age when youngest relative's tumour was diagnosed
Moderate–high risk		
2 first-degree relatives, average age <50 years	3–5-yearly colonoscopy	Begin age 30–35; refer to genetics
3 close relatives (not AC)		
High risk		
3 close relatives AC +ve (HNPCC)	2-yearly colonoscopy	Age 25–65; refer to genetics
(FAP)	Annual sigmoidoscopy from teens	and counselling

AC, Amsterdam criteria; FAP, familial adenomatous polyposis; HNPCC, hereditary non-polyposis colorectal cancer.

In 2006, bowel cancer screening using faecal occult blood (FOB) tests was introduced in England. It is estimated that if the uptake of FOB testing reaches 60% by the year 2026, 20 000 deaths from bowel cancer will be prevented. For every 1000 faecal occult blood tests completed, 20 will be abnormal and 16 patients will proceed to a colonoscopy, six of these will have polyps, two will have cancer, and eight a normal colonoscopy. The cost estimate equation for FOB testing is £1000 for each life-year saved. FOB testing will miss tumours and lead to a number of false positive findings. Colonoscopy is a more accurate means of detecting cancers but requires full bowel preparation, seda-tion and carries a risk of perforation (around one in 1500). Although the costs of colonoscopy for screening normal populations is, unfortunately, not economic, it is the investigation of choice for high-risk populations (Table 12.2).

New treatment

This is one group of tumours where we are delighted to report that a host of golden opportunities for our patients have arisen. The development of drugs targeting angiogenesis such as bevacuvimab and the EGFRs such as cetuximab have led to real improvements is survival.

Chapter 13

Genitourinary cancers

The treatment of testicular cancer is one of the few solid cancers in adults that may be successfully cured even in the presence of metastases. This has only been achievable in the last 40 years, since the introduction of cisplatin chemotherapy. Cisplatin was discovered serendipitously by Barnett Rosenberg, a physicist at Michigan State University, in 1965. He studied the effects of electric currents on *Escherichia coli* using platinum electrodes in a water bath and found that they stopped dividing but not growing, leading to bacteria up to 300 times longer than normal. This was found to be due to cisplatin, a product from the platinum electrodes, which was interfering with DNA replication. Following this, Professor Sir Alexander Haddow, the then head of the Chester Beatty Institute in London, showed that cisplatin was active against melanoma in mice, and clinical trials with human patients began in 1972.

The genitourinary tract is one of the most frequent sites of cancer in men and includes prostate cancer, which has emerged as the most common tumour in men (excluding non-melanomatous skin cancers). Table 13.1 shows the registration data for these tumours for southeast England in 2001 and the five-year survivals.

Cancer of the genitourinary tract includes cancers of the kidneys, bladder, prostate and testes, which are discussed in more detail in the next four chapters.

Table 13.1 Genitourinary cancer registration data for the UK and five-year survival rates.

Tumour	Percentage of registrations		Rank of registrations		Lifetime risk of cancer		Change in ASR, 1997–2006	5-year survival
	Male	Female	Male	Female	Male	Female		
Prostate	25%	–	1st	–	1 in 14	–	+37%	61%
Testis	2%	–	17th	–	1 in 210	–	+5%	96%
Kidney	3%	2%	9th	11th	1 in 89	1 in 162	+12%	44%
Bladder	5%	2%	4th	12th	1 in 30	1 in 79	–30%	66%

ASR, age-standardized rate.

Lecture Notes: Oncology, 2nd edition. By M. Bower and J. Waxman. Published 2010 by Blackwell Publishing Ltd.

Chapter 14

Kidney cancer

Epidemiology and pathogenesis

Renal carcinoma is not a particularly common cancer and causes approximately 3% of deaths from malignancy in the UK. In 2006 about 7840 people developed renal cancers in the UK per year and there were approximately 3700 deaths. Renal cancers may arise from the kidney nephrons or from the collecting systems. The histology is different for these two tumours and is described, respectively, as 'renal cell' for tumours arising from the nephrons and 'transitional cell' for tumours arising from the transitional cell epithelium of the collecting system. There is evidence for a genetic predisposition to this disease in a small percentage of patients. Renal cell cancer has an increased incidence in patients with von Hippel–Lindau disease and tuberous sclerosis. Transitional cell tumours may be caused by tobacco.

There has been increasing interest in the molecular genetics of renal cell cancer. This is concentrated around the importance of the loss of heterozygosity at chromosome 3p and the inactivation of the von Hippel–Lindau gene. Both are associated with the development of renal cell cancers. In one recent study there was loss of heterozygosity around chromosome 3p in 96% of conventional histology renal cell cancers, although in tumours with less common pathologies, such as the papillary and chromophobe variants, these changes are far less frequent. It is therefore likely that the loss of heterozygosity represents the loss of a specific tumour suppressor gene for renal cell cancer, and this fits in with conventional models for the development of malignancy. There are chromosomal changes in non-clear cell tumours too. The PTEN/MMAC1 tumour suppressor gene is lost in up to 90% of patients with chromophobe renal cell carcinoma, and so the molecular pathology of renal cell cancer defines a specific phenotype. Other changes have also been noted, involving chromosome 16q and 14q. A stepwise progression of molecular changes similar to those that are well described in colorectal tumours seems to characterize renal cell cancer. These molecular changes are completely different from those seen in papillary tumours, which are characterized by loss of the Y chromosome and multiple trisomy. In clear cell renal cancer, 3p loss leads to inactivation of hypoxia-inducible factors. This in turn leads to activation of vascular endothelial growth factor (VEGFR) and epidermal growth factor receptor (EGFR), with resultant new vessel formation and tumour development. VEGFR and EGFR upregulation are features of renal cell cancer that have been exploited for treatment, and this will be discussed in more detail below.

Lecture Notes: Oncology, 2nd edition. By M. Bower and J. Waxman. Published 2010 by Blackwell Publishing Ltd.

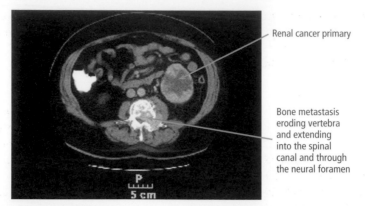

Renal cancer primary

Bone metastasis
eroding vertebra
and extending
into the spinal
canal and through
the neural foramen

Figure 14.1 Renal cancer. This CT scan shows a left renal inferior pole mass. In addition there is erosion of the vertebral body and posterior elements of the third lumbar vertebra. This is associated with extension into the spinal canal causing cauda equine compression and through the neural foramen into the psoas muscle.

Presentation

Patients with renal cancers commonly present with pain in the loins or blood in the urine. Other symptoms include joint pains, symptoms due to anaemia, a varicocele, generalized symptoms of malignancy, such as weight loss and cachexia, and symptoms due to a spread of the disease to metastatic sites such as brain, lung or bone. If a diagnosis of renal carcinoma is suspected, the patient should be referred to a urologist. Renal cell cancers are characteristically associated with paraneoplastic syndromes, which include polycythemia and pyrexia of unknown origin.

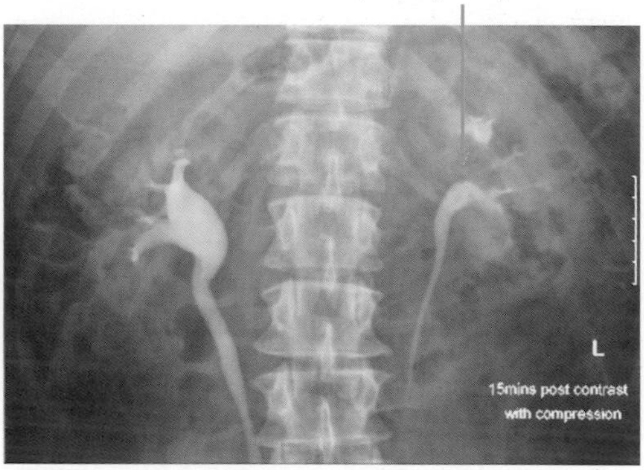

Outpatient diagnosis

The urologist will assess the patient in the outpatient clinic, taking a full medical history and examining the patient. Investigations to be organized will include full blood count, liver and renal function tests and a chest X-ray. Further investigation will also include a CT scan of the abdomen (Figure 14.1) and the thorax to define operability. Angiography and an intravenous urogram (IVU) (Figure 14.2) may also have to be performed.

Staging and grading

The majority of renal tumours are adenocarcinomas of renal cell origin. Approximately 2% of renal

Filling defect in
pelvicalyceal system

Figure 14.2 An IVU image demonstrating obstruction of the left pelvicalyceal system at the level of the pelviureteric junction with a filling defect. These appearances were due to a transitional cell carcinoma of the renal pelvis. Transitional cell cancer (TCC) of the renal pelvis arises in the collecting system and may be associated with TCC of the bladder and ureter. The biology, prognosis and treatment are similar to those of bladder cancer.

cancers are of transitional cell histology, arising from the collecting system rather than from the renal parenchyma. Both adenocarcinomas and transitional cell tumours are described as well, poorly or moderately differentiated. Nuclear grading, into four Fuhrman categories, is strongly correlated with prognosis. Only rarely is the kidney involved, either with a primary lymphoma or as the site of the spread of other cancers. The kidney can be the site of a rare non-metastasizing malignancy called an oncocytoma. The patient with renal cell carcinoma is staged according to the spread of the disease, using the TNM staging criteria.

Treatment

Surgery

If the patient has no evidence of spread of the disease, then the urological surgeon will arrange for the patient to be admitted for nephrectomy. At operation, the kidney and vascular pedicle and associated lymph nodes are removed, together with the ureter and adrenal. Renal tumours have a propensity to invade along the renal vein. This invasion may extend into the inferior vena cava (IVC) and right atrium. It does not represent a true invasion but a tumour thrombus. If this is suspected, then a combined approach involving a urologist and a vascular surgeon is advised in an attempt to fully resect the tumour.

Management of an inoperable primary tumour

Locally advanced, inoperable kidney cancer may cause significant symptoms, which may be poorly controlled by systemic palliative measures. These local symptoms can include haematuria, which may be so profound that regular blood transfusion is required, as well as loin pain, which may not respond to opiate analgesia. These symptoms can be treated by angioinfarction, where agents are introduced into the renal artery to occlude the tumour's blood supply. A number of different agents can be introduced into the renal artery. These include steel coils and chemotherapy pellets. By these means, successful symptom palliation is achieved in approximately 70–80% of all patients. The procedure does have significant morbidity, which includes a transient increase in pain, fever and, occasionally, shock due to the release of tumour products into the circulation. These symptoms peak a few hours after the procedure but may continue for up to 10 days. There is a specific mortality associated with the procedure, ranging up to

5%. In hospitals where it is not possible to treat by angioinfarction, radiation to the kidney may be given.

Adjuvant treatment

Local radiotherapy to the tumour bed following nephrectomy leads to no survival advantage in patients with adenocarcinoma and has morbidity. This is therefore not recommended. Similarly, adjuvant chemotherapy has no survival advantage. The value of adjuvant immunotherapy continues to be investigated; findings reported up to and including the year 2005, however, have shown no benefit. This includes treatment with interleukin 2 (IL-2) for poor prognosis tumours. The situation may possibly be different in transitional cell tumours. The outlook is very poor for these cancers, so adjuvant chemotherapy is given in some centres.

Management of metastatic kidney cancer

Where there are single sites or limited numbers of metastases, there is a surgical option that needs to be considered. The removal of limited numbers of pulmonary metastases, or brain or bone metastases, leads to a chance for cure. Where there are multiple metastases the situation is different. There have been significant changes in the management of metastatic disease as a result of our understanding of the molecular biology of this group of tumours.

Chemotherapy

Chemotherapy is generally ineffective in the treatment of adenocarcinoma of the kidney. The most active of the agents, which include the vinca alkaloids, produce responses in less than 10% of patients. Chemotherapy is given in the treatment of transitional cell tumours. The response rate of 60–70% is similar to that seen in patients with transitional cell cancer of the bladder. Unfortunately, these responses are transient and last for a median time of six to seven months.

Hormonal therapy

Initial reports of the efficacy of hormonal treatments in the management of renal cell cancer have proven to be incorrect. The use of hormonal therapies for renal cell cancer was based upon the observation over 30 years ago of a response to orchiectomy in Syrian golden hamsters bearing renal cell tumours. The leap of logic from this observation to the use of medroxyprogesterone acetate is rather dizzy, but response rates of up to 30% were described to medroxyprogesterone acetate. This order of response has, however, not been confirmed, and the true response rate to hormonal agents is probably less than 2%. A wide variety of hormonal treatments has been used in this condition, including tamoxifen and flutamide in addition to the progestogens. Transitional cell tumours do not respond to hormonal therapy.

Immunotherapy

Until recently, the most important therapy used for metastatic adenocarcinoma of the kidney was immunotherapy. The first agents used were bacillus Calmette–Guerin (BCG) and *Corynebacterium parvum*, but these have now been replaced by the interferons and interleukin 2. The overall order of response to interferon therapy is 15%. Approximately 5% of patients have a complete response, and the median duration of a complete response is 7 months. There is no incremental rise in response with dosages over three mega units weekly of interferon, merely increased toxicity. In 1985, the results of treatment with IL-2 were first published, and 60% of patients with kidney cancer were reported to respond to treatment. This high response rate was not confirmed in subsequent studies, which were nevertheless encouraging in that, overall, approximately 20% of patients were seen to respond to treatment.

The most significant aspect to IL-2 treatment is that responses are durable. Those lucky patients who achieve a complete response may be cured of their malignancy. In the original dosage regimen, treatment had significant toxicities. These toxicities are lower with subcutaneous low-dose schedul-

ing of IL-2 treatments. Currently, IL-2 is given with interferon. Cytokine treatment may be improved by combination with chemotherapy, but this is controversial. Transitional cell tumours do not respond to immunotherapy.

New treatment

Unfortunately the effective treatment of patients with renal cell cancer has been held back in the United Kingdom by the action of the National Institute for Health and Clinical Excellence (NICE). The bureaucratic processes that regulate NICE have delayed by at least three years effective treatment for this condition, and caused the unnecessary and early death of many patients. In finally coming to a view as to the efficacy of modern therapies for renal cell cancer, false cost calculations were made, and the opinion issued by NICE was changed three times before final agreement to allow some effective treatment for renal cancer patients in the UK. Therapy targets VEGFR and EGFR and the tyrosine kinases that affect receptor activation using drugs such as sunitinib and sorafenib. Response rates approach 40%, and those patients who respond do appear to have responses that are sustained. Treatment does have toxicity, but these toxicities are generally mild. Because treatment targets VEGFR, gastrointestinal bleeding and bowel perforation may occur.

Other new treatments for renal cell cancer include temsirolimus and everolimus, which inhibit mTOR (mammalian target of rapamycin) that is integral to various signal transduction pathways. Unfortunately these agents, which are effective, have also been rejected for use by our patients by NICE as a result of what we and most of our colleagues believe to be false cost calculations. These agents appear to have the same order of efficacy as sunitinib and sorafenib, but are kept as second-line therapies for kidney patients after progression on sunitinib or sorafenib.

Prognosis

The prognosis for localized adenocarcinoma of the kidney is variable. The survival rate for patients with good prognosis tumours is 60–80%, but if there is vascular or capsular invasion, only 40% survive 1 year. The median survival for patients with metastatic disease is nine months. These statistics have significantly changed as a result of the development of new treatments for kidney cancer. Where treatment is allowed, the median survival for patients with metastatic disease has been extended to two years. Kidney cancer survival is significantly longer for those that live in the least deprived areas of the UK compared to those who live in areas of greater material deprivation. Overall, 10% of patients with metastatic renal cell cancer survive five years from diagnosis, and this group represents a curious feature of the malignancy. Even in the absence of metastases at presentation, the outlook for patients with transitional cell tumours is very poor, with 10% surviving for one year, and 5% for two years.

Chapter 15

Bladder cancer

Epidemiology and pathogenesis

Carcinoma of the bladder is common in the United Kingdom. Each year in the UK, approximately 1020 men and women are registered with the disease and 4900 die. Worldwide more than one-third of a million people are diagnosed each year with bladder cancer. The average age at which patients with this condition present to their clinician is 65 years. The most important cause of bladder cancer is cigarette smoking. Workers in the dye, paint and rubber industries are also at increased risk of bladder cancer.

There have been many developments in our understanding of the molecular biology of bladder cancer, and, although these developments have not translated directly into treatment advances, they do provide significant prognostic information. Bladder tumours are thought to progress from a localized, superficial tumour to invasive and then metastatic disease. They are often multifocal. In an attempt to define the molecular events categorizing progression, it was originally noted that there was identical loss of heterozygosity in multifocal bladder tumours. This original description, however, of what was thought to be a primary genetic event in this cancer, has not been confirmed. Multiple loss of genetic material has been described, with the most common losses centred on chromosome 9q22, which is the site of a gene called *patched* (PTC). This is thought to be a tumour suppressor gene in basal cell carcinoma and medulloblastoma. There are other sites of chromosomal loss, particularly within chromosomes 3, 7 and 17. This loss of material can be used to follow up patients with bladder cancer, using fluorescence *in situ* hybridization (FISH) methodologies on urine cytology.

By far the most important of the recent findings in bladder cancer, however, has been the observation of overexpression of the human epidermal growth factor receptor (EGFR). This is reported in around 40% of the tumours of patients with bladder cancer. Overexpression correlates with a poor prognosis, and treatments directed against EGFR may well have some future role as therapies for this malignancy.

Presentation

The initial symptoms include haematuria, dysuria and frequency of micturition. These symptoms are, unfortunately, sometimes treated with antibiotics by GPs for a period of time, prior to referral to a specialist. New urinary tract infections in older women should always be investigated actively, and symptoms occurring in a man should always be

Lecture Notes: Oncology, 2nd edition. By M. Bower and J. Waxman. Published 2010 by Blackwell Publishing Ltd.

considered to be pathological and a referral made. There is of course a differential diagnosis, but one should have a very high index of suspicion of malignancy. Referral should be promptly organized to a specialist urological surgeon. The patient will be seen in an outpatient clinic. A careful history should be taken and an examination made. The patient's symptoms should be investigated further by performing a blood count, renal function tests, liver function tests and bacteriological and cytological examination of urine, to examine for the presence of infection and malignancy. An intravenous pyelogram (IVP) may be ordered to examine the urothelial tract radiologically or an ultrasound investigation carried out.

Outpatient diagnosis

These investigations should be organized promptly and the patient reviewed with the result within two to three weeks. A flexible cystoscopy is then generally organized and this takes place in the outpatient setting. If there is any suspicious appearance to the bladder, arrangements should then be made for a formal cystoscopy. The patient is anaesthetized for this procedure and the urethra and bladder carefully examined using a fibreoptic cystoscope. Any abnormal areas within the bladder

should be biopsied together with areas of surrounding, apparently normal-looking bladder. The urologists at cystoscopy may describe a normal-looking bladder or the presence of a papilloma or solid tumour. The suspicious areas are treated by diathermy and the pelvis carefully examined in order to describe the clinical staging of the tumour.

Staging and grading

The tumour should then be examined pathologically and be given a grade according to differentiation. These grades are as follows:
- G1: well differentiated tumour
- G2: moderately differentiated tumour
- G3: poorly differentiated tumour.

Lesions are further characterized pathologically by their microscopic appearance as either transitional cell carcinoma or squamous carcinoma. Approximately 90% of patients in the UK have transitional cell carcinomas. The rest are squamous carcinomas or adenocarcinomas. There may be squamous metaplasia present within a transitional cell carcinoma, and this is indicative of a poor prognosis.

The tumour should also be staged according to the T (tumour), N (node) and M (metastatic categories) system (Table 15.1).

Table 15.1 TNMstaging of bladder cancer.

T (primary tumour)	N (nodal status)	M (metastatic status)
Tis Carcinoma *in situ*	N0 No lymph node involvement	M0 No evidence of metastases
TA Papillary non-invasive tumour	N1 Single regional lymph node involvement	M1 Distant metastases
T1 Superficial tumour, not invading	N2 Bilateral regional lymph node beyond the lamina propria involvement	
T2 Tumour invading superficial	N3 Fixed regional lymph nodes muscle	
T2A Tumour invading superficial muscle	N4 Juxtaregional lymph node involvement	
T2B Tumour penetrating through superficial muscle		
T3A Invasion of deep muscle		
T3B Invasion through bladder wall		
T4A Tumour invading prostate, uterus or vagina		
T4B Tumour fixed to the pelvic wall		

A subscript 'P' is given to describe the pathological staging of the tumour.

Treatment

Treatment of superficial bladder cancer

The majority of transitional cell carcinoma of the bladder present as superficial tumours. After resection by diathermy at cystoscopy, approximately 60% of these will recur. The recurrence rate is greater where there are multiple tumours, associated carcinoma *in situ* or poorly differentiated tumours. The outlook is best for solitary tumours, tumours with good histology and tumours without invasion of the lamina propria. There is controversy as to whether or not a solitary superficial but clearly non-invasive tumour should be followed up, because recurrence or further papilloma development is unusual. There is also debate as to whether or not these papillomas should be classified as malignant.

The recommendation for follow-up is slightly controversial, but in most practices cystoscopy is performed three-monthly until the patient is tumour free and thereafter six-monthly for two years and yearly for three years. Practice varies throughout the UK.

If tumours are poorly controlled by cystoscopic diathermy but remain superficial, agents may be instilled into the bladder to try and control the disease. A number of different compounds are used, including bacillus Calmette–Guerin (BCG), interferon, thiotepa, adriamcyin, mitomycin C, mitrozantrone and epodyl. BCG is the treatment of choice for carcinoma *in situ*, and mitomycin C is the most popular treatment of multifocal superficial tumours. Maintenance BCG reduces recurrence rates.

Treatment of invasive bladder cancer

The treatment of muscle-invasive carcinoma of the bladder is by radiation or with surgery. Both have similar efficacy in terms of the control of the disease. This varies according to clinical staging: 40–60% of T2 tumours, 25% of T3 tumours and 5% of T4 tumours are controlled by radiotherapy or surgery. In the UK, radiotherapy is the most widely practised treatment, because the patient keeps his or her bladder at the end of therapy. Radical cystectomy has a mortality of up to 3%, depending on which centre it is performed in. After cystectomy, patients must be nursed either in intensive care or in high-dependency beds. Continent bladders may be fashioned by the surgeon so that the patient does not require an ileostomy. Men are invariably rendered impotent by cystectomy. Little is known of the effects of cystectomy on female sexual function. There are well-known electrolyte disorders associated with ileostomies.

Radical radiotherapy is generally given to a total dose of 6500 cGy over a six-week period. Treatment may be given to the whole pelvis, focusing down upon the bladder towards the end of treatment, or may be given to the bladder alone. There is a clear rationale for treating the bladder alone. Treatment of the whole pelvis is given with the aim of shrinking nodal disease, but this is unlikely in the dosage regimens used. If nodes in the pelvis are involved, there is a significant chance of distant nodal spread and so radiation of pelvic node is pointless. Whole pelvis radiotherapy has significantly greater toxicity than treatment to the bladder alone, and there is no logical reason for using whole pelvis radiotherapy.

During radiotherapy, the patient may get cystitis or proctitis. At the end of treatment, he or she may suffer from a small, shrunken bladder as a consequence of radiation fibrosis. Both cystitis and proctitis are common after radiotherapy to the bladder, occurring in up to 30% of patients.

Chemotherapy has been given to patients with bladder cancer. Response rates seem to be similar to radiotherapy and surgery. The advantage to the patient is the avoidance of the long-term side effects of radiotherapy and retention of the bladder.

Treatment of metastatic bladder cancer

When bladder cancer has spread beyond the bladder it is conventionally treated with chemotherapy. Recent advances in the treatment of this disease mean that new hope is now offered to patients with metastatic cancer. A number of different treatment schedules are used for treatment, including regimes which have the acronyms CMV, MVAC and MVMJ. New agents have become available for the treatment of bladder cancer. These include gemcitabine. The standard treatment currently is combination therapy with gemcitabine and cisplatin, chosen for efficacy and comparative lack of toxicity (Figure 15.1).

Prognosis

The consensus view is that diathermy and intravesical chemotherapy prevent the progression of superficial to locally advanced or metastatic disease in 40% of cases. Overall, however, approximately 30% of patients with superficial tumours develop invasive disease. If there is associated carcinoma *in situ*, over 60% of patients will develop invasive cancer. Poorly differentiated superficial bladder cancers have a particularly poor prognosis and are treated aggressively. Despite treatment, just 20% of patients survive five years.

The results of treatment vary from centre to centre, but the overall expectation is for an initial response in approximately 50% of patients with metastatic disease, for a median duration of 9 months. During the terminal phases of illness,

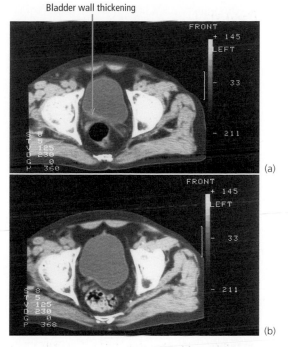

Bladder wall thickening

Figure 15.1 (a) CT scan demonstrating thickening of the posterior bladder wall due to invasive bladder cancer and (b) the same image after four cycles of platinum-based combination chemotherapy showing a reduction in bladder wall thickening.

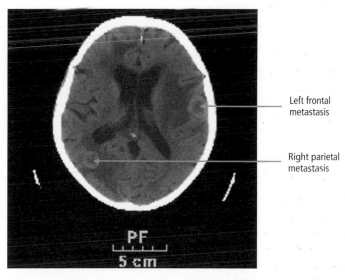

Left frontal metastasis

Right parietal metastasis

Figure 15.2 A man with a 3-year history of invasive bladder cancer treated with radical radiotherapy developed morning headaches and numbness of his right arm. His CT scan shown here shows two ring-enhancing metastases in the left frontal and right parietal regions with marked surrounding oedema.

patients require specialist care for symptom pallia-tion. The disease may spread to bone, lung or liver, and opiate analgesia or local radiotherapy may be helpful in easing symptoms (Figure 15.2).

New treatment

The major prospects for the development of new treatments for bladder cancer are targeted at methods of inhibiting the activity of the epidermal growth factor receptor. The first in development is gefitib (Iressa), but this is just one of a family of at least six EGFR targeting therapies in development.

Chapter 16

Prostate cancer

Epidemiology and pathogenesis

Carcinoma of the prostate is the second most common cancer of men in the Western world. The latest incidence figures suggest that in the UK, 35000 men were diagnosed as having prostate cancer and that there were over 10000 deaths. Prostate cancer death rates have trebled in the last 30 years, and the incidence figures have increased so strikingly that the number of men affected by this cancer has overtaken lung cancer as the most common of all male cancers in the UK. This is also the case in the US, where prostate cancer has replaced lung cancer as the most common cancer of males.

How do we explain this increase in prostate cancer incidence? It is very unlikely that there is a genetic basis to this dramatic recent change in incidence. What is likely is that there is an environmental risk factor. This can be seen from studies on the incidence of cancer in the succeeding generations of migrating populations – as well as from dietary evidence, we believe. There were huge waves of migration from South East Asia to North America and Hawaii at the turn of the 19th century. Prostate cancer has a very low incidence in Asia. The incidence of prostate cancer in the generations

that followed these waves of migration increased, so that in two generations the incidence of prostate cancer was almost equivalent to that occurring in their Caucasian neighbours.

The second line of evidence comes from dietary studies, where it has been clearly shown that the incidence of prostate cancer in vegetarians is 50–75% that of the incidence in omnivores. There are striking correlates between prostate cancer and diets containing smoked foods and dairy produce, and protective benefits from diets that are rich in yellow beans.

The genetic basis to prostate cancer has not been clearly elucidated and the reason for this is that it is unlikely that there is one. There are links between familial breast cancer and prostate cancer, and overall the risk of developing prostate cancer is increased by just 1.3-fold if you have an affected father with the condition and by 2.5-fold if you have a brother affected. No consistent genetic defect has been described in prostate cancer. Most have a multiplicity of observed changes. These include a loss of heterozygosity around a number of chromosomes, the most common of which is a loss of genetic material on chromosome 10p. The tumour suppressor genes are infrequently mutated in prostate cancer – for example, the retinoblastoma (RB) gene is mutated in just 5% of patients' tumours. No specific cell surface molecular identity has been demonstrated to occur consistently in prostate cancer. Epidermal growth factor

Lecture Notes: Oncology, 2nd edition. By M. Bower and J. Waxman. Published 2010 by Blackwell Publishing Ltd.

receptor (EGFR) positivity is described in up to 40% of tumours.

Prostate cancer is strikingly hormone dependent. This is because the growth of prostatic tumours is regulated by the androgen receptor, which is a member of the steroid superfamily of transcription factors, and the majority of treatments for prostate cancer have their effect through this receptor.

Presentation

Patients with prostate cancer commonly present with urinary frequency, a poor urine flow or difficulty with starting and stopping urination. Other associated symptoms on presentation include bone pain and general debility. Weight loss is rare. The patient with symptoms such as these should be referred by his GP to a urologist.

Patients with a potential diagnosis of prostate cancer are diagnosed in general practice as a result of prostate-specific antigen (PSA) screening and referred directly to oncology. In the UK between 2% and 6% of men are screened. PSA levels are not necessarily diagnostic of prostate cancer. Where levels are raised above the normal range of 4 μg/l to between 4 and 10 μg/l, the chance of the patient having prostate cancer is approximately 25%. At levels over 10 μg/l, the chance of diagnosing prostate cancer increases to 40%. Levels of this antigen may be elevated in benign prostatic hypertrophy. PSA is a serine protease and acts like drain cleaner for the prostate, dissolving the prostatic coagulum.

In outpatients, a careful history should be taken, a full examination made, routine blood tests performed and levels of acid phosphatase and PSA assessed. In addition, plain X-rays of the chest and pelvis should be performed and a transrectal ultrasound and bone scan booked (Figures 16.1 and 16.2; see Figure 1.8).

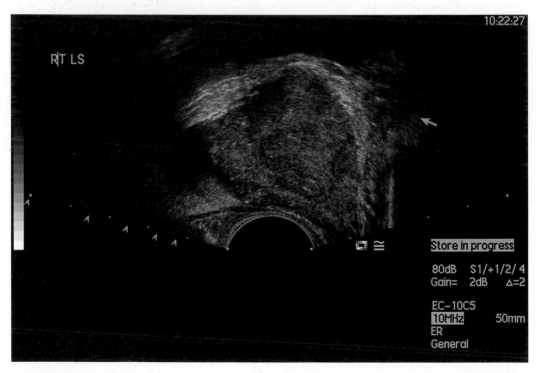

Figure 16.1 Transrectal ultrasound of the prostate gland showing extension of the primary tumour through the prostatic capsule (T3 disease).

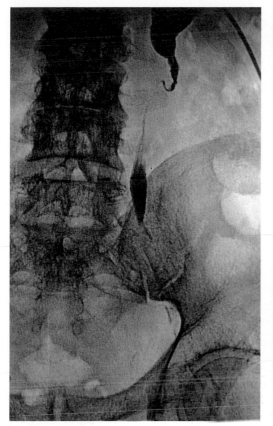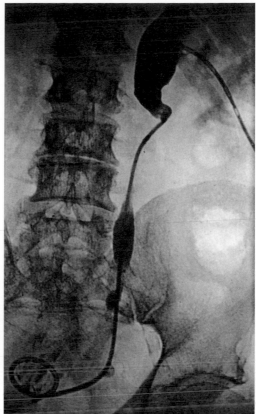

Figure 16.2 Antegrade nephrostogram showing irregular tapering and lack of contrast due to ureteric obstruction and hydronephrosis before and after the passage of a JJ stent to relive obstruction that was due to external compression by prostate cancer.

Staging and grading

From the clinical findings an assessment can be made of the degree of prostate enlargement. If the prostate is malignant, it is staged as in Table 16.1.

The tumour grade can be described as well, moderately or poorly differentiated. This is elaborated in the Gleason scoring system. The Gleason system scores prostatic tumours on a 1–10 scale, where 10 is the most poorly differentiated. The combined Gleason grade describes the appearances of the two most common areas of prostatic malignancy. High-grade PIN, an acronym that coasts off the tongue with greater ease than prostatic intraepithelial neoplasia, has been suggested as a premalignant condition leading to invasive cancer, as CIN leads to invasive cervical cancer. However, the

evidence for this is very poor and surgeons should be discouraged from operative procedures in patients with this condition.

If the X-rays show no evidence of metastases, a bone scan should be carried out. Transrectal ultrasound has low specificity for defining malignancy but a high specificity for describing the integrity of the prostatic capsule. In many centres, magnetic resonance is used as an adjunct to this procedure and has a reasonable specificity for describing prostatic staging. A CT scan should be used to define lymph node spread. Transrectal ultrasonography should be combined with needle biopsy. As a standard, six cores are taken in general. Since diagnostic certainty is increased by carrying out more biopsies, 8 or even 12, needle cores are taken in many centres. Where the diagnosis is difficult and

Table 16.1 TNM staging of prostate cancer.

T (primary tumour)	N (nodal status)	M (metastatic status)
T0 No tumour palpable	N0 No nodes	M0 No metastases
T1 Tumour in one lobe of the prostate	N1 Homolateral nodes	M1 Metastases
T2 Tumour involving both prostate lobes	N2 Bilateral nodes	
T3 Tumour infiltrating out of the prostate to involve seminal vesicles	N3 Fixed regional nodes	
T4 Extensive tumour, fixed and infiltrating local structures	N4 Juxtaregional nodes	

PSA levels are high, saturation biopsies are carried out but this procedure, which may involve 20 or more biopsies, may lead to yet further difficulties in defining treatment if a focus of low-grade cancer is found.

Treatment

Treatment of early-stage prostate cancer

The treatment of prostate cancer depends upon clinical stage and is surrounded by controversy. Early-stage small bulk prostate cancer, that is T1 and T2 disease, may be treated by observation, radiotherapy or radical prostatectomy if there is no evidence of spread. The options for treatment depend upon the patient's overall state and preference. Observation involves regular follow-up without treatment. Radiotherapy involves approximately 6 weeks of attendance at hospital for prostatic irradiation, which is given in an attempt to sterilize the tumour. Radiotherapy has morbidity. Acutely, it may be associated with symptoms of cystitis and proctitis; post-treatment it may produce impotence in up to 70% of patients. Radical prostatectomy involves major pelvic surgery, with removal of the prostate and associated lymph glands. Modern anaesthetic techniques and surgical advances have meant that the morbidity is limited, but a degree of incontinence is reported in up to 25% of patients, and a degree of impotence, which is under-reported by surgeons, occurs in up to 90% of patients. It is agreed that morbidity has been reduced by the introduction of nerve-sparing techniques. There is an operative mortality of less than 1%. Surgeons delight in new toys, and have been allowed to play with the Da Vinci robot; radical prostatectomy carried out by this procedure is said to lead to fewer problems with potency, and certainly less blood loss than with standard open surgery.

The reason the patient can be offered the prospect of choice in determining what therapy he should have for early-stage disease is that observation, radiotherapy and radical surgery have all been shown to offer the patient with good or moderate histology tumours the same overall chance of long-term survival. For younger patients, with poor histology, surgery offers a better survival chance than radiotherapy. The survival advantage is minimal. There has, however, been no randomized comparison of these three options involving significant patient numbers: hence this subject remains a matter for vociferous debate. A recent study of approximately 600 patients randomized to receive either watchful waiting or radiotherapy showed a better outlook for patients treated surgically.

In the early 1990s, investigations were initiated into the value of hormonal therapy given in addition to radiotherapy and surgery. No advantage to such 'neoadjuvant' hormonal therapy has been found in those patients proceeding to radical surgery. A number of randomized studies have shown an advantage to neoadjuvant hormonal therapy in patients receiving radiotherapy. The majority of studies have found a decreased risk of local relapse with hormonal therapy, and two major trials reported improved survival. There is controversy as to the suitable duration of treatment with adjuvant hormonal therapy.

Brachytherapy is a radiotherapy technique where the local intensity of radiation is increased by the

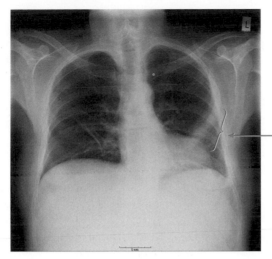

Sclerotic expanded left third rib due to metastatic prostate cancer

Figure 16.3 The chest X-ray shows a sclerosis and expansion of the anterolateral aspect of left third rib. This appearance was due to metastasis from prostate cancer, although the differential radiological diagnosis would include lymphoma, osteopetrosis and Paget's disease.

implantation of radioactive seeds or wires. This technique has been applied to localized prostate cancer. Excellent results have been claimed, but not proven in any randomized trial. Recent publications have shown that the incidence of major side effects of brachytherapy is the same as for conventional radiation, and the efficacy of brachytherapy is no doubt similar to conventional radiation treatment. Brachytherapy has additional side effects to radiotherapy and these include a 12% instance of urethral stricture requiring surgical intervention.

Treatment of locally advanced or metastastic prostate cancer

When patients have locally advanced, that is T3 or T4, prostate cancer or metastatic disease (Figures 16.3 and 16.4), the treatment involves the use of hormonal therapy. Again, this area is one of considerable debate and controversy. Hormonal therapy for this condition was first described in the 1940s, when the disease was found to be dependent upon testosterone. For this reason, the first treatments offered in the 1940s were orchiectomy, that is, removal of the testes, or oestrogen therapy.

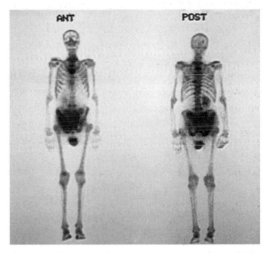

Figure 16.4 Bone scan showing multiple hot spots in the axial skeleton due to bone metastases and a non-functioning left kidney due to long-standing obstruction. The patient had locally advanced and metastatic prostate cancer.

The results of treatment were first analyzed in the 1960s by the Veterans Administration Cooperative Urological Research Group (VACURG). In their studies, the VACURG randomized patients to treatment with oestrogens or placebo, or with orchiectomy or placebo, respectively. The overall survival of patients treated or untreated was the same, but there was an excess mortality rate from cardiovascular deaths in the oestrogen-treated group. The reason for this is that oestrogens cause an increased coaguability of blood and increased blood volumes.

Because orchiectomy is barbaric and oestrogen therapy is associated with morbidity and mortality, medical treatments for this condition have been sought which are not so invasive and have no side effects. The most effective of these new treatments, which has the least morbidity associated with its use, is a group of compounds called the gonadotrophin-releasing hormone agonists. These include leuprorelin acetate, goserelin acetate and buserelin. These are currently given subcutaneously by monthly or three-monthly injection.

Prostate cancer is very responsive to treatment, and 80% of patients improve subjectively. After a period of approximately one year, however, most patients with metastatic cancer on presentation have PSA evidence of relapse. In relapse, treatment is palliative and hinges upon the use of radiotherapy and steroids. Blood transfusion is often necessary. Chemotherapy is increasingly popular in patients with prostate cancer. The reason for this popularity is that patients respond to docetaxel chemotherapy. The median survival in patients starting treatment with docetaxel is 18.7 months, which provides a benefit of three months over conventional therapy using mitoxantrone, a regimen which was introduced in the late 1980s.

Effects of treatment delay

Later analyses of the VACURG study showed that all the patients who were initially given placebos were eventually treated with hormonal therapies by their primary care physicians. As survival of both groups of patients, 'treated' and 'untreated', was the same, the real conclusion of the study is that early, as compared with late, treatment offers the same prospect for survival. This important issue was investigated by the Medical Research Council (MRC) in a randomized prospective trial. The MRC trial was published, and initial analysis showed both an increased risk of disease complica-

tions and a more rapid rate of death in those patients who had delayed treatment. It would appear that this increased risk of complications and of death is confined to patients with metastatic cancer. In a review of the MRC trial in 2002, however, the principal author revised his conclusions and considered it to be uncertain whether or not there is a survival advantage and a reduced complication rate to early treatment.

Prognosis

Prognosis for small bulk localized disease

The outlook for small bulk localized disease depends upon grade. Observation, radiotherapy and surgery all lead to an equivalent survival of 80% at 10 years for patients with well or moderately differentiated tumours. Patients with poorly differentiated, high Gleason grade tumours have a worse outlook with observation and radiotherapy than with surgery. Only 15% of patients survive 10 years, compared with 60–80% undergoing the latter treatment. It is argued that patient selection influences this result, as fitter patients, who will invariably do better than less well patients, are selected for surgery.

Prognosis for metastatic and large bulk localized disease

It has been shown in clinical trials that the addition of an anti-androgen to gonadotrophin-releasing hormone agonist therapy leads to an improvement in survival rate. The median survival for patients with metastatic tumours treated with combination anti-androgen therapy is three years, as opposed to 2.5 years for patients treated with single-agent gonadotrophin-releasing hormone agonist or by orchiectomy. The prospects for survival for a patient with locally advanced disease without metastases are much better. The median survival of this group is 4.5 years. It is not known whether there is an advantage to combination gonadotrophin-releasing hormone agonist and anti-androgen therapy in this patient group.

Screening

There is controversy also regarding the value of screening. Two recent reports, one from the Institute of Cancer Research, and the other from the University of York Health Economics Unit, have published findings similar to each other. Both reports conclude that there is little value to screening because of the poor specificity of the diagnostic tools and the lack of a proven survival advantage to early treatment.

Recently two major trials results were published, one showing a survival advantage, the other, no advantage. Both trials involved many thousands of patients. The European study that showed a survival gain to screening, also demonstrated that one patient's life was 'saved' for every 48 cancers detected.

New treatment

When biopsies from patients with recurrent tumour are examined and compared with biopsies on presentation, it is striking that up to 50% will show androgen receptor mutations. This is in contradiction to the situation in breast cancer, where hormone receptor amplification is the most commonly observed change. Over 700 mutations of the androgen receptor have been described, and these changes are a clue to the probable reason for the response to second-line hormonal therapy. The most commonly used second-line treatment is the withdrawal of anti-androgen therapy. Cessation of treatment with flutamide, for example, given in combination with an LHRH (luteinizing hormone-releasing hormone) agonist will lead to a response in up to 40% of patients. This response is transient and is thought to occur because the mutation has led the tumour to depend upon the anti-androgen as a growth factor. New treatments will thus have as their basis a molecular design that takes advantage of known androgen receptor changes.

Chemotherapy has become more important in the treatment of recurrent disease, following work in the early 1990s that showed good symptom palliation from the use of mitoxantrone chemotherapy given with concurrent steroids. New treatments with drugs such as docetaxel have shown promise and become a standard. Newer taxanes are in development and are effective as second line chemotherapy. Responses have been seen to anti-angiogenesis agents such as thalidomide and to steroids such as calcitriol. Dendritic cell therapy and vaccination approaches are also being trialled.

Recent work has shown major responses to vitamin D given orally to patients in dosages normally used as food supplementation. The reason for response to vitamin D is of great interest, but at present is not known. The oncogene SRC is upregulated in prostatic cancer cell lines and, for this reason, trial work with a new drug, dasatinib, is under current investigation. The synthesis of androgenic steroids takes place most in the adrenal, where hydroxylase enzymes are responsible for the grand passage of cholesterol to androstenedione and 4-hydroxyandrostenedione. Treatments such as with ketoconazole were aimed at blocking this pathway. However, whilst doing so, transiently, ketoconazole also causes significant side effects. Abiraterone, a new steroid hydroxylase inhibitor, has been found to be an effective treatment of prostate cancer in relapse.

As time goes by, we have become more aware of the side effects of hormonal therapy. The use of anti-androgen treatment is associated with osteoporosis, loss of muscle bulk, anaemia and neurological change, which includes both dementia and Parkinsonism. At present, the consensus view is that osteoporosis is best managed with bisphosphonates.

Until recently, men with prostate cancer represented a rather passive but extremely brave group of individuals who accepted their fate. The last two decades have seen significant changes in the way that men deal with their cancers, and prostate cancer has now become, quite rightly, politicized with the cause championed to good effect.

Chapter 17

Testis cancer

Epidemiology and pathogenesis

The treatment of testis cancer represents one of the major and wonderful triumphs of oncology. The application of modern treatments has led to a fall in death rates by 70% over the last 10–15 years, and in 2007 only 58 men died of this condition in the UK compared to over 2000 patients that were diagnosed. The major predisposing factor to the development of testicular cancer is maldescent of the testes. There have been significant advances in the understanding of the molecular biology of adult male germ cell tumours. It is over 15 years since the original identification of the characteristic cytogenetic marker of adult male germ cell tumours: isochromosome 12p. An extra copy of chromosome 12p is present in 85% of all tumours, and in the remaining percentage there are tandem duplications embedded within other chromosomal material. The cyclin D2 gene, which is concerned with the regulation of the cell cycle, is mapped to this area. This suggests that the aberrant expression of cyclin D2 leads to the dysregulation of the normal cell cycle and tumour development. This abnormality is present in both seminoma and teratoma. Testicular tumours also express c-KIT, stem cell factor receptor and platelet-derived growth factor (PDGF) α-receptor gene. Mutations in the KIT gene occur in 8% of all testicular germ cell tumours but are seen in 93% of patients with bilateral disease. These changes in the KIT gene appear to be specific to seminoma. These molecular findings suggest possible therapeutic options.

Presentation

Media campaigns have led to public awareness of testicular cancer as a curable condition and of the importance of early diagnosis. Generally, patients noticing testicular masses present to their GPs and are referred immediately to urology outpatients. There remain, however, a number of alarming instances where GPs have treated patients with testicular tumours for epididymitis rather than referring them on. Patients with teratoma present during the second and third decades of their lives, generally with swelling of the testes and less frequently with pain. Men with seminoma may present in their third to fifth decades. Men with testicular cancer may have gynaecomastia. This is due to the production of steroid hormones by the malignancy, and clearly not to α-fetoprotein (AFP) or human chorionic gonadotrophin (HCG) synthesis.

In urology outpatients, after examination, the patient should proceed to initial staging by routine haematology, biochemistry and measurement of AFP and HCG. A chest X-ray should be requested and an ultrasound examination of the testes ordered. The ultrasound will show features sugges-

Lecture Notes: Oncology, 2nd edition. By M. Bower and J. Waxman. Published 2010 by Blackwell Publishing Ltd.

tive of testicular cancer, such as increased vascularity accompanying a mass. There may be additional features of microlithiasis, suggesting that the tumour has developed from carcinoma *in situ*. Carcinoma *in situ* is a bilateral condition with a 3% subsequent chance of development of a second testicular tumour.

Following these investigations, arrangements should be made for the patient to proceed to orchiectomy. This is performed through a groin rather than a scrotal incision, which would lead to an increased risk of the scrotal spread of testicular cancer, particularly in cases where there are embryonal elements to the tumour. The testis is removed by the surgeon, cut in half, examined and sent for pathological examination (Figure 17.1).

Staging and grading

There are four main types of testicular tumour: seminoma, teratoma, lymphoma and small cell. Teratoma constitutes approximately 75% of all testicular malignancies and appears cystic when examined by the naked eye. Pure seminoma constitutes 20% of tumours and is uniform in appearance. Approximately 5% of all testicular tumours are lymphoma, the appearance of which is generally uniform but with some areas of necrosis. Less than 1% of tumours are of small cell origin. These tumours have no specific macroscopic features.

Microscopically, teratomas constitute a variety of different elements which may include cartilage, muscle, bone and virtually any other tissue. Subtypes of teratoma are described, and they are called undifferentiated, differentiated or choriocarcinoma. Seminoma consists of uniform and large cells with darkly standing nuclei.

Having made a histological diagnosis, treatment is initiated and depends upon the stage to which the tumour has advanced. The following stages are described and determined by CT imaging of the chest, abdomen and pelvis:
- Stage I: tumour confined to testes
- Stage II: tumour spread to abdominal lymph nodes
- Stage III: tumour spread to lymph nodes above the diaphragm

- Stage IV: tumour invading organs other than lymph nodes such as liver or lung.

The disease is further sub-staged according to the size of the metastatic deposits and the number of pulmonary metastases. In the US, retroperitoneal lymph node dissection is undertaken to stage testicular cancer, although this practice is disappearing. In our view, node dissection is not indicated as a routine staging procedure because of the major morbidity of the operation and also because of the side effects, which include retrograde ejaculation. Node dissection for staging purposes is not part of medical practice in the UK, which relies on imaging.

Retrograde ejaculation is the ejaculation of sperm backwards into the bladder rather than forwards into the urethra. This phenomenon does not necessarily mean that the patient is functionally sterile, because sperm can be collected and artificial insemination techniques employed to successfully fertilize the patient's partner. In modern times, such IVF programmes require aspiration of sperm from the testes or testicular biopsy with sperm retrieval if collection of urine post-ejaculation with sperm retrieval is unsuccessful.

Treatment

Treatment of Stage I testicular cancer

The tumour stage of testicular cancer defines its treatment. If the tumour is localized to the testis, two actions are available to the clinician. The first activity for both seminoma and teratoma is observation without further therapy. If this policy is followed in the absence of poor prognosis pathology features, then the likelihood of any further treatment being required is 13% for testicular teratoma and 17% for seminoma. It should be noted that almost all patients who develop progressive disease during the period of observation without treatment are salvageable by chemotherapy.

In the UK, the majority of urologists refer patients with stage I seminoma for radiotherapy, following which the prognosis is excellent, with virtually no chance of relapse. The option of two courses of single-agent carboplatin might also be offered. A randomized trial has shown that

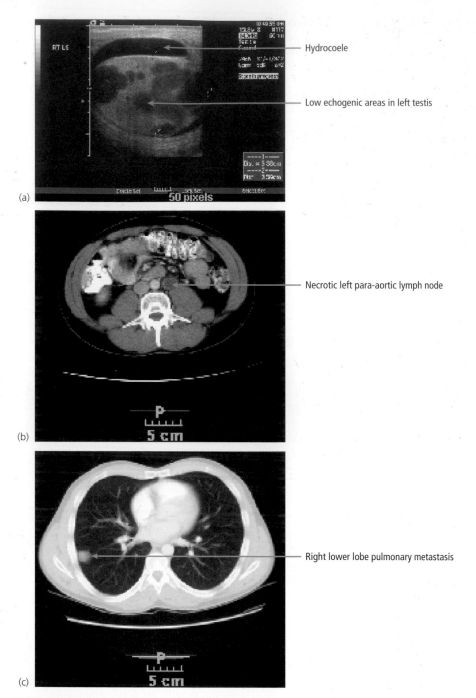

Hydrocoele

Low echogenic areas in left testis

(a)

Necrotic left para-aortic lymph node

(b)

Right lower lobe pulmonary metastasis

(c)

Figure 17.1 Testicular cancer. A 24-year-old Australian bar man presented with a swollen testicle. (a) His ultrasound examination showed an enlarged left testicle with multiple low echogenicity areas and a small hydrocoele. (b) His body CT scan showed an enlarged and necrotic left para-aortic lymph node, and (c) a right lower lobe peripheral lung nodule. His tumour markers were raised (serum AFP = 670 ng/ml; serum HCG = 56 IU/ml). Despite having metastatic disease at presentation, his chances of cure are over 80%.

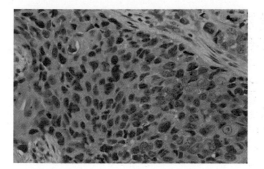

Plate 1.1 Histology of invasive ductal carcinoma of the breast with neoplastic cells invading the breast stroma.

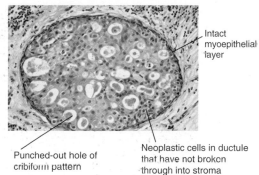

Intact myoepithelial layer

Punched-out hole of cribiform pattern

Neoplastic cells in ductule that have not broken through into stroma

Plate 1.2 Histology of intraductal carcinoma *in situ* of the breast, demonstrating neoplastic cells in a breast ductule with an intact myoepithelial layer.

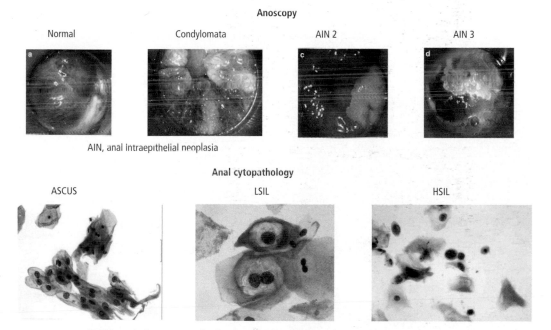

Anoscopy

Normal | Condylomata | AIN 2 | AIN 3

AIN, anal intraepithelial neoplasia

Anal cytopathology

ASCUS | LSIL | HSIL

ASCUS, atypical squamous cells of undetermined significance
LSIL, low-grade squamous intraepithelial lesions
HSIL, high-grade squamous intraepithelial lesions

Plate 1.3 Progression of pre-invasive anal cancer with associated cytopathology changes.

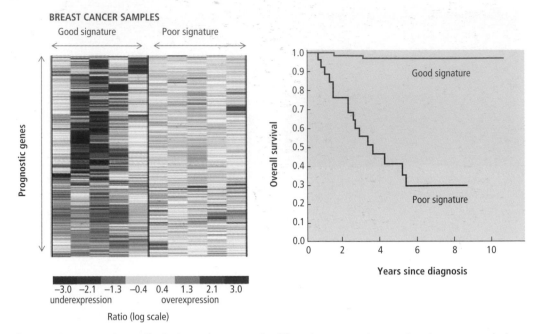

BREAST CANCER SAMPLES

Good signature   Poor signature

Prognostic genes

−3.0 −2.1 −1.3 −0.4 0.4 1.3 2.1 3.0
underexpression   overexpression
Ratio (log scale)

Overall survival

Good signature

Poor signature

Years since diagnosis

Plate 1.4 Gene expression profiles for breast cancer samples differentiate tumours into good- and poor-prognosis signatures that predict survival.

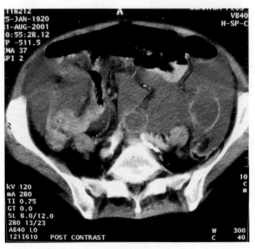

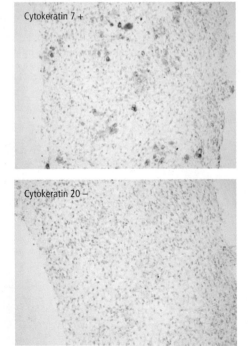

Cytokeratin 7 +

Cytokeratin 20 −

A 78-year-old woman presents with bowel obstruction and ascites. The CT scan shows extensive ascites and omental thickening. CT-guided biopsy of peritoneal deposits demonstrates adenocarcinoma, immunocytochemistry for cytokeratins (CK7+ and CK20−) suggests an ovarian rather than colonic primary

Plate 1.5 Cytokeratin immunohistochemistry in a patient with disseminated peritoneal metastases.

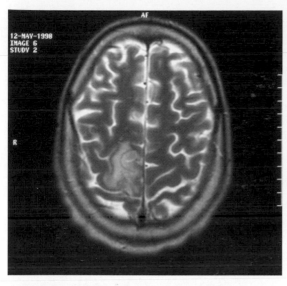
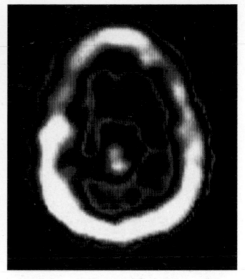

Plate 1.6 MRI (left) and FDG-PET (right) scan of a patient with a parietal primary cerebral lymphoma lesion.

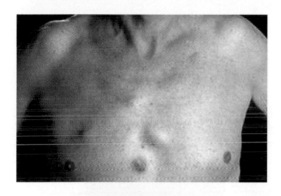

Plate 2.1 Patient with multiple cutaneous metastases from non-small cell lung cancer.

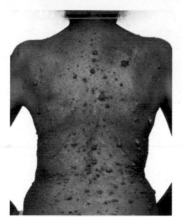

Multiple cutaneous neurofibromata

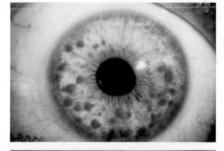

Lisch nodules (iris hamartomas)

Café au lait spot

Plate 2.2 Multiple dermal neurofibromata typical of peripheral neurofibromatosis or type 1 NF, previously known eponymously as von Reckling hausen's disease. It is due to hereditary mutation of the NF1 neurofibromin gene on chromosome 2p22, which encodes a guanosine triphosphatase (GTPase) activating protein involved in the signal transduction cascade.

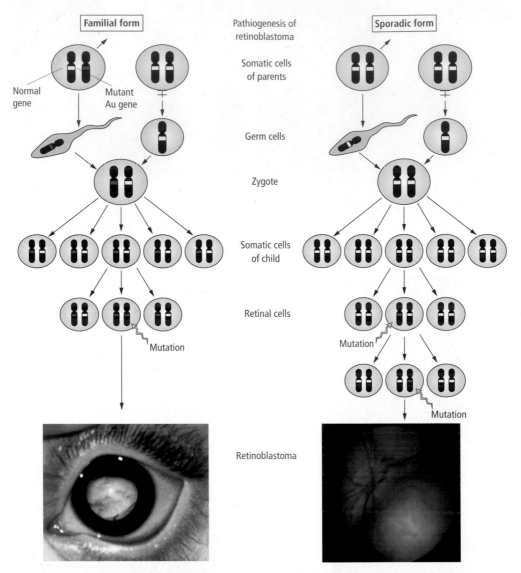

Plate 2.3 Knudson's two hit hypothesis of familial and sporadic retinoblastoma.

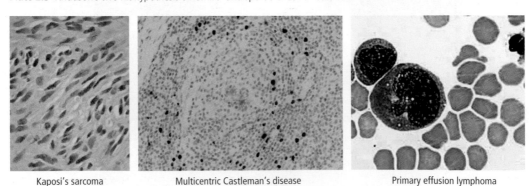

Plate 2.4 KSHV-related tumours. Immunohistochemistry staining for KSHV latent nuclear antigen (LANA) shows the presence of the virus in spindle cells of Kaposi's sarcoma and the plasmabalsts in multicentric Castleman's disease.

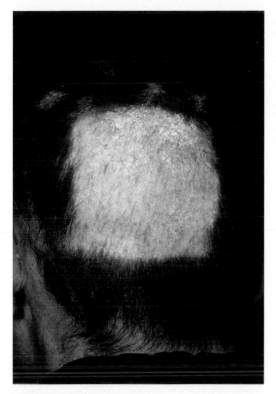

Plate 3.1 Clearly demarcated scalp alopecia due to radiotherapy.

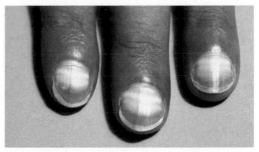

Plate 3.2 Beau lines. This image shows a man with Beau lines, transverse ridges that form as a result of temporary interference with nail growth, here shown following several cycles of chemotherapy.

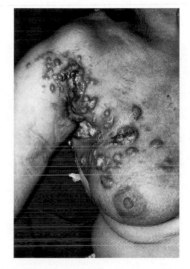

Plate 5.1 Local recurrence of breast cancer showing multiple ulcerating skin nodules.

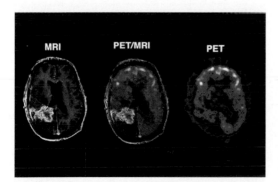

Plate 6.1 Co-registered and separate MRI and 18-fluoro-deoxyglucose PET scan images from a patient with a par-aventricular high-grade glioma demonstrating high glucose utilization by the tumour.

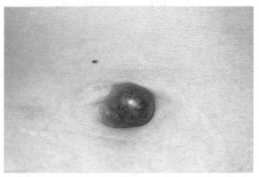

Plate 22.1 Umbilical nodule metastasis known as Sister Mary Joseph nodule, which usually denotes transcoelomic spread from an ovarian or gastric primary. The eponym appears to have been given for Sister Mary Joseph Dempsey (1856–1929) who was a surgical assistant to Dr William Mayo. This eponym is one of very few given for a nurse.

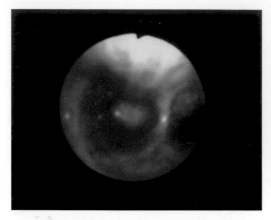

Plate 31.1 Appearance at bronchoscopy of a primary non-small cell lung tumour blocking the right main bronchus.

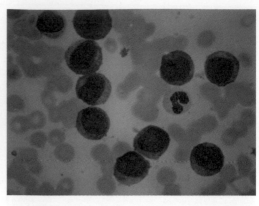

Plate 34.3 Bone marrow aspirate showing acute myeloid leukaemia with monocytic differentiation (AML-M5). This acute myelomonocytic subtype of AML is occasionally associated with gum infiltration and hypertrophy.

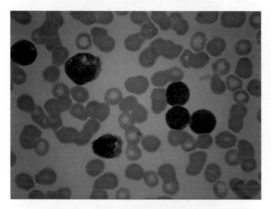

Plate 34.1 Peripheral blood film of acute myeloid leukaemia demonstrating myeloblasts. Occasionally Auer rods, needle-like granules in the cytoplasm, are seen.

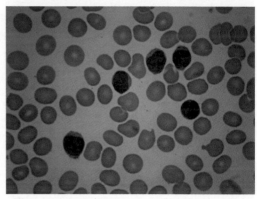

Plate 34.4 Peripheral blood film of chronic lymphocytic leukaemia showing multiple small B-cell lymphocytes with dense nuclei.

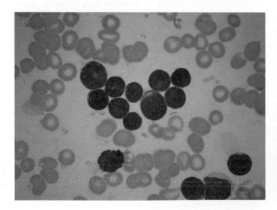

Plate 34.2 Peripheral blood film of acute lymphoid leukaemia demonstrating lymphoblasts with a very high nuclear to cytoplasmic ratio.

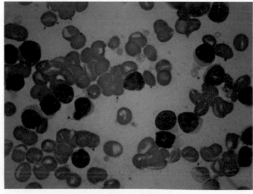

Plate 34.5 Bone marrow aspirate of an elderly asymptomatic man with a total white cell count of 28×10^9/l. There are many small lymphocytes present which were CD19- and CD5-positive B cells.

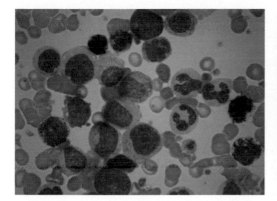

Plate 34.6 Peripheral blood film showing chronic myeloid leukaemia with a spectrum of myeloid cells including eosinophils, basophils, and segmented neutrophils as well as immature myeloid cells.

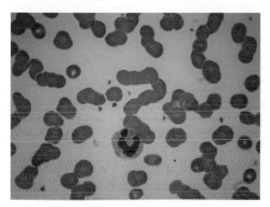

Plate 37.1 Peripheral blood film showing rouleaux formation with erythrocytes stacked up on each other, and a single neutrophil. Rouleaux are found at high levels in the blood of proteins such as fibrinogen or γ-globulin. They are particularly prominent in diseases that cause a very high erythrocyte sedimentation rate (ESR), such as multiple myeloma, cancers, chronic infections (e.g. TB) and connective tissue diseases.

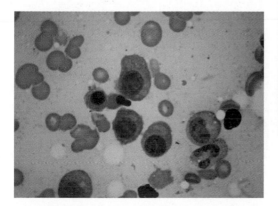

Plate 37.2 Bone marrow aspirate of myeloma showing plasma cells with large eccentric nuclei and basophilic cytoplasm.

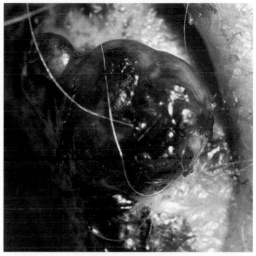

Plate 39.1 A large, raised, bleeding skin lesion on the pinna, a common site for squamous cell cancers of the skin. These tumours are related to UV exposure and may be preceded by actinic or solar keratoses.

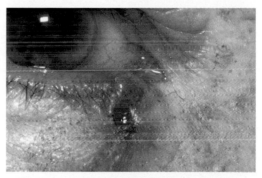

Plate 39.2 A pearly edged, ulcerated lesion characteristic of a basal cell cancer of the skin.

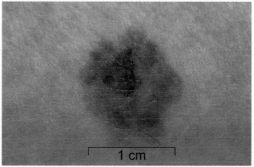

Plate 40.1 Atypical or dysplastic naevi are large naevi (moles) with irregular boarders and varied pigmentation. Atypical naevi are the precursors of melanomas.

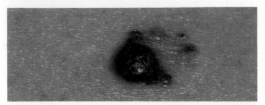

Plate 40.2 A pigmented nodular lesion with an irregular edge and adjacent satellite lesions. This was a nodular melanoma.

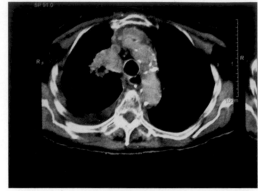

(a)

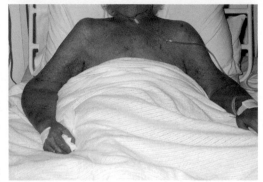

(b)

Plate 46.1 An 80-year-old woman presented with shortness of breath, headaches and swollen arms. (a) The CT scan shows a large right hilar mass that was small cell lung cancer compressing the superior vena cava and collateral circulation. (b) The clinical image also shows dilated veins on the anterior chest wall due to collateral circulation. The flow of blood in these veins will be from above as the blood is bypassing the obstructed superior vena cava to return via the patent inferior vena cava.

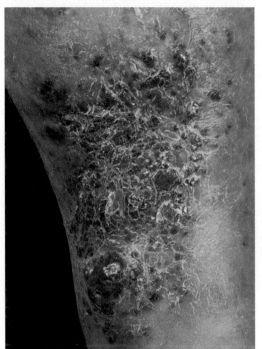

Plate 40.3 Irregular nodular pigmented lesion on the skin at the site of a previously excised malignant melanoma. This represents local recurrence of the melanoma.

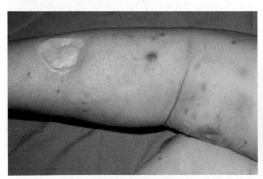
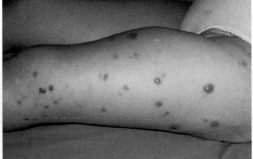

Plate 40.4 Multiple nodular skin metastases arising from a melanoma of the left calf that had been widely excised 2 years earlier, requiring a skin graft.

chemotherapy with carboplatin is as effective as radiation therapy and without the morbidity, two infusions being given at four-weekly intervals in contrast to three weeks of daily radiation therapy. Patients with stage I teratoma are generally referred for adjuvant chemotherapy using BEP (bleomycin, etoposide and cisplatin) chemotherapy: two to four courses are given. Treatment in certain circumstances might be modified, dropping bleomycin from the treatment programme to reduce the risk of lung damage.

Treatment of stage II testicular cancer

For stage IIa seminoma, that is, with a nodal mass of less than 2 cm in diameter as defined by CT scanning, many clinicians in the UK advise treatment with radiotherapy. A consensus of opinion is now emerging, which follows the view that two courses of cytotoxic chemotherapy are equally as effective as radiation treatment in the control of this stage of disease. For stage IIb seminoma, that is, for patients with a disease mass of less than 5 cm, some clinicians, particularly radiotherapists, still treat with radiotherapy, but this is not generally advised in view of the side effects of large field radiotherapy. Chemotherapy should be given using either single-agent or combination therapy.

For all patients with greater than stage IIb disease, whether it is seminoma or teratoma, cytotoxic chemotherapy is given. Before the advent of cytotoxic chemotherapy for teratoma, the disease was invariably fatal. The development of effective chemotherapy programmes has bought about a revolution in the management of patients with malignancy, and now virtually all patients are cured by treatment.

Treatment of advanced testicular cancer

Treatment with cytotoxic agents was originally introduced into medical practice by Li in the early 1960s. As a result, approximately 8% of patients with advanced disease were cured, using a combination of agents that included actinomycin and chlorambucil. In the early 1970s, Samuels treated patients with vinblastine and bleomycin and pro-

duced remissions in approximately 50% of men treated. This treatment was of considerable toxicity because of the large dosages of vinblastine and bleomycin used and the relative lack of support programmes for patients with neutropenic sepsis and thrombocytopenia, which occur as a result of the use of these agents. In 1976, Einhorn introduced the BVP (bleomycin, vinblastine and cisplatinum) programme for the treatment of malignant testicular tumours. This regimen was enormously successful, and 70% of patients with advanced disease were cured. By substituting etoposide for vinblastine, less toxicity resulted with equivalent effect.

Over the last decade, there have been further refinements in the way that treatment has been given. Drug treatment that initially required six courses of five-day treatments has now been reduced to four courses of three-day treatments. Substitution of drugs within this programme to produce the modern three-day JEB (bleomycin, etoposide and carboplatin) programme has meant that toxicity has been limited, and the expectation is that 95% of patients with good-prognosis tumour are cured with this regimen, and 48% of patients with poor-prognosis disease are cured with BEP chemotherapy. Extraordinarily, there has been further change in the collective view with regard to chemotherapy for testicular cancer, and many oncologists have reverted back to the original five-day BEP programme. This is based upon analyses of huge numbers of patients and the realization of the superiority of this standard programme.

Treatment of residual tumour masses

At the end of treatment, one problem may be that of a persistent mass. By this we mean a residual tumour at the site of the original metastatic disease. The approach to this problem is to proceed to surgery. Surgery may be very extensive and involve both thoracotomy and laparotomy. At surgery, the residual mass of tumour is excised as completely as possible, and this may require dacron grafting of major vessels or removal of a kidney in order to take away the tumour completely. This operative procedure is extremely intricate. Histological examination of the excised mass shows that in one-third of cases there is necrotic tumour, in one-third of cases there is differentiated teratoma and in one-third of cases there is undifferentiated cancer. If necrotic tumour is found, no further action is taken. If undifferentiated tumour is found, further chemotherapy is given and 30–40% of patients will be cured by a combination of chemotherapy and surgery. In those patients who have residual differentiated tumour, it is important to remove the residual mass of the disease because over a five-year period approximately 50% of differentiated tumours undergo further malignant change, transforming to undifferentiated malignancy.

Unfortunately, a significant number of patients still have progressive or unresponsive tumours, and for these patients there is still a possibility of cure, which is in the range of 20–40%. Treatment programmes such as VIP (vinblastine, iphosphamide and cisplatin) or high-dose therapy with stem cell rescue are used to treat such patients.

Monitoring treatment

The effects of treatment are very closely monitored by measuring the serum levels of AFP, PLAP and HCG. These are hormones secreted by teratoma and seminoma. If the tumour is being treated effectively, then the levels of these hormones in the blood will decay over a known period: 3–5 days for AFP and approximately 12–36 hours for HCG.

Side effects of treatment

There are specific toxicities that relate to treatment. Cisplatin will cause renal damage, deafness and a peripheral neuropathy, which may manifest as numbness in the fingers or toes or complete loss of motor and sensory function in the limbs. Bleomycin unfortunately causes pulmonary toxicity, that is, an irreversible and progressive loss of lung function, which is fatal in approximately 2% of patients treated (see Figure 3.13). Testicular cancer and the drug regimen that is used generally causes sterility; by this we mean loss of functional spermatogenesis. In 80% of patients, however, there is recovery of spermatogenesis, which generally

occurs at 18 months from the completion of treatment.

Prognosis

The treatment of teratoma and seminoma is highly complex and requires patient management in centres of excellence, where the delivery of chemotherapy and the maintenance of patients during neutropenic and thrombocytopenic episodes can be successfully achieved. In the best centres, 95% of patients with good-prognosis tumours are cured, which is without doubt a significant advance in medical science, as young men with this malignant tumour can be returned to an active life within the community after treatment.

Prognostic indices have been described in detail by many authors. One of the more commonly used is described by the International Germ Cell Cancer Collaborative Group. Patients with non-seminoma are classified as having good-prognosis disease with a five-year survival of 92–95%, intermediate-prognosis tumours with a 72–80% five-year survival and poor-prognosis tumours with a 48% five-year survival. Patients with pure seminoma are described as having either good- or intermediate-prognosis disease. The classification into these categories is based on the presence or absence of non-nodal visceral metastases and serum levels of tumour markers. The influence of delay on prognosis is variably reported. Some authors link delay in excess of one year to a good prognosis, although this is described as being associated with a poor prognosis by other authors.

New treatment

Testicular cancer remains an exclusively chemosensitive disease even at progression, and for this reason almost every new drug that has been developed for oncology has been applied to this condition. Amongst this new group of chemotherapy agents, the taxanes and gemcitabine have shown promise. Imatinib (Glivec), a c-KIT antagonist, has been applied to the treatment of testicular cancer. There are case reports of activity but no major trial evidence for a response to imatinib.

Chapter 18

Gynaecological cancers

In 1951, George and Margaret Gey and Mary Kubicek developed HeLa, the first human cancer continuous cell line. It proliferates in tissue culture and has been the basis of a great deal of research into cancer biology and drug development. The sample originated from the cervical cancer of a young black woman, Henrietta Lacks of Baltimore. Many thousands of tons of HeLa cells are now found in the incubators and freezers of laboratories around the world. Unfortunately the patient died less than a year after the cell line was established, and her family are said to be shocked by the development and proliferation of the cell line, which was obtained presumably without consent at the time. Gynaecological tumours are not restricted to humans; female Asian elephants and rhinos are particularly susceptible to uterine fibromata.

Gynaecological cancers range from gestational trophoblastic tumours, which are associated with probably the highest survival of any malignant tumour, to ovarian cancers where fewer than a third of women will survive five years. The registration and prognosis data for the commoner tumours are shown in Table 18.1.

Gynaecological cancers include gestational trophoblastic disease, cervical cancer, endometrial cancer and ovarian cancer and will be discussed in more detail in the following four chapters.

Table 18.1 Gynaecological cancer registration data for UK and five-year survival rates.

Tumour	Percentage of female registrations	Rank of female registrations	Lifetime chance of cancer	Change in ASR, 1997–2006	5-year survival
Cervix	2%	12th	1 in 136	−16%	66%
Endometrium	4%	5th	1 in 73	+20%	77%
Ovary	5%	6th	1 in 48	−7%	41%

ASR, age-standardized rate.

Lecture Notes: Oncology, 2nd edition. By M. Bower and J. Waxman. Published 2010 by Blackwell Publishing Ltd.

Chapter 19

Gestational trophoblastic disease

Gestational trophoblastic tumours originate from placental tissues and are among the few human cancers that can be cured, even in the presence of widespread metastasis. The term gestational trophoblastic disease (GTD) covers hydatidiform molar pregnancies, invasive moles, choriocarcinomas and placental site trophoblastic tumours. Half of the women with choriocarcinoma develop GTD after a molar pregnancy; the remainder have previously had non-molar gestations. Since GTD is relatively rare but can be treated with very high cure rates, all patients should be referred to specialist national units.

Epidemiology and pathogenesis

The incidence of GTD varies geographically, with the highest rates reported from Asia, and the risk rises with maternal age and a history of prior molar pregnancy. In the UK, hydatidiform moles account for one in 1000 pregnancies and about 10% of these will progress to persistent trophoblastic disease requiring chemotherapy. Cytogenetic and molecular analysis of hydatidiform moles has provided a clue as to their origin (Figure 19.1). The majority of complete moles have a 46XX karyotype, with both X-chromosomes of paternal origin

(androgenetic). They are believed to originate from fertilization of an empty ovum by a haploid sperm that then underwent duplication. In contrast, partial moles contain both maternal and paternal DNA and are typically triploid 69XXY, presumably as a result of fertilization of a single ovum by two sperm. It is thought that this developmental abnormality affecting uniparental diploid cells (in this case androgenetic, 46XX) is due to genomic imprinting. The expression of some genes is determined by their parental origin – whether the allele was inherited from the mother or father – and this persists through multiple rounds of DNA amplification. This parent-of-origin effect is known as genomic imprinting and only affects a minority of genes. Genomic imprinting is an epigenetic phenomenon that does not rely on changes to the DNA base sequence but rather on methylation of individual bases. One example of imprinting in humans is the insulin-like growth factor 2 (IGF2) gene. Only the paternal copy of IGF2 is expressed in foetal life; the maternal gene is said to be 'imprinted'. The relaxation of this maternal imprinting results in congenital Beckwith–Weidemann syndrome: gigantism, macroglossia, exophthalmos, neonatal hypoglycaemia and predisposition to childhood cancers, including Wilms' tumour, rhabdomyosarcoma and adrenal tumours. Imprinting is also responsible for paired congenital syndromes on chromosome 15q11. This region is differently imprinted in maternal

Lecture Notes: Oncology, 2nd edition. By M. Bower and J. Waxman. Published 2010 by Blackwell Publishing Ltd.

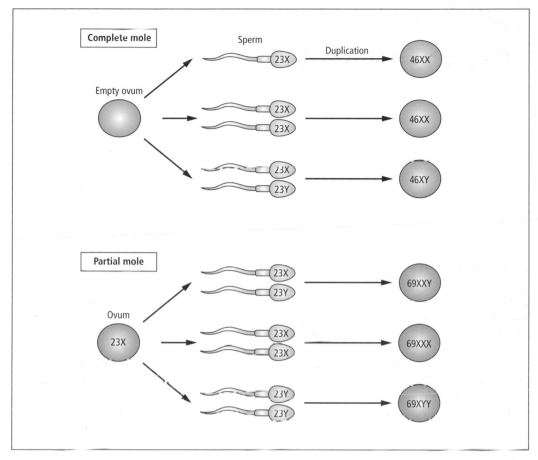

Figure 19.1 Possible chromosomal origin of complete and partial hydatidiform moles.

and paternal chromosomes, and both imprintings are needed for normal development. In a normal individual, the maternal allele is methylated, while the paternal allele is unmethylated. Some individuals fail to inherit a properly imprinted 15q11 from one parent, either due to deletion of the 15q11 region from that parent's chromosome 15 or rarely due to uniparental disomy (in which both copies have been inherited from the one parent). If neither copy of 15q11 has paternal imprinting, the result is Prader–Willi syndrome (characterized by hypotonia, obesity and hypogonadism). If neither copy has maternal imprinting, the result is the Angelman syndrome (characterized by epilepsy, tremors and a perpetually smiling facial expression).

Presentation

Women with trophoblastic disease usually present with antepartum haemorrhage, passing grape-like particles during early pregnancy, anaemia and hyperemesis. Hyperthyroidism may occur because human chorionic gonadotrophin (HCG) acts as a weak thyroid-stimulating hormone (TSH) receptor agonist, due to homology between β-subunits of HCG and TSH, which has been called molecular mimicry. Metastases are typically haemorrhagic. The most frequent sites are the lungs and brain, where they mimic pulmonary thromboembolic disease and subarachnoid haemorrhage. It is therefore always worthwhile performing a pregnancy test in women with these presentations, since normal serum or urine HCG levels exclude this diagnosis. Choriocarcinoma, although rare, is an important diagnosis, as the tumour is exquisitely sensitive to chemotherapy and over 95% of women with this diagnosis can be cured. The definitive diagnostic investigations are a quantitative serum HCG assay and pelvic ultrasonography with colour Doppler flow measurement. Most cases of choriocarcinoma follow a hydatidiform molar pregnancy, although it may also occur after either spontaneous abortion or normal-term pregnancy. If choriocarcinoma follows a molar pregnancy, molecular analysis reveals that the tumour DNA is entirely androgenetic, being derived from the father, with the loss of all maternal alleles. In contrast, post-term choriocarcinoma has a biparental genotype. Nonetheless, all cases of choriocarcinoma include paternal DNA sequences that are absent from the patient's genome and may be used to confirm the diagnosis genetically if necessary.

Treatment

Gestational trophoblastic disease was the first cancer to be cured by chemotherapy alone in the early 1960s. A scoring scheme has been devised that determines the risk of developing drug resistance to methotrexate, and women at low risk can be successfully treated with single-agent methotrexate, with very high success rates and very few long-term sequelae. Women at higher risk of resistance require combination chemotherapy schedules, which, although still highly successful, run a small risk of second malignancy. Serum HCG acts as the ideal tumour marker in this disease. HCG can be used to screen women following a molar pregnancy, to identify persistent trophoblastic disease that requires chemotherapy. Serum HCG can be used as a diagnostic investigation and in some circumstances obviates the need for a tissue diagnosis. Serum HCG levels form part of the prognostic scoring index and can be used to follow treatment: to determine the effectiveness of treatment and to detect remission or chemoresistance. Finally, HCG can be used in follow-up to identify relapse.

Prognosis

The prognosis of gestational trophoblastic tumours is excellent, with the rare exceptions of placental site histological subtype. The cure rates exceed 95%, and much of the current focus of clinical research is aimed at minimizing the long-term side effects of any treatment rather than attempts to increase the cure rates.

Chapter 20

Cervical cancer

Epidemiology and pathogenesis

Cancer of the cervix is thought to affect over one-third of a million women worldwide and represents 10% of all female cancers. Eighty percent of all cases of cervical cancer occur in the developing world. The incidence in the UK, as in many developed countries, is decreasing. In 2007, 2800 women were diagnosed and 941 women died of cervical cancer in the UK. In the UK, cervical cancer is the seventh most common of all female cancers, representing 2.5% of all cancer cases.

Invasive cervical cancer is believed to be the final stage in a continuum that starts with cervical infection by high-risk genotypes of human papillomavirus (HPV) and progresses via cervical intraepithelial neoplasia (CIN) to invasive cancer. CIN is a cytological diagnosis and is divided into three grades (CIN1–3). The histological equivalent of CIN is the squamous intraepithelial lesion (SIL), which is divided into low-grade SIL (LGSIL) that is similar to CIN1, and high-grade SIL (HGSIL) analogous to CIN2 and CIN3.

The decline in incidence of cervical cancer is associated with the development of the screening programmes, which began in 1964. Screening is based upon cervical smear assessment, and the current recommendation is for three-yearly screening. Four and a half million women are screened annually in the UK, and there has been a decline of 40% in the age-specific incidence over the last 20 years. Mortality has also decreased, falling from 11.2 deaths per 100000 women in 1950 to 2.4 in 2007. Screening is currently a subjective process, which, although well regulated, may be subject to human error. The accuracy of screening is likely to improve with the integration of molecular biological approaches to the process such as screening for the HPV genome.

Cervical cancer is associated with smoking, promiscuity, low socioeconomic status, the use of oral contraceptives, genital warts, herpes simplex virus 2 infection and, most particularly, infection with HPV 16 and 18. The average age of women with cervical cancer ranges from 35 to 44 years.

Presentation

Women with cervical cancer may present to their doctors with inter-menstrual bleeding, post-coital bleeding or painful intercourse. There may frequently be a vaginal discharge that can be bloody or offensive or symptoms suggestive of a urinary infection such as urinary frequency or urgency. When the cancer has spread, common symptoms include back pain due to enlarged abdominal lymph nodes or referred pain in the legs due to involvement of the nerve plexuses of the pelvis. These symptoms may be accompanied by loss of

Lecture Notes: Oncology, 2nd edition. By M. Bower and J. Waxman. Published 2010 by Blackwell Publishing Ltd.

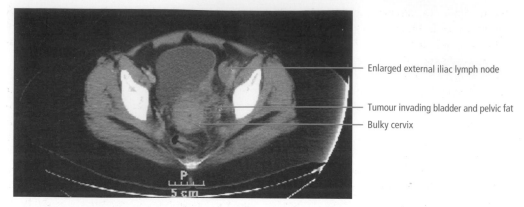

Figure 20.1 Cervical cancer with extensive, locally infiltrating tumour. This CT scan of a 65-year-old woman who had never had a cervical smear shows a bulky cervix with loss of the normal fat plane that separates it from the bladder. There is extension of the invasive cervical cancer into the posterolateral bladder wall anteriorly and into the pelvic fat laterally. There is also an enlarged left external iliac lymph node. The staging was therefore T4N1M0 (IVA).

weight. The examination should include an assessment of the patient's general state of health together with palpation of the abdomen and a vaginal assessment. This may confirm the presence of a discharge and reveal a cervical mass (Figure 20.1).

Outpatient diagnosis

The GP should refer the patient to a gynaecologist who will repeat the examination, take smears from the cervix for cytological examination and then organize admission for examination under anaesthesia and cervical biopsy. Colposcopy should be performed as an outpatient procedure prior to admission. This technique allows direct visualization of the cervix with properly directed biopsies. After these assessments have been performed and a histological diagnosis has been obtained, staging investigations should be organized. These should include a full blood count, profile, chest X-ray and a CT or magnetic resonance scan of the abdomen and pelvis.

Staging and grading

Carcinoma of the cervix is staged as a result of these findings as follows:
• Stage 0: carcinoma *in situ*. Intraepithelial carcinoma grades 1–3

• Stage 1A: microscopic disease confined to the cervix
• Stage 1B: disease confined to the cervix and greater than stage 1A
• Stage 2A: carcinoma extending beyond the cervix without parametrial involvement
• Stage 2B: parametrial involvement
• Stage 3A: extension to the pelvic side wall
• Stage 3B: extension to the pelvic wall with hydronephrosis or a non-functioning kidney
• Stage 4A: extension beyond the true pelvis to adjacent organs
• Stage 4B: spread to distant organs.

Sixty-six percent of cervical cancers are squamous cell tumours. These are graded as G1, G2 or G3 tumours, according to their microscopic appearance: G1 tumours are well differentiated, G2 tumours moderately and G3 tumours poorly differentiated. Fifteen percent are adenocarcinomas, and these are also graded G1–3. Other rarer tumours include small cell cancers and lymphomas. Carcinomas *in situ* are graded I–III and abbreviated to CIN or CGIN, depending on whether squamous or adenocarcinoma cells are present.

Treatment

The treatment of cervical cancer depends upon the stage of disease. Stage 0 carcinoma of the cervix should be treated by cone biopsy or by surgical excision. Stage 1A disease can sometimes be managed by cone biopsy or local excision but usually by hysterectomy. Stage 1B and 2A cervical cancer is usually treated by either radical hysterectomy with pelvic lymphadenectomy or by pelvic irradiation. Both methods are equally effective in the long-term control of the disease. Stage 2B and 3 carcinoma of the cervix should be treated by pelvic radiotherapy and stage 4 carcinoma with chemotherapy.

Patients treated with pelvic radiotherapy with curative intent are frequently prescribed additional concurrent adjuvant chemotherapy. Typically, patients will be treated with weekly courses of single-agent cisplatin. Chemoradiation has been subjected to a number of randomized trials, and it has been concluded that concomitant chemoradiation appears to improve overall survival and progression-free survival in locally advanced cervical cancer. Progressive or metastatic cervical carcinoma is treated with combination chemotherapy usually using a PMB regimen that contains cisplatin, methotrexate and bleomycin.

Carcinoma *in situ*

As a result of treatment, virtually 100% of patients with CIN disease are cured. Approximately 0.05–0.3% of treated women subsequently develop invasive carcinoma. If CIN is left untreated, then over a 30-year follow-up period, 10–40% of patients will develop invasive cancer. The evidence for this is based on data from a single study carried out in New Zealand of untreated patients with CIN, by a clinician who apparently was convinced that CIN did not progress.

Prognosis

Approximately 5% of patients treated for stage 1A carcinoma of the cervix will progress to develop advanced disease. 65 to 85% of all patients with stage 1B and 2A carcinoma of the cervix survive five years after treatment by a radical hysterectomy or radiation. The chance for a cure is smaller in stage 2B disease, and the expectation is that approximately 50–65% survive with radiotherapy

alone. About 40–60% of patients with stage 3A disease, and 25–45% of patients with stage 3B disease, survive five years and are treated with radiotherapy and frequently with chemotherapy.

These statistics are relevant to patients with squamous cancers or adenocarcinomas. Variant histologies, such as small cell carcinomas, are associated with a poor prognosis, with the expectation that, even at an early stage, survival is less than 5% at 5 years.

Patients with stage 4 cervical cancer do very poorly. In this situation, it is very unlikely that a cure will be achieved. Chemotherapy is the treatment of first choice. A number of agents have activity in the order of 15% and their combination is accompanied by some synergy of effect. The most commonly applied treatment programme involves the combination of cisplatin, methotrexate and bleomycin. About 30–40% of patients will respond to treatment, but durable cures are rare. Chemotherapy is associated with toxicity, and this includes nausea and vomiting, hair loss, infections and kidney failure. Because of the toxicities of treatment, an alternative approach is to palliate symptoms with pain killers alone.

Terminal care

In the terminal phases of illness, patients with cervical cancer may have a number of problems that prove difficult to manage. These include fistulae from the vagina to bladder and from the rectum to vagina or bladder, as a result of local progression of the tumour. Obstruction of kidney function may occur as a result of blockage of the ureters, either by enlarged lymph nodes or by tumour from the cervix growing within the pelvis, blocking the ureters. These situations can be treated surgically, in which case a colostomy or ileostomy may be formed, relieving bowel or ureteric obstruction, or radiologically by the passage of a stent to reverse obstructive damage to the kidneys.

New treatment

We hope that with the successful introduction of HPV vaccination and the institution of public health measures to eliminate smoking, there will be no need for treatment of cervical cancer in the future. In the developing world this utopian view may be a little optimistic. A number of vaccines have become available for the prevention of cervical cancer. It is estimated that there will be a significant reduction in cervical cancer rates, but only when 90% of all girls aged 11–12 years have been vaccinated for many years. New quadrivalent vaccines given to women who are seropositive for HPV lead to major increases in antibodies directed against HPV 16 or 18, and it may be that this initiative prevents the development of invasive cervical cancer in HPV seropositive patients.

Chapter 21

Endometrial cancer

Epidemiology and pathogenesis

The key to endometrial function lies in the effects of oestrogen and progesterone on the endometrium, enabling it to progress through the normal menstrual cycle and to prepare for embryo implantation. Oestrogen stimulates proliferation in the glands and stroma. Progesterone inhibits mitotic activity and stimulates secretion in the glands and decidualization of the stroma, where the cells acquire more cytoplasm. It is therefore perhaps not surprising that unopposed oestrogens will promote continuous mitotic activity, leading to cancers. Endometrial cancer is associated with elevated endogenous levels of free oestrogens due to falls in sex hormone-binding globulin or to increased aromatization and sulphation of androgens (androstenedione to oestrone). Thus, endometrial cancer is ten times more common in obese women due to peripheral conversion of androstenedione to oestrone by extraglandular aromatization in adipose tissue. Exogenous oestrogens also increase the risk of endometrial cancer. The use of unopposed oestrogens carries a 4–8-fold relative risk, especially in hormone replacement therapy, which is abrogated almost completely by combining progesterone with oestrogen. A great

deal of attention has been paid to the induction of endometrial cancer by tamoxifen and has led to the development of new selective oestrogen receptor modulators (SERMs), including raloxifene. Although the benefit of tamoxifen therapy for breast cancer outweighs the potential increase in endometrial cancer, the relative risk is six to seven-fold. Screening for endometrial cancer in women with breast cancer taking tamoxifen has no proven benefit, but abnormal bleeding should prompt rapid investigation. Endometrial cancer is a feature of hereditary Lynch type II non-polyposis colon cancer.

Endometrial cancer is the fifth most common cancer in women in England and Wales (see Table 18.1). It rarely develops before the menopause, and, since it causes abnormal vaginal bleeding, it can usually be diagnosed at an early stage.

Presentation

These tumours present in postmenopausal women as uterine bleeding. Postmenopausal bleeding is always abnormal and requires prompt investigation. Hysteroscopy, which allows visual inspection of the uterine lining, is often used for diagnosis and can detect abnormalities in 95–100% of cases. The probability of endometrial cancer among women with postmenopausal bleeding who do not use hormone replacement therapy (HRT) is 10%. If

Lecture Notes: Oncology, 2nd edition. By M. Bower and J. Waxman. Published 2010 by Blackwell Publishing Ltd.

the transvaginal ultrasound scan is normal, this probability falls to 1%, so ultrasound allows the majority of women to be quickly reassured. Outpatient endometrial biopsy methods are now as accurate as dilatation and curettage (D&C), which requires a general anaesthetic.

Treatment and prognosis

The optimum treatment for endometrial cancer depends on the stage and grade of the disease and on the risk of tumour in lymph nodes. When the cancer is confined to the inner third of the myometrium, the lymph nodes are likely to be clear and total hysterectomy is usually sufficient as treatment. This applies to about 90% of women with endometrial cancer, and their 5-year survival exceeds 70%. In women with tumour that extends beyond the inner half of the myometrium or with regional lymph node involvement, adjuvant pelvic radiotherapy is widely used. This has been shown to reduce the rate of local recurrence but may have long-term sequelae, including lymphoedema.

It would appear that endometrial cancer can be divided into two different classes of disease, with contrasting outlook. One group of endometrial cancer patients have tumours that are strongly hormone receptor positive and have an excellent prognosis, whilst a second variant develops in the elderly, has atypical histology, is poorly responsive to hormonal therapy and has a poor outlook. Endometrial cancer of typical histology expresses receptors for oestrogen, progesterone and gonadotrophin-releasing hormone. The expression of these receptors leads to opportunities for hormonal treatment.

Patients with endometrial cancer do respond to chemotherapy and the current standard is for the use of combination therapy with carboplatin and paclitaxel, and this is of particular use in the atypical histology patient. Nevertheless, hormonal therapy is of use in the treatment of endometrial carcinoma, and excellent palliation is seen with treatments such as progestogens.

New treatment

There appears to be little benefit from the use of new chemotherapy agents for patients with recurrent disease who have previously received chemotherapy. Response rates to investigational drugs, such as the exotically named ixabepilone, are in the order of 10%. In the situation of recurrent disease, chemotherapy should only be administered with palliative intent. As in so many tumour groups, there is interest in the possibility of an effect of tyrosine kinase inhibitors. Uterine carcinomas stain positively for epidermal growth factor receptor in up to 60% of cases, suggesting that this receptor could be targeted for treatment. The tumour suppressor gene, PTEN, and the oncogene, PIK3CA, are frequently mutated in endometrial carcinoma, suggesting again a target for therapy. The steroid sulphatase enzyme is involved in the hydrolysis of oestrone sulphate and dehydroepiandrosterone sulphate to oestrone and dehydroepiandrosterone, and this is an important step in the formation of oestrodial. Inhibitors of the steroid sulphatase enzyme have been developed and shown to be of value in breast cancer. It is likely that these inhibitors would also have potential activity in endometrial cancer.

Chapter 22

Ovarian cancer

Epidemiology and pathogenesis

Carcinoma of the ovary is a common tumour affecting nearly 6600 women annually and leading to the death of 4300 women each year in the UK. Ovarian cancer is the fourth most frequent cause of cancer death in women. The average age at which the disease occurs is approximately 65 years. By far the most common pathological subtype of ovarian cancer is epithelial, and this chapter concentrates virtually exclusively upon ovarian epithelial malignancy. There is a familial association between breast and ovarian cancer. This relates to germline mutations in the BRCA1 and BRCA2 genes, which are associated with a risk approaching 60% of developing ovarian cancer. In an analysis of benign, borderline and malignant ovarian cancers, somatic loss of heterozygosity for BRCA1 was demonstrated in none of the benign, in 15% of the borderline and in 66% of the malignant cancers. There is controversy as to other associated risk factors of the development of ovarian cancer. For example, long-term oestrogen replacement therapy may be associated with the development of these tumours, and in one prospective study of over 31 000 postmenopausal women, the increased risk of the development of ovarian cancer was 1.7-fold. As in many other tumours HER-2 overexpression is significantly associated with poorer survival prospects. HER-2 expression occurs in a minority of tumours; that is, in approximately 20% of patients.

Because ovarian cancer patients generally present with late-stage tumours, attempts have been made to reduce this risk by population screening. One of the largest published studies involved the prospective screening of nearly 4000 women by annual ultrasound examination and measurement of the serum tumour marker CA-125. This led to the identification of approximately 350 women with abnormalities, and 330 of these proceeded to laparotomy. In this group, there were 30 patients with ovarian tumours, the majority of which were at an advanced stage; so it seems that the value of screening using current technologies is low. Future screening programmes may benefit from a more refined approach. One technique involves the use of surface-enhanced laser absorption and ionization protein mass spectra. This rather complicated terminology describes the simple process of the separation of proteomic spectra from sera by electrophoresis. A number of protein patterns were identified in women with ovarian cancer, leading to a specificity of almost 90% in the identification of ovarian cancer. This would seem to be of interest in the development of more accurate screening technologies, particularly if the protein identities could be targeted using a rapid diagnostic test. This approach, of course, assumes that ovarian cancer progresses by an orderly process according to early and late stage. This is by no means clear, however, and there is genetic evidence that early- and late-

Lecture Notes: Oncology, 2nd edition. By M. Bower and J. Waxman. Published 2010 by Blackwell Publishing Ltd.

Omental cake of metastatic ovarian cancer

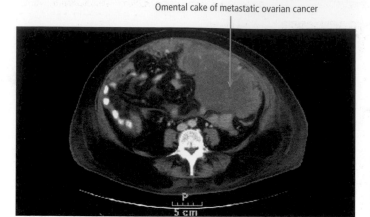

Figure 22.1 CT scan showing an omental cake of metastatic ovarian cancer deposits anteriorly with a large lobulated mass that extends from the midline to the left flank.

stage ovarian cancers may be different diseases that do not progress from one to the other.

Presentation

Patients with ovarian cancer usually present to their GPs with non-specific abdominal symptoms such as abdominal discomfort and swelling. There may be associated urinary frequency, alteration of bowel habit, tenesmus, colicky abdominal pain or postmenopausal bleeding. Patients with disseminated disease may have loss of appetite and weight. Early repletion is another common finding in the history. A patient with these symptoms should be examined by her GP, and if there is abdominal swelling or a pelvic mass, the patient should be referred on to a specialist gynaecologist for his or her views as to the patient's management. It is unfortunately the nature of ovarian cancer to present late, and almost 70% of patients have advanced disease at diagnosis. Patients with early-stage, localized tumours are often diagnosed as a result of the investigation of another medical condition.

The specialist should see the patient in outpatients and take a full clinical history and examine the patient. The examination should include a pelvic assessment. If the patient is thought clinically to have ovarian cancer, the investigations organized should include a full blood count, routine biochemistry, chest X-ray, a pelvic ultrasound and an abdominal and pelvic CT scan,

Lobulated heterogeneous ovarian cancer mass extending from the pelvis

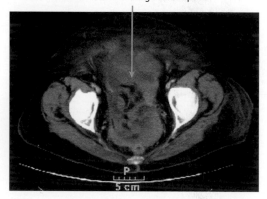

Figure 22.2 Ovarian cancer: pelvic mass. The CT scan shows a huge, lobulated, heterogenous pelvic mass that extends anteriorly. This mass was due to epithelial ovarian cancer.

together with measurement of serum levels of CA-125 (Figures 22.1–22.3 and see Plate 22.1). Ovarian cancer secretes CA-125, which is a glycoprotein. Approximately 80% of patients with advanced ovarian cancer have elevated CA-125 levels. Raised CA-125 levels may also occur in patients with almost any gynaecological, pancreatic, breast, colon, lung or hepatocellular tumour. CA-125 levels are elevated in a number of benign conditions including endometriosis, pancreatitis, pelvic inflammatory disease and peritonitis. Changing levels may be used to monitor treatment. If the tumour is operable, the patient should then be booked for a laparotomy. Surgery should be under-

Extensive mass of para-aortic lymph nodes

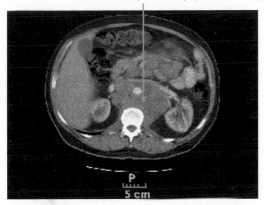

Figure 22.3 Lymph node metastases from ovarian cancer.

taken in specialist centres by a surgical gynaeco-logical oncologist. At operation, the abdominal contents are examined and, where possible, tumour debulking should be undertaken. This should include removal of the omentum, ovaries, fallopian tubes and uterus, with excision of all visible peritoneal deposits. The aim of surgery is to remove as much tumour as possible, optimally reducing the maximum diameter of any tumour deposit to 1 cm or less.

Staging and grading

Ninety-five percent of ovarian cancers are epithelial tumours. The classification of tumours is as in Table 22.1.

An attempt should be made to stage the patient's tumour. The staging used is the FIGO classification, which is as follows:
- Stage 1: growth limited to the ovaries
- Stage 1A: one ovary, no malignant ascites
- Stage 1B: both ovaries, no malignant ascites
- Stage 1C: tumour on ovarian surface or capsular rupture or ascites positive for malignant cell
- Stage 2: growth involving one or both ovaries with pelvic extension
- Stage 3: growth involving one or both ovaries with peritoneal implants or superficial liver metastases or abdominopelvic lymph node involvement
- Stage 4: tumour metastazing to liver parenchyma, pleura or other visceral metastatic sites.

Table 22.1 Pathological classification of ovarian tumours.

A. Epithelial	Serous
	Mucinous
	Endometrioid
	Clear cell
	Brenner
	Mixed
	Undifferentiated
	Unclassified
B. Sex cord/stromal	Granulosa
	Androblastoma
	Gynandroblastoma
	Unclassified
C. Lipid cell	
D. Gonadoblastoma	
E. Soft tissue	
F. Germ cell	Dysgerminoma
	Endodermal sinus
	Embryonal
	Polyembryonal
	Teratoma
	Mixed
G. Unclassifiable	
H. Metastatic	

Treatment

Treatment is defined by the FIGO staging system. If the tumour is confined to one ovary, the gynaecological oncologist may choose to observe the patient after definitive surgery. For stage 1A and 1B ovarian cancer, patients derive no benefit from adjuvant chemotherapy, and studies suggest that all patients with more advanced stages can be offered chemotherapy with benefit. Most specialists would agree that stage 1A or 1B well differentiated tumours can be observed, but adjuvant chemotherapy is increasingly offered to most patients with grade 2 and upwards disease irrespective of stage, and stage 1C and upwards irrespective of grade. Patients with early-stage ovarian cancer are usually offered single-agent carboplatin as adjuvant chemotherapy. Ovarian cancer is chemosensitive, and there is a long history of the use of chemical agents in the treatment of this condition. The discovery of responsiveness to single-agent treatments led to the use of combination chemotherapy programmes. Intensive treatment using multiple drug regimens was advocated throughout the 1970s and early 1980s.

For patients with advanced ovarian cancer it was thought during the early 1990s that single-agent therapy carboplatin was just as effective as combination treatments in terms of overall survival, although it was thought that there might be a minor advantage in terms of initial response rates and response duration to combination programmes. In the late 1990s, fashions changed again and treatment involved the use of combination therapy. There was evidence from randomized studies that combination therapy with cisplatin and paclitaxel had the highest response rates and in two high-profile studies showed superiority over another platinum-based regimen in terms of disease-free result and overall survival. In this century, treatment recommendations have come full cycle, and in the results of the ICON 3 study, a large trial conducted in the UK and Italy, single-agent carboplatin was not shown to be inferior to carboplatin and paclitaxel together. Ovarian cancer is, however, a highly heterogenous condition of many entities, and current advice from the National Institute for Health and Clinical Excellence (NICE) is that the patient and oncologist should discuss whether better benefit might be obtained from single-agent carboplatin or carboplatin and paclitaxel on a case-by-case basis.

Non-epithelial ovarian cancer is treated initially, where possible, by surgery. The procedures may range from oophorectomy to extensive tumour debulking. In relapse, or where a patient has presented with gross metastatic disease, treatment may involve similar chemotherapy programmes to those used for testicular cancer. Occasional responses are seen to hormonal therapy, using luteinizing hormone-releasing hormone (LHRH) agonists for those patients with ovarian malignancies secreting sex steroids.

Prognosis

Localized ovarian cancer constitutes 24% of all presenting patients. Patients with stage 1A and 1B ovarian cancer have an excellent outlook, with a 95% chance of survival. The survival of patients with stage 1C disease with ovarian cyst rupture is variably reported and depends on tumour grade. In one series, just 63% of patients survived five years. Approximately 60–80% of patients with advanced ovarian cancer respond to suitable chemotherapy. The median survival for this group of patients is 2.5 years, with less than 30% of patients surviving for five years.

New treatment

At present the main 'new' treatment for ovarian cancer consists of new lines of chemotherapy. Agents such as pemetrexed, gemcitabine, topotecan, oxaliplatin and ixabepilone have been shown to be effective. Chemotherapy resistance is one of the major features of patients with end-stage ovarian cancer, and this may be due to clonal evolution with gains of chromosomal material on the chromosomes 1 and 17 and losses at chromosome 3.

However, the explosion of targeted biotherapies informed by the results of the Human Genome Project is beginning to find its way into ovarian cancer clinical trials. The main targets under consideration currently are the epidermal growth factor (EGF) receptor's tyrosine kinase intracellular domain and its extracellular ligand-binding component, the vascular endothelial growth factor (VEGF) and its receptor, and the IGF/PI3 kinase pathway. Treatments are being developed from an understanding of platinum resistance, which may take its origin from BRCA1 mutant states and MSH4 suppressed states, which may respectively mediate platinum sensitivity and resistance.

Other targets for the modern therapy of ovarian cancer include small molecular weight inhibitors ('nibs') and monoclonal antibodies ('mabs'), and treatment with these agents has in some senses undergone a renaissance. The early antibody studies, with radioisotope-labelled antibodies directed against the human milk fat globulin given intraperitoneally as an adjuvant to systemic chemotherapy, produced some exciting, but non-reproducible, survival data. The development of new antibodies that are relatively specific to ovarian cancer is now offering real promise.

Chapter 23

Head and neck cancers

To the oncologist, the head and neck comprises six regions: the nasopharynx (the area behind the nose and pharynx), the oral cavity (including the lips, floor of the mouth, tongue, cheeks, gums and hard palate), the oropharynx (the base of the tongue, the tonsillar region, the soft palate and pharyngeal walls), the hypopharynx (the lower throat), the larynx (including the vocal cords and both supraglottis and subglottis) and the nasal cavity (the ethmoid and maxillary sinuses and the parotid, submandibular and minor salivary glands) (Figure 23.1). Although lymphomas, sarcomas, melanomas and other tumours may affect these regions, the term 'head and neck cancers' generally refer to squamous tumours, which make up 90% of cancers at these sites. Cancers of the nasopharynx include not only squamous cancers but also non-keratinizing transitional cell cancers and undifferentiated lymphoepitheliomas. The latter are the most common, and, unlike most other head and neck cancers, they frequently spread to distant sites. Tumours of the salivary glands are the most heterogeneous group of tumours of any tissue in the body, with almost 40 histological types of salivary gland tumours. Salivary gland tumours are more often benign than malignant. Sigmund Freud succumbed to cancer of the head and neck in 1939, attributed to smoking.

Epidemiology and pathogenesis

Head and neck cancers comprise 5% of all cancers in the UK and account for 2.5% of cancer deaths. They are twice as common in men as women and generally occur in those over 50 years old. The sites in order of frequency are: the larynx, oral cavity, pharynx and salivary glands. Over 90% are squamous carcinomas. Cancer of the head and neck is often preventable, and, if diagnosed early, is usually curable. Patients, however, often have advanced disease at the time of diagnosis. This is incurable or requires aggressive treatment, which leaves them functionally disabled. The optimum management of these tumours requires a multidisciplinary approach, including oncologists, otorhinolaryngologists, oromaxillofacial surgeons and plastic surgeons, along with clinical nurse specialists, speech and language therapists, dieticians and prosthetics technicians.

The incidence of head and neck cancers varies geographically, as does the most common anatomical site of these cancers. Smoking, high alcohol intake and poor oral hygiene are well-established risk factors for the development of head and neck tumours. In addition, Epstein–Barr virus is implicated in the aetiology of nasopharyngeal carcinoma in southern China, betel nut chewing in oral cancer in Asia, and wood dust inhalation by furniture makers, who may contract nasal cavity adenocarcinomas. In the UK, the incidence and mortality are greater in deprived populations, most notably for carcinoma of the tongue.

Lecture Notes: Oncology, 2nd edition. By M. Bower and J. Waxman. Published 2010 by Blackwell Publishing Ltd.

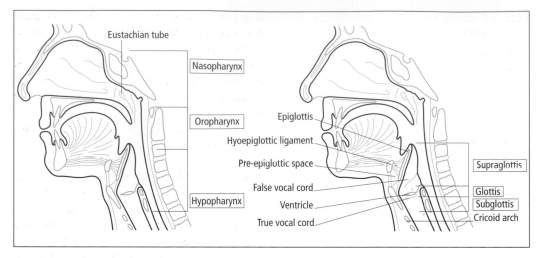

Figure 23.1 The head and neck.

Primary prevention by smoking cessation and alcohol abstention are the most effective methods of reducing the risk of head and neck cancers. Increasing awareness of head and neck cancers may encourage earlier referral and diagnosis at a stage when the cancer is still curable. In this respect, dentists play an important role in examining the oral mucosa. Retinoids may reduce the risk of both recurrence and second primary tumours in patients following primary therapy. Moreover, they may reduce malignant transformation in precancerous conditions such as leukoplakia.

Students who are concerned about biodiversity or just simply fans of the Looney Tunes cartoon character Taz may be concerned to learn that the carnivorous marsupial the Tasmanian devil has become an endangered species because of a head and neck tumour that threatens the survival of the whole species. Devil facial tumour disease is a parasitic tumour allograft transmitted between individual devils. The tumours are all derived from the same original cells. Transmissible cancer is extremely rare. The only other well-described example is canine transmissible venereal tumour in dogs, where again it is the actual cancer cells themselves that are spread from animal to animal rather than transmission of an infection that causes the cancer. Occasional similar cancer transmission has been described in humans. For example, organ transplant recipients very rarely develop cancers that are shown genetically to derive from the donor. Transplacental transmission of malignancy has also been described with spread of melanoma from mother to child.

Clinical presentation

Most head and neck tumours present as malignant ulcers with raised indurated edges on a surface mucosa. Oral tumours present as non-healing ulcers with ipsilateral otalgia. Oropharyngeal tumours present with dysphagia, pain and otalgia. Hypopharyngeal tumours present with dysphagia, odynophagia, referred otalgia and neck nodes. Laryngeal cancers present with persistent hoarseness, pain, otalgia, dyspnoea and stridor. Nasopharyngeal cancers present with a bloody nasal discharge, nasal obstruction, conductive deafness, atypical facial pain, diplopia, hoarseness and Horner's syndrome. Nasal and sinus tumours present with a bloody discharge or obstruction. Salivary gland tumours present as painless swellings or facial nerve palsies. Cervical lymph node enlargement as the presenting feature is not uncommon, particularly when the primary tumour lies in certain hidden sites, such as the base of the tongue, supraglottis and nasopharynx. Systemic metastases are uncommon at presentation

Table 23.1 Indications for urgent referral for suspected head and neck cancer.

Hoarseness persisting for >6 weeks
Ulceration of oral mucosa persisting for >3 weeks
Oral swellings persisting for >3 weeks
All red or red-and-white patches on the oral mucosa
Dysphagia persisting for >3 weeks
Unilateral nasal obstruction, particularly when associated with purulent discharge
Unexplained tooth mobility not associated with periodontal disease
Unresolved neck masses for >3 weeks
Cranial neuropathies
Orbital masses

(10%). Synchronous or metachronous tumours of the upper aerodigestive tract occur in 10–15% of patients.

A number of criteria for urgent referral have been established (Table 23.1). Diagnostic surgical resection of cervical nodes, without first determining the site of the primary tumour, may compromise subsequent therapy, increases the morbidity and worsens the outcome.

Treatment

The approach to managing these tumours varies according to their site, but in general the primary site and potential for cervical lymph node metastases should be considered. Small early stage 1 and 2 tumours, where there are no regional lymph node metastases, should be treated with surgery or radiotherapy, with 60–69% cure rates. The decision between surgery and radiotherapy is often determined by the anatomical site and the long-term morbidity. Function is generally better after radiotherapy but requires daily attendance for four to six weeks, whilst surgical treatment is quicker, but patients need to be fit for anaesthesia.

More advanced tumours are usually managed surgically, providing that the tumour is resectable. This is followed by adjuvant radiotherapy if the margins are insufficient, or if there is extranodal spread, multiple lymph node involvement or poorly differentiated histology. The resection of large tumours may leave sizeable defects, requiring myocutaneous flaps. Inoperable or recurrent disease may be treated with combinations of chemotherapy and radiotherapy, but outcomes generally remain poor, and in many cases of advanced disease symptomatic palliation is a more valued approach.

If cervical lymph node metastases are present, surgical resection is recommended, and, recently, more limited and selective neck dissection has been advocated. This preserves function, especially in relation to the accessory nerve, which, if sacrificed, usually gives rise to a stiff and painful shoulder. A scoring index can be used to predict the likelihood of metastasis to cervical lymph nodes. If the expected incidence of lymph node involvement exceeds 20%, neck dissection is usually recommended.

The addition of chemotherapy to radiotherapy, the use of hyperfractionated radiotherapy as well as intensity-modulated radiotherapy have all improved the delivery of radiotherapy for patients with advanced head and neck tumours, resulting in modest improvements in survival and declines in morbidity. The addition of the monoclonal antibody cetuximab, which targets epidermal growth factor receptor (EGFR), to radiotherapy has been shown to double survival in advanced head and neck cancer, especially tumours of the oropharynx. However, this widely quoted landmark phase III trial did not use cisplatin chemoradiotherapy, the gold standard therapy, as the control arm. Recurrent or metastatic tumour may be palliated with further surgery or radiotherapy to aid local control, and systemic chemotherapy has a response rate of around 30%. Second malignancies are frequent in patients who have been successfully treated for head and neck tumours, with an annual rate of 3%, and all patients should be encouraged to give up smoking and drinking to lower this risk. In addition, a number of studies have addressed the role of retinoids and β-carotene as secondary prophylaxis, but none have proved to have any significant effect.

Quality of life issues are especially important in head and neck cancers, given the anatomical site of the disease and the consequences of treatment, which can affect facial appearance, speech, swallowing and breathing. These cancers have enormous sociopsychological impact and may result in physical disability. These concerns must be addressed sympathetically with patients. Rehabilitation following treatment for head and neck cancers needs input from many professionals, particularly speech and language therapists, dieticians and prosthetics technicians. Rehabilitation, furthermore, requires enormous patience and effort on behalf of the patient. For example, 40% of patients will achieve communication by oesophageal speech following total laryngectomy.

Prognosis

Five-year survival rates for patients with head and neck tumours are listed in Table 23.2.

Salivary gland tumours

Salivary gland tumours represent around 5% of all head and neck cancers and affect both genders equally. They are most common in the sixth and seventh decades of life. Over half of the tumours are benign, and 80% originate in the parotid gland. Approximately 25% of parotid tumours, 40% of submandibular tumours and over 90% of sublingual gland tumours are malignant. Histologically, the most common benign tumour is the pleomorphic adenoma, and the most common malignant tumour is the mucoepidermoid carcinoma. Most patients present with painless swelling of the parotid, submandibular or sublingual glands.

Table 23.2 Five-year survival rates for head and neck tumours.

Tumour	5-year survival
Larynx	68%
Larynx (glottic)	85%
Larynx (supraglottic)	55%
Oral cavity	54%
Oropharynx	45%
Nasopharynx	45%
Hypopharynx	25%
Salivary glands	60%

Facial numbness or weakness due to cranial nerve involvement usually indicates malignancy and is an ominous sign. Pleomorphic adenomas, although not malignant, often recur if not completely excised, and a small proportion may become malignant if left untreated. Early-stage, low-grade malignant salivary gland tumours are usually curable by surgical resection alone. The prognosis is best for parotid tumours, then submandibular tumours; the least favourable sites are the sublingual and minor salivary glands. Larger or high-grade tumours require postoperative radiotherapy. Complications of surgical treatment for parotid neoplasms include facial nerve palsy and Frey's syndrome. Frey's syndrome is gustatory flushing and sweating of the ipsilateral forehead because the sympathetic nerve fibers to the sweat glands of the scalp and parasympathetic fibers to the parotid gland have reconnected wrongly after the auriculotemporal branch of the trigeminal nerve has been severed in surgery; instead of salivating the patient sweats.

New treatment

Conventional radiotherapy is delivered by photons or occasionally electron beams (β-radiation) for superficial tumours. However, particle beam radiotherapy uses hadrons (colour charge neutral collections of quarks bound by the strong nuclear force) usually protons, neutrons or positive ions. Proton beam therapy is the most commonly used of these techniques but is only available in one institution in the UK currently. The theoretical advantage of proton beam radiotherapy is that the higher mass of protons results in less scatter and a more concentrated delivery of energy to the tumour and greater sparing of normal adjacent tissues. Proton beam therapy offers promise in the management of head and neck cancers as well as other tumours located in anatomically challenging sites such as intraocular melanoma and retinoblastoma. In recent times it has been suggested that antiprotons (a fermion formed of two anti-up quarks and one anti-down quark) and pi-mesons (formed of an up and an anti-down quark) could be used as particle beam radiotherapy (Box 23.1).

Box 23.1: A brief lesson in fundamental particles

According to the standard model of quantum theory, the universe is made up of fermions (quarks and leptons) and bosons (force carriers). There are three sets of quark pairs and three sets of lepton pairs and for every particle there is a corresponding antiparticle, denoted by a bar over the symbol. Quarks are named after a quote in James Joyce's *Finnegan's Wake* 'Three quarks for Muster Mark!' and they carry three types of colour charge (which have nothing to do with visible colours). Quarks do not exist in isolation but are confined in colour charge neutral hadrons. Two types of hadrons exist, mesons that are formed from a combination of a quark and an antiquark, and baryons that are formed of three quarks. Protons are baryons formed of three quarks (uud) that carry a net +1 electrical charge, whilst neutrons are baryons with no net electrical charge (udd), and pi-mesons are formed by a quark (u) and an antiquark ([d̄]) and carry a +1 electrical charge.

Four forces or interactions are known, strong force, weak force, electromagnetic force and gravitational force. The force carriers or bosons for all but gravity have been identified. The strong nuclear force (also known as the colour charge) that holds protons and neutrons together in atomic nuclei is mediated by gluons exchanging colour charges with quarks. The weak nuclear force is responsible for lepton decay and β-radiation and is mediated by W^+, W^- and Z bosons. The electromagnetic force is, of course, mediated by photons whilst the force carrier particle for gravity has not been observed but nevertheless has been named graviton.

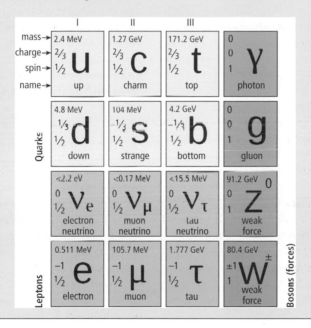

Chapter 24

Endocrine cancers

Endocrine cancers are a group of tumours whose clinical manifestations seem to delight old-fashioned physicians almost as much as they are concerned for the patients with these cancers. In particular, the products that they secrete give rise to many unusual syndromes. The majority of endocrine tumours are rare, with an incidence of 0.5 per million of population per annum. But others are more common, such as carcinoid tumours, which have a reported incidence of 1.5 per 10^5 of people per annum. These tumours are frequently listed as occurring in the context of multiple endocrine neoplasia (MEN). MENs are due to gene mutations. The MEN 1 gene is encoded at chromosome 11q13. The gene product is called, imaginatively, menin and encodes a nuclear protein that partners with JunD, NF-κB and many other proteins. The function of menin is, however, not known, and is lost in MEN 1. Mutations in MEN 2 lead to changes in the RET proto-oncogene.

The RET gene encodes a receptor tyrosine kinase and mutations at different sites within the RET gene are associated with MEN type 2A and type 2B, Hirschsprung's disease (congenital aganglionic megacolon) and medullary thyroid carcinoma. This one-gene source of multiple diseases is of course a blow to traditional paradigms of genetic disease but should perhaps be seen in the context of the shrinking genome. The number of genes postulated for the human genome has steadily fallen from the early days of the Human Genome Project, when it was speculated that 50 000–75 000 genes were present in the human genome, to the present 'post-genomic' era, when estimates have decreased to 25 000 genes only.

The MEN syndromes are described in Table 24.1.

Thyroid cancer, adrenal cancers and carcinoid tumours are discussed in detail in the following three chapters.

Lecture Notes: Oncology, 2nd edition. By M. Bower and J. Waxman. Published 2010 by Blackwell Publishing Ltd.

Table 24.1 Features of multiple endocrine neoplasia syndromes.

	MEN 1 (Werner's syndrome)	MEN 2A (Sipple's syndrome)	MEN 2B (also known as MEN 3)
Components	Parathyroid hyperplasia or adenoma (90%)	Medullary thyroid cancer (100%)	Mucosal neuromas (100%)
	Pancreatic islets adenoma, carcinoma or more rarely diffuse hyperplasia (80%)	Phaeochromocytoma (50%)	Medullary thyroid cancer (90%)
	Pituitary anterior adenomas (65%)	Parathryoid hyperplasia or adenoma (40%)	Marfanoid habitus (65%)
	Adrenal cortex hyperplasia or adenoma (40%)		Phaeochromocytoma (45%)
Genetic locus	Chromosome 11q13 Menin gene	Chromosome 10q11 RET gene	Chromosome 10q11 RET gene

Chapter 25

Thyroid cancer

Epidemiology and pathogenesis

Thyroid cancers are relatively uncommon malignancies. There were 1933 patients registered a year in the UK with this condition and 341 deaths reported in the last national statistics publication. There is a 3 to 1 ratio of women to men affected with thyroid malignancies. Radiation exposure is the most common predisposing factor to the development of thyroid cancer, and it was reported for many thousands of people across Europe following the Chernobyl disaster and in Japanese populations after the atomic bomb devastations.

Thyroid cancer includes a number of clinical entities, ranging from the classical papillary, follicular and anaplastic tumours to the atypic Hurthle and medullary cell carcinomas, as well as thyroid lymphoma. Mutations in BRAF(V599E) are seen in 40% of papillary carcinomas. Cyclin D1 overexpression is observed in approximately 50% of papillary carcinomas, while the transcription factor E2F1, which is part of the Rb oncogene signalling pathway, is upregulated in 80% of papillary and anaplastic thyroid carcinomas. Medullary thyroid carcinoma is associated with multiple endocrine neoplasia (MEN) types 2A and 2B (see Table 24.1). The RET gene encodes a transmembrane tyrosine kinase receptor. This gene is mutated in almost 100% of all MEN 2A patients and in 85% of patients with familial medullary thyroid carcinoma families.

Presentation

The most common presentation of thyroid malignancy is with a thyroid nodule or with cervical lymphadenopathy. Much less frequently, patients will present with features suggestive of advanced disease, such as vocal cord paralysis or with symptoms due to metastases.

Investigations

The diagnosis of a thyroid malignancy is made following routine investigations, which should include thyroid function, thyroid isotope scanning and thyroid ultrasound. Under ultrasound control, fine needle aspiration biopsy is used to obtain a cytological diagnosis and thereby define treatment. Other staging investigations should include CT scanning of the neck and thorax. Serum calcitonin levels are measured in patients with medullary thyroid carcinomas, while serum thyroglobulin can be used to monitor relapse in well differentiated carcinomas after thyroid ablation.

Lecture Notes: Oncology, 2nd edition. By M. Bower and J. Waxman. Published 2010 by Blackwell Publishing Ltd.

Treatment

After initial staging, patients with thyroid malignancies proceed to surgery. In the majority of patients with thyroid cancers, the surgical options are either subtotal thyroid resection, removing the lobe bearing the tumour together with the thyroid isthmus, or total thyroidectomy. Generally, partial thryoidectomy is only considered in those patients with low-risk tumours, for example those with a single focus of papillary carcinoma measuring less than 1 cm in diameter. There is no evidence that routine lymph node dissection has any added survival advantage. Subsequent to surgery, patients are treated with thyroid replacement, aiming to suppress thyroid-stimulating hormone (TSH) completely, which may be a driver for the development of recurrence.

When patients with thyroid tumours develop recurrent disease, further options for management may include surgery or radiation therapy. Surgery is the treatment of choice for patients with recurrent medullary carcinoma of the thyroid, which is relatively resistant to radiation therapy and chemotherapy. Radiation treatment is given both by using external beam radiotherapy and by treating with radioiodine, which localizes to thyroid tissue. Thyroid lymphomas are treated with standard lymphoma chemotherapy. Their prognosis is said to be poor, but this information is based upon limited clinical studies and may not be true. These data, however, do lead most clinicians to recommend that chemotherapy is followed by adjuvant radiotherapy to the thyroid.

Table 25.1 Five-year survival rates for thyroid cancers.

Tumour	5-year survival
Papillary thyroid cancer	80%
Follicular thyroid cancer	60%
Anaplastic thyroid cancer	10%
Medullary thyroid cancer	50%

Prognosis

Table 25.1 shows the five-year survival rates for thyroid tumours according to histological subtype.

New treatment

New treatments for thyroid cancers target the molecular changes seen in this tumour, and in particular it is possible that the RET oncogenes could be a target for treatment with small molecule tyrosine kinase inhibitors such as sorafenib and sunitinib. Laboratory work is showing that this group of compounds is effective in inhibiting kinase activity of RET/PTC3 and leads to reversion of the malignant characteristics of transformed thyroid cell lines. Sunitinib also causes a dose-related inhibition of growth of rat thyroid cells. Supporting this theoretical basis for activity is very limited clinical trial work, which shows a response rate of up to 30%.

Chapter 26

Adrenal cancers

Epidemiology of adrenal cortical cancers

Adrenal cortical cancers are likely to occur with an incidence of approximately one per million of population per annum. Adrenal cortical cancers are derived from the adrenal cortex and may be secretory. The major adrenal hormone products of these tumours include androgens, aldosterone and cortisol. Serum levels of these hormones may be elevated, and 24-hour urinary cortisol secretion may be increased.

Presentation of adrenal cortical cancers

Patients with adrenal cortical cancers generally present with non-specific symptoms, such as weight loss and general fatigue, or specific symptoms relating to their anatomical position, which include abdominal or loin pain. Adrenal cortical cancers may also produce symptoms related to the hormones that they secrete. Women may be virilized by the excessive production of androgenic hormones. Occasionally, adrenal cortical cancers are picked up as a result of an abdominal ultrasound or CT scan carried out for another reason.

Investigations of adrenal cortical cancers

[The patient with a suspected diagnosis of adrenal cortical cancer will generally be investigated in an endocrinological or surgical outpatient setting where routine blood testing together with specific endocrinological investigations will be arranged. These will include measurement of the adrenal androgens, diurnal cortisol production, adreno-corticotrophic hormone (ACTH) levels, 24-hour urinary cortisol levels, plain X-rays and CT scans of the abdomen, pelvis and chest (Figure 26.1).

Initial treatment of adrenal cortical cancers

Once staging investigations have been completed, the patient with a suspected diagnosis of an adrenal cortical cancer should be referred on to a specialist endocrine surgeon. The patient will proceed to laparotomy, and an attempt is made to resect the tumour. Surgery is complex, and there may be a major morbidity and mortality associated with the procedure. There is no clinical advantage to any adjuvant treatment.

Treatment of metastatic or locally advanced adrenal cortical cancer

The secretory symptoms of adrenal cortical tumours are unpleasant. Secretory symptoms are

Lecture Notes: Oncology, 2nd edition. By M. Bower and J. Waxman. Published 2010 by Blackwell Publishing Ltd.

Right adrenal phaeochromocytoma

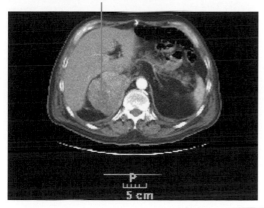

Figure 26.1 Adrenal tumour. This CT scan was performed on a 28-year-old man with hypertension and shows a lobulated heterogeneous right adrenal mass which was due to phaeochromocytoma.

most unpleasant in women because of a virilization caused by androgenic steroid production. These symptoms may include acne, hirsutism, change in habitus and increased libido. Attempts are made to block the production of hormones by an adrenal cortical cancer, using blocking agents such as metyrapone and ketoconazole, which inhibit steroidogenesis. Treatment may be given using OPDD, which is also called 'Mitotane'. Mitotane is a selective adrenal poison that is structurally related to the chlorinated insecticide DDT. DDT is a cheap insecticide developed in the 1940s that has cumulative toxicity in mammals. It is estimated that DDT saved 500 million people globally from malaria. In 1962, however, Rachel Carson published *The Silent Spring*, in which she attributed the declining song-bird population to widespread DDT use, and there since have been calls to ban DDT globally. The alternative insecticides are far more expensive, however, as they remain subject to patents owned by the pharmaceutical industry. Patients with adrenal cortical cancers are also pre-

scribed chemotherapy. Approximately 40% of patients will respond and the most effective agents include doxorubicin and cisplatin.

The secretory symptoms of adrenal carcinoma can be controlled with octreotide. This agent has no effect on survival and does not lead to reductions in tumour bulk.

Prognosis of adrenal cortical cancers

The outlook for the majority of patients with adrenal cortical cancers is very poor, except in the patient with localized, small bulk disease. For this group of patients, the expectation is for a 70% chance of complete cure following surgery. For patients with bulky tumours, the expectation is for a median survival of one year. Patients with metastatic tumours survive a median period of four months.

Adrenal medullary tumours

These uncommon tumours occurring in association with multiple endocrine neoplasia are a rare cause of hypertension. Phaeochromocytomas of the adrenal medulla produce their effects by the secretion of catecholamines, resulting in intermittent, episodic or sustained hypertension, anxiety, tremor, palpitations, sweating, flushing, headaches, gastrointestinal disturbances and polyuria. Twenty-four-hour urinary collection for urinary free catecholamines (epinephrine, norepinephrine and dopamine) is now the most widely employed diagnostic test, although some centres also measure catecholamine metabolites such as metanephrines and vanillylmandelic acid (VMA). The treatment is surgical and the results of treatment generally excellent. Metastatic phaeochromocytoma may be treated with ^{131}I-MIBG (meta-iodobenzyl guanidine), a catecholamine precursor, which may also be used to image the tumour.

Chapter 27

Carcinoid tumours

Carcinoid tumours are neuroendocrine tumours that may arise in numerous anatomical sites, particularly the gastrointestinal tract and lungs (Table 27.1). Much of their medical notoriety derives from their secretion of vasoactive compounds that give rise to the carcinoid syndrome. This usually follows the development of liver metastases, when first pass metabolism of these products is bypassed. Carcinoid tumours are much more common than previously recognized but the true incidence is not clearly known.

Presentation

Patients with carcinoid tumours may be asymptomatic or may present with symptoms due to the secretory products of their tumour, if there is significant metastatic disease. These metabolic products cause diarrhoea, flushing and occasionally bronchospasm. These symptoms are so specific that there is little difficulty in making a diagnosis, which is often achieved in general practice.

Investigations

The presence of symptoms is likely to indicate that the patient with a carcinoid tumour has metastatic

Lecture Notes: Oncology, 2nd edition. By M. Bower and J. Waxman. Published 2010 by Blackwell Publishing Ltd.

disease. The examination of such a patient should be confined to establishing the extent of disease and obtaining a histological diagnosis. The investigations that are required include a blood count, liver function test, chest X-ray and a CT scan of the chest and abdomen (Figure 27.1). Twenty-four-hour urinary 5HIAA (5-hydroxyindole-acetic acid) levels should be measured. This is because 5HIAA is the excretory product of the metabolites produced by carcinoids and results from the breakdown of 5HT (5-hydroxytryptamine or serotonin). There has been interest in the use of chromagranin A as a serum marker for carcinoid. This is a neurosecretory product that is of value because we can monitor carcinoid using this as a blood test, rather than having to carry out 24-hour urinary collections to measure 5HIAA.

Treatment

Pharmacological control

These agents act to block the synthesis, release and peripheral blockade of circulating tumour products. The list of drugs used in the treatment of carcinoid symptoms include inhibitors of 5HT synthesis such as parachlorphenylalanine, peripheral 5HT antagonists such as cyproheptadine, antihistamines, and inhibitors of 5HT release such as somatostatin and its long-acting analogues. The most frequently used somatostatin analogue is

Table 27.1 Comparison of carcinoid tumours by site of origin.

	Foregut	Midgut	Hindgut
Site	Respiratory tract, pancreas, stomach, proximal duodenum	Jejunum, ileum, appendix, Meckle's diverticulum, ascending colon	Transverse and descending colon, rectum
Tumour products	Low 5HTP, multihormones*	High 5HTP, multihormones*	Rarely 5HTP, multihormones*
Blood	5HTP, histamine, multihormones,* occasionally ACTH	5HT, multihormones,* rarely ACTH	Rarely 5HT or ACTH
Urine	5HTP, 5HT, 5HIAA, histamine	5HT, 5HIAA	Negative
Carcinoid syndrome	Occurs but is atypical	Occurs frequently with metastases	Rarely occurs
Metastasizes to bone	Common	Rare	Common

*Multihormones include tachykinins (substance P, substance K, neuropeptide K), neurotensin, PYY, enkephalin, insulin, glucagon, glicentin, VIP, somatostatin, pancreatic polypeptide, ACTH and α-subunit of human chorionic gonadotrophin. ACTH, adrenocorticotrophic hormone; 5HIAA, 5-hydroxyindole-acetic acid; 5HT, 5-hydroxytryptamine (serotonin); 5HTP, 5-hydroxytryptophan.

octreotide, and this leads to a relief of symptoms in 80% of patients for a median duration of 10 months.

Cytokines

Interferon has been used to treat patients with metastatic carcinoid tumours. Symptom relief will occur in between 50% and 60% of patients. Less than 5% of patients, however, achieve any significant tumour regression. Treatment with interferon is associated with significant side effects, which may include flu-like symptoms; for this reason, it is not generally given.

Complications of carcinoid hormone production

Carcinoid heart disease develops in patients with 5HT-producing neuroendocrine tumours. It is due to the formation of fibrous plaques within the heart, causing valvular dysfunction. Classically, the valves affected are right-sided. Right-sided heart failure due to valve disease is treated surgically by valve replacement. In view of the underlining excellent prognosis for carcinoid tumours, this condition is actively treated. Carcinoid tumours also lead, because of their secreted prod-

ucts, to fibrosis at other sites, such as in the retroperitoneum, where it may lead to small bowel obstruction.

Embolization

When metastatic disease in the liver is extensive, hepatic artery embolization may be considered. This involves selective cannulation of the artery with injection of embolic material. This will lead to sustained symptom relief in the majority of patients. There may be significant side effects from embolization, and so this procedure is not entered into without due consideration of the benefits. In some clinical series, mortality rates are 3–5%.

Prognosis

The prognosis for patients with metastatic carcinoid tumour is relatively good in comparison to that for most metastastic tumours. Patients with metastatic carcinoid tumour commonly survive a considerable time and the expectation, even in the presence of liver disease, is that approximately 36% of patients will survive five years and 20% for 10 years. In the absence of metastases and following resection of the primary, the outlook is excellent. Carcinoid tumours of different primary sites

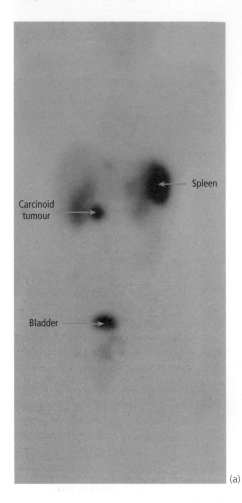

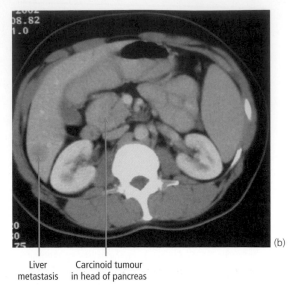

(b)

Liver   Carcinoid tumour
metastasis   in head of pancreas

(a)

Figure 27.1 (a) Indium-113-labelled somatostatin scan demonstrating a focus of carcinoid tumour in the pancreas as well as normal tracer uptake in the spleen and bladder. (b) Matched CT scan showing a tumour in the head of the pancreas and liver metastases.

are thought to have different outlooks, but this is very much debated.

New treatment

Carcinoid tumours highly express epidermal growth factor receptor (EGFR) but not ErbB. There is a potential therefore to treat this group of patients with EGFR inhibitors such as cetuximab or erlotinib. Neuroendocrine tumours express vascular endothelial growth factor (VEGF) and its receptor (VEGFR). Sunitinib, an agent that targets the tyrosine kinases of VEGF and VEGFR, has some minimal efficacy with up to 15% of patients improving and 70% having stable disease with treatment.

Chapter 28

Pituitary tumours

Pituitary tumours are common, and the most common are prolactinomas with an incidence of up to one in 3000 of the population per annum. Pituitary tumours arise from the anterior lobe and produce their effects by uncontrolled production of specific hormones, by destruction of normal pituitary tissues leading to hypopituitarism, or by compressing adjacent structures such as the optic chiasm, hypothalamus and bony structures (Table 28.1). Secretory tumours produce syndromes that cause gross clinical signs and symptoms. The local symptoms include headaches and visual field loss. The systemic symptoms produced depend upon the secreted product and range from acromegaly to pituitary Cushing's.

Treatment options include blocking agents, such as bromocriptine, neurosurgery and radiotherapy. The mainstay of therapy, however, is surgery,

Table 28.1 Comparison of clinical features of pituitary tumours.

Tumour	Percent of tumours	Morphology	Endocrine features	Neurological features
Prolactin-secreting adenoma	40%	Macroadenoma	Amenorrhoea, galactorrhoea, hypopituitarism in men	Headache, visual field defects
Non-secretory adenoma	20%	Macroadenoma	Hypopituitarism	Headache, visual field defects
Growth hormone-secreting adenoma	20%	Macroadenoma	Gigantism in children, acromegaly in adults	Headache, visual field defects
Corticotropin-secreting adenoma	15%	Microadenoma	Cushing's disease	Usually none
Gonadotropin-secreting adenoma	5%	Macroadenoma	Panhypopituitarism	Headache, visual field defects
Thyrotropin-secreting adenoma	<1%	Microadenoma	Hyperthyroidism	Usually none

Lecture Notes: Oncology, 2nd edition. By M. Bower and J. Waxman. Published 2010 by Blackwell Publishing Ltd.

which is important in establishing the histological diagnosis, in decompressing the optic chiasm and in relieving obstructive hydrocephalus, as well as in completely excising the tumour. A transfrontal approach is required for large tumours with extra-sellar extension, while a trans-sphenoidal approach is safer and tolerated better for smaller tumours. Radiotherapy may be used as the primary treatment for intrasellar tumours and as an adjunct to surgery for larger tumours. The outlook is generally excellent.

There are no classical oncogene mutations in pituitary tumours. However, there are clues to the development of this group of malignancies that come from dysregulation of the inhibitory components of the β-catenin pathway, and the relationship of this pathway to the cadherins. Both the Akt and MAPK pathways appear to be overexpressed in many pituitary tumours, and this causes an inhibition of the inhibitors of the cell cycle. This is equivalent to snapping the brake cable as you are bicycling down a steep hill.

Chapter 29

Parathyroid cancers

Parathyroid carcinomas are extremely rare, with an annual incidence of 0.5–1 per million of the population. Parathyroid cancers secrete parathormone, and for this reason the majority of patients present with hypercalcaemia. The hypercalcaemia is usually gross and, rather oddly, patients may be asymptomatic, with a calcium level that would normally be associated with death in the acute situation. The reason for this is that this condition generally has a long natural history and may have been present for many years prior to diagnosis. Calcium levels in excess of 4 mmol/l are frequently reported and the patient's cellular processes will have adapted to this level of hypercalcaemia. The primary treatment for this condition is surgical. The outlook for patients with metastatic disease is awful.

Lecture Notes: Oncology, 2nd edition. By M. Bower and J. Waxman. Published 2010 by Blackwell Publishing Ltd.

Chapter 30

Thoracic cancers

Table 30.1 Lung cancer registration data for southeast England from Thames in 2001 and five-year survival rates.

	Percentage of registrations		Rank of registrations		Lifetime risk of cancer		Change in ASR, 1997–2006		5-year survival
	Male	Female	Male	Female	Male	Female	Male	Female	
Lung cancer	15%	11%	2nd	3rd	1 in 13	1 in 23	−21%	+5%	6%
Mesothelioma	1%	0.2%	16th	>20th			+25%	+61%	8%

ASR, age-standardized rate.

In a celebrated television documentary *Death in the West*, produced in 1976 by Thames Television, the vice president of Philip Morris attempted to dismiss established links between tobacco and cancer. During the interview he said: 'Too much of anything can kill you. Too much apple sauce can kill you.' And: 'If there were something harmful in tobacco smoke, we could remove it'. Despite numerous court cases since, the tobacco industry continues to target the young and encourage smoking. It took until 1999 for the Royal Family to withdraw its royal warrant from the tobacco multinational Gallaher, which entitled them to display 'By Appointment' on packs of Benson & Hedges cigarettes. This was despite the death of the last

Table 30.2 Five-year survival rates for lung cancer and mesothelioma.

Tumour	5-year survival
Non-small cell lung cancer	8%
Small cell lung cancer	5%
Mesothelioma	5%

three kings from tobacco-related disease, including King George VI, who died of lung cancer.

Thoracic cancers include primary lung cancers and mesotheliomas, although a number of other cancers may occur in the thorax: particularly haematological cancers. Primary lung cancer has recently been pushed into second place in the ranking order of cancer registration in men (Table 30.1) and has a very poor overall survival rate (Table 30.2).

Lecture Notes: Oncology, 2nd edition. By M. Bower and J. Waxman. Published 2010 by Blackwell Publishing Ltd.

Chapter 31

Lung cancer

Epidemiology and pathogenesis

Carcinoma of the bronchus is the second most common tumour of men and the second most common cancer of women. The overall prospects for survival are poor: only between 5% and 8% of patients survive five years from diagnosis. Currently in the UK, there are approximately 39 000 men and women registered annually with carcinoma of the bronchus: 22 300 men and 16 600 women. The latest survival figures indicate that 34 500 of these people will die from their tumour.

The most important cause of carcinoma of the bronchus is smoking, and the incidence of lung cancer is directly related to the number of cigarettes smoked. Although the overall incidence of smoking is decreasing in the UK at a rate of a little under 1% per annum, there has been an increase in women smokers and in young smokers, and this bodes poorly for the future.

There are other risk factors for developing lung cancer. These include exposure to asbestos and heavy metals, such as nickel, and fibrotic disease of the lung. Air pollution is a significant factor in the development of lung cancers, and it is often said that living in London has the equivalent effect on lung cancer incidence to smoking five cigarettes a

SHIT!

day. Similarly, proximity to industrial pollution has a significant impact upon mortality rates.

As with so many other tumour groups, there is significant interest in the molecular biology of lung cancer. Amongst the first observations of the molecular changes in lung cancer were mutations in the Ras family of oncogenes, which have guanosine triphosphatase (GTPase) activity and are important as second messengers linking events between the cell membrane and nucleus. The history of the molecular biology of lung cancer reads almost like a contemporaneous commentary on the development of our understanding of the molecular biology of cancer, and the next to be discovered were mutations in the tumour suppressor genes Rb and p53 present in at least 80% of all small cell lung cancers. Loss of heterozygosity of a number of chromosomes has been observed in small cell lung cancer. These include chromosomes 3, 9, 12, 13 and 17. The changes in chromosome 17 involve the c-erb-B2 oncogene and this has led to the development of new therapeutic approaches to the management of lung cancer.

More recently, observations of abnormal DNA methylation of the cyclin D2 gene has been described in approximately 60% of small cell cancer lines. The cyclin D2 gene has a primary function in cell cycle regulation and has recently been brought to the general public's attention because of the awards of the 2001 Nobel Prizes to the scientists involved in this discovery who

Lecture Notes: Oncology, 2nd edition. By M. Bower and J. Waxman. Published 2010 by Blackwell Publishing Ltd.

included Sir Paul Nurse. Sir Paul Nurse according to *The Sun* is 'the David Beckham of science'. He later became the director of CRUK (Cancer Research UK) but that did not stop him saying that Margaret Thatcher did 'a good job of ruining British science'.

Presentation

Patients with carcinoma of the bronchus generally present with a cough or haemoptysis. This may be associated with weight loss and symptoms of metastatic cancer, such as bone pain (Figure 31.1) or jaundice. Patients with chest symptoms suggestive of a diagnosis of carcinoma of the bronchus are generally referred promptly by general practitioners to a specialist chest physician. One of the concerns of oncologists in the 1990s was the lack of referral on from specialist chest physicians to oncologists, with patients regarded somewhat as property and their treatment proprietarily. One of the major changes that we have seen in this current decade has come about as a result of the central promotion of the philosophy of the multidisciplinary team. As a result, there is multispecialty input into the management of lung cancer patients and it is the view of these authors that the care of lung cancer patients has generally improved throughout the country.

The signs of carcinoma of the bronchus are many and of particular interest is the observation of clubbing of the fingers occurring in non-small cell carcinoma of the bronchus. The aetiology of finger clubbing, which is associated with hypertrophic osteoarthropathy and polyarthralgias, has been postulated as including the secretion of parathormone (PTH) by tumours and also, more recently, the ectopic secretion of platelet-derived growth factor (see Figures 45.2 and 45.3). Other clinical abnormalities may include Horner's syndrome (Figure 31.2) or hoarseness, which are pointers to inoperability as a result of nerve entrapment by the tumour, and dysphagia which comes as a result of mediastinal nodal enlargement. Paraneoplastic syndromes are commonly associated with lung cancer, particularly the small cell carcinoma variant. These include cutaneous syndromes of dermatomyositis and acanthosis nigricans, the neurological complications of peripheral neuropathy and the Eaton–Lambert syndrome. The endocrine features of ectopic PTH, adrenocorticotrophic hormone (ACTH) and antidiuretic hormone (ADH) secretion are all spectacular in their presentations.

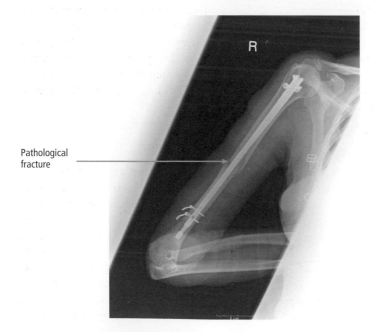

Pathological fracture

Figure 31.1 Pathological fracture of the mid-humerus in a patient with metastatic non-small cell lung cancer. The fracture has been pinned with an intramedullary nail.

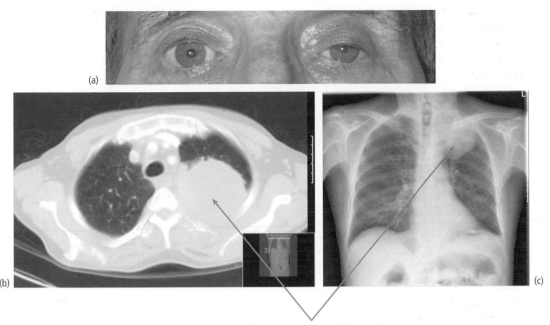

(a)

(b)

(c)

Non-small cell lung cancer at apex of left lung (Pancoast tumour)

Figure 31.2 (a) Unilateral ptosis and miosis (constricted pupil). The other features of Horner's syndrome are enophthalmos (sunken eye) and anhidrosis (no sweating). It is due to loss of sympathetic innervation due in this case to a Pancoast tumour of the left lung apex affecting the T1 nerve root (b, c) (also associated with ipsilateral wasting of the small muscles of the hand). Horner (1831–1886) was a Swiss ophthalmologist; Pancoast (1875–1939) was an American radiologist.

Investigations should include a full blood count, liver function tests, chest X-ray (Figure 31.3) and sputum cytology. Bronchoscopy is organized and should proceed within a few days (Plate 31.1). Biopsies and washings are then obtained and examined microscopically. By these means, a histological diagnosis will be achieved. Diagnosis may not be achieved in the context of peripheral lesions and if this is the case, then needle biopsies under CT scanning or fluoroscopic imaging should be arranged. (See also Figures 2.6, 45.1, 45.3, 46.1 and 46.5 and Plate 46.1.)

Pathology

There are a number of different variants of carcinoma of the bronchus, and these histological classifications are important in that they define the patient's further treatment. The main histological variants are squamous cell carcinoma, small cell carcinoma, adenocarcinoma and large cell carcinoma. For treatment purposes, tumours are described as either being small or non-small cell cancers. These constitute 95% of primary lung neoplasms. Squamous cell carcinoma accounts for approximately 40% of lung cancers, with adenocarcinoma accounting for 30% and small cell carcinoma for 25% of all lung tumours. Approximately 10% of lung cancers are of mixed histology. Rarer variants include carcinoid tumours, lymphomas and hamartomas.

Staging and grading

Lung cancer staging is usually by the TNM classification. Staging should include a CT scan of the chest and abdomen, a radioisotope bone scan, a liver ultrasound and ideally a positron emission tomography (PET) scan. Although not carried out routinely, examination of the bone marrow by aspiration and trephine in small cell lung cancer shows the presence of metastases in 95% of patients. Pulmonary function tests to assess vital capacity are essential, both to assess operability,

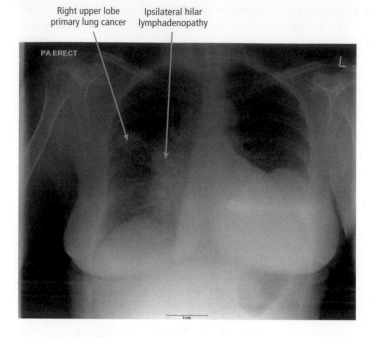

Right upper lobe primary lung cancer

Ipsilateral hilar lymphadenopathy

PA ERECT

Figure 31.3 Chest X-ray of a 67-year-old woman with T2N2M0 small cell lung cancer showing a right upper lobe primary lesion with extensive ipsilateral and contralateral hilar lymphadenopathy.

and to ensure that the patient is not left with profound breathlessness following lung resection.

Treatment

Treatment of non-small cell lung cancer

Non-small cell lung cancer may be treated with either surgery or with radiation treatment. Surgery is only possible for patients with limited stage disease; that is, T1N0M0 and T2N0M0 disease, and a small number with T2N1M0 tumours. There is increasing surgical enthusiasm for operating on more extensive tumours, and it is not uncommon to find patients with T3 disease proceeding to surgery. The results of this approach are poor, however.

The UK falls below the European average in terms of the number of people proceeding to surgery because of issues of resource availability in terms of scans and surgeons. Surgery has a significant morbidity and mortality, and operability depends upon lung function prior to resection, together with cardiac status and the presence of other major illnesses. It is estimated that approximately 30% of patients with non-small cell carcinoma of the lung

have operable tumours. The five-year survival for this group of patients is variably quoted at between 5% and 40%. A review of 2675 patients gave a five-year survival of 30%. There is a subgroup variation in survival, depending upon pathological staging and histology. For example, if those operable patients with adenocarcinoma are considered, the expectation for survival ranges between 38% and 79% and averages 65% at five years. If, on the other hand, operable patients under 40 years of age are considered, survival rises to 70%.

Radical radiotherapy, that is, radiotherapy given with curative intent, is considered for those patients who have inoperable disease by virtue of a poor medical state rather than spread of the cancer. Five-year survival figures of 6% were reported in a review of 1487 patients. Conventionally, patients receive 6000 cGy over a six-week period. More rapid treatment regimens are used, particularly in the north of England, and similar survival figures are found.

For the majority of patients with more advanced cancer, palliative radiotherapy is the only treatment option. This is given to patients who have symptoms as a result of their disease, which might include haemoptyses, breathlessness or chest pain.

Radiotherapy is given according to various pre-scriptions; some radiotherapists advise a single dose of 1000–1500 cGy, others 3000 cGy in 10 fractions over two weeks. Radiotherapy, too, has side effects, and these include tiredness, oesophagitis and skin changes.

There is a limited place for chemotherapy in this condition. Response rates for the most active regimens are in the range of 15–25%. The median survival of responding patients is six to seven months, offering only minor though statistically significant survival advantage over palliative therapy. Combination therapy using regimens such as MIC (mitomycin C, ifosfamide and cisplatin) is considered to be too toxic in view of the low response rates. Single-agent therapy using agents such as vinorelbine or platinum-based doublets have a role in the fitter patient, and may be used as primary neoadjuvant therapy in rendering operable the surgically inoperable patient and as adjuvant therapy following surgery.

Treatment of small cell lung cancer

Small cell lung cancer is an entirely different disease from non-small cell lung cancer. It is very rare for patients to have localized small cell lung cancer, and approximately 95% of patients with small cell lung cancer have metastatic disease at presentation.

The most important modality of treatment for small cell lung cancer is chemotherapy. The current chemotherapy programme of first choice is etoposide and cisplatin. Approximately 80% of patients have an initial response to chemotherapy with this and similar programmes, and this generally includes a complete remission rate of up to 60% of patients. However, the great majority of small cell lung cancers will recur after chemotherapy. Untreated, the median survival is three months. With treatment, 10–20% of patients will survive for two years and 5% for five years.

Treatment of paraneoplastic syndromes

Small cell lung cancer is associated with many paraneoplastic syndromes, due to secretion by the tumour of specific growth factors and hormones. One of the commonest is hyponatraemia, due to inappropriate secretion of ADH. This is treated by water restriction or tetracyclines. Steroids are prescribed in high dose for the treatment of polymyositis, Eaton–Lambert syndrome and the peripheral neuropathies associated with small cell lung cancer. Ectopic ACTH secretion may require high-dose therapy with adrenal enzyme-blocking drugs such as metyrapone and ketoconazole. Unfortunately, these two agents have toxicity in the dosages used and may make the patient feel awful. In this context, adrenalectomy may be rarely required.

New treatment

One of the most exciting developments of recent times has been that of specific therapies aimed at the molecular abnormalities expressed by cancer cells. The observation of aberrant epidermal growth factor receptor (EGFR) expression in non-small cell lung cancer has led to the hope that agents directed against this receptor may provide a therapeutic advance. The most interest recently has been around the use of gefitinib (Iressa) and erlotinib (Tarceva), which are EGFR tyrosine kinase inhibitors. There is some evidence of activity in non-small cell lung cancer, with disease stability being the best outcome. Women, non-smokers and patients with adenocarcinoma or bronchoalveolar carcinoma histologies are more likely to respond. These agents are used with a degree of optimism in patients with bronchioalveolar carcinomas and adenocarcinomas, with response rates of up to 30%. Response rates are highest in those patients with EGFR mutations reaching up to 80%. The proteasome inhibitor, bortezomib, has some efficacy in non-small cell carcinoma, but the best hope for this agent in terms of outcome is for stable disease. Future investigations of these agents hinge around their combination with cytotoxic chemotherapy and radiotherapy. Side effects are reported, the most common of which is an erythematous skin reaction, and the occurrence of this rash seems to be associated with tumour responsiveness.

Chapter 32

Mesothelioma

Epidemiology and pathogenesis

The incidence of mesothelioma has been steadily increasing, and it is estimated that the lifetime risk is around 0.5–1%. This tumour was originally described by occupational health doctors working in the asbestos factories in the East End of London around the time of the end of the First World War. It would appear, however, that this information was suppressed, and it was not until the 1960s that the association between mesothelioma and asbestos exposure was clearly publicized.

The development of mesothelioma is generally related to asbestos exposure, but this is not always the case. The risk of mesothelioma is not related to the amount of exposure. It may not only occur in the asbestos worker but also in family members exposed to the fibres of asbestos brought home in their spouse's, father's or mother's clothes. There are no specific chromosomal changes associated with the development of mesothelioma, but there are a host of abnormalities that may occur, which are entirely non-specific. Different asbestos fibres have different properties and carcinogenicity. The most carcinogenic fibres tend to be the needle-shaped blue (crocidolite) and brown (amosite)

asbestos rather than the commoner corkscrew-shaped white asbestos (chrysotile) (Table 32.1).

Presentation

Mesothelial tumours take their origins in the pleura or peritoneum. Patients with mesothelioma characteristically present with pleural effusions or ascites.

Investigations

The diagnosis of mesothelioma may be suspected from a chest X-ray (Figure 32.1), where a patient may have pleural thickening and an effusion. CT scanning will show the extent of the pleural or peritoneal tumour. The next step in the investigatory process is to carry out a pleural or peritoneal biopsy. Multiple biopsies are usually required to make the diagnosis.

Possibly the most important aspect of the care of patients with mesothelioma is to ensure that the appropriate compensatory mechanisms are put in place. In the UK, industrial compensation is usually arranged for patients by their union officers and involves an examination of the tumour by a pathology panel. It is enormously important for the patient and his or her family that the clinician signposts this process.

Often a pleural biopsy may not be sufficient to obtain diagnostic material, in which case

Lecture Notes: Oncology, 2nd edition. By M. Bower and J. Waxman. Published 2010 by Blackwell Publishing Ltd.

Table 32.1 Types of asbestos and cancer risk.

Type	Colour	Morphology	Usage	Cancer risk	Location of mining
Crocidolite	Blue	Amphibole needles	10%	+++	South Africa, Australia
Chrysotile	White	Serpentine corkscrew	85%	+	Canada
Amosite	Brown	Amphibole needles	5%	++	South Africa

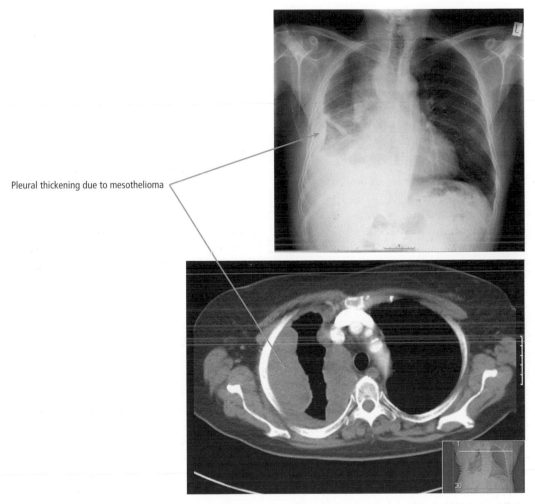

Pleural thickening due to mesothelioma

Figure 32.1 This chest X-ray and CT scan of a retired boiler-maker shows diffuse circumferential pleural thickening of the right hemithorax, extending to the mediastinal pleura. In addition there is substantial volume loss of the right hemithorax. The appearances are due to mesothelioma.

video-assisted thoracic screening may be required. Recurrent effusions are a dramatic problem for patients, and the intervention of a thoracic surgeon may be required to strip the pleura and provide an effective pleurodesis.

Treatment

Unfortunately, the majority of patients with mesothelioma present with incurable disease. Treatment options are limited. Chemotherapy is generally ineffective, with response rates in the order of less than 10% although newer combinations of cisplatinum and permetrexed offer promise. Radiation therapy may be helpful in controlling pain and is often given to pleural biopsy track sites to prevent the tumour growing down these channels. Multiple pleurodeses are often required, with installation into the pleural cavities of materials such as talc, tetracycline and bleomycin. There have been times when cytokine treatment was thought to be effective, with interferon being given into the thoracic cavity. This has, however, not proven to be a successful treatment option.

Prognosis

Unfortunately, the outlook for patients with mesothelioma is poor, with survival for patients with advanced disease ranging between 6 and 18 months.

New treatment

Recently, responses have been reported for pemetrexed, a dihydrofolate reductase inhibitor, and reductase. This is likely to become the standard. A 2009 analysis of survival in mesothelioma patients assessed 523 patients and defined progno-sis according to four risk groups, but for all these groups the median progression-free survival ranged from 2.1 to 5.3 months, an indication of how poorly responsive to chemotherapy mesothelioma is.

Mesothelioma patients have high circulating levels of vascular endothelial growth factor (VEGF), and mesothelioma tissue stains strongly positively for VEGF receptor 3. For this reason patients with mesothelioma have been treated with antibodies to VEGF, such as bevacizumab, and with angiogenesis inhibitors, such as thalidomide. Bevacizumab, a recombinant monoclonal antibody to VEGF, has not been effective but agents such as thalidomide have led to disease stabilization in patients with progressive mesothelioma. Approximately 25% of patients have stable disease for a period of more than six months as a result of treatment with thalidomide. Sorafenib, a multikinase inhibitor of VEGF receptor and platelet-derived growth factor receptors, has led to responses in heavily pretreated patients.

Mesothelioma is an awful tumour to have and there is limited hope for new therapeutic strategies. The one true hope that exists is in the reduction of risk to workers, which is little compensation for those currently suffering as a result of the global epidemic.

Chapter 33

Haematological cancers

Louis Leakey found possibly the oldest hominid malignant tumour in 1932 in the remains of either a *Homo erectus* or an *Australopithecus*. This tumour was suggestive of a Burkitt's lymphoma, although that nomenclature was certainly not in use then. The leukaemias, lymphomas and myeloma are amongst the success stories in cancer treatment, with major advances in the second half of the 20th century. Cancer chemotherapy started with the treatment of these malignancies in the 1940s, following the demonstration by Alfred Gilman and Louis Goodman at Yale of lymphoma regression in mice with nitrogen mustard and their treatment of the first patient in 1944. Shortly afterwards, Sidney Farber at Harvard began to use folate antagonists in children with acute leukaemia, and in 1947 he reported temporary remissions with aminopterin. Since that era, when childhood acute leukaemia was universally fatal, the long-term remission rate has risen to over 80%. Perhaps because of this success, medical oncologists and haematologists often fight over the management of haematological malignancies in the UK.

The leukaemias, lymphomas and myeloma are discussed in more detail in the following four chapters.

Lecture Notes: Oncology, 2nd edition. By M. Bower and J. Waxman. Published 2010 by Blackwell Publishing Ltd.

Chapter 34

The leukaemias

Epidemiology and pathogenesis

Leukaemias are relatively common with a preponderance of men affected. In the UK, the Office of National Statistics recently registered 4229 male and 3008 female leukaemia patients, with 2492 male and 1858 female deaths annually. The leukaemias are described generally as either acute or chronic. The main variants are lymphoid and myeloid leukaemia, which account for almost 95% of leukaemia. Acute lymphoid leukaemia is marginally more common than acute myeloid leukaemia (AML). Acute lymphoblastic leukaemia (ALL) is far more common in childhood than AML, and in adults approximately 80% of all the acute leukaemias are myeloid. Patients with Down's syndrome are at increased risk of leukaemia, as are patients with certain other conditions with a chromosomal basis, such as Klinefelter's syndrome, Fanconi's syndrome and ataxia telangiectasia.

The biology of leukaemia has been studied intensively over the last 20 years. With this investigation, the idea of a monoclonal origin of leukaemias has developed. The leukaemic clone is thought to have a survival advantage over normal haematological cells. One of the first leukaemias to be characterized at a molecular level was chronic myeloid leukaemia (CML), where there is a fusion between chromosomes 9 and 22 that juxtaposes the BCR and ABL genes, which is observed cytogenetically as the 'Philadelphia' chromosome. This molecular abnormality may be seen in other haematological cells, such as platelet and red cell precursors. The protein product of a fusion gene may have aberrant function. For example, the BCR-ABL protein is thought to provide protection from chemotherapy drugs by interfering with apoptosis.

Other hybrid genes of interest occur in the leukaemias. For example, acute promyelocytic leukaemias (APMLs) are characterized by a translocation between chromosomes 15 and 17. The resultant fusion gene is formed between part of the PML gene and the retinoic acid alpha receptor gene, RARA. This hybrid gene interacts with chromosomal histone deacetylase complexes. Treatment with retinoic acid leads to dissociation of this complex and a transient remission of the leukaemia. Some examples of the fusion genes seen in leukaemia are described in Table 34.1.

Point mutations and gene deletions are also seen in leukaemias involving oncogenes such as p53 and RAS. P53 mutations are seen in ALL and blast crisis of CML, and N-RAS and c-KIT mutations are found in AML. It should be noted that the predominant molecular change in leukaemia is chromosomal translocation. This is in contrast with solid tumours, where the predominant changes are gene deletions and amplifications.

Lecture Notes: Oncology, 2nd edition. By M. Bower and J. Waxman. Published 2010 by Blackwell Publishing Ltd.

Table 34.1 Chromosomal abnormalities and their products.

Abnormalities	Disease	Fusion gene
Altered transcription regulators		
t(12;21)	ALL	*TEL/AML1*
t(8;21)	AML	*AML1/ETO*
t(15;17)	APML	*PML/RARA*
Activated kinases		
t(9;22)	CML, ALL	*BCR/ABL*
t(5;12)	CMML	*TEL/PDGFRB*

Table 34.2 The FAB classification of acute leukaemia.

M0	Acute myeloid leukaemia with minimal evidence of differentiation
M1	Acute myeloid leukaemia without maturation
M2	Acute myeloid leukaemia with maturation
M3	Acute promyelocytic leukaemia
M4	Acute myelomonocytic leukaemia
M5	Acute monocytic leukaemia
M6	Acute erythroleukaemia
M7	Acute megakaryoblastic leukaemia
L1	Small, monomorphic
L2	Large heterogeneous
L3	Large homogeneous (Burkitt)

Although there is a greater understanding of the molecular biology of leukaemia, the reason for the genetic changes observed is not known. The exceptions are those rare leukaemias that occur in the context of exposure to radiation or as secondary events following chemotherapy. Such secondary leukaemias are commonly associated with chromosome 5 and 7 abnormalities (see Figure 3.11).

Presentation

The presentation of patients with acute leukaemia is remarkable in its dramatic onset. It is usual to obtain a history that dates back only a few days, with features of anaemia, thrombocytopenia and leucopenia, although some people date their symptoms back for much longer periods. Chronic leukaemia may be diagnosed as an incidental finding, for example when a blood count is performed as part of a routine screen for another medical problem. Patients with chronic leukaemia may have abdominal discomfort due to splenomegaly or present with anaemia or lymphadenopathy. Such presentations generally tend to be insidious; this is particularly the case for chronic lymphocytic leukaemia (CLL). The situation is a little different for CML, which progresses from a chronic to an accelerated to a blast phase. The diagnosis can be made at any point in this clinical course.

Investigations and classification

The diagnosis of acute leukaemia is made by an examination of the peripheral blood and bone marrow (see Plates 34.1–34.3). In ALL, a lumbar puncture will be performed in order to investigate the possibility of CNS infiltration. Two common cytochemical stains are used to distinguish between acute myeloid and acute lymphoblastic leukaemias. These are the Sudan black, which is usually positive in AML and negative in ALL, and the periodic acid Schiff (PAS) test, which is usually positive in ALL and negative in AML. The PAS stain is outmoded and has been largely replaced by immunophenotyping.

The classification of acute leukaemias usually follows the French–American–British (FAB) classification, which essentially describes the degree of differentiation and maturation. The myelogenous leukaemias are described as M1 to M7, and acute leukaemias as L1 to L3 (Table 34.2).

Immunophenotyping is also carried out in suspected acute lymphoblastic leukaemias, where the presence of B- and T-cell markers is sought out. More than 70% of adult acute lymphocytic leukaemias are of B-cell origin. Following immunophenotyping, cytogenic and molecular analysis is carried out in order to define chromosomal and molecular abnormalities, which provide prognostic information. Cytogenetic analysis is useful in the diagnosis of CML but may not be particularly helpful in CLL.

The 8;21 translocation in AML is associated with a good prognosis and occurs in about 8% of patients. The inversion or reciprocal translocation t(16;16) of chromosome 16 is associated with the M4 phenotype and again confers a favourable

Table 34.3 Chronic lymphocytic leukaemias.

B cell	T cell
B-cell chronic lymphocytic leukaemia/small lymphocytic lymphoma	T-cell chronic lymphocytic leukaemia (large granular lymphocytic leukaemia)
B-cell prolymphocytic leukaemia	T-cell prolymphocytic leukaemia
Hairy-cell leukaemia and variant	Adult T-cell leukaemia/lymphoma
Splenic marginal zone lymphoma, including splenic lymphoma with villous lymphocytes	Leukaemic phase of mycosis fungoides/Sézary syndrome
Leukaemic phase of mantle cell lymphoma	
Leukaemic phase of follicular lymphoma	
Leukaemic phase of lymphoplasmacytoid lymphoma	

response. Translocation with an 11q23 breakpoint is a poor prognostic feature. The presence of the Philadelphia chromosome is found in about 5% of childhood and 25% of adult ALL, and is thought to perhaps indicate transformation from a chronic myeloid leukaemia phase: this is an adverse prognostic feature. Chronic lymphocytic leukaemia (Table 34.3 and see Plates 34.4–34.6) is a tumour of B-cell origin in 95% of patients.

Cytogenetic changes are described in up to 80% of patients with CLL. Although there is no particular pattern that emerges to characterize this leukaemia, five or six abnormalities are usually observed. Trisomy 12, for example, the most common cytogenetic abnormality, is found in just one-third of patients. Patients with CLL are classified using a number of different systems, most of which are helpful in describing survival related to lymphocytosis, lymph node involvement and the presence or absence of anaemia or thrombocytopenia.

Treatment

The management of acute leukaemia is complex. It requires psychological support of the individual and of the family, and active and urgent treatment, particularly for the acute leukaemias. Initial treatment involves attempts to stabilize the patient by transfusion of red cells and platelets, combined with treatment of infection by antibiotics to limit the complications that may occur with the initiation of chemotherapy. These mainly revolve around the tumour lysis syndrome. Rehydration is

required, and the patient is started on allopurinol to prevent the metabolic abnormalities that are described in detail in Chapter 46 of this book.

The chemotherapy that is given to patients with leukaemia has evolved as a result of many clinical trials over very many years, involving the Medical Research Council (MRC) in the UK, and the Cancer and Leukaemia Group B in the USA. The mainstay of induction chemotherapy in adult has been the use of daunorubicin and cytosine arabinoside given in a daily schedule, the dosage and duration of which is varied and repeated upon recovery of haematological parameters.

During treatment, patients require supportive therapies with blood products such as platelets and red cells. Platelet support is given to keep platelet counts above 10×10^9/l, which limits the risk of spontaneous haemorrhage. There is a risk of immunization against platelets, which may require human leucocyte antigen (HLA) matched transfusions rather than random donor platelet transfusion. Patients are of course at risk from neutropenic sepsis, which is treated with intravenous antibiotics. Prolonged neutropenia may be associated with fungal infection. In the context of persistent fever, particularly following transplantation, antifungal therapy is instituted. CT scanning may be appropriate in order to diagnose *Aspergillus* pneumonia. There is little evidence to suggest that any prophylactic antifungal treatment is of value, but randomized studies have shown that prophylaxis with antibiotics such as co-trimoxazole reduces the risk of *Pneumocystis* infection.

With recovery of the marrow, a further bone marrow examination is carried out. The majority of patients will have entered complete remission just before the second course of chemotherapy. Generally, four to six cycles of treatment are given in all, and this may be followed by post-remission treatment using an allogenic autologous stem cell transplant. These approaches are used in younger patients who have entered their first remission. Approximately 50–55% of patients who receive a transplant will be cured, but there is no evidence of better survival after transplantation in the good-prognosis patients.

The management of patients in transplant programmes is, of course, highly specialized, and medical training is focused on the recognition of the problems associated with profound and prolonged immunosuppression. The management of transplant patients has completely changed in recent years, because of the availability of recombinant growth factors. The use of granulocyte colony-stimulating factor (G-CSF) in transplant programmes has reduced the period of profound neutropenia such that the average duration of stay on a transplant ward has decreased from 28 to 17 days.

The management of chronic phase CML has evolved over the years from the use of single-agent alkylating agents, such as busulfan and hydroxyurea, to the use of interferon alpha and then allogeneic stem cell transplantation. Real hopes of cure came with the application of transplant programmes to CML. In the last few years, the introduction of imatinib (Glevec), a novel compound that acts to inhibit the tyrosine kinase activity of the BCR-ABL oncoprotein, has been most encouraging. Between 80% and 90% of patients respond to imatinib. In about half of these responding patients, a cytogenic response is also seen. There have been no serious adverse side effects from treatment with this agent, which offers a dramatic improvement over conventional therapy. Unfortunately, late relapses do occur, although at present we do not know the median duration of response.

CLL may be an entirely indolent disease with an excellent prognosis, and for many patients treatment may not be necessary. Therapy, when it is required, is similar to treatment given for low-grade lymphoma, with single-agent chlorambucil, steroids and occasionally combination therapy, all being helpful.

Treatment of recurrent disease

Although 50% of patients with good-prognosis acute leukaemia survive, the majority of patients still die. Relapse generally occurs within the first two years. Patients are usually re-treated with chemotherapy, with a 50% chance of re-entering remission and a 10% chance of cure. It is usual in these situations to use a different induction drug regimen, which is frequently more intensive, with a greater risk of treatment complications and death. Recurrence in chronic leukaemia may require stem cell transplantation, but this is not the practice for CLL.

Leukaemia in young children

Acute lymphocytic leukaemia is the commonest childhood leukaemia. Overall, the prospects for cure are very good, with a chance in excess of 80% of a sustained remission. The treatment of acute childhood leukaemia owes a great debt to the MRC-organized trials, which have examined issues such as the duration of therapy both for induction and maintenance, the need for cranial irradiation to prevent central nervous system relapse and the value of the individual drugs within the treatment programmes. Because of the high likelihood of a cure, recent clinical trials have concentrated on trying to moderate the side effects of treatment, and these are particularly important in limiting neurological toxicity, such as the effects upon intelligence, personality and pituitary function, and the effects on growth and fertility.

New treatment

In many ways, the future is 'here and now' for leukaemia. The treatment of CML has recently been transformed by the development of imatinib. Imatinib binds to the BCR-ABL protein, inhibiting its kinase activity and effectively controlling disease driven by this kinase. Remissions in CML are seen with clearance of the Philadelphia chromosome, as shown by cytogenetic analysis. Imatinib resistance emerges as a consequence of mutations in the kinase domains of BCR-ABL and new inhibitors including dasatinib and nilotinib, which are more potent, may overcome imatinib resistance. In other leukaemias where there is a major genetic base, such as those arising in the context of Fanconi's anaemia, haematopoietic stem cells using target effectors may offer hope for cure. Haematological malignancies offer a solid chance for targeted delivery of molecular therapies, with the possibility that naked DNA strategies or interfering mRNA therapeutic approaches may reach their target and help us cure leukaemia.

One of the major complications of transplantation is the development of graft versus host disease (GVHD), which is associated with a significant morbidity and mortality rate. New drugs to suppress GVHD have been developed over the last decade including sirolimus, tacrolimus and mycophenolate. Sirolimus, also known as rapamycin, was first discovered as a product of the bacterium *Streptomyces hygroscopicus* in a soil sample from Rapa Nui, one of the Easter Islands. Both sirolimus and tacrolimus inhibit mTOR (mammalian target of rapamycin), which is a cellular protein kinase that acts as a common step in many signal transduction pathways.

There have been major advances in cytogenetics and molecular biology, and these have been applied to leukaemia and are a significant aid to diagnosis, and define prognosis. One of the challenges in this area is in defining new markers for AML, where 50% of patients lack a characteristic cytogenetic signature.

Chapter 35

Hodgkin's disease

Epidemiology and pathogenesis

Hodgkin's disease is a relatively uncommon tumour, affecting approximately 1600 people each year in UK. Currently, there are about 310 deaths annually, including, in 2002, the original Albus Dumbledore actor Richard Harris. More men than women present with Hodgkin's disease, and there is a bimodal age distribution with peaks in the third and seventh decades. Little is known of the risk factors for the development of Hodgkin's disease, although there are minor associations with Down's syndrome and smoking. Geographical clustering has been noted, and there have been a few familial cases of Hodgkin's disease. Hodgkin's disease is also associated with sarcoidosis. The Epstein–Barr virus (EBV) genome is found incorporated within Reed–Sternberg cells, but we do not know for certain whether this virus is a causal agent for Hodgkin's disease. The Reed–Sternberg cell is pathognomonic for the diagnosis of Hodgkin's lymphoma and is thought to originate from lymphocytes affected by EBV. In HIV there is a tenfold increase in Hodgkin's disease. There is significant interest in the origins of the Reed–Sternberg cells, which are large cells with multinucleated or bilobed nuclei that according to histopathologists look like owl's eyes (Figure 35.1). Reed–Sternberg cells have a specific immunophenotype, express-ing CD15 and CD30, but not expressing CD20 or CD45. Immunoglobulin gene expression is mutated within Reed–Sternberg cells, and there are functional rearrangements that lead to abnormal immune function. This leads to defective apoptosis, prolonged B-cell survival and, ultimately, to the development of Hodgkin's disease. EBV proteins remain present in about 40% of Reed–Sternberg cells and there is a three-fold increased risk of Hodgkin's disease following infectious mononucleosis (glandular fever). This possibly suggests that EBV is a future target for immunotherapy.

Presentation

The presentation of Hodgkin's disease is usually with enlarged lymph nodes. This is generally painless and may be accompanied by constitutional symptoms that include profound sweating, sufficient to drench bedclothes, fevers greater than 38°C and weight loss exceeding 10% of body mass. These constitutional symptoms are prognostically important. There are other non-specific symptoms relating to the presentation of Hodgkin's disease, including alcohol-related pain and skin itching.

Investigations

In clinic, a careful history should be obtained and an examination made. Investigations will be organized which include a full blood count and erythrocyte sedimentation rate (ESR), liver and

Lecture Notes: Oncology, 2nd edition. By M. Bower and J. Waxman. Published 2010 by Blackwell Publishing Ltd.

RS cell

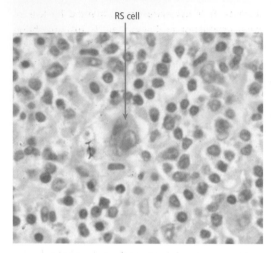

Figure 35.1 Histopathological sample demonstrating a Reed–Sternberg cell (a large binucleated cell with prominent nucleoli surrounded by a clear space or lacunae) diagnostic of Hodgkin's disease.

Mediastinal mass

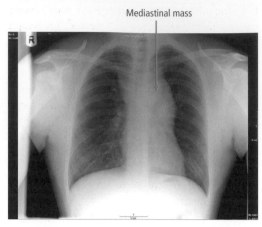

Figure 35.2 Hodgkin's disease with a mediastinal mass. This chest X-ray of a 20-year-old male student shows infilling of the aortopulmonary window and a wide left paratracheal stripe due to mediastinal lymph node enlargement from Hodgkin's disease.

renal function tests, a chest X-ray, CT scan of the chest and abdomen, bone marrow aspiration and trephine biopsy. The patient will be reviewed in outpatients with the results of these tests. Admission will then be organized for a biopsy of the lymph glands. The purpose of these investigations is to define the clinical stage of the disease and the purpose of the biopsy to make a histological diagnosis. The examination of bone marrow is commonly undertaken in the investigation of patients with Hodgkin's disease. Less than 5% of men and women with Hodgkin's disease have bone marrow involvement, however, and this is generally only present in patients with advanced tumours of stages greater than IIB. There are strong arguments against carrying out this assessment except in advanced-stage patients.

The investigation of Hodgkin's disease is a recapitulation of the history of imaging in the UK. Plain X-rays (Figure 35.2) remain helpful, but approaches such as lymphography have been replaced by CT and magnetic resonance imaging (MRI). There are significant errors in the accuracy of both CT and MRI in defining hepatic and splenic involvement, with an error rate of up to 60% in the specificity for indicating involvement by lymphoma. Staging laparotomy has long been aban-

doned as an investigative tool, and the saga of the downside to staging diagnostic splenectomy continues to this day. It includes an ever-enlarging list of infection susceptibilities for which antibiotic therapy and immunization are recommended.

Pathology

Four different histological variants of Hodgkin's disease are described: nodular sclerosing, mixed cellularity, lymphocyte-predominant and lymphocyte-depleted Hodgkin's disease. Nodular sclerosing Hodgkin's disease is subclassified as grade I or II. Lymphocyte-predominant Hodgkin's disease is rare, constituting less than 5% of all histological phenotypes. The nodular sclerosing variant occurs in about 70% of all cases and is even more common in Hodgkin's disease affecting young women. The mixed cellularity variant is commonly associated with HIV-related malignancy and will often be diagnosed in infradiaphragmatic presentations of Hodgkin's disease.

Staging

The results of the staging investigations will help the clinician to determine the clinical stage of the Hodgkin's disease, and this in turn defines treatment. In stage I Hodgkin's disease, one lymph node or two contiguous lymph node groups are affected. In stage II disease, two non-contiguous lymph node groups on the same side of the diaphragm are affected. In stage III Hodgkin's disease, lymph node groups on both sides of the diaphragm are affected. In stage IV disease, there is extranodal spread to the liver, lung or bone but rarely to other sites.

The tumour is further classified as A or B. 'A' defines a lack of constitutional symptoms and 'B' indicates the presence of the constitutional symptoms of Hodgkin's disease. Finally, the staging is defined by use of the subscript 'S', which indicates splenic involvement, or 'E', which defines extension to involve extranodal tissue in direct apposition to an enlarged lymph node group.

Treatment and side effects

The purpose of staging is to define treatment groups. The current recommendations for treatment are as follows. Stage I and IIA Hodgkin's disease is generally treated with radiation. The exceptions are where there is bulky lymphadenopathy or constitutional symptoms. In these instances, chemotherapy may be the preferred option. Stage IIB–IV disease is usually treated with combination chemotherapy.

Radiation

Radiation treatment is generally given according to two well-defined treatment plans. Lymphadenopathy above the diaphragm is treated with mantle radiation which includes the lymph node groups in the neck, axillae and chest to a total dosage of 3500 cGy given over a period of four to six weeks. Infradiaphragmatic radiation is generally given in the inverted Y distribution that includes the para-aortic and iliac nodal groups. Treatment is given to a total dosage of 3500 cGy over a four to six-week period.

Mantle radiotherapy may be complicated by radiation pneumonitis, which is characterized by a period of breathlessness and fever and responds to steroids. It is invariably accompanied by loss of saliva production and oesophagitis. Infradiaphragmatic radiotherapy may be complicated by some minor bowel disturbance but generally is well tolerated. Radiation is usually avoided in children and adolescents as it may lead to gross growth disturbance. Infradiaphragmatic radiation may cause sterility. In patients with good-prognosis disease the radiation fields may be reduced to lower toxicity. Thus extended field or mini-mantle treatments may be prescribed in order to reduce radiotherapy toxicity.

Chemotherapy

Combination chemotherapy for Hodgkin's disease was introduced in the mid-1960s. The original treatment regimen, which has the acronym MOPP, combined mustine, vincristine (Oncovin), prednisone and procarbazine. These drugs are given intravenously and orally for two weeks and repeated every four weeks. Six cycles are administered. Treatment is associated with acute nausea and vomiting, sterility in 90% of males and 50% of females, and the development of second tumours in approximately 5% of patients.

Chemotherapy treatments have been modified over the years in order to reduce side effects. Six is a 'magic number' in oncology, and it is possible that four cycles of therapy are as effective as six cycles. The most frequently used current programme is called ABVD which combines adriamycin, bleomycin, vinblastine and dacarbazine. These drugs cause neither sterility nor second malignancies and are of obvious advantage in a disease where there is a high expectation of cure. Randomized trials have shown an equivalence of ABVD to standard therapy with MOPP and to hybrid therapies.

Haemopoietic stem cell transplantation

High-dosage chemotherapy with either bone marrow transplantation or peripheral blood stem cell support is a relatively new and toxic treatment for drug-resistant Hodgkin's disease. The most commonly applied current programme in the UK uses 'mini-BEAM' or BEAM chemotherapy. Treatment is accompanied by either peripheral blood stem cell or bone marrow transplantation. Morbidity is high, and in certain groups, such as those pretreated with mediastinal radiotherapy, mortality reaches up to 30%. Long-term remissions occur in up to 40% of patients. The rationale for first-line treatment with high-dose chemotherapy and bone marrow product support is absent. There are no randomized trials comparing such treatment programmes with conventional approaches for first-line treatment of Hodgkin's disease.

Prognosis

The results of treatment of Hodgkin's disease are considered to be one of the miracles of modern oncology, in that approximately 90% of patients with small-volume, early-stage disease are curable with radiation and between 40% and 60% of patients with advanced disease are curable with chemotherapy. A poorer prognosis results from the presence of bulk disease, constitutional symptoms or poor-prognosis histology. The patient who is 'cured' as a result of treatment is unfortunately at risk from late relapse; this may occur 15–30 years after diagnosis. This risk of a late relapse is small and largely confined to lymphocyte-predominant Hodgkin's disease.

Complications of chemotherapy

Hodgkin's disease is a tumour with significant cure rates, occurring in young people with an expectation of prolonged survival. This leads to a significant onus for providing a therapy that is without major long-term toxicity. Conventional chemotherapy and radiotherapy for Hodgkin's disease using alkylating agents is associated with the development of second tumours. The incidence of second tumours reaches approximately 5%, with staggering increases in the rates of acute leukaemias and lymphomas. The leukaemias present early, two to four years after the completion of

chemotherapy. The solid tumours, such as breast, colorectal and lung cancer, occur late, sometimes 15–20 years after diagnosis. Sterility is also an important consequence of treatment with any alkylating agent-containing regimen, reaching up to 80% in males and 50% in females.

New treatment

The most important prospect for Hodgkin's disease remains the development of immunization programmes for EBV. EBV antigens are present in up to 40% of patients with Hodgkin's disease, and it is thought that this herpes virus might be a significant cause for the development of this 'B-cell' malignancy. Vaccination strategies have been developed, and it is hoped that these may lead to the elimination of a proportion of cases of Hodgkin's lymphoma. Other attempts have been made to develop cytotoxic lymphocyte-based immunotherapy for Hodgkin's disease. They have, however, not been successful, because of the facility of EBV to use multiple strategies to avoid detection. Attempts at immunotherapy have included downregulation of immunodominant antigens, together with cytokine secretion.

Combination chemotherapy regimens using hybrid treatment programmes have been investigated for the treatment of advanced Hodgkin's disease for the reason that, in this group of patients, a significant proportion of patients remain incurable. Although some studies have shown a small advantage to such hybrid regimens, the treatment carries the disadvantage of increased long-term toxicity from the alkylating agent-containing regimens. A recent trial of 850 patients which compared ABVD with MOPP/ABVD has shown an identical complete remission and failure-free survival rate.

Where there is predominant CD20 expression, there are prospects for treatment with immunotherapy directed to this surface antigen, such as rituximab, which in a recent study has shown a response rate of 86% in a small group of patients.

Chapter 36

Non-Hodgkin's lymphoma

Epidemiology and pathogenesis

Non-Hodgkin's lymphoma is relatively common. In the UK there are just over 4500 deaths each year and 10500 patients presenting with this condition. There have been many descriptions of the pathological classification of this disease. Rather than achieving clarity, however, most have tended to confuse the situation further because of their complexity. In terms of clinical practice, the most significant divisions are into high- and low-grade lymphoma.

High-grade lymphoma is much more common than low-grade lymphoma. About 1000 people with low-grade lymphoma present each year. Slightly more men are affected than women. Lymphomas arise from lymphoid organs or lymphatic tissue associated with other systems that contain lymphatic tissue. The latter, the so-called 'extranodal lymphomas', constitute up to 30% of all non-Hodgkin's lymphoma.

There have been extraordinary advances in the molecular biology of lymphoma, and from this we have begun to understand some of the aetiological features involved in this condition. It is thought that Epstein–Barr virus infection is linked to the development of African Burkitt's lymphoma,

certain other B-cell lymphomas, HIV-associated lymphomas and almost all lymphomas associated with the immunosuppression consequent to the transplantation of heart, kidneys and lung.

The human T-cell leukaemia lymphoma virus type 1 (HTLV-1) causes adult T-cell lymphoma and leukaemia and both are endemic in the Caribbean and Japan. Other viruses associated with the development of lymphoma include hepatitis C and human herpesvirus 8 (HHV 8). *Helicobacter* infection in the stomach leads to a proliferation of gastric lymphoid tissue and the development of low-grade mucosa-associated tumours. Such tumours may respond to *H. pylori* eradication treatment, but unfortunately they may evolve into classical lymphoma despite eradication.

Presentation

Patients present with nodal enlargement which may be accompanied by constitutional symptoms including weight loss, sweating and fever. These symptoms – where weight loss is in excess of 10% of pre-morbid weight, sweating is sufficient to drench night clothes, and fever exceeds 38°C – are described as 'B' symptoms. 'B' symptoms are less common in high-grade lymphoma than low-grade malignancies. Patients with such symptoms should be referred to specialist centres where the chance for survival and the quality of survival are significantly better than in peripheral non-

Lecture Notes: Oncology, 2nd edition. By M. Bower and J. Waxman. Published 2010 by Blackwell Publishing Ltd.

specialist centres. The care of patients with lymphoma should be by oncologists or haematologists, depending upon the specialist interests of the clinicians.

Staging and grading

In outpatients, a careful history is obtained from the patient who is then examined. The investigations organized should include a blood count, renal and hepatic function tests, chest X-ray, bone marrow aspiration and trephine, and CT scan of the abdomen and chest (Figures 36.1–36.4). These investigations are done in order to define the extent of the disease. From these investigations the clinical staging is obtained. This is defined as follows:

• Stage I: disease confined to one lymph node or two contiguous lymph node groups
• Stage II: disease on one side of the diaphragm in lymph node groups that are separate
• Stage III: disease on both sides of the diaphragm
• Stage IV: extranodal spread of the lymphoma.

Preliminary investigations having been organized, the patient should then proceed to a lymph node biopsy. Lymph node biopsies used to be required to describe the architectural arrangement of the tumour. In modern times, they are no longer

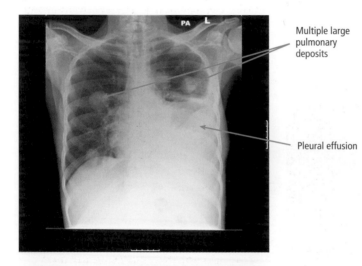

Multiple large pulmonary deposits

Pleural effusion

Figure 36.1 Chest radiograph showing multiple large pulmonary nodules and a left sided pleural effusion due to diffuse large B-cell non-Hodgkin's lymphoma.

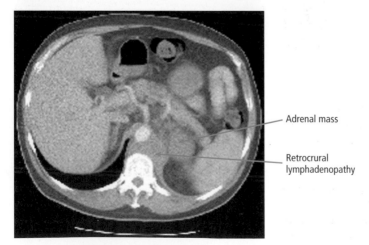

Adrenal mass

Retrocrural lymphadenopathy

Figure 36.2 CT scan showing extensive left retrocrural adenopathy and a left adrenal mass due to high-grade B-cell non-Hodgkin's lymphoma.

Extradural mass displacing and compressing spinal cord

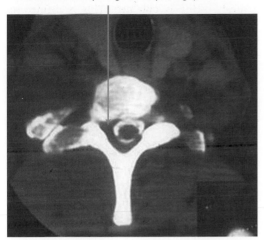

Figure 36.3 Spinal cord deviation and compression at T1 vertebra by an extradural mass of high grade non-Hodgkin's lymphoma.

Liver   Spleen

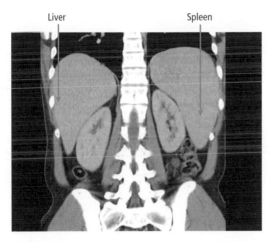

Figure 36.4 CT scan showing hepatosplenomegally due to follicular non-Hodgkin's lymphoma.

always considered to be necessary. Sufficient material can often be obtained from core needle biopsies to define the pathological diagnosis. There are many classification systems for non-Hodgkin's lymphoma, which include the WHO classification (Table 36.1), the Kiel classification, the Working Formulation and the Revised European and American Lymphoma Classification (REAL).

For the purposes of defining treatment, the most practical classification, however, is to describe the

tumour as being low or high grade. A low-grade tumour tends to have a follicular nature and to contain relatively inactive cells. A high-grade tumour contains cells that have a high index of mitotic activity and there is no follicular structure to the lymph node. An intermediate-grade tumour, which generally behaves clinically like a high-grade tumour, has some of the features of both high- and low-grade tumours. There are variant lymphomas, such as mantle cell and Burkitt's lymphomas, which are clinical entities with poor prognosis.

Many modern techniques have been applied to the pathological diagnosis of lymphoma. Immunophenotyping using monoclonal antibodies is the most helpful, firstly, in initially distinguishing between a lymphoma or a carcinoma by using antibodies to the leukocyte common antigen (CD45), and secondly, in defining the lymphoma by using antibodies that are specific for B or T lymphocytes, such as CD20 or CD4, CD2 and CD3. T-cell receptor and immunoglobulin gene rearrangements are also carried out, and are helpful in describing tumour clonality. Fluorescent *in situ* hybridization is also useful. This is because of the observed cytogenetic abnormalities that are relatively specific for non-Hodgkin's lymphoma. Some of these are outlined in Table 36.2.

Treatment

Low-grade non-Hodgkin's lymphoma

Low-grade tumours are generally disseminated at diagnosis. If they are localized, that is stage I, small bulk, peripheral and without B symptoms, the treatment should be radiotherapy. For stage II–IV disease, treatment is with chemotherapy with oral alkylating agents such as chlorambucil or with an intravenous chemotherapy programme known as CVP which uses cyclophosphamide, vincristine and prednisone. Chlorambucil has very little early toxicity but at high total dosages causes sterility, secondary myelodysplasia (MDS) and acute myeloid leukaemia (AML). CVP leads to hair loss, but apart from this it is without significant morbidity. Both regimens may be associated with marrow toxicity which results in admissions with neutropenic

Table 36.1 World Health Organization (WHO) classification of lymphomas. (More common lymphomas are shown in italics.)

B-cell neoplasms	T-cell and NK-cell neoplasms
Precursor B-cell neoplasms	**Precursor T-cell neoplasms**
B-lymphoblastic leukaemia/lymphoma	*T-lymphoblastic leukaemia/lymphoma*
Mature B-cell neoplasms	**Mature T-cell and NK-cell neoplasms**
B-cell chronic lymphocytic leukaemia/small lymphocytic lymphoma	*T-cell prolymphocytic leukaemia/lymphoma*
B cell prolymphocytic leukaemia	T-cell large granular cell lymphocytic leukaemia
Lymphoplasmacytic lymphoma	NK-cell leukaemia
Splenic marginal zone B-cell lymphoma	Adult T-cell leukaemia/lymphoma (± villous lymphocytes)
Hairy cell leukaemia	Extranodal NK-/T-cell lymphoma, nasal type
Plasma cell myeloma/plasmacytoma	Enteropathic-type intestinal T-cell lymphoma
Extranodal marginal zone lymphoma (of MALT type)	Hepatosplenic γ/δ T-cell lymphoma
Nodal marginal zone lymphoma	Subcutaneous panniculitis-like T-cell lymphoma
Follicular lymphoma	*Mycosis fungoides/*Sézary syndrome
Mantle cell lymphoma	Primary cutaneous anaplastic large cell lymphoma
Diffuse large B-cell lymphoma	*Peripheral T-cell lymphoma, not otherwise characterized*
Subtypes: *mediastinal (thymic),* intravascular, primary effusion lymphoma	Angioimmunoblastic T-cell lymphoma
Burkitt's lymphoma/Burkitt's cell leukaemia	*Systemic anaplastic large cell lymphoma*
MALT, mucosa-associated lymphoid tissue.	

sepsis or with thrombocytopenic bleeding. The monoclonal antibody rituximab that targets CD20 is frequently added to these cytotoxic agents.

Patients with stage I non-Hodgkin's lymphoma have a 70–95% chance of cure with radiotherapy. The patient with disseminated low-grade lymphoma is not cured by treatment. Although 85% of patients achieve a complete response to therapy, this response is transient. After a median period of 18 months, the patient relapses and requires re-treatment. The average patient has four such episodes of response and relapse. Finally after a median period of 7.5 years, there is transformation to high-grade lymphoma.

High-grade and intermediate-grade non-Hodgkin's lymphoma

Paradoxically, high-grade and intermediate-grade lymphomas are more likely to be confined to one lymph node group than low-grade tumours and are curable. Stage I disease may be treated with radiotherapy. Some clinicians will then proceed to treat with adjuvant chemotherapy. Patients with small bulk stage I non-Hodgkin's lymphoma have a 95% chance of cure with radiation, and this chance is only minimally improved with chemotherapy. If the stage I disease is bulky, chemotherapy alone may be given. Treatment is with the R-CHOP regimen, and there is little evidence that more complex regimens add to the chance of cure. Of all patients, 70–80% enter remission, which is sustained in about 40–60% of cases. CHOP consists of cyclophosphamide, doxorubicin (hydroxydaunorubicin), vincristine (oncovin) and prednisolone and was introduced in the 1970s. It has remained the gold standard therapy for many high-grade lymphomas ever since with the addition of rituximab for CD20-expressing lymphomas in the 1990s. In 1993 a pivotal trial compared CHOP with several newer chemotherapy regimens with less memorable but more exotic names (e.g. m-BACOD, ProMACE-CytaBOM, MACOP-B); CHOP emerged as the regimen with the least toxicity but similar efficacy.

Table 36.2 Recurrent chromosomal translocations in non-Hodgkin's lymphoma subtypes, resulting in oncogene dysregulation.

Histology	Translocation	Alteration of gene function	Mechanism/features of translocation	Frequency
Follicular lymphoma	t(14;18)(q32;21)	Upregulation of BCL2 (inhibitor of apoptosis)	BCL2 relocates to IgH locus. Error in physiological IgH rearrangement. Seen rarely in normal B cells	80%
Burkitt's lymphoma	t(8;14)(q24;q32); t(2;8)(p12;q24); t(8;22)(q24;q11)	Upregulation of c-MYC (transcription factor for cell cycle progression/ proliferation)	c-myc relocates to IgH locus or to one of the light chain gene loci	100%
Mantle cell lymphoma	t(11;14)(q13;q32)	Upregulation of cyclin D1 (G1 cyclin)	Cyclin D1 relocates to IgH	>90%
Diffuse large B-cell lymphoma*	t(3;14)(q27;32) and several others involving 3q27	Deregulation of BCL6 (zinc finger transcription factor)	BCL6 relocates to IgH, IgL, IgK or one of many other non-Ig loci	30–40%
Extranodal marginal zone lymphoma (MALT)	t(11;18)(q21;q21)	Gene fusion of AP12 and MLT/MALT1 genes (AP12 is inhibitor of apoptosis)	Gene fusion	20–35%
Extranodal marginal zone lymphoma (MALT)	t(1;14)(q22;q32)	Deregulation of BCL10 (apoptosis regulatory protein)	BCL10 relocates to IgH locus	<5%
Lymphoplasmacytic lymphoma	t(9;14)(q13;q32)	Deregulation of PAX5 (paired homeobox transcription factor)	PAX5 relocates to IgH locus	50%
Anaplastic large cell lymphoma	t(2;5)(p23;q35) and others involving 2p23	Gene fusion of ALK (anaplastic lymphoma kinase, a receptor tyrosine kinase) and NPM (located at 5q35) or other gene malignant transforming capacity *in vitro* and *in vivo*	Gene fusion	ALK-NPM, 50% Others, 15%

*BCL2 (30%) and c-myc (10%) rearrangements are also frequently seen in diffuse large B-cell non-Hodgkin's lymphoma. Ig, immunoglobulin; MALT, mucosa-associated lymphoid tissue.

High-dose therapy

Patients with poor-prognosis lymphomas at presentation or with recurrent high-grade lymphomas may be considered for high-dose chemotherapy with auto- or allogeneic bone marrow or other stem cell support. These programmes may be linked with attempts to purge the marrow or peripheral blood stem cells of specific cell populations. Immunosuppression is required for patients receiving allografts. Prognosis depends on a number of risk factors. There is an associated mortality rate to these procedures that may exceed 10%.

New treatment

New agents have become available for the treatment of lymphoma. Amongst the most interesting are antibody treatments directed against B-cell antigens, such as rituximab. Rituximab is directed against CD20 and usually has very little toxicity apart from the possibility of a hypersensitivity response. It has been used mainly in the treatment of recurrent lymphoma. In more recent trials, however, rituximab has been prescribed as first-line therapy for patients with B-cell lymphomas. These trials have been successful, and rituximab in combination with chemotherapy is considered to be standard first-line treatment for patients with B-cell lymphomas. There are other anti-CD20, -CD40 and -CD8 antibody treatments, which show some promise and these have been combined with radioisotopes such as iodine-131. Vaccine trials using patient-specific immunization with immunoglobulin idiotype are also underway. There is new hope for lymphoma patients!

Chapter 37

Myeloma

Epidemiology and pathogenesis

Myeloma is a relatively common haematological malignancy affecting 3987 people each year in the UK, and leading to 2695 deaths per year. There is an equal sex distribution and an increasing incidence with age. The rate of myeloma is higher amongst black populations, and the disease is associated with industrial and radiation exposure.

Multiple myeloma is a B-cell neoplasm characterized by the proliferation of plasma cells that synthesize and secrete monoclonal immunoglobulins or fragments thereof. The molecular basis of the transformation that characterizes this tumour is not clearly known. Karyotypic abnormalities have been identified in up to 50% of myeloma patients, but there is no clear, unifying change that underlies this transformation. Several molecular events have been described. These involve 14q32 translocations, chromosome 13 deletion and fibroblast growth factor receptor 3 (FGFR3) activation. These abnormalities are seen in no more than 20% of all myeloma patients. The translocations that have been described mostly involve the switch rearrangements of the heavy chain locus with partner genes such as FGFR3. Mutations have been observed in tumour suppressor genes and abnormalities of expression in apoptosis-related genes

such as BCL-2. T cells secrete interleukin 6 (IL-6), which appears to be an essential growth factor for myeloma cells in culture. Excessive secretion of IL-6 occurs in myeloma and this may be a primary cause for the condition.

The destructive bone lesions that are seen in myeloma are thought to be due to dysregulation of the osteoprotegerin Rankl system. Rankl is the ligand for osteoprotegerin and is released in myeloma by the malignant plasma cells and bone marrow stroma, leading to osteoclast activation and hence osteolysis. The osteolytic bone lesions of myeloma are best seen on plain X-rays rather than bone scans as they generally lack osteoblastic activity. They appear as punched-out lesions, including the classical 'pepper pot' appearance of the skull X-ray, and the bone breakdown releases calcium and may cause hypercalcaemia.

Presentation

Patients with myeloma often present in a dramatic fashion with significant bone pain due to the lytic lesions that characterize this disease (Figure 37.1). Vertebral collapse is often a feature of presentation, and this may lead to symptoms of cord compression. Patients with myeloma may present with symptoms of hypercalcaemia, which every medical student reading this chapter is able to describe. Hypercalcaemia can be one of the precipitating factors for renal failure commonly observed in myeloma. The other causes include amyloidosis

Lecture Notes: Oncology, 2nd edition. By M. Bower and J. Waxman. Published 2010 by Blackwell Publishing Ltd.

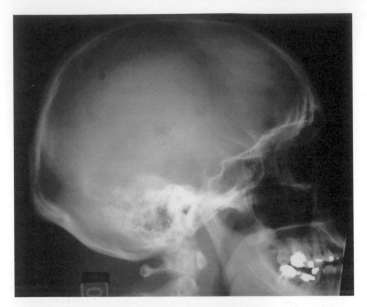

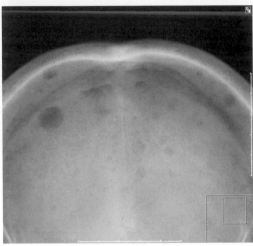

Figure 37.1 Skull radiograph of a 52-year-old man with multiple myeloma showing multiple, well-defined lucencies that are fairly uniform in size, unlike bone metastases which usually vary in size.

(AL amyloid containing immunoglobulin light chains), precipitation of Bence–Jones protein (urinary free light chain papprotein), direct infiltration and infection. An excess of immunoglobulin may cause the hyperviscosity syndrome, which is more common with an IgG myeloma than an IgM myeloma. This is explained by the fact that a far greater proportion of patients have IgG than have IgM myelomas, which represents just 0.5% of all myeloma cases.

The raised paraprotein levels may cause other problems, including peripheral neuropathy. Mar-row infiltration with an excess of plasma cells leads to a decrease in numbers of other marrow constituents, causing anaemia, thrombocytopenia and neutropenia. This in turn has consequences for both the presentation and the clinical features of the disease as it evolves.

Investigations

The investigation of myeloma is relatively simple. It requires the examination of the peripheral blood, paraprotein levels, blood count, β_2-

microglobulin levels, renal function and calcium levels (see Plates 37.1 and 37.2), assessment of the bone marrow, examination of the urine for Bence–Jones protein urea and a skeletal survey. Bone scanning is of low diagnostic value in myeloma. Myeloma is staged, and the staging has prognostic value (Table 37.1). Two systems are used, that of Durie and Salmon and that of the Medical Research Council (MRC) (Tables 37.2 and 37.3).

Treatment

The initial treatment of myeloma requires stabilization of the patient and correction of renal function abnormalities and hypercalcaemia (Table 37.4). The patient is started on allopurinol and may require hydration or transfusion. Hypercalcaemia is treated with bisphosphonates, steroids and rehydration. Where there is significant bone pain, which is poorly responsive to opiates, radiotherapy may be required. A single fraction treatment will alleviate bone pain in approximately 80% of patients. Anaemia may require transfusion and significant hyperviscosity needs plasmaphoresis.

Chemotherapy for myeloma has a 50-year history, beginning with the use of alkylating agents such as melphalan and cyclosphosphamide. Nowadays, the initial treatment of multiple myeloma depends on the patient's age and co-morbidities. High-dose chemotherapy with hematopoietic stem cell transplantation has become the preferred treatment for patients under the age of 65. Prior to stem cell transplantation, these patients receive an initial course of induction chemotherapy. The most common induction regimens used are thalidomide–dexamethasone, bortezomib-based regimens, and lenalidomide–dexamethasone. Unfortunately, many patients are older and frailer

Table 37.1 Diagnostic criteria for myeloma.

Major criteria	
I	Plasmacytoma or tissue biopsy
II	Bone marrow plasmacytosis >30%
III	Monoclonal (M) spike on electrophoresis:
	>35 g/l (IgG peaks)
	or >20 g/l (IgA peaks)
	or κ or λ light chain excretion >1.0 g/24 hours

Minor criteria	
	Distant metastases
a	Bone-marrow plasmacytosis 10–30%
b	M spike present but less than in major criteria
c	Lytic bone lesions
d	Normal immunoglobulin levels decreased:
	IgM < 0.05 g/l
	or IgA < 0.01 g/l
	or IgG < 0.60 g/l
	Diagnosis of myeloma requires a minimum of one major plus one minor criteria or three minor criteria

Diagnostic criteria for MGUS	
I	Monoclonal gammopathy
II	Bone marrow plasma cells <10%
III	Monoclonal (M) component level:
	IgG < 35 g/l
	or IgA < 20 g/l
	or κ or λ light chains <1.0 g/24 hours
IV	No overt bone lesions
V	No symptoms to suggest myeloma

MGUS, monoclonal gammapathy of uncertain significance.

Table 37.2 Durie and Salmon staging system for myeloma.

Cell mass category: Requirements:		High (stage III) One of A, B, C or D	Low (stage I) All of A, B, C and D	Intermediate (stage II)
Haemoglobin (pre-transfusion)	A	<85 g/dl%	>10 g/dl%	
Serum calcium	B	>12 mg%	Normal	Neither
M component	C	IgG >nbsp;7 g/dl%	<5 g/dl%	I or III
IgA >nbsp;5 g/dl%	<3 g/dl%			
Bence–Jones >12 g/day	<4 g/day			
Bone lesion on skeletal survey	D	Advanced lytic disease	None/solitary lesion	

Table 37.3 MRC staging system.

		Poor prognosis (stage III) A, C or B, C	Good prognosis (stage I) All of A, B, C and D	Intermediate (stage II) Not in I or III
Blood urea concentration	A	>10 mM/l	=8 mM/l	Not in I or III
Haemoglobin	B	=7.5 g/dl	>10.0 g/dl	Not in I or III
Performance status	C	Restricted activity	Minimal symptoms or asymptomatic	Not in I or III

Table 37.4 Southwest Oncology Group myeloma response criteria.

A. Responsive patients who satisfy all the following criteria are considered to have achieved definite objective improvement:

　1. A sustained decrease in the synthesis index of serum monoclonal protein to 25% or less of the pre-treatment value, and to less than 25 g/l on at least two measurements separated by 4 weeks. For IgA and Ig$_3$M proteins, the synthetic index is the same as the serum concentration. For IgG proteins of subclasses 1, 2 and 4, the synthetic index must be estimated using a nomogram

　2. A sustained decrease in 24-hour urine globulin to 10% or less of the pre-treatment value, and to less than 0.2 g/24 hours on at least two occasions separated by 4 weeks

　3. In all responsive patients the size and number of lytic skull lesions must not increase, and the serum calcium must remain normal. Correction of anaemia (haematocrit >27 vol%) and hypoalbuminaemia (>3.0 g/dl) is required if they are considered to be secondary to myeloma. With equivocal data (e.g. non-secretors or L-chain producers for whom the pre-treatment urine collection was lost), the following two points support the conclusion that an objective response has occurred

　4. Recalcification of lytic skull lesions

　5. Significant increments in depressed normal immunoglobulins (e.g. increments >200 mg/l IgM, >400 mg/l IgA, and >4000 mg/l IgG)

B. Improved patients show a decline in the serum M protein synthesis rate to less than 50%, but not less than 25%, of the pre-treatment value

C. Unresponsive patients fail to satisfy the criteria for responsive or improved patients

patients and here the standard of care has been chemotherapy with melphalan and prednisone. Bortezomib and lenalidomide are suitable treatments at relapse. Bortezomib inhibits proteosome, the cellular organelles that identify tagged proteins in the cytoplasm, and breaks them down. It is not quite clear how thalidomide and lenalidomide work but they seem to have both immunomodulatory and anti-angiogenic actions. Both are potent teratogens and it is essential that they are not prescribed to women who could become pregnant.

New treatment

Because myeloma is a clonal disease that expresses a unique surface immunoglobulin, it was thought possible that patients might mount an immune defense against these myeloma cells if they were somehow used as a vaccine. Myeloma cell/dendritic cell fusions have been examined as a vaccination strategy for multiple myeloma and have been found to induce myeloma-specific cell death. Similarly, antisense oligonucleotides have been shown to have some efficacy in patients with recurrent myeloma. *In vitro*, IL-6 causes the proliferation of myeloma cells, and a monoclonal antibody that blocks the IL-6 receptor is being used in trials as treatment for myeloma.

Chapter 38

Skin cancer

Cinema has wide-ranging influence on fashion trends and one of the most striking examples was the mid-20th century trend towards sun tanning. The fashion of the Victorian era was sun avoidance; the upper classes stayed pale in part to distinguish themselves from lower class workers who had to toil in the sun. Yet by the 1950s, the beach culture of southern California spread worldwide via the movies. The ill effects of chronic exposure to ultraviolet radiation on skin ageing are well demonstrated by Clint Eastwood. The carcinogenic effects of sunlight led to the removal of a basal cell carcinoma from the former actor, US President Ronald Reagan, whilst his eldest daughter Maureen Reagan died of melanoma.

The following two chapters discuss both non-melanoma skin tumours and melanomas.

Lecture Notes: Oncology, 2nd edition. By M. Bower and J. Waxman. Published 2010 by Blackwell Publishing Ltd.

Chapter 39

Non-melanoma skin tumours

Epidemiology and pathogenesis

Non-melanoma skin cancers probably comprise more than one-third of all cancers in the UK and have been described as a worldwide epidemic. The term includes two major types: basal cell carcinoma (BCC) and squamous cell carcinoma (SCC). Other less common non-melanoma skin cancers include Kaposi's sarcoma, cutaneous lymphoma and Merkel cell carcinoma. Despite their frequency, these tumours account for only 2% of cancer deaths.

BCC is four times more common than SCC. Sun damage is the major cause of both cancers, especially the ultraviolet B (UVB) spectrum (290–320 nm wavelength). The UV radiation produces DNA mutations, particularly thymidine dimers in the p53 tumour suppressor gene. The incidence of skin cancer rises with latitudes approaching the equator. Light-exposed areas of the body are the most frequent sites for tumours, and occupations with high sun exposure like farming have an increased incidence of BCC and SCC. Ozone absorbs UVB, and progressive destruction of the ozone layer by fluorinated hydrocarbons may lead to increased rates. Melanin absorbs UV light, and its lower levels in melanocytes of white people

accounts for the higher incidence of skin cancers in white people. The benefits of melanin in areas of high UV exposure are offset against the reduced production of vitamin D3, which requires UV light, so in regions of low sunlight, black people are prone to rickets. This delicately balanced system of biological geodiversity has been abused to justify some of the most inhumane behaviour. Genetic predispositions to skin cancers include xeroderma pigmentosum, Gorlin's basal cell naevus syndrome and familial melanoma syndromes. Patients with xeroderma pigmentosa are unable to repair the UV-induced DNA damage and develop both BCC and SCC under the age of 10 years old. Gorlin's basal cell naevus syndrome patients develop BCC in their teens and brain tumours later in life; it is caused by a mutation of a patched gene involved in the Hedgehog pathway signal transduction. The gene name *Hedgehog* was originally coined because mutations lead to spikes on *Drosophila* fruit flies. Humans have three homologues of the gene named after the two common varieties of hedgehogs, 'Indian' and 'Desert'. The third human gene was named *Sonic* after Sega's game character. Familial melanoma is caused by inherited mutations of the CDKN2 (p16) gene (chromosome 9p21) and of CDK4 (chromosome 12q13), both implicated in insensitivity to cell cycle checkpoints. Chemical carcinogens, including arsenic, are associated with SCC. Sir Percival Pott's description in 1775 of scrotal cancers in chimney sweeps

Lecture Notes: Oncology, 2nd edition. By M. Bower and J. Waxman. Published 2010 by Blackwell Publishing Ltd.

is thought to be due to industrial exposure to coal tar. Radiation is associated with an increased incidence of SCC, BCC and Bowen's disease (SCC *in situ*). Allogeneic organ transplant recipients are at greatly increased risk of SCC, with as many as 80% having SCC within 20 years of the graft. This may be related to the finding of genotypes five and eight of human papillomavirus in some skin SCC.

Presentation

BCC begins in the basal cell layer of the epidermis, usually develops on chronically sun-exposed areas of the skin, rarely metastasizes, and is usually slow growing. If left untreated, however, BCC may spread locally to the bone or other tissues beneath the skin. BCC starts as painless, translucent, pearly nodules with telangiectasia on sun-exposed skin. As they enlarge, they ulcerate and bleed and develop a rolled shiny edge sometimes referred to as a 'rodent ulcer' (see Plate 39.1). They may progress slowly over many months to years, but less than 0.1% metastasize to regional lymph nodes. They occur mostly on the face, especially the nose, nasolabial fold and inner canthus, usually in elderly people and are more common in men than in women.

SCC arises from more superficial layers of the epidermis and tends to be more aggressive. SCC can invade tissues beneath the skin and 1–2% spread to the lymph nodes. These cancers typically appear on sun-exposed areas of the body, such as the face, ears, neck, lips and backs of the hands (see Plate 39.2). Marjolin ulcers are SCCs arising in long-standing, benign ulcers, such as venous ulcers, or scars, such as old burns. SCCs are irregular, red hyperkeratotic tumours that ulcerate and crust. Unlike BCCs, SCCs grow more rapidly over months rather than years and occasionally bleed. Precursors to SCC include actinic keratosis and SCC *in situ*, which is also called Bowen's disease. SCC *in situ* is a full-thickness malignant transformation of the epidermis that, by definition, has not invaded the dermis.

Merkel cell carcinoma is a highly malignant tumour in the basal layer of the epidermis, most commonly found in elderly, white patients. It consists of rapidly growing, painless and shiny purple nodules that may occur anywhere on the body. These tumours are thought to arise from neuroendocrine cells and are positive for neuron-specific enolase staining. They resemble small cell lung cancer in their clinical course. In 2008, a polyomavirus (Merkel cell polyomavirus, MCV) was identified in most of these tumours and represents the first of a new class of human oncogenic viruses. Max Perutz, who won the Nobel Prize for his work on crystallography and who was Watson and Crick's PhD supervisor whilst they were discovering the structure of DNA, died of Merkel cell tumour. Distant metastases are common, and treatment is with combination chemotherapy, although relapses are frequent and the prognosis is poor. Other, rarer non-melanoma skin cancers include Kaposi's sarcoma, which usually starts within the dermis but can also develop in internal organs. This cancer, once extremely rare, has become more common due to its association with HIV/AIDS. It is caused by infection with an oncogenic herpesvirus, HHV8 (human herpesvirus 8). Primary cutaneous lymphoma or mycosis fungoides is a low-grade lymphoma that primarily affects the skin. Generally, it has a slow course and often remains confined to the skin, but progression of the tumour to a more aggressive, life-threatening stage is more likely the longer it has been present. Adnexal tumours, which start in the hair follicles or sweat glands, are extremely rare and usually benign.

Treatment

The goal of treatment for BCC and SCC is to eradicate local disease and achieve the best cosmetic appearance. For BCC, a complete skin examination is indicated because of the increased risk of actinic keratosis or cancers located at other skin sites in persons presenting with a suspicious lesion. For SCC, regional lymph nodes should also be examined. The main options include: (i) surgery, which offers a single brief procedure and histological confirmation of completeness of excision; (ii) curettage, which is suitable for small, nodular lesions of less than 1 cm and yields good cosmesis; and (iii) cryotherapy, which can be used for lesions of less than 2 cm but may leave an area of depigmentation, and radiotherapy. Mohs' micrographic surgery is a specialized form of excisional surgery that provides 100% microscopically controlled histological margins. The technique involves tumour excision, mapping of the removed tissue and immediate microscopic assessment of the surgical specimen. If occult tumour extension is detected microscopically, the process is repeated until a tumour-free margin is attained. Frederick Mohs developed this surgical approach whilst still a medical student and, according to at least one of our surgical colleagues, it is analogous to peeling rather than chopping a vegetable. Mohs' surgery is curative for 99% of primary BCCs and for 97% of primary SCCs, the highest documented cure rates. Radiotherapy has the advantages of no pain, no hospitalization and no keloids or contracture; it preserves uninvolved tissue and produces smaller defects. It does, however, require multiple visits and results in depigmentation and loss of hair follicles and sweat glands at the treated site. The decision between surgery and radiotherapy is based on size and site, histology, age of patient, recurrence rates and anticipated cosmetic results. Topical 5-fluorouracil chemotherapy may be used for actinic keratosis and small, superficial, non-invasive tumours. Side effects include progressive inflammation, erythema, erosions and contact dermatitis. Systemic chemotherapy is reserved for treating locally advanced and metastatic disease. The most widely used regimens include cisplatin in combination with 5-fluorouracil or doxorubicin.

Prevention remains the most important aspect of the management of skin cancers and requires campaigns to increase public awareness. Children should not get sunburnt, and white-skinned people should limit their total cumulative sun exposure. The public should be encouraged to look out for new skin lesions, and those that are not obviously benign should be seen and removed in their entirety for pathological examination within four weeks.

Prognosis

The prognosis of five-year survival for patients with non-melanoma skin tumours is given in Table 39.1.

Table 39.1 A prognosis of five-year survival for patients with non-melanoma skin tumours.

Tumour	5-year survival
Basal cell carcinoma	95–100%
Squamous cell carcinoma	92–99%

Chapter 40

Melanoma

Epidemiology and pathogenesis

Melanoma is a tumour of melanocytes: the pigmented cells of the skin. The incidence of melanoma has increased by a factor of 4 since 1971. More than 10 000 people were diagnosed with melanoma in the UK in 2006. The primary cause is thought to be an increase in exposure to sunlight. Risk factors for the development of melanoma, however, include being Caucasian and having dysplastic naevi or familial melanoma. It is encouraging to note that recently there has been a stabilization of the increase in melanoma incidence. One hopes that with all the publicity, the risks of exposure to sun are at last entering into the public consciousness.

Less than 10% of all melanoma cases constitute families with an inherited predisposition to melanoma. Mutations in two genes, CDKN2A and CDK4, have been shown to confer increased risk of melanoma, but these mutations only constitute about one-fifth of all familial cases. The melanocortin receptor gene, *MC1R*, influences skin pigmentation and polymorphisms in this gene are linked to an increased risk of melanoma. In other families, there is linkage around the 1p22 chromosomal region. Loss of the transcription factor AP-2 is also thought to have some tumour suppressor-like role in melanoma progression.

Presentation

Patients with malignant melanoma generally present with a history of a growing mole, which may bleed or itch (see Plates 40.1 and 40.2). Because of the public awareness of melanoma, generally there is quite rapid self-referral to GPs with these symptoms. Specialist referral to plastic surgery or dermatology is also quick, and many hospitals now offer walk-in skin lesion clinics. In clinic, the specialist will on initial examination seek to confirm the diagnosis. If there is no evidence for metastases, he will make arrangements to excise the primary lesion. This proceedure requires specialist surgery with wide excision of the surrounding normal tissue. The reasons for this are, firstly, concerns about the incidence of local recurrence following inadequate resection (see Plates 40.3 and 40.4) and, secondly, the need for good cosmesis. Although wide excision is practised, there is no evidence from a randomized trial that supports this practice.

Staging and grading

There are four main clinical descriptions of melanoma and these are the superficial spreading, nodular, lentigo maligna and acral lentiginous subtypes (Table 40.1).

Lecture Notes: Oncology, 2nd edition. By M. Bower and J. Waxman. Published 2010 by Blackwell Publishing Ltd.

Table 40.1 Clinicopathological features of four common forms of melanoma.

Type	Location	Age (median)	Gender and race	Edge	Colour	Frequency
Superficial spreading	All body surfaces, especially legs	56 years	White females	Palpable, irregular	Brown, black, grey or pink; central or halo depigmentation	50%
Nodular	All body surfaces	49 years	White males	Palpable	Uniform bluish black	30%
Lentigo maligna	Sun exposed, areas, especially head and neck	70 years	White females	Flat, irregular	Shades of brown or black, hypopigmentation	15%
Acral lentigenous	Palms, soles and mucous membranes	61 years	Black males	Palpable, irregular nodule	Black, irregularly coloured	5%

Following excision and confirmation of the diagnosis histologically, staging investigations, which should include CT scanning, should be performed. As a result of surgery and staging procedures, the clinical stage can be defined as follows:

• Stage 1a: localized melanoma less than 0.75 mm thick
• Stage 1b: localized melanoma 0.76–1.5 mm thick
• Stage 2a: localized melanoma 1.6–4 mm thick
• Stage 2b: localized melanoma greater than 4 mm thick
• Stage 3: limited nodal metastases involving only one regional lymph node group
• Stage 4: advanced regional metastases or distant metastases.

There are additional, widely practised staging systems, which are not included in this book. For prognostic purposes, however, pathological staging is significant and includes the Breslow thickness and Clark's levels:

• Clark's level I: melanoma confined to the epidermis
• Clark's level II: penetration into the papillary dermis
• Clark's level III: extension to the reticular dermis
• Clark's level IV: extension into the deep reticular dermis
• Clark's level V: invasion of the subcutaneous fat.

Breslow's staging system measures the vertical thickness of the primary tumour, grouping melanomas into 'Breslow's thickness', as less then 0.75 mm, 0.76–1.5 mm, 1.51–3.99 mm and greater than 4 mm.

Treatment

Adjuvant therapy

There have been many studies of the use of adjuvant immunotherapy in melanoma. Adjuvant immunotherapy using the interferons has led to some conflicting findings. Some studies have been positive and others not. In patients with poor-prognosis melanoma the consensus now is that treatment with adjuvant interferons may have a slight survival benefit. Cancer vaccines have been developed, enhancing antitumour immune responses, and in some recent studies prolonged survival has been reported. Treatment with adjuvant chemotherapy has largely been without any benefit at all and has produced remarkable levels of toxicities without any effect.

Management of local skin metastases and nodal disease

The treatment of this pattern of relapse is primarily surgical. Localized recurrence is excised and nodal metastases are managed by radical lymph node dissection. There are advocates of regional infusional programmes using cytotoxic chemotherapy, but the value of this is contentious. Radiotherapy may be used where localized disease is inoperable or as an adjuvant to surgery, reducing the bulk of disease prior to definitive surgery.

Treatment of metastatic melanoma

The outlook for patients with metastatic melanoma is poor. Patients generally have disease in multiple sites, and the median survival is approximately four to six months. Treatment depends upon the patient, on his or her fitness and on the disease site. Patients with multiple disease sites are treated with chemotherapy or biological therapies or a combination of the two. The most effective chemotherapeutic drugs are dacarbazine, the nitrosoureas and vindesine. The response rate to these compounds is in the range of 5–10%. Prolonged survival is very rare, and the consensus view is that there is no advantage to the combination of single agents. New chemotherapy agents are being developed for melanoma, and there is interest in the role of temozolomide.

It is clear that biological therapies are effective in melanoma. Within this group, the interferons lead to response rates of 10%. The median duration of a partial response is approximately four months, and of a complete response seven months. More recently, adoptive immunotherapy using interleukin 2 and LAK (lymphokine activated killer) cells has been evaluated in melanoma. The high response rates initially reported have not been confirmed, and the true response rates are in the order of 10% with a median duration of 3 months. Very rarely, spontaneous regression of metastatic disease occurs.

Prognosis

The most important prognostic factor is clinical stage, as reported in a group of 4000 patients treated in America and Australia. Approximately 90% of stage 1 patients, 60% of stage 2 patients and 30% of stage 3 patients survive for 10 years. The survival of stage 4 patients depends upon the metastatic site. Median survival for patients with metastases in the skin is seven months, in the lung is one year, in the brain is five months, in the liver is two months and in bone is six months. The depth of tumour invasion is the most important prognostic factor for localized melanoma. This can be described according to Clark's stage and Breslow's thickness. Ten-year survival for a lesion less than 0.75 mm thick or for a Clark's level I melanoma is 90%, for a lesion 0.75–1.5 mm thick or Clark's level II is 80%, for a lesion 1.6–2.49 mm thick or Clark's level III is 60%, for a lesion 2.5–3.99 mm thick or Clark's level IV is 50%, and for a lesion greater than 4 mm or Clark's level V is approximately 30%.

Other important survival factors have been described from multifactorial analyses. They include the type of initial surgical management, pathological stage, ulceration, presence of satellite nodules, a peripheral anatomical location and, to a much lesser extent, the patient's sex, age and tumour diameter.

The American Joint Committee on Cancer, in a study involving 17 600 patients, has provided recent information on survival. This ranges from 90% survival at five years for early-stage disease to, as might be expected, the usual miserable outlook of only 5% survival at five years for metastatic disease.

New treatment

Angiogenesis inhibitors such as thalidomide are currently under evaluation and responses have been reported. Antitumour vaccination programmes have also been developed, based on the initial observation by Morton and others.

Chapter 41

Paediatric solid tumours

Epidemiology and pathogenesis

Cancer is a leading cause of death in children in England and Wales, second only to accidental injury. It is responsible for around 10% of deaths in childhood. Cancer in children is nonetheless relatively rare, affecting 1 in 600 children, and includes a different spectrum of cancers than adults. The solid tumours encountered in childhood are often embryonal in origin, and many are associated with an inherited predisposition. There are few areas of medicine that can rival the advances made in paediatric oncology in the second half of the 20th century. 7 in 10 children with cancer are now cured, compared with fewer than three in ten in 1962–1966. It is estimated that in 2000, 55000 young adults in Britain aged 16–40 years were survivors of childhood cancer.

Many paediatric tumours are associated with recognized familial predispositions that are due to inherited mutations of tumour suppressor genes and therefore are inherited as autosomal dominant traits. Examples are hereditary retinoblastoma (mutations of the RB gene on chromosome 13q14) and familial Wilms' tumours (mutations of the WT1 gene on chromosome 11p13). In contrast, environmental oncogenic factors have been less

readily identified for paediatric solid tumours; one example, however, is the excess of papillary thyroid cancers in children following the nuclear explosion at Chernobyl (see Chapter 2).

After leukaemias, which account for 22% of childhood malignancies or 440 cases per year in the UK, central nervous system (CNS) tumours are the most common (20% or 330 cases), accounting for 2.5 in 100000 persons under 18 years old, followed by lymphoma (non-Hodgkin's lymphoma, 8%; Hodgkin's lymphoma, 6%), neuroblastoma (8%), Wilms' tumour (6%) and bone tumours (6%).

Presentation and management of CNS tumours

Tumours in the CNS occur throughout childhood; the age distribution of paediatric CNS tumours is 15% between birth and two years old, 30% from two to five years old, 30% from 5 to 10 years old, and 25% from 11 to 18 years old. In contrast to adult brain tumours, most (60%) are infratentorial and 75% are midline, involving the cerebellum, midbrain, pons and medulla. The most common tumours, accounting for 45%, are astrocytomas of varying grades. They include optic nerve gliomas, which are usually well differentiated tumours. A further 20% are medulloblastomas, a small round cell tumour of childhood, of neuroectodermal

Lecture Notes: Oncology, 2nd edition. By M. Bower and J. Waxman. Published 2010 by Blackwell Publishing Ltd.

origin. Medulloblastomas usually arise in the posterior fossa and may seed metastases in the neuraxis by dropping them down the subarachnoid space into the spinal canal. Craniopharyngiomas make up 5–10% of CNS tumours of childhood and cause raised intracranial pressure, visual defects and pituitary dysfunction: usually reduced growth hormone, thyroid-stimulating hormone (TSH), antidiuretic hormone (ADH: diabetes insipidus) or luteinizing hormone/follicle-stimulating hormone (LH/FSH) abnormalities (precocious puberty or delayed secondary sexual characteristics). Suprasellar calcification is a characteristic X-ray finding. A further 1–2% are pineal region tumours that present with Perinaud's syndrome (failure of conjugate upward gaze). Histologically, most pineal tumours are extragonadal germ cell tumours (teratomas and germinomas). Naturally, the management of these children will be determined both by the histological diagnosis and the anatomical location of the tumour and frequently involves surgery, radiotherapy and (occasionally) chemotherapy. The overall five-year survival rates according to the histology are shown in Table 41.1.

Presentation and management of neuroblastoma

Neuroblastoma is the most common malignancy in infants and often is clinically apparent at birth. About 100 new cases of neuroblastoma are diagnosed each year in the UK. Tumours often have

Table 41.1 The 5-year survival rates for paediatric CNS tumours.

Tumour	5-year survival
Any paediatric CNS tumours	56%
Low-grade glioma	80%
High-grade glioma	25%
Optic glioma	80%
Brainstem glioma	5–50%
Medulloblastoma	60%
Ependymoma	60%
Pineal germinoma	90%
Pineal teratoma	65%
Craniopharyngioma	90%

amplification of the n-Myc oncogene on chromosome 1, either as small 'double minute' (DM) chromosomes, or as 'homogenously staining regions' (HSR). They may arise from any site along the craniospinal axis derived from neural crest. The sites include abdominal sites (55%) such as the adrenal medulla (33%), pelvis (25%), thorax (13%) and head and neck (7%). In the case of head and neck neuroblastoma, these occur most commonly in the sympathetic ganglion or olfactory bulb (the latter are more common in adults). The most common finding is a large, firm and irregular abdominal mass that crosses the midline. Tumours may present with non-specific symptoms such as weight loss, failure to thrive, fever and pallor of anaemia, especially if widespread metastases are present. 70% are disseminated at diagnosis via lymphatic and haematogenous spread. Metastases to bones of the skull are common, and orbital swelling is a frequent presentation. Paraneoplastic opsoclonus or myoclonus is a rare feature. These tumours have the highest spontaneous regression rate of any tumour, usually by maturation to ganglioneuroma. Plain abdominal X-ray may show calcification: this occurs in 70% of neuroblastoma and 15% of Wilms' tumours. Other diagnostic investigations include [131]-I-labelled MIBG (meta-iodobenzyl guanidine) scan and urinary catecholamines including VMA (vanillylmandelic acid), serum NSE (neuron-specific enolase) and ferritin. Localized disease has a high cure rate with surgery and radiotherapy. On account of the high rate of disseminated disease at presentation, which is 70%, however, the overall five-year survival rate for neuroblastoma is 55%.

Presentation and management of Wilms' tumours

This highly malignant embryonal tumour of the kidney is the most common malignant lesion of the genitourinary tract in children. It was named after Dr Max Wilms, who first described it, and is also known as nephroblastoma. Most occur in children under five years old, and some are hereditary. Only about 75 children develop a Wilms' tumour each year in Britain. Wilms' tumours are associated with congenital abnormalities including aniridia and the WAGR syndrome (Wilms' tumour, aniridia, gonadoblastoma and mental retardation), Denys–Drash syndrome (Wilms' tumour, male pseudohermaphroditism and diffuse glomerular disease) and Beckwith–Wiedemann syndrome (organomegaly, hemihypertrophy, increased incidence of Wilms' tumour, hepatoblastoma and adrenocortical tumours). Wilms' tumours present in usually healthy children as abdominal swellings with a smooth, firm, non-tender mass. A quarter have gross haematuria, and occasionally children present with hypertension, malaise or fever. Up to 20% have metastases at diagnosis; lungs are the most common site of metastases. The main stay of treatment is surgical resection with adjuvant radiotherapy to the tumour bed, reserved for children with a high risk of relapse. The five-year survival for Wilms' tumours now exceeds 80%, and one of the goals of more recent trials is to reduce the long-term morbidity of treatment.

Presentation and management of liver tumours

Fewer than 10 children in the UK develop liver tumours each year. Liver cancers are divided into hepatoblastoma (66%), which usually occurs before the age of three years, and hepatocellular cancers (33%), which occur at any age. Hepatoblastoma occurs as part of the Beckwith–Widemann syndrome and is also associated with familial adenomatous polyposis. Hepatoblastoma is the third most common intra-abdominal malignancy in young children – after neuroblastoma and Wilms' tumours. It most frequently affects the right lobe of the liver, and 10% have disseminated disease at presentation with regional lymph node involvement or lung metastases. Hepatocellular carcinoma is associated with hepatitis B and C infection, tyrosinaemia, biliary cirrhosis and α_1-antitrypsin deficiency. Surgical resection with or without neoadjuvant chemotherapy has dramatically improved the prognosis in hepatoblastoma, where the five-year overall survival is now 70%. In contrast, the prognosis for hepatocellular carcinoma in children is not greatly different from that for

adults, with five-year overall survival rates of around 25%.

Presentation and management of retinoblastoma

Retinoblastoma most often occurs in children under five years old and in a third of cases is bilateral. There are about 40 new cases of retinoblastoma diagnosed each year in the UK. Up to 40% are hereditary due to germline mutations of the retinoblastoma (RB) gene, and these children frequently have bilateral retinoblastoma and present at a younger age. Hereditary retinoblastoma was the basis of Knudsen's two-hit model of tumour suppressor genes. These tumours present with whitening of the pupil, squint or secondary glaucoma. Retinoblastoma is usually confined to the orbit, and hence the cure rate with enucleation is high. Smaller tumours may be treated with localized cryotherapy, laser treatment or a radioactive iodine plaque stitched to the outer surface of the eye. Overall, 90% of children with retinoblastoma are cured. Hereditary retinoblastoma, however, is also associated with other malignancies, especially osteosarcoma, soft tissue sarcoma and melanoma. Genetic counselling is an integral part of therapy for retinoblastoma. All siblings should be examined periodically: DNA polymorphism analysis may identify relatives at high risk.

Presentation and management of bone tumours and sarcomas

Osteosarcoma

The incidence of bone tumours is highest during adolescence, although they only represent 3% of all childhood cancers. Only about 30 children develop these tumours each year in the UK. Most tumours occur in areas of rapid growth in the metaphysis near the growth plate, where cellular proliferation and remodelling are greatest during long bone growth. The most active growth plates are in the distal femur and proximal tibia. These are also the most common sites for primary bone cancers. Known risk factors include hereditary retinoblastoma, Li–Fraumeni syndrome and prior radiotherapy. Most primary bone tumours present as painful swellings which may cause stiffness and effusions in nearby joints. Occasionally, tumours present as pathological fractures. The radiological appearances are a lytic or sclerotic expansile lesion, associated with a wide transition zone, cortical destruction, a soft tissue mass, periosteal reaction and calcification. The clinical management of bone tumours requires a specialist multidisciplinary unit including orthopaedic surgeons, plastic surgeons and oncologists. Clinical management should happen in the context of an adolescent oncology unit, since the majority of patients fit into this age group, with all its special needs. Neo-adjuvant chemotherapy plays an important role in localized osteosarcoma and Ewing's sarcoma to shrink the tumour and hopefully allow limb sparing surgery without increasing relapse rates. Postoperative adjuvant chemotherapy and radio-therapy are useful in some tumours. The five-year survival has steadily risen from under 20% in the late 1960s to over 60%.

Ewing's sarcoma

Ewing's sarcoma is named after Dr James Ewing, who described the tumour in the 1920s. Ewing's sarcoma is a childhood bone malignancy of uncertain cellular origin that is associated with the t(11;22) chromosomal translocation that juxtaposes the EWS and Fli-1 genes, resulting in a hybrid transcript from these two transcription factor genes. This same chromosomal translocation occurs in peripheral neuroectodermal tumours (PNETs) and Askin lung tumours, suggesting a possible common origin. PNETs are thought to arise from peripheral autonomic nervous system tissue and stain for NSE as well as S-100. Morphologically, all three tumours are small round blue cell tumours – a group that also includes embryonal rhabdomyosarcoma, non-Hodgkin's lymphoma, neuroblastoma and small cell lung cancer. About 30 children each year in the UK develop Ewing's sarcoma. It most frequently occurs in the teenage years. Ewing's sarcoma is very rare in African and Asian children and is not associated with familial

syndromes or prior radiotherapy. It usually starts in a bone at the diaphysis or, less frequently, the metaphysic – most commonly in one of the bones of the hips, upper arm or thigh, although it can also develop in soft tissue. The most common symptom is pain and swelling, but systemic symptoms such as pyrexia, weight loss and night sweats may also occur. X-rays usually demonstrate ill-defined medullary destruction, small areas of new bone formation, periosteal reaction and soft tissue expansion. Approximately a fifth of patients have metastases in their lungs or bones at presentation. Multimodality treatment including surgery, radiotherapy and chemotherapy is standard practice for Ewing's sarcoma, and the five-year survival rate is 55%.

Rhabdomyosarcoma

Rhabdomyosarcoma is the most common paediatric soft tissue sarcoma, although only 60 children are diagnosed with this tumour in the UK each year, and most are under 10 years old. Rhabdomyosarcoma may be divided into alveolar (25–30%), embryonal (50–60%) and pleomorphic (5%). The embryonal type occurs in the first decade, most often in the head and neck and genitourinary tract. The alveolar type occurs in adolescents, in the forearms and trunk. The pleomorphic type occurs in adults. Consistent chromosomal translocations have been found in a number of soft tissue sarcomas, both benign and malignant. These chromosomal rearrangements may be of help diagnostically; for example, 75% of alveolar rhabdomyosarcomas harbour the t(2:13)(q35:q14) chromosomal translocation that fuses the PAX3 gene and the FKHR (forkhead) gene. The consequence of many of these translocations is the transcription of chimeric mRNA, containing 5′ sequences of one gene and 3′ sequences from another gene, and translation to hybrid proteins. Many of the genes involved with these translocations are themselves transcription factors, and it is postulated that the consequence of these translocations is the aberrant expression of a number of downstream genes. Rhabdomyosarcomas present as masses that grow and may become hard and painful. Approximately 15% have metastases at presentation; most frequently in the lungs, bones and lymph nodes. Treatment involves both surgery and chemotherapy but is risk stratified, with radiotherapy reserved for those at higher risk of relapse in order to save those at low risk of recurrence from the late effects of radiotherapy. The five-year overall survival is 75%.

Langerhans' cell histiocytosis

Langerhans' cell histiocytosis (LCH), previously known as histiocytosis X, is not strictly a cancer but may behave in an aggressive fashion and is often treated by oncologists. About 30 children develop LCH in the UK each year; most of them are under two years old. LCH is a proliferation of epidermal histiocytes or Langerhans' cells, which are antigen-presenting dendritic cells named after Paul Langerhans, who first described them in 1868 when he was a 21-year-old medical student in Berlin. LCH comprises three overlapping syndromes: unifocal bone diease (solitary eosinophilic granuloma), multifocal disease of bone (Hand–Schüller–Christian disease) and multifocal, multisystem disease (Letterer–Siwe disease). Letterer–Siwe disease occurs mainly in boys under two years old; Hand–Schüller–Christian syndrome has a peak of onset in children aged 2–10 years; whilst solitary eosinophilic granuloma occurs in those aged 5–15 years. Solitary eosinophilic granuloma occurs at any site in bones, is usually asymptomatic and is frequently an incidental finding. Patients with Hand–Schüller–Christian syndrome often present with recurrent episodes of otitis media and mastoiditis or with polyuria and polydipsia due to diabetes insipidus. Letterer–Siwe disease presents with symptoms suggestive of a systemic infection or malignancy with a generalized skin eruption, anaemia and hepatosplenomegaly and other protean manifestations (Table 41.2). This eponymous classification of LCH has in part been abandoned, and a simpler classification into either restricted LCH (skin or bone lesions) or extensive LCH (visceral organ involvement) has been introduced. The diagnosis is confirmed histologically; the characteristic cytological features are

Table 41.2 Clinical manifestations of extensive Langerhans' cell histiocytosis.

System	Clinical manifestations
Systemic effects	Pyrexia, weight loss, fatigue
Bone	Painful swelling (skull (50%), femur (17%), ribs (8%), pelvis, vertebrae), associated soft tissue swelling (proptosis, mastoiditis and deafness, gums)
Skin	Scaly, erythematous, seborrhoea-like brown to red papules (behind the ears and in the axillary, inguinal and perineal areas) (50%)
Endocrine glands	Diabetes insipidus (20%) due to involvement of the hypothalamus or pituitary stalk
Bone marrow	Pancytopenia
Lymph nodes	Lymphadenopathy (30%)
Liver and spleen	Hepatosplenomegaly
Gastrointestinal tract	Failure to thrive, malabsorption, diarrhoea, vomiting (5–10%)
Lungs	Dyspnoea, honey-comb lungs, bullae, spontaneous pneumothorax, emphysema (20%)
Central nervous system	Progressive ataxia, dysarthria, intracranial hypertension, cranial nerve palsies (10%)

CD1a surface antigen expression and cytoplasmic Birbeck granules. Localized bone disease is treated surgically or, less frequently, with radiotherapy, whilst systemic disease requires chemotherapy with cladribine often with desmopressin for the management of the diabetes insipidus. Survival exceeds 95% in unifocal disease and 80% in multifocal bone disease, but is only 50% in patients with systemic multiorgan disease.

Complications of treatment

Although many of the delayed effects of chemotherapy and radiotherapy in children are similar to those in adults, the effects on developing organs also produce unique late side effects, particularly on the skeleton, brain and endocrine systems.

These delayed effects of multimodality therapy on the developing child are substantial and the late sequelae cause considerable morbidity in this group of patients where the long-term survival rates are high. Radiotherapy retards bone and cartilage growth, and causes intellectual impairment, gonadal toxicity, hypothalamic and thyroid dysfunction, as well as pneumonitis, nephrotoxicity and hepatotoxicity. Late consequences of chemo- therapy include infertility, anthracycline related cardiotoxicity, bleomycin-related pulmonary fibrosis and platinum-related nephrotoxicity and neurotoxicity. Up to 5% of children cured of this cancer will develop a second malignancy as a consequence of an inherited cancer predisposition or the late sequelae of cancer treatment. Second malignancies occur most frequently following combined chemotherapy and radiotherapy.

Chapter 42

Bone cancers and sarcomas

Epidemiology and pathogenesis

Bone tumours are amongst the oldest cancers discovered in humans according to palaeopathological evidence. A Bronze Age woman with bone metastases in her skull has been dated to 1600–1900 BC, whilst Saxon bones from Standlake in Oxfordshire, UK, demonstrate features of osteosarcoma in a young adult warrior. St Peregrine, born in 1260 at Forlì, Italy, is the patron saint of cancer sufferers (the feast day is on 4 May). He was due for an amputation for a sarcoma of the leg, but the cancer was cured on the night prior to surgery, following a vision of Christ. He lived a further 20 years and was canonized in 1726. The presumed origins of primary bone tumours are shown in Table 42.1.

Sarcomas are tumours of the connective tissue, which supports the body and includes bone muscle, tendon, fat and synovial tissue. These tumours represent less than 1% of all malignancies. They have an incidence of approximately 1–2 per 100 000 per annum. There are no known associated aetiological factors, although sarcomas rarely occur as second malignancies in areas of the body that have been previously irradiated. The most common bone tumours are osteosarcoma (see Figure 2.12) and Ewing's sarcoma.

Ewing's sarcoma occurs in childhood and in early adult life. Molecular biology studies have shown the presence of a specific chromosomal translocation between chromosomes 22 and 11. This translocation is present in a group of small, round, blue cell tumours which include peripheral neuroectodermal tumours (PNETs), classic Ewing's and extraosseous Ewing's sarcoma; these are now grouped together for treatment purposes. In patients with this group of tumours there may be difficulty in obtaining a histopathological diagnosis. Modern advances in molecular biology have led to the identification of the EWS/FLI-1 translocation present in patients with Ewing's sarcoma. The presence of this translocation is identifiable by fluorescence *in situ* hybridization (FISH).

Osteosarcoma occurs in two groups of patients: firstly in adolescence or early adult life and secondly in old age, where osteosarcoma complicates Paget's disease. p53 mutations are commonly seen in osteosarcoma, as are mutations in the retinoblastoma gene.

Presentation

Most soft tissue sarcomas occur in the limbs, and patients present to their GPs with localized swelling. Patients with Ewing's tumours and sarcomas generally present with pain, and the diagnosis

Lecture Notes: Oncology, 2nd edition. By M. Bower and J. Waxman. Published 2010 by Blackwell Publishing Ltd.

usually comes as a result of the classic X-ray appearances of these tumours. Fractures are common and nerve palsies may be seen where there is a cranial presentation. Patients may also present with metastases. Because of the rarity of these tumours and the requirement for a multidisciplinary specialist approach, patients with a suspected diagnosis of sarcoma should be referred on to specialist centres, where results have been shown to be vastly superior to those achieved by peripheral clinics. These tumours are usually diagnosed after a significant delay.

Tables 42.2–42.4 list the clinical features of the different types of bone cancers and sarcomas, some of which are illustrated in Figures 42.1–42.4.

Investigations and management

In a patient where a diagnosis of soft tissue sarcoma is suspected, an initial biopsy should be carried out by the surgeon who is to perform definitive surgery. Fine needle aspiration cytology, core needle biopsy and incisional biopsies are all techniques that are considered by the surgeon and, for those patients with rare abdominal or thoracic soft tissue sarcomas, CT-guided biopsies may be required. After the pathological diagnosis has been established, definitive surgery can be planned. This requires a

Table 42.1 Origins of primary bone tumours.

Origin	Benign tumour	Malignant tumour
Cartilage	Enchondroma Osteochondroma Chondroblastoma	Chondrosarcoma
Bone	Osteoid osteoma Osteoblastoma	Osteosarcoma
Unknown origin	Giant cell tumour	Ewing's sarcoma Malignant fibrous histiocytoma

Table 42.2 Clinical features of cartilage-derived bone tumours.

	Enchondroma	Osteochondroma (exostosis)	Chondroblastoma	Chondrosarcoma
Age	10–50 years	10–20 years	5–20 years	30–60 years
Site	Hands, wrist Diaphysis	Knee, shoulder, pelvis Metaphysis	Knee, shoulder, ribs Epiphysis prior to fusion	Knee, shoulder, pelvis Metaphysis or diaphysis
X-ray	Well-defined lucency, thin sclerotic rim, calcification	Eccentric protrusion from bone, calcification	Well-defined lucency, thin sclerotic rim, calcification	Expansile lucency, sclerotic margin, cortical destruction, soft tissue mass
Notes	Ollier's disease = multiple enchondromas	1% transform to chondrosarcoma		

Table 42.3 Clinical features of osteoid-derived bone tumours.

	Osteoid osteoma	Osteoblastoma	Osteosarcoma
Age	10–30 years	10–20 years	10–25 years and >60 years
Site	Knee Diaphysis	Vertebra Metaphysis	Knee, shoulder, pelvis Metaphysis
X-ray	<1 cm central lucency, surrounding bone sclerosis, periosteal reaction	Well-defined lucency, sclerotic rim, cortex preserved, calcification	Lytic/sclerotic expansile lesion, wide transition zone, cortical destruction, soft tissue mass, periosteal reaction, calcification

Table 42.4 Clinical features of bone tumours of uncertain origins.

	Giant cell tumour	Ewing's sarcoma	Malignant fibrous histiocytoma
Age	20–40 years	5–15 years	10–20 years and >60 years
Site	Long bones, knee	Knee, shoulder, pelvis	Knee, pelvis, shoulder
	Epiphysis and metaphysis post closure	Diaphysis, less often metaphysis	Metaphysis
X-ray	Lucency with ill-defined endosteal margin, cortical destruction, soft tissue mass, eccentric expansion bone/lung metastases	Ill-defined medullary destruction, small areas of new bone formation, periosteal reaction, soft tissue expansion,	Cortical destruction, periosteal reaction, soft tissue mass

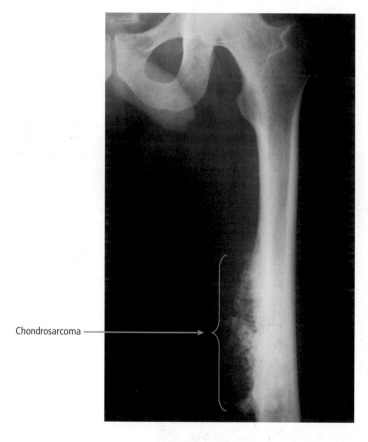

Chondrosarcoma

Figure 42.1 Femur chondrosarcoma showing an expansile lesion with sclerotic margin, cortical destruction and punctuate internal calcification and an associated soft tissue mass. These tumours are most common in middle age and occur around the knee, shoulder or pelvis.

multidisciplinary approach that takes place in the context of magnetic resonance (MR) staging of the local tumour and CT definition of the metastatic sites. The surgical approach requires the removal of the muscle compartment to include the fascia. This limits the risk of local relapse.

In those patients with Ewing's sarcoma and osteosarcoma, initial staging will include CT assessment of the chest, abdomen and pelvis, and MR imaging of the primary tumour site. The initial management option for Ewing's sarcoma includes the consideration of either primary surgery or

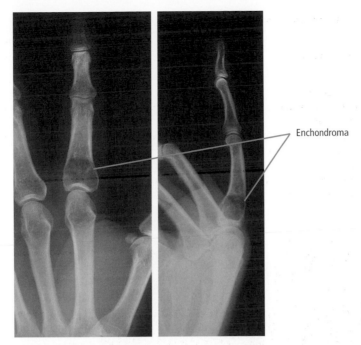

Enchondroma

Figure 42.2 Enchondroma of the ring finger proximal phalynx showing well-defined lucency and a thin sclerotic rim with preserved cortex. These cartilage-derived tumours occur in 10–50-year-olds most frequently in the diaphyses of the hand or wrist. Multiple enchondromas occur in Ollier's disease, a non-hereditary condition that is associated with an increased risk of chondrosarcoma.

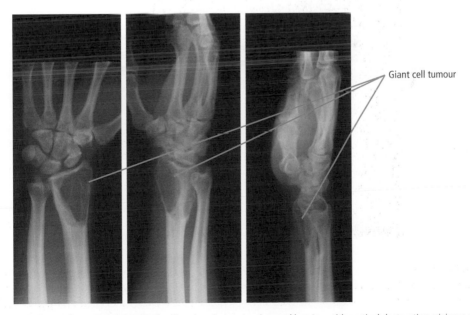

Giant cell tumour

Figure 42.3 Giant cell tumour of the distal radius showing expansion and lucency with cortical destruction giving a multi-loculated appearance. These tumours occur most commonly in 20–40-year-olds in long bones at the epiphyses and metaphyses after closure.

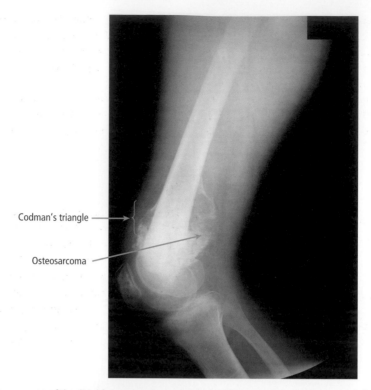

Codman's triangle

Osteosarcoma

Figure 42.4 Osteosarcoma of the distal femur showing an expansile soft tissue mass with internal calcification and cortical destruction. There is a marked periosteal reaction with lifting of the periosteum that is described as Codman's triangle, which is almost always due to an aggressive malignant bone tumour extending into adjacent soft tissues.

radiotherapy to control the local lesion. If the lesion is small and it is possible to have substantial resection margins, surgery is the best option with immediate endoprosthetic replacement. For the majority of patients, however, radiotherapy remains the most important treatment modality for the control of local disease.

Osteosarcomas are rare and for this reason also best managed in specialist centres. This is particularly important for teenage patients with sarcomas. For these patients, chemotherapy, radiation, surgery and counselling all have a significant role in management. Patients with osteosarcomas are generally managed well because of the excellent results achieved using multidisciplinary specialist approaches. In osteosarcoma, bone scanning as well as CT and MR scanning are essential in the initial work up of a patient. Biopsy of the tumour is required with the open approach preferred. Surgi-

cal advances have meant that bone tumours are managed much better than they were, with the aim of limb-sparing prosthetic surgery.

Pathology

The most helpful classification of soft tissue tumours is into tumours of fibrous tissue, fibrohistiocytic tumours, adipose tissue tumours including liposarcomas, tumours of muscle, tumours of blood vessels, tumours of lymph vessels, tumours of synovium, tumours of mesothelium, tumours of peripheral nerves, tumours of autonomic ganglia, tumours of paraganglionic structures, tumours of cartilage and bone-forming tissue, tumours of pleuripotential mesochyme, tumours of uncertain histogenesis and unclassified soft tissue tumours. This latter tumour group is extremely diverse, with at least 50 different subtypes.

These groups may in turn be divided into benign and malignant conditions. Benign tumours do not generally metastasize, and microscopic examination shows a low mitotic rate. Malignant tumours have a high mitotic rate and do tend to metastasize. Approximately one-third of tumours are low grade and two-thirds are high grade. Osteosarcomas are described as being of low, intermediate and high grade.

Treatment of soft tissue sarcomas

The clinical features of soft tissue sarcomas are listed in Table 42.5, along with the primary therapy.

Treatment of the primary tumour

There is considerable discussion as to the appropriate management of a soft tissue sarcoma. Low-grade tumours, which by definition should not spread, should be treated by surgical excision alone. Local control should result in 85–100% recovery in these patients. The situation is different for those patients with high-grade tumours, and there is debate as to whether surgery alone, surgery combined with radiation, or surgery, radiation and chemotherapy in combination is the correct approach.

Surgery

There is little argument that surgery is necessary, and the operation of first choice should be one that allows a reasonably wide margin of normal tissue to be excised with the tumour. If a good procedure is carried out, such as muscle compartmental excision, the local failure rate is 7–18%. If less radical procedures such as excision biopsy are performed, then the local failure rate is approximately 50%. More radical procedures such as amputation have a

Table 42.5 Clinical features of soft tissue sarcomas.

Tumour	Age (years)	Commonest sites	Primary therapy	5-year survival
Fibrosarcoma	20–50	Thigh, arm, head and neck	Wide excision and adjuvant radiation	90% (well differentiated) 50% (poorly differentiated)
Liposarcoma	40–60	Thigh, head and neck (rarely arise from lipoma)	Wide excision and adjuvant radiation	66% (myxoid) 10% (pleomorphic)
Embryonal rhabdomyosarcoma	0–10	Head and neck, genitourinary (botyroid)	Neoadjuvant chemoradiation and surgery	40%
Alveolar rhabdomyosarcoma	10–20	Thigh	Neoadjuvant chemoradiation and surgery	60%
Pleomorphic rhabdomyosarcoma	40–70	Thigh, upper arm	Wide excision and adjuvant radiation	10%
Synovial sarcoma	20–40	Leg	Wide excision and adjuvant radiation	40%
Angiosarcoma	50–70	Skin, superficial soft tissues	Wide excision and adjuvant radiation	15%
Leiomyosarcoma	45–65	Retroperitoneal, uterine	Wide excision and adjuvant radiation	40%

lower local recurrence rate, of approximately 5%. Over the last decade, there has been a trend toward radical compartmental excision with limb-sparing procedures.

Adjuvant chemotherapy and radiation

After definitive surgery has been performed, the need for radiation and chemotherapy is assessed. Radiation is not given for low-grade tumours. In high-grade tumours, radiotherapy to the tumour bed has an advantage in terms of reduced local recurrence rates in extremity lesions where effective dosages can be given without risking vital structures. Local radiation has no effect upon the progression of distant metastases. Because patients with high-grade sarcomas are at great risk from the progression of their cancer to a metastatic state, adjuvant chemotherapy has been investigated in a number of trials. The original studies, which were non-randomized, showed an advantage to combination chemotherapy. This result has not held up, and the consensus view now is that adjuvant chemotherapy has no advantage in terms of five-year survival. This remains very much a subject for debate, however, and in many centres adjuvant chemotherapy is still administered.

Treatment of metastatic sarcoma

The treatment of metastatic soft tissue sarcoma requires the use of chemotherapy. The most effective single-agent treatments lead to responses in 15–35% of patients. Attempts are made to capitalize on this by the use of combination chemotherapy programmes. A slight increase in response rates has been found by some groups of clinicians. This supposed advantage is, however, much debated. Many cancer doctors would advocate the administration of single-agent chemotherapy to their patients simply because combination therapies maximize toxicities and do not provide a significant advantage.

Treatment of Ewing's sarcomas

For patients with Ewing's tumours, the last 20 or 30 years have seen a significant evolution of treatment protocols. One type of management generally consists of treatment with induction chemotherapy, followed by local treatment to the primary site with either surgery or radiotherapy or both. This will be followed by further consolidation chemotherapy.

Treatment of osteosarcomas

Similarly in sarcomas, primary chemotherapy to debulk the tumour is followed by surgery. Both chemotherapy and surgery are complex and highly specialized, requiring immense technical skill and input from many areas of medical and paramedical expertise. Patients with metastatic osteosarcoma can be cured, and, once more, surgery is enormously important. Surgical excision of pulmonary mestastases is considered and may be curative in a limited number of patients.

New treatment

Although there have been some developments in chemotherapy, it is not thought that chemotherapy will be the future for patients with sarcomas. Oncologists and their patients have been most encouraged by the development of imatinib (Glevec), which is an agent that inhibits the function of the BCR-ABL oncogene and of the KIT and platelet-derived growth factor (PDGF) tyrosine kinases. This agent is active in chronic myeloid leukaemia and is described in the leukaemia section of this book. It also has activity in gastrointestinal stromal sarcomas, which are rare sarcomas of the bowel. Patients who have gross metastatic disease have been seen to respond to this agent without any significant toxicity. This is clearly a wonderful development and may have a role in the management of bone tumours.

Chapter 43

Unknown primary cancer

Epidemiology and pathogenesis

For most patients who present with metastatic disease, routine examination and investigation will quickly disclose the underlying primary tumour. Occasionally, the primary tumour may be more elusive, and a number of clinical, histopathological and serological clues may help to establish the site. For 1–5% of patients, however, the primary site remains undisclosed because it is too small to be detected or has regressed. The usual histological diagnosis in these patients with an unknown primary site is adenocarcinoma or poorly differentiated carcinoma. The benefits of establishing the primary site include diagnosing treatable disease (Table 43.1), avoiding overtreating unresponsive disease and hence iatrogenic morbidity in resistant disease, preventing complications that relate to occult primary disease, such as bowel obstruction, and, finally, clarifying the prognosis. The methods commonly used to aid in the hunt for a primary site are described below.

Clinical sites of metastatic spread

Different tumours follow different patterns of metastatic spread. This may be related to chemokine

and chemokine receptor expression by tumours and stromal cells (see Part 1).

Brain and meningeal metastases

Up to 30% of solid tumours develop parenchymal brain metastases. Carcinomatous meningitis is less common. Carcinomatous meningitis presents with multiple, anatomically distant, cranial and spinal root neuropathies. The diagnosis may be confirmed by finding malignant cells in the cerebrospinal fluid. Treatment usually involves a combination of intrathecal chemotherapy and craniospinal radiotherapy. Carcinomatous meningitis most frequently occurs with leukaemias and lymphomas and occasionally with breast cancer. Parenchymal brain secondaries that may occur with any solid tumour are usually treated with whole-brain radiotherapy, although surgery may be considered for patients with solitary brain metastases and limited systemic disease (see Figure 15.2).

Bone metastases

Bone metastases are a major source of morbidity in patients with cancer and often have a prolonged course. Bone metastases cause pain, reduced mobility, pathological fractures, hypercalcaemia, myelosuppression and nerve compression syndromes. The tumours that commonly metastasize to bone

Lecture Notes: Oncology, 2nd edition. By M. Bower and J. Waxman. Published 2010 by Blackwell Publishing Ltd.

are lung, breast, prostate, renal and thyroid tumours and sarcomas. Metastases usually occur in the axial skeleton, femur or humerus. If they are found elsewhere, then renal cancer and melanoma should be considered as possible primary tumour sites. Most bone metastases are lucent, lytic lesions; occasionally dense, sclerotic deposits are seen in prostate, breast, carcinoid tumours and Hodgkin's disease. The diagnosis of bone metastases is rarely complicated. The differential diagnosis is outlined in Table 43.2. (See also Figures 1.7, 16.1, 16.2 and 31.3.)

Lung metastases

The lungs are the second most common site for metastases via haematogenous spread. Tumours that commonly metastasize to the lung include lung, breast, renal, thyroid, sarcoma and germ cell tumours. Surgical resection of pulmonary metastases is occasionally undertaken where the primary site is controlled and the lungs are the sole site of metastasis. (See also Figures 2.7 and 17.1c.)

Liver metastases

Of all patients with liver metastases, 60% have a colorectal primary tumour, 25% have melanoma, 15% lung cancer and 5% breast cancer. Hepatic resection for patients with up to three metastases from colorectal cancer results in five-year survivals of 30% and is the best treatment available for selected patients.

Malignant effusions

Eighty percent of malignant pleural effusions are due to lung and breast cancer, lymphoma and

Table 43.1 Treatable unknown primary diagnoses.

Chemosensitive tumours	Hormone-sensitive tumours
Non-Hodgkin's lymphoma	Breast cancer
Germ cell tumours	Prostate cancer
Neuroendocrine tumours (including small cell lung cancer)	Endometrial cancer
Ovarian cancer	Thyroid cancer

Table 43.2 Differential diagnosis of bone metastases.

Diagnosis	Pain	Site	Age	X-ray	Bone scan, CT/MRI	Biochemistry
Metastases	Common	Axial skeleton	Any	Discrete lesions, pathological fracture, loss of vertebral pedicles	Soft tissue extension on MRI/CT	Raised ALP and Ca
Degenerative disease	Common	Limbs	Old	Symmetrical	Symmetrical uptake on bone scan	Normal
Osteoporosis	Painless (unless pathological fracture)	Vertebrae	Old (female)	Osteopenia	Normal bone scan/MRI	Normal
Paget's disease	Painless	Skull (often)	Old	Expanded sclerotic bones	Diffusely hot bone scan	Raised ALP and urinary hydroxyproline
Traumatic fracture	Always	Ribs	Any	Fracture	Intense linear uptake on bone scan	Normal

ALP, alkaline phosphatase; Ca, calcium; CT, computed tomography; MRI, magnetic resonance imaging.

leukaemia. Malignant pericardial effusion is rarer than pleural effusions; breast and lung cancer account for 75%. Metastases to the heart and pericardium are 40 times more common than primary tumours at these sites, but only 15% will develop tamponade. Malignant ascites is a common complication of ovarian, pancreatic, colorectal and gastric cancers and lymphoma. Measures for long-term control of malignant effusions include sclerosis with talc, bleomycin or tetracycline for pleural effusions, drainage by pericardial window for pericardial effusions and peritoneovenous shunts for malignant ascites (see Figure 46.6).

Clinical unknown primary syndromes

Five highly treatable subsets of unknown primary site have been identified, which have more favourable outcomes and require distinct management:
1. Women with isolated axillary lymphadenopathy (adenocarcinoma or undifferentiated carcinoma) usually have an occult breast primary and should be managed as stage II breast cancer. They have a similar prognosis (five-year survival is 70%).
2. Women with peritoneal carcinomatosis (often papillary carcinoma with elevated serum CA-125) should be managed as stage III ovarian cancer.
3. Men with extragonadal germ cell syndrome or atypical teratoma present with features reminiscent of gonadal germ cell tumours. They occur predominantly in young men with pulmonary or lymph node metastases. Germ cell tumour markers (α-fetoprotein (AFP) and human chorionic gonadotrophin (HCG)) may be detected in the serum and in tissue by immunocytochemistry. Cytogenetic analysis for isochromosome 12p (see Box 1.4) is positive in 90% of cases. Empirical chemotherapy with cisplatin-based combinations yield response rates of over 50% and up to 30% long-term survival.
4. Patients with neuroendocrine carcinoma of an unknown primary site overlap with extrapulmonary small cell carcinoma, anaplastic islet cell carcinoma, Merkel cell tumours and paragangliomas. Immunocytochemical staining for chromogranin, neuron-specific enolase, synapto-

physin and epithelial antigens (cytokeratins and epithelial membrane antigen) are usually positive. Patients often present with bone metastases and diffuse liver involvement. These tumours are frequently responsive to platinum-based combination chemotherapy.
5. Patients with high cervical lymphadenopathy containing squamous cell carcinoma may have occult head and neck tumours of the nasopharynx, oropharynx or hypopharynx. Radical neck dissection followed by extended field radiotherapy that includes these possible primary sites may yield five-year survival rates of 30%. Adenocarcinoma in high cervical nodes and lower cervical adenopathy containing either histology, however, have a much worse prognosis and should not be treated in this aggressive fashion.

Unfortunately, the majority of unknown primary tumours do not fit into any of these subsets, and the response rates to chemotherapy are below 20%. These responses are usually of brief duration, with no impact on overall survival. The median survival is under 12 months. The exception to this rule is in the group of patients who are under 45 years old. In this group, treatment with BEP (bleomycin, etoposide and cisplatin) or a taxane combination is worthwhile. For this group of patients, 50% survive in excess of two years. Tumours from patients such as these do not have the characteristics of testicular cancer, that is, their tumours do not stain positively for HCG or AFP.

Histopathological characterization

The histopathological characterization of unknown primaries to establish their origin includes a number of techniques: light microscopy, immunocytochemical staining, immunophenotyping, electron microscopy, cytogenetics and molecular analysis. These are described in detail in Part 1.

Serological characterization

Tumour markers are proteins produced by cancers that are detectable in the blood of patients. Ideally, serum tumour markers should be quick and cheap

Table 43.3 The most common serum tumour markers and their uses.

Name	Natural occurrence	Tumour	Comments	Screening	Diagnosis	Prognosis	Follow-up
Carcino embryonic antigen (CEA)	Glycoprotein found in intestinal mucosa during embryonic and fetal life	Colorectal cancer (especially liver metastases), gastric, breast and lung cancer	Elevated in smokers' cirrhosis, chronic hepatitis, UC, Crohn's, pneumonia and TB (usually <10 ng/ml)	No	Yes	Yes	Yes
Alpha-fetoprotein (AFP)	Glycoprotein found in yolk sac and fetal liver	Germ cell tumours (GCTs) (80% non-seminomatous GCTs), hepatocellular cancer (50%), neural tube defects, Down's pregnancies	Role in screening in pregnancy not cancer Only prognostic for GCT not HCC Transient increase in liver diseases	No	Yes	Yes	Yes
Prostate-specific antigen (PSA)	Glycoprotein member of human kallikrein gene family. PSA is a serine protease that liquefies semen in excretory ducts of prostate	Prostate cancer (95%), also benign prostatic hypertrophy and prostatitis (usually <10 ng/ml)	Tissue specific but not tumour specific although a level of >10 ng/ml is 90% specific for cancer	*	Yes	No	Yes
Cancer antigen 125 (CA-125)	Differentiation antigen of coelomic epithelium (Muller's duct)	Ovarian epithelial cancer (75%), also gastrointestinal, lung and breast cancers	Raised in cirrhosis, chronic pancreatitis, autoimmune diseases and any cause of ascites	*	Yes	No	Yes
Human chorionic gondadotrophin (HCG)	Glycoprotein hormone, 14 kD α subunit and 24 kD β subunit from placental syncytiotrophoblasts	Choriocarcinoma (100%), hydatidiform moles (97%), non-seminomatous GCT (50–80%), seminoma (15%)	Screening post-hydatidiform mole for trophoblastic tumours, also used to follow pregnancies and diagnose ectopic pregnancies	Yes	Yes	Yes	Yes

Table 43.3 *Continued*

Name	Natural occurrence	Tumour	Comments	Screening	Diagnosis	Prognosis	Follow-up
Calcitonin	32 amino acid peptide from C cells of thyroid	Medullary cell carcinoma of thyroid	Screening test in MEN 2	Yes	Yes	Yes	Yes
Beta-2-microglobulin	Part of HLA common fragment present on surface of lymphocytes, macrophages and some epithelial cells	Non-Hodgkin's lymphoma, myeloma	Elevated in autoimmune disease, renal glomerular disease	No	No	Yes	Yes
Thyroglobulin	Matrix protein for thyroid hormone synthesis in normal thyroid follicles	Papillary and follicular thyroid cancer		No	Yes	No	Yes
Placental alkaline phosphatase (PLAP)	Isoenzyme of alkaline phosphatase	Seminoma and ovariandysgerminoma (50%)		No	Yes	No	Yes

* See Part 3.

HCC, hepatocellular carcinoma; HLA, human leucocyte antigen; TB, tuberculosis; UC, ulcerative colitis.

to measure, have high sensitivity (of more than 50%) and specificity (over 95%) and yield a high predictive value of positive (PPV) and negative (NPV) results. Under these circumstances, tumour markers may be used for population screening, diagnosis, as prognostic factors, for monitoring treatment, diagnosing remission and detecting relapse and for imaging metastases. A large number of serum tumour markers are available, and each may be valuable for any of screening, diagnosis, prognostication and monitoring treatment (Table 43.3).

Approach to investigation of metastatic disease to establish primary site

There is a worrying tendency to over-investigate patients with unknown primary cancer while at the same time ignoring their palliative care needs. So often the greater the eminence and number of consultants whose advice is sought, the larger the number of esoteric investigations ordered, and the less well the patient and their family are informed. Investigations should be restricted to those that will alter clinical management. It is estimated that in the absence of a localizing sympton, extensive radiological investigation leads to the identification of a primary site in less than 5% of all patients. The prognosis is generally poor, with a median survival of three to four months. Less than 25% of patients survive to one year, and less than 10% are alive after five years. The site of the primary is usually on the same side of the diaphragm as the metastases, and 75% of tumours are infradiaphragmatic; of the 25% that arise above the diaphragm, nearly all arise from the lung. Where identified, the most common primary sites, in order of frequency, are: lung, pancreas, liver, colorectal, stomach, kidney, prostate, ovary, breast, lymphoid and testis. A good performance status is the most important predictor of survival, while extensive weight loss and older age are adverse prognostic factors. With the exception of the five clinical syndromes listed above, treatment other than symptom palliation is rarely appropriate.

Chapter 44

Immunodeficiency and cancer

Hereditary or primary immunodeficiency

Primary immunodeficiencies are mainly single-gene inherited disorders that present in early childhood. They include nearly 100 syndromes, three-quarters of which have been characterized genetically. One important exception is common variable immunodeficiency (CVID), a complex, polygenic disease that is often first manifest in early adulthood. Classically, primary immunodeficiency disorders are classified into B-lymphocyte, T-lymphocyte, phagocytic cell and complement deficiencies. This classification is useful, as it helps us establish the clinical manifestations. For example, B-cell deficiencies usually present after the age of 6 months, when maternal antibodies are exhausted, and the most common pathogens are encapsulated bacteria (like *Streptococcus* and *Haemophillus*), fungi (such as *Giardia* and *Cryptosporidia*) and enteroviruses. In contrast, primary T-cell deficiencies usually present within the first 6 months of life, with opportunistic infections such as *Mycobacterium*, *Candida*, *Pneumocystis jiroveci* and cytomegalovirus. Both B-cell and T-cell primary immunodeficiency may be associated with an increased risk of malignancy (Table 44.1). An increased risk of cancer has not been found with complement deficiencies or phagocyte abnormalities.

Acquired or secondary immunodeficiency

Two forms of acquired immunodeficiency have dominated the last quarter of the 20th century and are responsible for the majority of cancers in the immunosuppressed. Both human immunodeficiency virus (HIV) and iatrogenic immunosuppression following allogenic transplantation are associated with cancers that are linked with oncogenic viruses. The first renal transplant was performed between identical twins by Joseph Murray at Boston's Brigham Hospital in 1953. The development of azathioprine by George Hitchins and Gertrude Elion 10 years later enabled successful allogeneic transplantation and began an era of transplantation medicine dependent upon iatrogenic immunosuppression. The allogeneic organ transplant recipients who received immunosuppressant therapy were found to be prone to post-transplantation lymphoproliferative diseases (PTLDs) and other tumours. The emergence of post-transplant tumours is widely quoted as evidence to support Burnet's immune surveillance theory that states that the immune system acts to remove abnormal clones of cells. In 1949, Frank Macfarlane Burnet described a theory of acquired

Lecture Notes: Oncology, 2nd edition. By M. Bower and J. Waxman. Published 2010 by Blackwell Publishing Ltd.

Table 44.1 Description of primary immunodeficiency syndromes.

Syndrome	Inheritance and incidence	Genetic defect	Immunological defect	Clinical manifestations	Cancer risk
B-cell/antibody deficiency					
X-linked (Bruton's) agammaglobulinemia (XLA)	X-linked recessive (1 in 200000 male live births)	Defect of btk Bruton's (B-cell progenitor tyrosine kinase) intracellular signalling path involved in pre-B cell development. Less often, the mutation is of the mu heavy chain gene	There are virtually no immunoglobulins present in the serum and the number of residual B lymphocytes in blood is very low	Recurrent pyogenic bacterial infections starting aged 6 months after maternal IgG is exhausted. Chronic sinusitis and bronchiectasis may follow	Small increased risk of lymphoma
Common variable immunodeficiency (CVID)	Polygenic, most common primary immunodeficiency (1 in 30000)		Characterized by variably decreased concentrations of all immunoglobulin classes	Recurrent bacterial infections of the respiratory tract. These disorders are also associated with autoimmune diseases (e.g. Crohn's)	Increased risk of lymphomas and digestive carcinomas
Selective IgA deficiency	(1 in 700 live births)	Mapped to chromosome 6p21	No secreted IgA but surface IgA present on B cells	Common mild onset in childhood. Sinusitis and recurrent lung infections	No increased risk
Hyper IgM syndrome (HIM)	X-linked (CD40 ligand = CD154; <1 in 1 000 000 male live births), autosomal recessive (CD40 or activation induced deaminase)	Three defects causing lack of isotype class switching from IgM to IgG, IgA and IgE	Excess IgM production but no IgG, IgA or IgE	Prone to opportunistic infections particularly *Pneumocystis carinii* and *Cryptosporidium parvum*. The latter may progress to sclerosing cholangitis and cirrhosis	Liver cancer in X-linked HIM
Hyper IgE syndrome (HIE)	Autosomal dominant	Gene not identified yet. Mapped to chromosome 4q	Elevated IgE, defective neutrophil chemotaxis, impaired lymphocyte response to *Candida* antigen	Recurrent bacterial skin and lung infections, chronic mucocutaneous candidiasis, craniofacial abnormalities, scoliosis and bone fractures	No increased risk

X-linked lymphoproliferative syndrome (XLPS; Duncan's syndrome)	X-linked signalling lymphocyte-activating molecule (SLAM)-associated protein (SAP) (<1 in 1 000 000 male live births)	SLAM activates cytotoxic T cells and this action is regulated by SAP	Overproduction of polyclonal CD8+ cytotoxic T cells in response to EBV infection	EBV-induced T-cell proliferation causes severe organ damage, progressive or hypogammaglobulinaemia	Increased risk of EBV-associated lymphomas
T-cell deficiency					
DiGeorge syndrome (thymic aplasia)	Most have deletions of 22q11; 1 in 3500 live births	The third and fourth branchial pouches fail to form properly	Moderate to severe lack of T cells	Tetany and cardiac malformations just after birth. Lack of T cells may lead to fungal, viral or other infection in infancy. Increased risk of autoimmune diseases (e.g. thyroiditis)	No increased risk
Severe combined immunodeficiency (SCID) syndromes	Nine genetic (8 autosomal recessive, 1 X-linked) defects of T-cell maturation; 1 in 30000 live births	Genetic defects affect purine metabolism (e.g. adenosine deaminase), VDJ recombination (e.g. recombinase activating genes) and lymphocyte signalling (e.g. common γ chain of interleukin receptors)	A variety of profound deficiencies of both T-cell and B-cell function	Failure to thrive and repeated infections caused by opportunistic infections by 6 months old. Protracted diarrhoea and death by 2 years in the absence of treatment	None known

Table 44.1 *Continued*

Name of syndrome	Inheritance and incidence	Genetic defect	Immunological defect	Clinical manifestations	Cancer risk
DNA-repair defects (see Chapter 1)					
Ataxia telangiectasia (AT; Louis–Bar syndrome)	Autosomal recessive ataxia-telangiectasia mutated (ATM), a protein kinase that reacts to DNA damage and affects the accumulation of p53 (1 in 60 000 live births)	Chromosomal instability due to defective DNA repair may interfere with immunoglobulin and T-cell receptor gene rearrangement	Most have IgA deficiency. Other hypoimmunoglobulinaemia and T-cell function deficits occur	Progressive cerebellar ataxia, skin telangiectasia. Most die in third decade of respiratory infections or tumours	Increased risk of acute leukaemias and lymphomas
Nijmegen breakage syndrome	Autosomal recessive	Chromosomal instability due to defective DNA repair may interfere with immunoglobulin and T-cell receptor gene rearrangement	Lymphopenia	As for AT but in addition have progressive microcephaly ('bird-like face')	Increased risk of acute leukaemias and lymphomas
Other					
Wiskott–Aldrich syndrome	X-linked recessive	Defective gene for WASP (Wiskott–Aldrich syndrome protein) involved in cytoskeleton reorganization following activation of platelets and T cells	Low IgM and raised IgE levels	Thrombocytopenia, eczema and increased autoimmune diseases (including vasculitis). Usually die by age 10 years	Increased risk of EBV-associated lymphomas

immunological tolerance, proposing that lymphocytes that were able to respond to self-antigens were deleted in prenatal life. This hypothesis was confirmed experimentally by Peter Medawar who shared the Nobel Prize with Burnet in 1960. Peter Medawar also wrote several wonderful books and collections of essays and I would encourage anyone who is thinking of doing scientific research to read *Advice to a Young Scientist*. In the 1960s, however, in a *volte face* that signalled a paradigm shift, Burnet began to champion the view that a major function of the immune system is to eliminate malignant cells. This was based upon evidence that animals can be immunized against syngeneic transplantable tumours. This theory of immune surveillance led to the identification of tumour antigens and of immunotherapy strategies to treat tumours.

Tumours in allograft recipients

The risk of cancer following an organ transplant varies with both the organ that has been transplanted and the type of cancer. The greatest risks numerically are with heart and heart–lung transplants, which often require a more aggressive regimen of immunosuppression to prevent graft rejection. In addition to PTLD that is caused by the Epstein–Barr virus (EBV), the risks of Kaposi's sarcoma (caused by Kaposi sarcoma herpesvirus (KSHV)), cervical cancer (caused by human papillomavirus (HPV)) and non-melanoma skin cancers are most dramatically increased. In the case of PTLD and post-transplantation Kaposi's sarcoma, reducing the immunosuppression may cause regression of the tumours – but this of course increases the risk of graft rejection.

Tumours in HIV patients

Studies by the World Health Organization (WHO) estimated that by December 2007, over 25 million people had died of acquired immune deficiency syndrome (AIDS) and 33 million people are living with the virus. The number of people newly infected with HIV worldwide is approximately 2.5

million per year. Along with opportunistic infections, tumours are a major feature of HIV infection. The most frequent tumours in this population are Kaposi's sarcoma (KS), non-Hodgkin's lymphoma and cervical cancer, and these three are AIDS-defining illnesses. The management of cancer in the immunodeficient host requires careful attention to the balance between antitumour effects and the toxicity associated. Combination antiretroviral treatment has both dramatically reduced the incidence of opportunistic infections and prolonged the survival of people with HIV infection. In addition, this highly active antiretroviral therapy (HAART) has reduced the incidence of AIDS-defining malignancies and improved their prognosis. Less than five million of the estimated 33 million people infected with HIV worldwide, however, are receiving HAART, as the majority of affected people live in developing countries. In addition, even in the established market economies with access to medical treatment, many individuals remain undiagnosed and consequently do not receive HAART.

Tumours in primary immunodeficiency

The cancers that occur with primary immunodeficiency syndromes are rare, and as a consequence treatment protocols and outcome data are scarce. Most patients succumb to infections, and these continue to pose a major threat to life during treatment of associated tumours.

Management of immunodeficiency-associated malignancies

The incidence of congenital immunodeficiency-associated tumours is sufficiently low for there to be little consensus upon their clinical management. In contrast, the incidence of both PTLD and KS has risen dramatically in recent years with the spread of the HIV pandemic and the marked increase in transplant surgery. The management of PTLD relies upon enhanced immunity against EBV by reducing immunosuppression and infusing

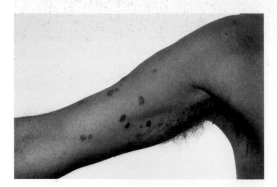

Figure 44.1 Multiple pigmented Kaposi sarcoma skin lesion in a man with HIV infection. Following antiretroviral therapy alone there was a marked regression of these lesions.

cytotoxic T lymphocytes against EBV. In addition, antiviral agents, low-dose chemotherapy and anti-CD20 monoclonal antibodies may be useful. The introduction of HAART has reduced the incidence of HIV-associated KS in established market economies where this treatment is available. Moreover, early-stage KS may be successfully treated with HAART alone, leading to regression of KS (Figure 44.1). Visceral KS is usually treated with systemic liposomal anthracycline chemotherapy with concomitant HAART. Other tumours that arise in immunodeficient individuals are generally treated along conventional lines, with extra attention to the risk of infectious complications of therapy.

Part 3

The Practice of Oncology

Chapter 45

Paraneoplastic complications of cancer

Paraneoplastic complications of malignancy are remote effects of cancer that arise without local spread. Most of these paraneoplastic syndromes arise due to secretion by tumours of hormones, cytokines and growth factors. Paraneoplastic syndromes also arise when normal cells secrete products in response to the presence of tumour cells. For example, antibodies produced in this fashion are responsible for many paraneoplastic neurological syndromes including cerebellar degeneration, Lambert–Eaton myasthenic syndrome and paraneoplastic retinopathy. Paraneoplastic neurological complications always appear on the list of differential diagnoses. However, just as viewers of *House MD* will know that 'it's not lupus', it is rarely paraneoplastic either.

Paraneoplastic endocrine complications

Cushing's syndrome

Cushing's syndrome is a clinical disorder resulting from prolonged exposure to excess glucocorticoids and should not be confused with Cushing's disease which refers exclusively to those cases that arise

Lecture Notes: Oncology, 2nd edition. By M. Bower and J. Waxman. Published 2010 by Blackwell Publishing Ltd.

due to an adrenocorticotrophic hormone (ACTH) secreting pituitary adenoma (Table 45.1). Clinically overt Cushing's syndrome caused by ectopic secretion of ACTH by non-endocrine-derived tumours is rare. Approximately 20% of cases of Cushing's syndrome are caused by ectopic ACTH secretion by a tumour that is frequently occult at presentation. For this reason the differential diagnosis between pituitary adenoma and ectopic ACTH is important clinically but biochemical overlap often makes this difficult. More than half the cases of ectopic ACTH syndrome are due to small cell lung cancer, with carcinoid tumours and neural crest tumours (phaeochromocytoma, neuroblastoma, medullary cell carcinoma of the thyroid) accounting for a further 15%. The typical presentation is of a middle-aged smoker with features of severe hypercortisolism and hypokalaemic metabolic alkalosis. Patients have muscle weakness or atrophy, oedema, hypertension, mental changes, glucose intolerance and weight loss. When ectopic ACTH production arises from a more benign tumour (e.g. bronchial carcinoid or thymoma), the other classic features of Cushing's syndrome may be present including truncal obesity, moon facies and cutaneous striae (Figure 45.1).

The diagnosis of Cushing's syndrome may be confirmed by elevated urinary free cortisol, loss of diurnal variation of plasma cortisol and failure of

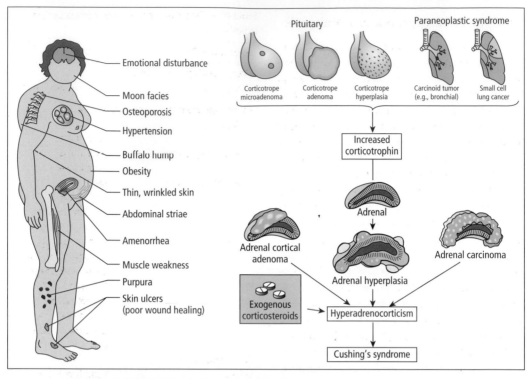

Figure 45.1 Causes and clinical features of Cushing's syndrome.

Table 45.1 Aetiology of Cushing's syndrome.

Type	Example
ACTH dependent	Pituitary adenoma (Cushing's disease)
	Ectopic ACTH secretion
	Ectopic CRH secretion (very rare)
ACTH independent	Exogenous glucocorticoid administration
	Adrenal adenoma
	Adrenal carcinoma
	Nodular adrenal hyperplasia

ACTH, adrenocorticotrophic hormone; CRH, corticotrophin-releasing hormone.

cortisol suppression in the low-dose dexamethasone (2 mg) test. After establishing the diagnosis, an elevated plasma ACTH supports the diagnosis of pituitary adenoma or ectopic ACTH syndrome. Failure of cortisol suppression following high-dose dexamethasone (2 mg four times daily for two days, or 8 mg overnight) and very high levels of ACTH (>200 pg/ml) suggest an ectopic source of ACTH. In difficult cases, a corticotrophin-releasing hormone (CRH) stimulation test, selective venous catheterization of the inferior petrosal sinus with ACTH estimations, somatostatin analogue scintigaphy and technetium-99 methoxyisobutylisonitrile (MIBI) imaging may be necessary to determine the source of ACTH.

The mainstay of palliative therapy for Cushing's syndrome due to ectopic ACTH production is inhibition of steroid synthesis, although inhibition of ACTH release and blocking glucocorticoid receptors have also been attempted. Several steroid synthesis inhibitors are available and successful use in these circumstances has been reported with aminoglutethamide, metyrapone, mitotane, ketoconazole and octreotide. On rare occasions laparoscopic bilateral adrenalectomy or adrenal artery embolization may be necessary to control symptoms.

Syndrome of inappropriate antidiuresis

Hyponatraemia is a common finding in association with advanced malignancy and many factors may contribute including cardiac and hepatic failure, hyperglycaemia and diuretics. However, the detection of concentrated urine in conjunction with hypo-osmolar plasma suggests abnormal renal free water excretion and the presence of the syndrome of inappropriate antidiuresis (SIAD). This acronym is better than the previous term 'SIADH' (syndrome of inappropriate antidiuretic hormone) since there is no vasopressin (ADH) secretion in approximately 15% of cases. In malignancy-related SIAD, tumours secrete ectopic arginine vasopressin or vasopressin-like peptides. In many respects SIAD is the opposite of diabetes insipidus; patients with SIAD are waterlogged with low plasma osmolality and sodium and high urine osmolality, whilst patients with diabetes insipidus are dehydrated with high plasma osmolality and sodium and low urine osmolality. SIAD is most frequently associated with small cell lung cancer or carcinoid tumours but has also been described in pancreatic, oesophageal, prostatic and haematological malignancies. Nonetheless many factors may contribute to SIAD (Table 45.2).

Significant symptoms of hyponatraemia appear at plasma sodium levels below 125 mmol/l, with confusion progressing to stupor, coma and seizures as levels fall. Nausea, vomiting and focal neurological deficits may also occur. The clinical features depend on both the levels of plasma sodium and the rate of decline. With gradual falls in sodium, the brain cells are able to compensate against cerebral oedema by secreting potassium and other intracellular solutes. Asymptomatic hyponatraemia therefore suggests chronic SIAD rather than acute SIAD. The division into chronic and acute SIAD is of therapeutic importance as their management differs. The diagnosis of SIAD requires the demonstration of plasma hyponatraemia and hypo-osmolality in the presence of concentrated urine and normal extracellular fluid volume (Table 45.3).

The management of SIAD depends upon the rate of onset of hyponatraemia and the presence of neu-

Table 45.2 Causes of the syndrome of inappropriate diuresis (SIAD).

Source of ADH	Examples
Ectopic ADH production	
Malignancy	Small cell lung cancer
Inappropriate pituitary secretion of ADH	
Malignancy	Lung cancer
	Lymphoma
Inflammatory lung disease	Pneumonia
	Lung abscess
Neurological disease	Meningitis
	Head injury
	Subdural haematoma
	Surgery
Drugs	Antidepressants
	(tricyclics, SSRIs)
	Carbamazepine
	Chlorpropamide
	Phenothiazines
	Vincristine
	Cyclophosphamide
	Ecstasy*
Postoperative	
Others	Hypothyroidism
	Porphyria
	Addison's disease

*Excessive water consumption may contribute to the development of hyponatraemia with ecstasy.
ADH, antidiuretic hormone; SSRI, selective serotonin reuptake inhibitor.

rological complications. Acute SIAD with an onset over two to three days and falls in serum sodium in excess of 0.5 mmol/l per day are associated with neurological sequelae and require prompt correction by intravenous hypertonic saline. In contrast, the mainstay of therapy for chronic asymptomatic SIAD is fluid restriction and inhibition of tubular reabsorption of water with drugs including the tetracycline antibiotic demeclocycline, which causes nephrogenic diabetes insipidus.

Non-islet cell tumour hypoglycaemia

Tumour-related hypoglycaemia is a frequent complication of β-islet cell tumours of the pancreas which secrete insulin (insulinomas), but occurs

Table 45.3 Diagnosis of the syndrome of inappropriate diuresis (SIAD).

Essential criteria to establish diagnosis

Plasma hypo-osmolality (plasma osmolality <275 mosmol/kg water and plasma sodium <135 mmol/l)

Concentrated urine (plasma osmolality >100 mosmol/kg water)

Normal plasma/extracellular fluid volume

High urinary sodium on a normal salt and water intake (urine sodium>20 mmol/l)

Exclude (i) hypothyroidism, (ii) hypoadrenalism and (iii) diuretics

Supportive criteria for diagnosis

Abnormal water load test (unable to excrete >90% of a 20 ml/kg water load in 4 hours and/or failure to dilute urine to osmolality <100 mosmol/kg water)

Elevated plasma arginine vasopressin levels

---

uncommonly with non-islet cell tumours. Most non-islet cell tumours produce hypoglycaemia through increased glucose use or by secreting insulin-like growth factors (IGF1 and IGF2). Non-islet cell tumours associated with hypoglycaemia are usually large retroperitoneal or intrathoracic sarcomas. Unlike other endocrine complications of malignancy, hypoglycaemia is very rarely associated with lung cancer. The clinical manifestations are due to cerebral hypoglycaemia and secondary secretion of catecholamines; they include agitation, stupor, coma and seizures that may follow exercise or fasting. Tumour-related hypoglycaemia should be differentiated from other causes of hypoglycaemia including drugs (e.g. sulphonylureas), hypoadrenalism, hypopituitarism and liver failure. In advanced malignancy the most common cause of hypoglycaemia is continued oral hypoglycaemic medication in long-standing diabetics.

Enteropancreatic hormone syndromes

Enteropancreatic hormone production is relatively uncommon in malignant disease. A variety of clinical syndromes occur associated with hormone secretion by endocrine tumours of the pancreas and less frequently tumours arising in other organs

(Table 45.4). The majority of pancreatic islet cell tumours are malignant (with the exception of most insulinomas) and metastases are frequently present at diagnosis. For many patients the distressing clinical manifestations arising from excessive secretion of gastrointestinal peptides require palliation and this may be difficult to achieve. These tumours often secrete more than one polypeptide hormone and may switch their hormone production during follow-up.

Carcinoid syndrome

Carcinoid tumours arise from enterochromaffin cells principally in the gastrointestinal tract, pancreas and lungs but occasionally in the thymus and gonads (Table 45.5). One in ten patients with carcinoid tumours develop the carcinoid syndrome after the development of hepatic metastases. This avoids the first pass metabolism of 5-hydroxytryptamine (serotonin, 5HT) and kinins in the liver so that the systemic symptoms occur. The acute symptoms are vasomotor flushing (typically of upper body lasting up to 30 minutes), fever, pruritic wheals, diarrhoea, asthma/wheezing, borborygmi and abdominal pain. Chronic complications include tricuspid regurgitation, arthropathy, pulmonary stenosis, mesenteric fibrosis, cirrhosis, pellagra (due to secondary deficiency of trytophan) and telangiectasia. The diagnostic investigation is 24-hour urinary collection of 5-hydroxyindoleacetic acid (5HIAA), a metabolite of 5HT. Somatostatin analogues are considered by most physicians to be the first-line treatment of choice for patients with carcinoid syndrome and indeed most enteropancreatic hormone syndromes. Palliation of the clinical manifestations of carcinoid syndrome includes symptomatic therapy of diarrhoea (codeine phosphate, loperamide or diphenoxylate), β_2-adrenergic agonists for wheezing, and avoiding precipitating factors to reduce flushing (including alcohol and some foods).

Phaeochromocytoma

Phaeochromocytomas arise from the chromaffin cells of the sympathetic nervous system, most

Table 45.4 Clinical manifestations of secretory endocrine tumours.

Tumour	Major feature	Minor feature	Common site	Percentage that are malignant	Percentage that are associated with MEN	Palliative treatments
Insulinoma	Neuroglycopenia (confusion, fits)	Permanent neurological deficits	Pancreas (β cells) >99%	10%	4–5%	Frequent feeding Glucose Glucagon Diazoxide Octreotide
Gastrinoma (Zollinger–Ellison syndrome)	Peptic ulceration	Diarrhoea Weight loss Malabsorption Dumping	Pancreas (D cells) 25% Duodenum 70%	>50%	20–25%	Gastrectomy Proton pump inhibitor H2 receptor antagonists Octreotide
VIPoma (Werner–Morrison syndrome)	Watery diarrhoea Hypokalaemia Achlorhydria	Hypercalcaemia Hyperglycaemia Hypomagnesaemia	Pancreas (A–D cells) 90% Neuroblastoma SCLC Phaeochromocytoma	>50%	6%	Octreotide Glucocorticoids
Glucagonoma	Migratory necrolytic erythema Mild diabetes mellitus Muscle wasting Anaemia	Diarrhoea Thromboembolism Stomatitis Hypoaminoacidaemia Encephalitis	Pancreas (α cells) 99%	>70%	1–20%	Octreotide Oral hypoglycaemics
Somatostatinoma	Diabetes mellitus Cholelithiasis Steatorrhoea Malabsorption	Anaemia Diarrhoea Weight loss Hypoglycaemia	Pancreas (β cells) 55% Duodenum and jejunum 45%	>60%	Case reports only	

H2, histamine type 2; MEN, multiple endocrine neoplasia; SCLC, small cell lung cancer; VIP, vasoactive intestinal polypeptide.

Table 45.5 Comparison of carcinoid tumours by site of origin.

Features	Foregut	Midgut	Hindgut
Frequency of occurrence	2–33% carcinoid tumours	75–87% carcinoid tumours	1–8% carcinoid tumours
Site	Respiratory tract, pancreas, stomach, proximal duodenum	Jejunum, ileum, appendix, Meckle's diverticulum, ascending colon	Transverse and descending colon, rectum
Tumour products	Low 5HTP, multihormones*	High 5HTP, multihormones*	Rarely 5HTP, multihormones*
Blood	5HTP, histamine, multihormones*, occasionally ACTH	5HT, multihormones*, rarely ACTH	Rarely 5HT or ACTH
Urine	5HTP, 5HT, 5HIAA, histamine	5HT, 5HIAA	Negative
Carcinoid syndrome	Occurs but is atypical	Occurs frequently with metastases	Rarely occurs
Metastasizes to bone	Common	Rare	Common

*Multihormones include tachykinins (substance P, substance K, neuropeptide K), neurotensin, PYY, enkephalin, insulin, glucagon, glicentin, vasoactive intestinal polypeptide, somatostatin, pancreatic polypeptide, ACTH and α-subunit of human chorionic gonadotrophin.
ACTH, adrenocorticotrophic hormone; 5HIAA, 5-hydroxyindole-acetic acid; 5HT, 5-hydroxytryptamine (serotonin); 5HTP, 5-hydroxytryptophan.

frequently in the adrenal medulla but occasionally from sympathetic ganglia. Phaeochromocytomas commonly secrete norepinephrine (noradrenaline) and epinephrine (adrenaline) but in some cases significant quantities of dopamine are also produced. Phaeochromocytomas are associated with a number of familial inherited cancer syndromes including multiple endocrine neoplasia (MEN) 2a, MEN 2b, von Hippel–Lindau syndrome and neurofibromatosis. The catecholamines cause intermittent, episodic or sustained hypertension and other clinical manifestations including anxiety, tremor, palpitations, sweating, flushing, headaches, gastrointestinal disturbances and polyuria. These symptoms are all attributable to excessive adrenergic stimulation.

24-hour urinary collection for urinary free catecholamines (epinephrine, norepinephrine and dopamine) is now the most widely employed diagnostic test although some centres also measure catecholamine metabolites such as metanephrines and vanillylmandelic acid (VMA). The tumour may be localized by radiolabelled meta-iodobenzyl guanidine (MIBG) scintography.

Initial treatment should be α-blockade to control hypertension followed by β-blockade to control tachycardia. This combination will control symptoms in most patients with malignant phaeochromocytoma. If palliation is not achieved, high-dose ^{131}I-MIBG may be used as therapy for phaeochromocytoma and neuroblastoma as it reduces catecholamine synthesis. This may only have a chance of success if the patient has small volume metastases, because ^{131}I-MIBG is β-emitting and β-particles have poor tissue penetration.

Gynaecomastia

Gynaecomastia results from elevation in the oestrogen : androgen ratio, which may be either a consequence of decreased androgen production or activity or increased oestrogen formation (usually by peripheral aromatization of circulating androgens to oestrogens). In men with advanced cancer, gynaecomastia is most often a consequence of drug therapy, either chemotherapy (alkylating agents, vinca alkaloids, nitrosoureas), anti-emetics (metoclopramide, phenothiazines), anti-androgens

Box 45.1: Oncological mnemonics

Causes of hypercalcaemia: GRIM FED

Granulomas (TB, sarcoid)
Renal failure
Immobility
Malignancy
Familial (familial hypocalciuric hypercalcaemia)
Endocrine **PATH** (**p**haeochromocytoma, **A**ddison's, **t**hyrotixicosis, **h**yperparathyroidism)
Drugs (thiazides, lithium, vitamins A and D, milk alkali syndrome)

Causes of SIADH: SIADH

Surgery
Intracranial (infection, head injury, cerebrovascular accident)
Alveolar (pus, cancer)
Drugs **ABCD** (**a**nalgesics: opiates, non-steriodal anti-inflammatory drugs, **b**arbiturates, **c**yclophosphamide/**c**arbamazepine/**c**hlorpromazine, **d**iuretic: thiazides))
Hormonal (hypothyroid, Addison's)

Causes of Cushingoid features: CUSHINGOID

Cataracts
Ulcers
Striae
Hypertension, hirsutism
Infections
Necrosis (avascular necrosis of femoral head)
Glycouria, glycaemia
Osteoporosis, obesity
Immunosuppression
Diabetes

Phaeochromocytoma: rule of 10s

This mnemonic applies to *adults* with phaeochromocytomas.
10% are extra-adrenal
10% are bilateral or multiple
10% are malignant
10% are familial

Phaeochromocytoma symptoms: 5 Hs

Headache
Hypertension
Hypotension (postural)
Heartbeat (palpitations)
Hyperhidrosis (sweating)

Causes of gynaecomastia: GYNAECOMASTIA

Genetic (Kleinfelter's, Kallman's)
Youth (puberty)*
Neonate*
Antifungals (ketoconazole)
Estrogen
Cirrhosis/cimetidine
Old age*
Marijuana
Alcoholism
Spirolonactone/stilboestrol
Tumours (testicular, adrenal)
Isoniazid
Alkylating agents

Causes of clubbing: CLUBBING

Cyanotic congenital heart disease
Lung disease (abscess, bronchiectasis, cystic fibrosis, empyema, fibrosing alveolitis)
Ulcerative colitis/Crohn's disease
Biliary cirrhosis
Birth defect (hereditary pachydermoperiostosis)
Infective endocarditis
Neoplasia (non-small cell lung cancer, mesothelioma, gastrointestinal lymphoma)
Goitre (thyrotoxicosis)

Features of MEN

MEN 1: 3Ps
Pituitary adenoma
Pancreatic islet cell tumours
Parathyroid

MEN 2: 2Cs
Catecholamines (phaeochromocytoma)
Cell carcinoma (medullary) of thyroid
Plus:
MEN 2a: parathyroid tumours
MEN 2b (also known as MEN 3): mucocutaneous neuromas

* Physiological causes.

(cyproterone acetate, flutamide, bicalutamide) or gonadotrophin-releasing hormone analogues (goserelin, leuprorelin). Occasionally other tumour secretion of oestrogens or gonadotrophins may be responsible. Tumours may either secrete oestrogens (Leydig cell testicular tumours and feminizing adrenocortical tumours), promote the conversion of androgens to oestrogens (Sertoli cell testicular tumours and hepatoma) or secrete human chorionic gonadotrophin (HCG) stimulating oestradiol production in the testes (testicular tumours, non-small cell lung cancers, hepatoma and islet cell tumours of the pancreas).

Paraneoplastic neurological conditions

In contrast to the metabolic and endocrine paraneoplastic conditions where products secreted by the tumours are responsible, most neurological paraneoplastic syndromes are immune mediated. Moreover with neurological paraneoplastic syndromes, the tumour may be asymptomatic or occult. It is thought that antibodies reacting to antigens on the surface of cancer cells cross-react with neural antigens and are the basis of these syndromes. The antibodies may be directed at ion channels, for example the presynaptic P-type voltage-gated calcium channel in the case of Lambert–Eaton myasthenic syndrome and the nictonic acetyl choline receptor in myasthenia gravis. Alternatively, antibodies may bind intracellular proteins such as Hu, a neuronal nuclear RNA-binding protein, and Yo, a cytoplasmic protein in Purkinje cells of the cerebellum. The most common paraneoplastic neurological manifestations are described in association with small cell lung cancer (Table 45.6).

Paraneoplastic dermatological conditions

A number of paraneoplastic dermatological manifestations have been described, and some are listed in Table 45.7. Amongst the most common paraneoplastic dermatological manifestation is clubbing

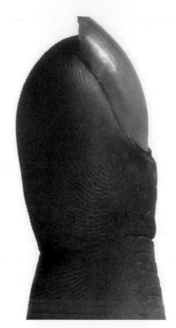

Figure 45.2 Finger nail clubbing is characterized by increased longitudinal curving of the nail, loss of the angle between the nail and its bed and bogginess of the nail fold.

(see Figure 45.2), a clinical sign beloved of physicians and first described by Hippocrates over 2400 years ago. It is characterized by softening of the nail bed and periungual erythema with loss of the normal 15 degree angle at the hyponychium. As this advances, bulging of the distal phalynx and curvature of the nail lead to a drumstick end appearance. Clubbing may be associated with hypertrophic osteoarthropathy with new subperiosteal cancellous bone formation at the distal ends of long bones, particularly the radius and ulna or tibia and fibula (Figure 45.3). A hereditary form of clubbing with hypertrophic osteo-arthropathy, Touraine–Solente–Golé syndrome, has recently been shown to be due to germline mutations of the 15-hydroxyprostaglandin dehydrogenase gene that catabolizes prostaglandin E2. Whether paraneoplastic clubbing is due to elevated levels of prostaglandin E2 or tumour-related secretion of growth factors, including PDGF (platelet-derived growth factor) and HGF (hepatocyte growth factor), remains unclear.

Table 45.6 Paraneoplastic neurological manifestations.

Condition	Clinical features	Antibodies	Percentage that are paraneoplastic	Underlying malignancy
Dermatomyositis	Erythematous rash, arthralgia	Anti-Jo-1	20%	NSCLC, SCLC, lymphoma
Encephalomyelitis	Fluctuating confusion, anxiety, depression, impaired short term memory	Anti-Hu, anti-CV2	10%	SCLC, thymoma
Lambert–Eaton syndrome	Proximal muscle weakness sparing eyes; power increases with repetition	Anti-VGCC	60%	SCLC
Myasthenia gravis	Muscle fatigability, ptosis, ophthalmoplegia	Anti-AChR	5%	Thymoma
Opsoclonus–myoclonus syndrome	Opsoclonus (irregular, rapid, horizontal and vertical eye movements) and myoclonus (brief, shock-like muscle spasms), intention tremor, unsteady gait	Anti-Hu, anti-Ri	20 50%	Neuroblastoma, breast
Polymyositis	Proximal muscle weakness, rash	Anti-Jo-1	10%	NSCLC, SCLC, lymphoma
Retinopathy	Night blindness, ring scotomas, photosensitivity	Anti-recoverin		SCLC, melanoma
Sensory neuropathy	Rapid progressive loss of all sensory modalities especially proprioception	Anti Hu	10–20%	SCLC
Subacute cerebellar degeneration	Ataxia, nystagmus, dysarthria	Anti-Yo, anti-Hu, anti-VGCC, anti-Tr	50%	SCLC, ovary, Hodgkin's

NSCLC, non-small cell lung cancer; SCLC, small cell lung cancer.

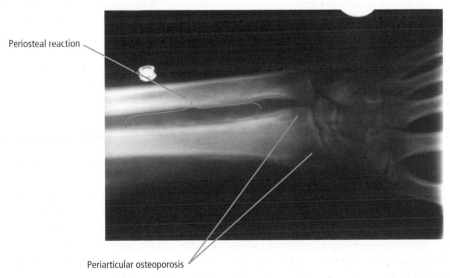

Figure 45.3 Forearm radiograph showing a periosteal reaction in the metaphysis and diaphysis of the radius and ulnar and periarticular osteoporosis due to hypertrophic osteoarthropathy secondary to non-small cell lung cancer (squamous cell).

Table 45.7 Paraneoplastic dermatological conditions.

Condition	Clinical features	Underlying malignancy
Acanthosis nigricans	Grey-brown, symmetrical, velvety plaques on neck, axillae and flexor areas	Adenocarcinoma, predominantly gastric
Acquired ichthyosis	Generalized dry, cracking skin; hyperkeratotic palms and soles	Hodgkin's disease, lymphomas, myeloma
Acrokeratosis paraneoplastica (Bazex syndrome)	Symmetrical psoriasiform hyperkeratosis with scales and pruritis on toes, ears and nose; nail dystrophy	Squamous carcinoma of oesophagus, head and neck, and lungs
Bullous pemphigoid	Large tense blisters; antibodies to desmoplakin	Lymphomas and others
Cushing's syndrome	Broad purple striae; plethora; telangiectasia; mild hirsutism	Small cell lung cancer, thyroid, testis, ovary and adrenal tumours, pancreatic islet cell tumours, pituitary tumours
Dermatitis herpetiformis	Pleomorphic, symmetrical, subepidermal bullae	Lymphoma and others
Dermatomyositis	Erythema or telangiectasia of knuckles and periorbital regions	Miscellaneous tumours
Erythema annulare centrifugum	Slowly migrating annular red lesions	Prostate tumours, myeloma and others
Erythema gyratum repens	Progressive scaling erythema with pruritis	Lung, breast, uterus and gastrointestinal tumours
Exfoliative dermatitis	Progressive erythema followed by scaling	Cutaneous T-cell lymphoma, Hodgkin's disease and other lymphomas
Flushing	Episodic reddening of face and neck	Carcinoid syndrome, medullary cell carcinoma of the thyroid
Generalized melanosis	Diffuse grey-brown skin pigmentation	Melanoma, ACTH-producing tumours
Hirsutism	Increased hair in male distribution	Adrenal tumours, ovarian tumours
Hypertrichosis lanuginosa	Rapid development of fine, long, silky hair	Lung, colon, bladder, uterus and gallbladder tumours
Muir–Torre syndrome	Sebaceous gland neoplasm	Colon cancer, lymphoma
Necrolytic migratory erythema	Circinate area of blistering and erythema on face, abdomen and limbs	Islet cell tumour of the pancreas (glucagonoma)
Pachydermoperiostosis	Thickening of skin folds, lips and ears; macroglossia; clubbing; excessive sweating	Lung cancer
Paget's disease of the nipple	Red keratotic patch over areola, nipple or accessory breast tissue	Breast cancer
Pemphigus vulgaris	Bullae of skin and oral blisters	Lymphomas, breast cancer
Pruritis	Generalized itching	Lymphoma, leukaemia, myeloma, central nervous system tumours, abdominal tumours
Sign of Leser–Trelat	Sudden onset of large number of seborrhoeic keratoses	Adenocarcinoma of the stomach, lymphoma, breast cancer
Sweet's syndrome	Painful, raised, red plaques; fever; neutrophilia	Leukaemias
Systemic nodular panniculitis (Weber–Christian disease)	Recurrent crops of tender, violaceous, subcutaneous nodules, which may be accompanied by abdominal pain and fat necrosis in bone marrow and lungs	Adenocarcinoma of the pancreas
Tripe palms	Hyperpigmented, velvety, thickened palms with exaggerated ridges	Gastric and lung cancer

ACTH, adrenocorticotrophic hormone.

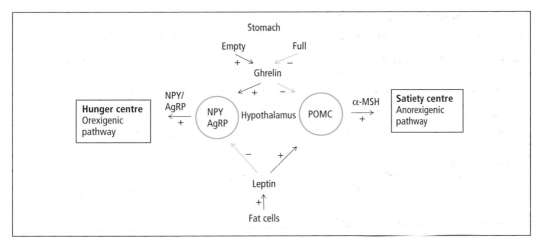

Figure 45.4 Schematic diagram of the hypothalamic control of hunger (see text for abbreviations).

Cachexia

Cachexia or severe protein-calorie malnutrition is one of the most debilitating and life-threatening aspects of cancer. This highly distressing symptom severely impairs the quality of life of many patients with cancer but is the focus of relatively little research. The normal balance between hunger and satiety, anorexia and obesity in humans is maintained by equilibrium between adipose-derived hormones including leptin and gut-derived hormones including ghrelin. An empty stomach stimulates ghrelin release which acts to promote neuropeptide Y (NPY) and Agouti-related peptide (AgRP) secretion in the hypothalamus, resulting in stimulation of the hunger centre. At the same time, ghrelin inhibits the release of pro-opiomelanocortin (POMC) hormones including α-MSH (melanocyte-stimulating hormone) from the hypothalamus, thus inhibiting the satiety centre and blocking anorexigenic pathways. Leptin, which is produced by fat cells, antagonizes ghrelin's actions on the hypothalamus by inhibiting NPY and AgRP release and stimulating α-MSH secretion (Figure 45.4). Amongst the mechanisms invoked in cancer cachexia is disruption of this delicate homoeostatic mechanism. In addition, tumour-related secretion of pro-inflammatory cytokines including interleukin-1 (IL-1) and interleukin-6 (IL-6), interferon gamma (IFN-γ) and tumour necrosis factor alpha (TNF-α) are thought to play a role in the pathogenesis of cancer cachexia. These effects may be mediated partly via the hypothalamic leptin/gherlin axis. Another clue to cancer cachexia has been found with the identification of proteolysis-inducing factor (PIF) and lipid-mobilizing factor (LMF). PIF causes breakdown of muscle proteins in skeletal muscle by activating the ubiquitin proteosome pathway and levels of PIF are raised in cancer patients with wasting. LMF, which is produced by tumour cells, causes lipolysis by raising the levels of the mitochondrial uncoupling proteins that turn brown fat into heat in hibernating animals.

The severe weight loss shortens survival and decreases quality of life substantially, indeed for many malignancies weight loss of >10% body weight is an independent adverse prognostic factor. The two major options for pharmacological therapy that aim to enhance appetite are progestogens, such as megestrol acetate, and corticosteroids. Neither these drugs nor enteral or parenteral nutrition has proved universally beneficial and both approaches are associated with appreciable toxicity. This is particularly so for corticosteroids, which, although they stimulate appetite, are catabolic in effect, leading to muscle loss. As the molecular aetiology of cancer cachexia is unveiled, novel therapeutic strategies are emerging.

Chapter 46

Oncological emergencies

Hypercalcaemia

One in ten cancer patients develop hypercalcaemia and malignancy accounts for about half the cases of hypercalcaemia amongst hospital inpatients. Hypercalcaemia occurs most frequently with myeloma, breast, lung and renal cancers, and 20% of cases occur in the absence of bone metastases. Most patients with hypercalcaemia of malignancy have disseminated disease and 80% die within one year. Thus hypercalcaemia is usually a complication of advanced disease and its treatment should be directed at palliation as it may produce a number of distressing symptoms (Table 46.1). The treatment of hypercalcaemia of malignancy frequently ameliorates these symptoms, and for this reason the diagnosis should always be sought.

In recent years there have been significant advances in our understanding of the biochemical processes that cause hypercalcaemia in malignancy, such that the factors involved in local osteolysis and in the evolution of humoral hypercalcaemia have now been delineated. A number of different cytokines have been implicated in the development of hypercalcaemia as a result of local osteolysis. These osteoclast-activating factors, which are released locally by metastatic tumour and stimulate osteoclastic resorption of

Lecture Notes: Oncology, 2nd edition. By M. Bower and J. Waxman. Published 2010 by Blackwell Publishing Ltd.

bone, include prostaglandin E2, tumour necrosis factors alpha (TNF-α) and beta (TNF-β), epidermal growth factor and transforming growth factor beta (TGF-β). It is probable that interleukin 1, epidermal growth factor and the tumour necrosis factors are the most important of these aetiological agents as the release of macrophage colony-stimulating factor by osteoblasts is enhanced by these factors. Since osteoclasts are derived from a haematopoietic stem cell progenitor, this release of macrophage colony-stimulating factor may be fundamental to oestoclastic bone resorption.

Humoral hypercalcaemia was described in 1941 by Albright but it was only in the late 1980s that the humoral factor causing hypercalcaemia was characterized. In the 1970s hypercalcaemia was thought to result from the ectopic production of parathyroid hormone (PTH) but this hypothesis remained unproven because the use of PTH antisera failed to demonstrate excessive secretion of PTH in patients with humoral hypercalcaemia. In addition, low serum concentrations of 1,25-vitamin D3 and urinary cyclic adenosine monophosphate (AMP) levels failed to reflect excess PTH activity and no PTH mRNA was found in the tumours of patients with humoral hypercalcaemia.

In the late 1980s polyadenylated RNA from a renal carcinoma from a patient with this syndrome was used to construct a cDNA library which was screened with a codon-preference oligonucleotide, synthesized on the basis of a partial *N*-terminal

Table 46.1 Clinical features of hypercalcaemia of malignancy.

General	Gastrointestinal	Neurological	Cardiological
Dehydration	Anorexia	Fatigue	Bradycardia
Polydipsia	Weight loss	Lethargy	Atrial arrhythmias
Polyuria	Nausea	Confusion	Ventricular arrhythmias
Pruritis	Vomiting	Myopathy	Prolonged P-R interval
	Constipation	Hyporeflexia	Reduced Q-T interval
	Ileus	Seizures	Wide T waves
		Psychosis	
		Coma	

amino acid sequence from a human tumour-derived peptide and a 2.0 kilobase cDNA was identified. The cDNA encoded a 177 amino acid prohormone, which consisted of a 36 amino acid leader sequence that is cleaved to produce a 141 amino acid, mature peptide and PTH-related peptide. The first 13 amino acids of the mature peptide have a sequence homology with PTH, and the N-terminal sequence is thought to be the PTH receptor binding region. PTH-related peptide was found to be expressed in most normal human tissue, where its role is undetermined. The gene for PTH-related peptide has been mapped to the short arm of chromosome 12 and this is in contrast to the PTH gene which has been mapped to the short arm of chromosome 11. The gene for PTH-related peptide is complex and contains a six exon, 12 kilobase, single copy sequence, encoding up to five mRNA species. Exons 2, 3 and 4 are similar to the PTH gene.

A radioimmunoassay for PTH-related peptide was used to screen patients with hypercalcaemia-associated malignancy and the results contrasted with patients who were normocalcaemic and had malignant disease, patients with primary hyperparathyroidism and normal controls. PTH-related peptide was elevated in 19 of 39 (49%) patients with malignant hypercalcaemia, 12 of 74 (16%) normocalcaemic patients with malignancy, and four of 20 patients (20%) with hyperparathyroidism, but in none of 22 normal controls.

The clinical manifestations of hypercalcaemia are varied (Table 46.1) and many symptoms may be wrongly attributed to the underlying malignancy. A diagnosis of hypercalcaemia can only be made by biochemical investigation so all symptomatic patients with malignancy should have their corrected serum calcium measured if treatment is likely to be appropriate:

$$\text{Corrected calcium} = \text{measured calcium} + [(40 - \text{serum albumin (g/l)}) \times 0.02]$$

The mainstay of therapy is rehydration with large volumes of intravenous fluids followed by the administration of calcium-lowering agents, most commonly bisphosphonates. Low calcium diets are unpalatable, exacerbate malnutrition and have no place in palliative therapy. Drugs promoting hypercalcaemia (e.g. thiazide diuretics, vitamins A and D) should be withdrawn. The cornerstone of the re-establishment of normocalcaemia is treatment with a bisphosphonate. Bisphosphonates have multiple functions in hypercalcaemia. They reduce serum calcium levels by a direct effect on the osteoclast, by stabilizing hydroxyapatite crystals. There are two classes of effect of bisphosphonates. One group of bisphosphonates, which include clodronate and etidronate, acts through their incorporation into non-hydrolyzable analogues of adenosine triphosphate (ATP) that accumulate in osteoclasts and induce apoptosis. Alternately, agents such as pamidronate and zoledronate inhibit an enzyme called FPP synthase which functions in the mevalonate pathway. This leads to inhibition of protein prenylation. The bisphosphonates of choice are currently pamidronate, zoledronate and ibandronate. Approximately 80% of patients respond to hydration and bisphosphonate treatment by normalization of serum calcium levels. Calcium levels start to normalize within the first 24 hours of treatment with bisphos-phonates and reach normal levels usually within three days. It is a dogma that treatment with bisphosphonates has to be repeated, usually on a three to four-weekly cycle. However, there is some information that suggests that a single treatment may be sufficient with re-setting of the calcium-stabilizing mechanisms. As well as these actions, bisphosphonates have valuable analgesic activity in patients with metastatic bone pain and reduce skeletal morbidity in patients with breast cancer and myeloma. In 20% of patients with hypercal-caemia, bisphosphonates do not work. Alternative treatments include the use of a somatostatin ana-logue such as octreotide which acts to reduce serum levels of PTHr-related peptide. Other more old fashioned treatments include calcitonin and mithramycin.

Superior vena cava obstruction

Superior vena cava obstruction (SVCO) restricts the venous return from the upper body resulting in oedema of the arms and face, distension of the neck and arm veins, headaches and a dusky blue skin discoloration over the upper chest, arms and face. SVCO is caused by a mediastinal mass com-pressing the vessel with or without intraluminal

thrombus. Collateral circulation via the azygous vein may provide some drainage and over a period of weeks collaterals may form over the chest wall. In this case the flow of blood in these collateral veins will be from above downwards into the infe-rior vena cava circulation and this may be demon-strated clinically as an aid to confirm the diagnosis.

The presenting symptoms of SVCO include dys-pnoea, swelling of the face and arms, headaches, a choking sensation, cough and chest pain (see Plate 46.1). The most important clinical sign is loss of venous pulsations in the distended neck veins. This is usually accompanied by facial oedema, plethora and cyanosis, and tachypnoea. The sever-ity of the symptoms is determined by the rate of obstruction and the development of a compensa-tory collateral circulation. The symptoms may deteriorate when lying flat or bending, which further compromises the obstructed venous return. Careful assessment of the patient's history is fre-quently suggestive of a long period with minor symptoms of SVCO. In 9 out of 10 cases, the cause of SVCO is a malignancy, most often lung cancer (disproportionately more often small cell lung cancer) (Figure 46.1), lymphoma or metastatic breast or germ cell cancer. Rare non-malignant causes are listed in Table 46.2.

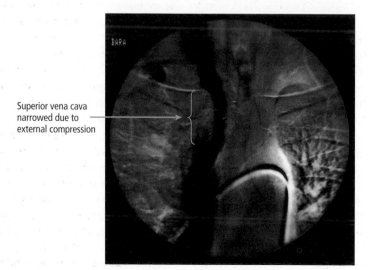

Superior vena cava narrowed due to external compression

Figure 46.1 Angiogram showing superior vena cava compression at the level of the carina due to small cell lung cancer.

Table 46.2 Non-maligant causes of superior vena cava obstruction (SVCO).

Mediastinal fibrosis	Idiopathic
	Histoplasmosis
	Actinomycosis
	Tuberculosis
Vena cava thrombosis	Idiopathic
	Behcet's syndrome
	Polycythemia vera
	Paroxysmal nocturnal haemoglobinuria
	Long-term venous catheters, shunts or pacemakers
Benign mediastinal tumours	Aortic aneurysm
	Dermoid tumour
	Retrosternal goitre
	Sarcoidosis
	Cystic hygroma

The management of SVCO depends upon the cause and severity, along with the patient's prognosis, and includes relieving symptoms as well as treating the underlying cause. SVCO is an oncological emergency in the presence of airway compromise and delays whilst histological findings are confirmed may adversely affect the outcome. In such circumstances patients are treated empirically with steroids and radiotherapy. However, when it is safe to do so, it is important to establish the diagnosis as this will determine the optimum treatment and a delay of one to two days to obtain a histological diagnosis is often appropriate, particularly in the context of a patient with minor symptoms and a long clinical history. Diagnostic procedures should include a plain chest X-ray (CXR), sputum cytology, bronchoscopy, thoracoscopy or mediastinoscopy, computed tomography (CT) scans or magnetic resonance imaging (MRI) and venography. A palpable lymph node may be amenable to biopsy, thereby providing a diagnosis.

Patients may respond to being sat upright with oxygen therapy and intravenous corticosteroids should be administered. In the majority of cases radiotherapy is the most appropriate treatment modality and relieves symptoms in up to 90% of patients within a fortnight. Where a diagnosis of lymphoma, small cell lung cancer or germ cell

tumour has been obtained chemotherapy may be the optimal initial treatment.

For patients with recurrent SVCO, or in those where other therapeutic modalities are unsuitable, insertion of expandable wire stents under radiological guidance can be effective (Figure 46.2). Studies report instantaneous symptomatic relief with an excellent response rate. Although bypass of the obstruction has been performed surgically, this is usually reserved for patients with benign disorders. For central venous access catheter-associated thrombosis, removal of the line and anticoagulation should be commenced. The administration of low-dose warfarin has been reported to reduce the incidence of thrombosis associated with central venous access catheters.

Spinal cord compression

Spinal cord compression is a relatively common complication of disseminated cancer and affects 5% of patients with cancer. Spinal cord compression occurs with many tumour types but is particularly frequent in myeloma and prostate cancer. Up to 30% of these patients will survive for one year, so it is essential to be spared paraplegia for this remaining time by making the diagnosis swiftly and instituting treatment quickly. In general, the residual neurological deficit reflects the extent of deficit at the start of treatment, so early treatment leaves less damage. Neoplastic cord compression is nearly always due to extramedullary, extradural metastases usually from breast, lung, prostate, lymphoma or renal cancers. Commonly compression occurs by posterior expansion of vertebral metastases or extension of paraspinal metastases through the intervertebral foramina. These result in demyelination, arterial compromise, venous occlusion and vasogenic oedema of the spinal cord, all contributing to myelopathy; 70% occur in the thoracic spine, 20% in the lumbar spine and 10% in the cervical spine.

The earliest symptom of cord compression is vertebral pain, especially on coughing and lying flat. Subsequent signs include sensory changes one or two dermatomes below the level of compression. A complaint of back pain with focal weakness and

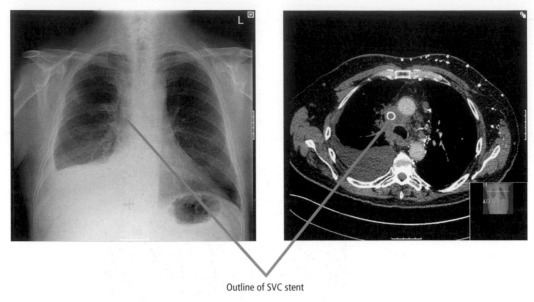

Outline of SVC stent

Figure 46.2 Chest X-ray and CT scan showing a superior vena cava (SVC) stent *in situ*.

bladder or bowel dysfunction with a sensory level requires urgent investigation in a patient with cancer. This will progress to motor weakness distal to the block and finally sphincter disturbance. If spinal cord compression is missed, or left untreated, patients can develop severe neurological deficits and double incontinence.

Spinal cord compression should be treated as a medical emergency. High-dose intravenous corticosteroids should be initiated on clinical suspicion alone to prevent further evolution of neurological deficit. Plain X-rays of the spine looking for vertebral collapse and MRI of the spinal axis to define the presence and level(s) of spinal cord compression should then be performed (Figures 46.3–46.5). 20 to 30% of patients have multiple levels of cord compression and imaging of the whole cord is therefore essential. If appropriate, a neurosurgical opinion should be obtained regarding the potential of surgical decompression, especially if there is vertebral instability or if the level of the compression has been previously irradiated. Otherwise, the definitive treatment is urgent local radiotherapy. It is important to provide adequate analgesia. Pretreatment ambulatory function is the main deter-

minant of post-treatment gait function, thus prompt diagnosis and treatment is the key to gait and continence preservation.

Malignant effusions

Pleural effusions

Although not strictly an emergency, approximately 40% of all pleural effusions are due to malignancy (Table 46.3) and it frequently indicates advanced and incurable disease. The pleural space is normally filled with 10-40 ml of hypoproteinaceous plasma that originates from the capillary bed of the parietal pleura and is drained through the parietal pleura lymphatics. A pleural effusion is often the first manifestation of malignancy, and lung cancer and breast cancer account for almost two-thirds of cases. Malignant pleural effusions may be asymptomatic or cause progressive dyspnoea, cough and chest pain which may be pleuritic in nature. Malignant pleural effusions are usually exudates and this may be confirmed by a fluid lactate dehydrogenase (LDH) of >200 U/ml, a fluid : serum LDH ratio >0.6, a fluid : serum protein

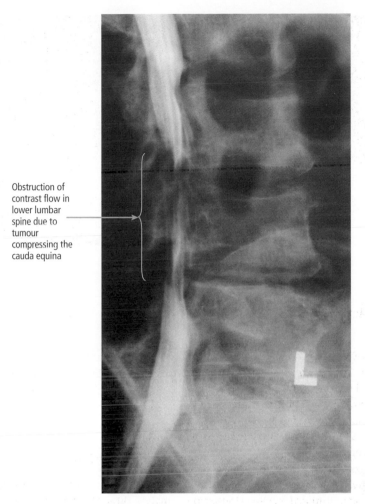

Obstruction of contrast flow in lower lumbar spine due to tumour compressing the cauda equina

Figure 46.3 Myelogram demonstrating cauda equine compression. This invasive technique has been largely replaced by CT and MRI.

ratio >0.5 and a fluid : serum glucose ratio of <0.5. The fluid may be blood stained and is typically hypercellular, containing lymphocytes, monocytes and reactive mesothelial cells; exfoliated tumour cells may be present also.

The management of malignant effusions should be tailored to the patient's symptoms as only half the patients will be alive at 3 months and over 90% of effusions will recur within 30 days of thoracocentesis. Reaccumulation of pleural effusions may be delayed by chemical pleurodesis (usually using talc or tetracycline) or video-assisted thoracic surgery (VATS) with pleurectomy and/or talc insufflation. Pleuroperitoneal shunts or chronic indwelling catheters may be considered for patients who fail pleurodesis, but this is rarely appropriate.

Pericardial effusions

The accumulation of fluid in the pericardial space around the heart may adversely affect cardiac function and like all effusions may be transudate, exudate or haemorrhage. Cardiac tamponade occurs when the pressure on the ventricles in

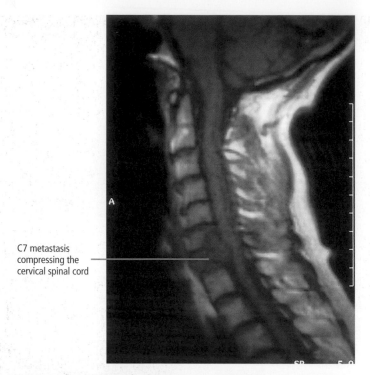

C7 metastasis compressing the cervical spinal cord

Figure 46.4 MRI scan demonstrating metastasis in a cervical C7 vertebral body with soft tissue extension posteriorly to cause compression of the cervical spinal cord.

diastole prevents them from filling, thus reducing the stroke volume and cardiac output. The classic sign of cardiac tamponade is Beck's triad of hypotension because of decreased stroke volume, jugular–venous distension due to impaired venous return to the heart, and muffled heart sounds due to fluid inside the pericardium (Figure 46.6).

Ascites

The most frequent malignancies causing ascites are primary tumours of the ovaries, pancreas, stomach and colon, breast and lungs. The distressing symptoms of ascites include abdominal distension or pain, dyspnoea due to diaphragmatic splinting, oedema of the legs, perineum and lower trunk, and a 'squashed stomach syndrome' leading to anorexia. If these symptoms are distressing, paracentesis is indicated – it offers rapid symptom relief but poor long-term control. Whilst anticancer therapy may reduce the subsequent reaccumulation of ascites, if this is not an option or is unsuccessful, diuretics may be helpful. Rarely a peritoneovenous shunt may be surgically placed under general anaesthetic if the ascites cannot be controlled.

Tumour lysis syndrome

The acute destruction of a large number of cells is associated with metabolic sequelae, and is termed the 'tumour lysis syndrome'. Cell destruction results in the release of different chemicals into the circulation, some of which may cause profound complications. Electrolyte release may cause transient hypercalcaemia, hyperphosphataemia and hyperkalaemia. The release of calcium and phosphate into the blood stream rarely causes any significant consequences. However, the calcium and phosphate may co-precipitate and cause some impairment of renal function. Hyperkalaemia can be a much more significant problem and may manifest as minor electrocardiograph (ECG) abnormal-

(a)

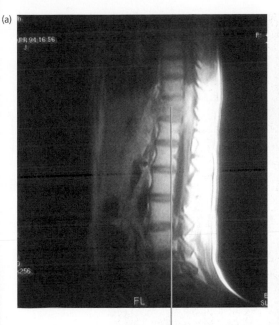

T11 metastasis compressing spinal cord

(b)

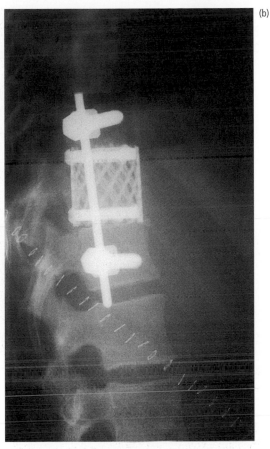

Figure 46.5 (a) MRI showing spine bone metastasis and cord compression at T11 due to vertebral metastasis with soft tissue extension. (b) A matched plain X-ray following surgical decompression and stabilization of the metastasis.

ities which, of course, all students reading this book can describe in intimate and complex detail (Table 46.4). Even more significant, however, are the cardiac arrhythmias, which may include ventricular tachycardia or ventricular fibrillation, and which may lead to the demise of the patient. Nucleic acid breakdown leads to hyperuricaemia and this, unless treated appropriately, can be complicated by renal failure due to the precipitation of uric acid crystals in the renal tubular system. So, of course, it is best that these things do not happen because we do not like our patients dying, least of all because of the complications of the treatment that we give them.

There are certain malignancies whose treatment is associated with a higher than usual risk of tumour lysis syndrome and these include acute promyelocytic leukaemia and high-grade lymphomas. Patients with acute promyelocytic leukaemia can develop the tumour lysis syndrome, with minor trauma to the patient, or even infection. In this instance there is a release of pro-coagulants from blast cells with the risk of a devastating coagulopathy. Patients with high-grade T-cell lymphomas may also be at risk from circumstances where one would not normally expect there to be a problem. For example, if these patients are started on steroids, they may develop tumour lysis because steroids have cytotoxic qualities in lymphoma. In these malignancies the risk of tumour lysis syndrome is pre-empted by a cunning pretreatment plan. Patients are started two days prior to

Table 46.3 Causes of pleural effusion.

Transudate	Cardiac failure
	Nephrotic syndrome
	Cirrhosis
	Protein-losing enteropathy
	Constrictive pericarditis
	Hypothyroidism
	Peritoneal dialysis
	Meig's syndrome (pleural effusion associated with ovarian fibroma)
Exudate	
Tumour	Primary: lung cancer, mesothelioma
	Secondary: breast or ovary cancer, lymphoma
Infection	Pneumonia
	Tuberculosis
	Subphrenic abscess
Infarction	Pulmonary embolus
Connective tissue disease	Rheumatoid arthritis
	Systemic lupus erythematosus
Others	Pancreatitis (usually left-sided pleural effusion)
	Dressler's syndrome (inflammatory pericarditis and pleurisy following myocardial infarction or heart surgery)
	Yellow nail syndrome (combination of discoloured hypoplastic nails, recurring pleural effusions and lymphedem; aetiology unknown)
	Asbestos exposure

chemotherapy or radiation therapy with allopurinol. The day before treatment intravenous hydration is started, and these efforts generally prevent the development of tumour lysis syndrome. Many clinicians advise alkalinization of the urine. However, in practice it is very difficult to achieve an alkaline urine and there are significant dangers inherent in the use of significant amounts of sodium bicarbonate. A proportion of patients will go on to develop tumour lysis syndrome despite these measures. For this reason patients who are treated require careful monitoring with two-hourly measurement of serum potassium levels for the first 8–12 hours of treatment. Many clinicians will also advise ECG monitoring but it is our experience that these monitors are generally not observed to best effect. A new drug has become recently available for the treatment of this condition. Recombinant urate oxidase (rasburicase) converts uric acid, which is insoluble, into allantoin, which is. Clinical trials have shown that urate oxidase controls hyperuricaemia faster and more reliably than allopurinol, and its use is indicated in children and haematological malignancy.

Hyperviscosity syndrome

Blood hyperviscosity can be caused by too much protein or too many cells in the blood. The clinical features include spontaneous bleeding from mucous membranes, retinopathy, headache, vertigo, coma and seizures. The most frequent causes of excess proteins are monoclonal paraproteinaemias such as Waldrenström's macroglobulinaemia (IgM) and myeloma (especially IgA and IgG3 myelomas). Hyperviscosity due to excess cell counts occurs in acute leukaemia blast crises. The retinopathy resembles retinal vein occlusion with dilated retinal veins and retinal haemorrhages. The serum viscosity may be measured (normal range: 0.14–0.18 cPa/s), but treatment of suspected hyperviscosity should be started before the results are available as they often take days to come back. Plasmapheresis should be used to decrease hyperviscosity related to excess proteins, whilst leukapheresis removes excess leukaemic blasts before definitive treatment can begin.

Myelosuppression

Neutropenia

We explain to our patients that chemotherapy puts them at risk of developing bone marrow suppression, as cancer treatments kill 'good' as well as 'bad' cells. In this case the 'good' cells are the haematological progenitor cells and patients are at risk of death if the effects of treatment upon the bone marrow are not recognized. Neutropenic sepsis is very common in cancer treatment and, if undiag-

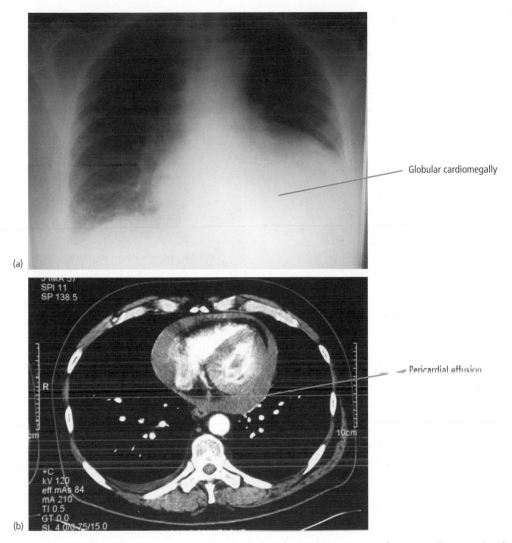

Globular cardiomegally

Pericardial effusion

(a)

(b)

Figure 46.6 (a) Chest X-ray showing a globular enlarged heart shadow and (b) CT scan confirming a malignant pericardial effusion due to metastatic non-small cell lung cancer. These effusions may present as a medical emergency with cardiac tamponade. The clinical symptoms include dyspnoea and cough and the signs are hypotension, tachycardia, pulsus paradoxus (fall of systolic blood pressure of >10 mmHg on inspiration), quiet muffled heart sounds and a raised jugular–venous pressure (JVP) with Kussmaul's sign (paradoxical rise in JVP on inspiration). The electrocardiograph may show pulsus alternans (alternating QRS voltages). The emergency treatment is by pericardiocentesis and a subsequent surgical formation of a pericardial window to prevent recurrence may be necessary.

nosed, leads to a mortality rate approaching 20–30%. Patients with neutropenic sepsis develop fevers and rigors with associated oral ulceration and candidiasis. It is standard practice for patients with neutropenic sepsis – which is defined by septic symptoms in the presence of a white count that is $<1.0 \times 10^9/l$ – to be admitted to hospital. The patient is resuscitated with intravenous fluids and blood cultures are taken. In the absence of any obvious focus of infection, such as the urinary tract, the advantage of culturing from sites other than blood is virtually zero. Cultures from other

Table 46.4 Electrocardiolgy for oncologists.

Oncological emergency	ECG features	Tracings
Hypercalcaemia	Short QT Broad-based, tall, peaked T waves wide QRS Low R wave Disappearance of P waves	
Pericardial effusion	Sinus tachycardia Low voltage complexes PR segment depression Alternation of the QRS complexes, usually in a 2 : 1 ratio (electrical alternans)	
Tumour lysis		
Hyperkalaemia	Peaked T waves Flattened P waves Prolonged PR interval Widened QRS complexes Deep S wave	
Hypocalcaemia	Long QT interval Narrow QRS Reduced PR interval Flat or inverted T waves Prominent U wave Ventricular arrhythmia	

sites merely act to swamp the microbiology lab with unnecessary requests for culture work without yielding any positive advantage. Just 20% of blood cultures from patients with neutropenic sepsis are positive for bacterial organisms. The cause for infection is generally not clear.

Antibiotic policies vary from hospital to hospital but there is good evidence that treatment with single-agent ceftazidime is as effective as treatment with combination antibiotic regimens. In the UK patients are generally admitted, though it is interesting to note that this conservative management policy is not strictly necessary. In one randomized study, treatment with oral ciprofloxacin in the community was compared with inpatient treatment with intravenous ceftazidime. The results were absolutely identical in terms of control of fever and patient outcome.

Over the last decade marrow growth factors have become available and granulocyte colony-stimulating factor (G-CSF), which stimulates the marrow to produce granulocytes, has entered wide use. There is no evidence that prophylactic use of G-CSF in any way prevents neutropenic sepsis or septic deaths. The evidence for its use in established infection is poor and the consensus view is that G-CSF is of value only in patients with established neutropenic sepsis who have a non-recovering marrow and in whom, additionally, an infective agent has been identified. G-CSF is of enormous value in transplantation programmes, where the mean period of time to engraftment has been reduced from 28 to 18 days by the use of these agents.

Anaemia

Anaemia is a very common complication of cancer and its treatment. It is estimated that up to 30% of all cancer patients will require a transfusion. In general, anaemia is cumulative and builds up over several cycles of chemotherapy. Recombinant erythropoietin is considered to be a valuable alternative to blood transfusion. The response of patients to erythropoietin is wide ranging and reported at between 20% and 60%. Haemoglobin levels increase after about six weeks of treatment with recombinant erythropoietin. The price of this agent used to be considered prohibitive, however it may become relatively more affordable as the cost of blood is widely predicted to increase significantly because of the increased costs of testing blood for infective agents such as Creutzfeldt–Jakob disease (CJD). The pharmaceutical industry markets erythropoietin for its effect upon the asthenia related to cancer treatment; claims are made for a far greater improvement in cancer fatigue than haemoglobin level.

Thrombocytopenia

Thrombocytopenia is not as significant a problem in the treatment of solid tumours as it is in the treatment of haematological malignancies. There is a significant risk of spontaneous major haemorrhage as the platelet count declines below 10–20 $\times$ 10^9/l and most oncologists advocate prophylactic platelet transfusions at this level or in the presence of bleeding. There are a number of regulatory molecules that stimulate early haematopoietic progenitors and these include the interleukins IL-1, IL-6 and IL-11. IL-1 and IL-6 have poor efficacy and significant toxicity, but IL-11 has been licensed for the prevention of chemotherapy-induced thrombocytopenia. The pharmaceutical industry continues to develop agents for the treatment of thrombocytopenia, and the focus recently has been on analogues of thrombopoietin, which appear to have more efficacy and less toxicity than the interleukins.

Cancer-related thromboses

Patients with cancer have an increased tendency to thrombosis, a problem that was first documented by Trousseau, who sadly went on to develop venous thromboses himself and died from cancer. Patients with cancer have an increased risk of developing thromboses for two major reasons. The first may be a pressure effect, where the primary tumour mass or secondary nodal masses impinge upon the vasculature, producing venous stasis and thrombosis. The second reason for the increased risk is the release from the tumour of pro-coagulants. A number of tissue pro-coagulants have been described, ranging from factors S and C to the current view that activated factor 10 is released by tumours, which sparks off the clotting cascade.

The incidence of venous thrombosis and thromboembolism in cancer patients is variably reported. One study looked at a group of patients presenting with deep venous thromboses (DVTs). Screening of these patients showed that almost 30% had a cancer that was most commonly a pelvic malignancy. As always in medicine, there is initial positive reporting, and later studies showed the true incidence of previously undetected cancer in patients presenting with venous thrombosis to be in the order of 5%. Once cancer has been diagnosed, thromboembolic events are remarkably common and described in about 10% of all patients. The incidence increases significantly

Thrombus in inferior vena cava

Metal filter in inferior vena cava

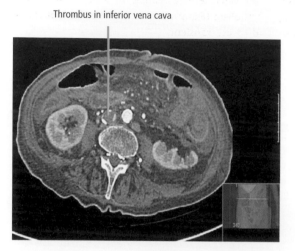 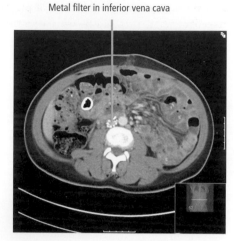

Figure 46.7 CT scan showing an inferior vena cava filter *in situ* in a woman with advanced ovarian cancer and recurrent thromboses.

Thrombus in left and right main pulmonary arteries suggesting saddle embolus

Ventilation scan

Perfusion scan

Large segmental perfusion defect

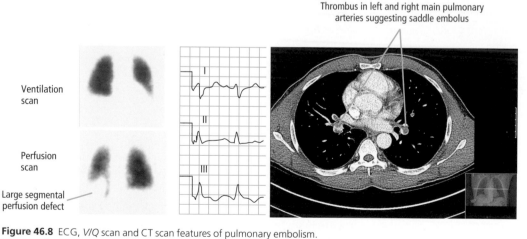

Figure 46.8 ECG, *V/Q* scan and CT scan features of pulmonary embolism.
V/Q scan showing large segmental perfusion defect in the left lower lung and normal ventilation.
ECG showing $Q_IS_{III}T_{III}$ pattern (S wave in lead I, Q save in lead III and inverted T wave in lead III).
CT scan shows filling defects occluding the central pulmonary artery and extending into all the lobar branches due to saddle embolus.

when long lines are inserted in cancer patients for the purposes of chemotherapy or supportive care. In this group of patients the incidence of thromboembolism increases to 20%. For this reason prophylaxis with low-dose warfarin is recommended and this decreases the risk of subsequent thrombosis to between 2% and 5%. These statistics, however, are considered controversial and are debated endlessly. Because of the high risk of thrombosis in cancer patients it has been suggested that anticoagulation should be prophylactically prescribed. Logically, the best way of preventing thromboembolism would be with a heparin-like compound rather than with a coumarin. At the moment the evidence is that the low molecular weight heparins are probably more effective than warfarin in the prophylaxis of thromboembolism. There is an additional unexpected benefit to anticoagulation with low molecular weight heparins, and this is a modest survival advantage for patients, as demonstrated by randomized clinical trials. In some patients with pelvic tumours and recurrent thromboses, filters may be inserted into the inferior vena cava to reduce the risk of pulmonary embolism (Figures 46.7 and 46.8). The benefits of filters are transient.

Chapter 47

End of life care

Amongst the most important elements of onco-logical care is recognizing shifting goals as the cancer progresses. The balance of benefit and side effects of any intervention should be carefully weighed up. Whilst neurosurgical resection of soli-tary metastases from melanoma may be appropri-ate in some circumstances, venepuncture for measuring the serum electrolytes in a dying patient is rarely justifiable. These decisions should involve the patients wherever possible and require skilful use of communication. Throughout the cancer journey patients often enquire about their life expectancy and there is a temptation for clinicians to pluck some figure out of the air. An intelligent doctor will recognize the pitfalls of prognostica-tion when applied to an individual and will appre-ciate that the median survival (the statistic most relevant in this circumstance) is the time when half the patients will still be alive. Stephen J. Gould, the evolutionary palaeontologist, explained this from a patient's perspective in the essay 'The median is not the message' published in the collec-tion *Bully for Brontosaurus*. During the patient's journey with cancer a number of emotions are experienced and these may follow a stepwise suc-cession originally described by the Swiss psy-chologist Elisabeth Kubler Ross. In her 1969 book

On Death and Dying she records the stages as denial, anger, bargaining, grieving and finally acceptance.

As the cancer progresses and the patient deterio-rates, it is important that reviews are frequent and that problems are anticipated. This close follow-up is often best undertaken in the community by community palliative care services rather than bringing patients up to hospital or GP surgeries for regular appointments, but this approach requires excellent communication between all the health professionals involved. This may be facilitated by patient-held records similar to those used in shared care obstetrics. The anticipation of symptoms, including pain and diminishing mobility, should be addressed in advance so that analgesia is quickly available to patients.

Pain control

Nerve endings, or nociceptors, exist in all tissues and are stimulated by noxious agents including chemical, mechanical and thermal stimuli, giving rise to pain (Table 47.1). These stimuli are relayed by Aβ, Aδ (fast transmitting fibres) and C (slow transmission of sensation) sensory nerve fibres to the dorsal horns of the spinal cord and different qualities of pain may use different sensory fibres.

Analgesic drugs form the mainstay of treating cancer pain and should be chosen based on the severity of the pain rather than the stage of the

Lecture Notes: Oncology, 2nd edition. By M. Bower and J. Waxman. Published 2010 by Blackwell Publishing Ltd.

Table 47.1 Definition of pain terms.

Term	Definition
Allodynia	Pain due to a stimulus that does not normally cause pain
Analgesia	Absence of pain in response to stimulation that would normally be painful
Dysesthesia	An unpleasant abnormal sensation, whether spontaneous or evoked
Hyperalgesia	Heightened response to a normally painful stimulus
Hyperpathia	An abnormally painful reaction to a stimulus, especially a repetitive stimulus, as well as an increased threshold
Hypoalgesia	Diminished pain in response to a normally painful stimulus
Neuralgia	Pain in the distribution of a nerve or nerves
Neuropathic pain	Pain initiated or caused by a primary lesion or dysfunction in the peripheral nervous system
Nociception	Nervous system activity resulting from potential or actual tissue damaging stimuli
Paraesthesia	An abnormal sensation, whether spontaneous or evoked

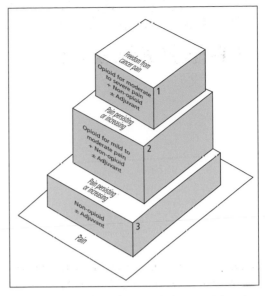

Figure 47.1 The World Health Organization's three step ladder to the use of analgesic drugs.

cancer. Drugs should be administered regularly to prevent pain using a stepwise escalation from non-opioid, to weak opioid and strong opioid analgesia (Figure 47.1). Adjuvant drugs may be added at any stage of the analgesic ladder as they may have additional analgesic effect in some painful conditions. Examples of adjuvant analgesics are corticosteroids, non-steroidal anti-inflammatory drugs, tricyclic antidepressants, anticonvulsants and some anti-arrythmic drugs. Morphine is the most commonly used strong opioid analgesic and whenever possible should be given by mouth. The dose of morphine needs to be tailored to each patient and be repeated at regular intervals so that the pain does not return between doses. There is no upper dose limit for morphine; however, a number of myths have arisen around opioid prescribing that may deter prescribers as well as patients. Firstly, opioid tolerance is rarely seen in patients with cancer pain and neither psychological dependency nor addiction is a problem in this patient group. The toxicity of opioids may prove to be an obstacle for some patients (Table 47.2). Sedation is common at the start of opioid therapy but resolves in most patients within a few days. Similarly, nausea and vomiting may prove troublesome at the start of regular opioid dosing but usually dissipate within a few days and may be controlled with anti-emetics. Constipation develops in almost all patients on opioids and this toxicity persists and necessitates routine prophylactic laxatives for almost everyone receiving opioids. A careful explanation of these issues will result in the acceptance of opioid analgesia by almost all patients.

Care of the dying patient

The continuing attention to the needs and comfort of a dying patient is as important as the care given to any other patient and part of that care includes reducing the distress of relatives. Many issues may be raised by relatives that pose ethical dilemmas and these may make you question the therapy that has been or should be given. Amongst the most

269

Table 47.2 Side effects of opiates.

Side effect	Comments
Constipation	This affects almost all patients and all patients require prophylaxis with a stimulant laxative (e.g. senna, bisacodyl) and a softener (e.g. docusate sodium) or as a combined preparation (e.g. co-danthramer, co-danthrusate)
Drowsiness	Generally remits after a few days
Nausea	Affects one-third of opioid naïve patients but usually resolves within 1 week. Consider prophylaxis for 1 week
Hallucinations	An uncommon side effect that often features images in the peripheral vision
Nightmares	Vivid and unpleasant but rare
Myoclonic jerks	Occur usually with excess doses and may be mistaken for fits
Respiratory depression	Not a problem in patients with pain

frequent scenarios is the role of intravenous hydration, evaluating the balance between painful cannulation and restriction of mobility versus an uncomfortable dry mouth and thirst. To address these questions you should consider whether death from the cancer is now inevitable, whether interventions would relieve symptoms and whether treatment would cause harm. Careful explanation to the relatives is essential; in this circumstance, for example, they need to be reassured that the patient is not dying because of dehydration but rather because of progression of the cancer.

Symptom control in the dying patient often requires a different route of administration as swallowing may be difficult and agitation and restlessness are often prominent features as death approaches. A number of factors may contribute to terminal agitation including physical causes such as pain, sore mouth and full bladder or rectum, along with emotional factors including fear of dying and the distress of relatives. The physical causes should be addressed appropriately and unnecessary medications should be stopped. Often the best method of delivering analgesia, anti-emetics and sedation, if appropriate, is via a subcutaneous syringe driver. Similarly, oral secretions accumulating in a patient who is too weak to cough may be distressing to the patient and family alike. Drug treatment for terminal secretions includes hyoscine hydrobromide and glycopyrronium bromide, which is less sedating. It is important to recall that not all patients wish to be sedated and this should be discussed with them and their families.

The last hours and days

For many patients with cancer the last hours and days are heralded by a deterioration to semiconsciousness. At this time patients are usually unable to take oral medication and prescriptions need to be reconsidered. Many medicines may be stopped altogether and alternative routes of administration, including subcutaneous, rectal and transdermal routes, may be employed for other necessary medications including analgesia. Although patients may no longer be receiving medicines by mouth, oral hygiene remains an important part of overall care. It is particularly important to avoid unnecessary unpleasant interventions at this time and to adopt a practical problem-oriented approach to symptom control. A practical guide to the care of the dying patient in a hospital was developed at the Royal Liverpool Hospital in conjunction with Marie Curie Cancer Care to transfer best practice learnt from hospice care. The Liverpool Care of the Dying Pathway helps members of the multidisciplinary team in making a decision about which medical interventions should be stopped and which continued (including anticipatory prescribing) and what comfort measures should be started. It also promotes psychological support of the patients, family and carers as well as addressing spiritual needs and bereavement. There has been debate recently about the value of the Liverpool Pathway, with some critics suggesting that it is a one-way road that sanitizes and precipitates the process of dying without allowing thought or revison of decisions.

When death is inevitable, as it is for all of us, and is approaching rapidly it is the policy in many UK hospitals to discuss resuscitation policies with patients and their relatives. Under these circumstances resuscitation is rarely appropriate and, if deemed futile, the lead clinician may make a DNAR (do not attempt resuscitation) decision. These DNAR decisions should be discussed with patients who wish to engage in advanced care planning. However, prolonged discussions about DNAR policies with patients who do not wish to contemplate their future are, in the view of these authors, distressing and irrelevant. The reason for our autocratic view is that cardiac resuscitation cannot return the patient who has died from cancer from his journey across the River Styx, and it causes distress in the relatives and the arrest team.

Bereavement

Bereavement care and support includes recognizing the physical and emotional needs of families and carers and continues after the patient's death. A number of features have been identified that are associated with the risk of severe bereavement reactions (Table 47.3), and the recognition of these risks prior to death can allow planning of care for those left behind after the death. Health professionals are not immune to bereavement, or at least the good ones are not, and our need for support should not be ignored.

The culture of death and dying

Just as different cultures, regardless of the scientific evidence, have developed distinct explanations for the origins of life ranging from Big Bangs and evolution to creationist genesis, similar cultural variations affect attitudes to death. For example, Christians, Jews (Box 47.1) and Sufis believe in resurrection whilst Hindi, Buddhists (Box 47.2) and Sikhs believe in reincarnation. These cultural discrepancies must be recognized and respected, particularly where patients' and carers' views differ.

Box 47.1: Jewish mourners' Kaddish prayer

Glorified and sanctified be God's great name throughout the world which He has created according to His will. May He establish His kingdom in your lifetime and during your days, and within the life of the entire House of Israel, speedily and soon; and say, Amen.

May His great name be blessed forever and to all eternity. Blessed and praised, glorified and exalted, extolled and honoured, adored and lauded be the name of the Holy One, blessed be He, beyond all the blessings and hymns, praises and consolations that are ever spoken in the world; and say, Amen.

May there be abundant peace from heaven, and life, for us and for all Israel; and say, Amen

He who creates peace in His celestial heights, may He create peace for us and for all Israel; and say, Amen.

With a strong belief in an afterlife, mourning practices in Judaism are extensive, but are not an expression of fear of death. Instead they aim to show respect for the dead and to comfort the living. As an expression of respect, following death the body is never left alone and on hearing of the death, friends and relatives tear a portion of their clothes. Burial is prompt, within 2 days, and is followed by 7 days of mourning (shiva). Mourners sit on low stools or the floor instead of chairs, do not wear leather shoes, do not shave or cut their hair, do not wear cosmetics, do not work and do not do things for comfort or pleasure, such as bathe, have sex or put on fresh clothing. Mourners wear the clothes that they tore at the time of learning of the death and mirrors in the house are covered. The Jewish Kaddish prayer is recited for the first 11 months following a death by identified mourners and on each anniversary of the death (Yahrzeit). It is remarkable that there is no reference to death in the prayer but rather it focuses on the greatness of God and on a call for peace.

Table 47.3 Risk factors for bereavement.

Patient	Young
Cancer	Short illness, disfiguring
Death	Sudden, traumatic (haemorrhage)
Relationship to patient	Dependent or hostile
Main carer	Young, other dependents, physical or mental illness, unsupported

Box 47.2: The *Tibetan Book of the Dead* (bardo thodol)

A fundamental tenet of Buddhism is that death is not something that awaits us in some distant future, but something that we bring with us into the world and that accompanies us throughout our lives. Rather than a finality, death offers a unique opportunity for spiritual growth with the ultimate prospect of transformation into an immortal state of benefit to others. Among Tibet's many and varied religious traditions are esoteric teachings that address compassionate death including the *Tibetan Books of the Dead*. These popular texts are manuals of practical instructions for the dying, who are immediately facing death; for those who have died, who are wandering in the intermediate state between lives; and for the living, who are left behind to continue without their loved ones.

Before death, friends and relatives are encouraged to bid farewell without excess drama so that neither regret nor longing is experienced by the dying as their state of mind at death must be positive. This may be facilitated by a spiritual master (lama) whispering guiding instructions from *Liberation Through Hearing during the Intermediate State* commonly known as the *Tibetan Book of the Dead* into the dying person's ear.

Tibetan Buddhism recognizes that spiritual growth may be derived from acknowledging death and proposes detailed meditation strategies that relate to the acceptance of death in order to comprehend the nature of human existence. Four human life cycle stages are recognized: birth, the period between birth and death, death, and the interval between death and rebirth (the bardo). This post-mortem bardo lasts seven weeks and is followed by rebirth into a worldly state that is influenced by past actions or karma. The cycle of rebirth (samsara) may be broken by enlightenment, culminating in the final liberation of buddhahood.

1. In a woman, what carries the greatest risk for breast cancer?
   a. family history of breast cancer
   b. previous contralateral breast cancer
   c. benign breast disease
   d. oral contraceptive usage
   e. nulliparity

2. A 30-year-old man receives BEP chemotherapy for a metastatic germ cell tumour. He develops interstitial lung disease. Which drug is most likely to be responsible?
   a. bleomycin
   b. etoposide
   c. cisplatin
   d. ondansetron
   e. filgrastim (G-CSF)

3. A 55-year-old woman had surgery, radiotherapy and adjuvant chemotherapy for breast cancer three years previously. She presents with lower back pain and mild leg weakness. An MRI scan reveals vertebral bone metastases and cord compression at L1. What is the most appropriate treatment?
   a. physiotherapy and mobilization
   b. surgical decompression and radiotherapy
   c. chemotherapy
   d. endocrine therapy
   e. non-steroidal anti-inflammatory drugs and bed rest

4. A 79-year-old smoker presented with dyspnoea. Investigations reveal a 10 cm lung mass and a serum sodium of 112 mmol/l. What histological subtype of lung cancer is most likely?
   a. small cell carcinoma
   b. adenocarcinoma
   c. squamous cell carcinoma
   d. large cell carcinoma
   e. carcinoid

5. A woman received extended field mantle radiotherapy for stage 2A Hodgkin's lymphoma; 10 years later, what malignancy is the most likely sequelae?
   a. thyroid carcinoma
   b. acute myeloid leukaemia
   c. non-Hodgkin's lymphoma
   d. breast cancer
   e. ovarian germ cell tumour

6. A 26-year-old man is treated with the CODOX-M/IVAC chemotherapy regimen for sporadic Burkitt lkymphoma. Which cytotoxic drug causes the least bone marrow suppression?
   a. cyclophosphamide
   b. doxorubicin
   c. ifosfamide
   d. etoposide
   e. vincristine

7. What is the most common site of spread of epithelial ovarian tumours?
 a. inguinal lymph nodes
 b. adnexae
 c. bone
 d. lungs
 e. liver

8. A 28-year-old woman presents with amenorrhoea, a large uterus and multiple rounded opacities on her chest X-ray. Which serum tumour marker is most helpful in establishing a diagnosis of choriocarcinoma?
 a. carcinoembryonic antigen
 b. human chorionic gonadotropin
 c. α-fetoprotein
 d. CA-125
 e. Ca199

9. A 60-year-old woman undergoing chemotherapy for acute myeloid leukaemia develops chemotherapy refractory disease. Which of the following is most likely to be overexpressed by the leukaemia cells and account for the chemotherapy resistance?
 a. P glycoprotein
 b. p53
 c. Bcl-2
 d. P450
 e. myc

10. Which cancer is most likely to produce bone metastases that are osteoblastic rather than osteolytic?
 a. choriocarcinoma
 b. endometrial cancer
 c. colorectal cancer
 d. ovarian cancer
 e. prostate cancer

11. What is the most common site of tumours in adults who present with myasthenia gravis?
 a. skeletal muscle
 b. stomach
 c. lung
 d. thymus
 e. thyroid

12. Red cell aplasia due to failure to produce erythrocytes is a paraneoplastic syndrome. What tumour type is most frequently associated with it?
 a. carcinoid
 b. glucagonoma
 c. insulinoma
 d. neuroblastoma
 e. thymoma

13. Which secretory endocrine islet cell tumour produces a distinctive, severe rash?
 a. gastrinoma
 b. glucagonoma
 c. insulinoma
 d. somatostatinoma
 e. VIPoma

14. Which of the following facts concerning the risk of mesothelioma is true?
 a. mesothelioma is more common in women than men
 b. the wives of asbestos workers have an increased risk of mesothelioma
 c. since the banning of asbestos in the 1980s the incidence of mesothelioma is falling
 d. the risk of mesothelioma decreases with age
 e. asbestos exposure is not a risk for peritoneal mesothelioma

15. The high incidence of hepatitis B infection in Africa and parts of Asia is thought to be causally associated with increased incidence of which malignancy?
 a. hepatocellular carcinoma
 b. oesophageal cancer
 c. Burkitt lymphoma
 d. gastric carcinoma
 e. Kaposi's sarcoma

16. Brachytherapy involves the delivery of radiation therapy locally by direct apposition to the treated tissue. What is the most common radioisotope used in this application?
 a. iodine-125
 b. carbon-14

c. hydrogen-3

d. phosphorus-34

e. fluorine-18

17. DNA viruses have been implicated in several human tumours. Evidence for a causative role exists for which of the following neoplasms?

a. Burkitt lymphoma

b. testicular germ cell tumour

c. mesothelioma

d. osteogenic sarcoma

e. oesophageal carcinoma

18. A woman of 63 years has advanced metastatic breast cancer and is confined to bed due to painful bone metastases. What is her ECOG (Eastern Co-operative Oncology Group) performance status?

a. 0

b. 1

c. 2

d. 3

e. 4

19. Childhood retinoblastoma occurs in both sporadic and familial forms. What feature occurs more often in the sporadic form?

a. bilateral retinoblastoma

b. later age at retinoblastoma onset

c. family history of retinoblastoma

d. germline mutation of the Rb gene

e. development of osteosracoma

20. A 45-year-old man with long-standing gastroesophageal reflux undergoes upper endoscopy that reveals patchy areas of epithelium resembling gastric mucosa extending 5 cm proximal to the oesophagogastric junction. Biopsies are obtained. The pathological report describes 'Barrett's epithelium'. Which of the following processes does this finding represent?

a. cellular hyperplasia

b. cellular hypertrophy

c. metaplasia

d. carcinoma *in situ*

e. cellular atrophy

21. What are the chances that you will die of cancer?

a. 1 in 4

b. 1 in 8

c. 1 in 9

d. 1 in 20

e. 1 in 40

22. Which skin condition is premalignant?

a. seborrhoeic keratosis

b. actinic keratosis

c. blue naevus

d. strawberry naevus

e. haemangioma

23. How much does it cost to develop a new cancer drug?

a. £1 billion

b. £750 million

c. £100 million

d. £10 million

e. £1 million

24. What is the current UK NHS budget?

a. £100 million

b. £200 million

c. £10 billion

d. £100 billion

e. Not enough

25. What proportion of the European average does the UK spend on cancer drugs?

a. 60%

b. 100%

c. 150%

d. 10%

e. 200%

26. What percentage of patients with humeral hypercalcaemia of malignancy respond to bisphosphonates?

a. 80%

b. 96%

c. 42%

d. 50%

e. 10%

27. What is the main obstacle to cancer cure?
   a. money
   b. love
   c. lifestyle
   d. big pharma
   e. doctors

28. What is the source of at least 95% of the drugs that we use for cancer treatment?
   a. big pharma
   b. universities

c. crackpot researchers
d. government
e. World Health Organization

29. What is the androgen receptor?
   a. an oncogene
   b. something that you take with a sip of water
   c. a transcription factor
   d. a source of embarrassment
   c. cytoplasmic and nuclear protein that trimerizes when activated

Answers to MCQs

1. b
2. a
3. b
4. a
5. d
6. e
7. b
8. b
9. a
10. e
11. d
12. e
13. b
14. b
15. a

16. a
17. a
18. e
19. b
20. c
21. a
22. b
23. b
24. d
25. a
26. a
27. c
28. a
29. d

Index

Page numbers in italic, e.g. *214*, refer to boxes, figures or tables.